Surgical Techniques in Ophthalmology

Strabismus Surgery

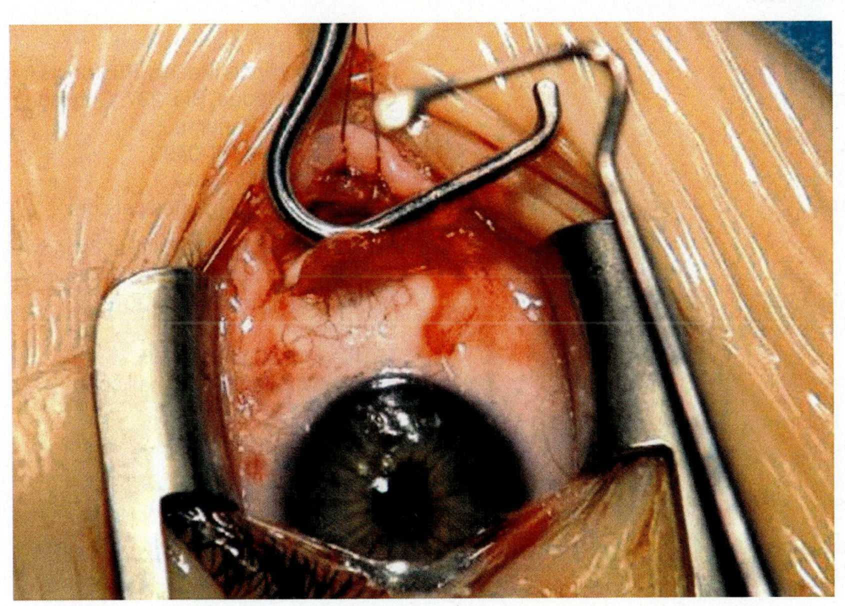

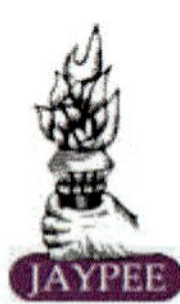

Jaypee Brothers Medical Publishers (P) Ltd

Headquarters

Jaypee Brothers Medical Publishers (P) Ltd
4838/24, Ansari Road, Daryaganj
New Delhi 110 002, India
Phone: +91-11-43574357
Fax: +91-11-43574314
Email: jaypee@jaypeebrothers.com

Overseas Offices

J.P. Medical Ltd
83 Victoria Street, London
SW1H 0HW (UK)
Phone: +44 20 3170 8910
Fax: +44 (0)20 3008 6180
Email: info@jpmedpub.com

Jaypee-Highlights Medical Publishers Inc
City of Knowledge, Bld. 237, Clayton
Panama City, Panama
Phone: +1 507-301-0496
Fax: +1 507-301-0499
Email: cservice@jphmedical.com

Jaypee Medical Inc
The Bourse
111 South Independence Mall East
Suite 835, Philadelphia, PA 19106, USA
Phone: +1 267-519-9789
Email: jpmed.us@gmail.com

Jaypee Brothers Medical Publishers (P) Ltd
17/1-B Babar Road, Block-B, Shaymali
Mohammadpur, Dhaka-1207
Bangladesh
Mobile: +08801912003485
Email: jaypeedhaka@gmail.com

Jaypee Brothers Medical Publishers (P) Ltd
Bhotahity, Kathmandu, Nepal
Phone: +977-9741283608
Email: kathmandu@jaypeebrothers.com

Website: www.jaypeebrothers.com
Website: www.jaypeedigital.com

Surgical Techniques in Ophthalmology (Strabismus Surgery)

First Edition: 2010
Revised Reprint: **2016**

ISBN 978-93-80704-24-1

Printed at Sanat Printers

Surgical Techniques in Ophthalmology

Strabismus Surgery

Editors-in-Chief

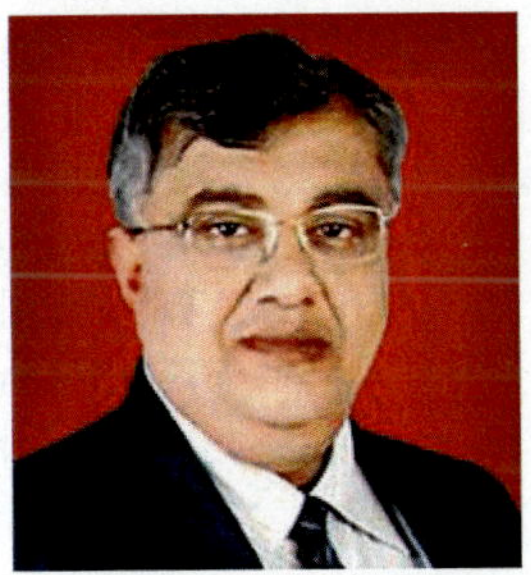

Ashok Garg
MS PhD FIAO (Bel) FRSM ADM FAIMS FICA
International and National Gold Medalist
Chairman and Medical Director
Garg Eye Institute and Research Centre
235 Model Town, Dabra Chowk
Hisar-125005, Haryana, India

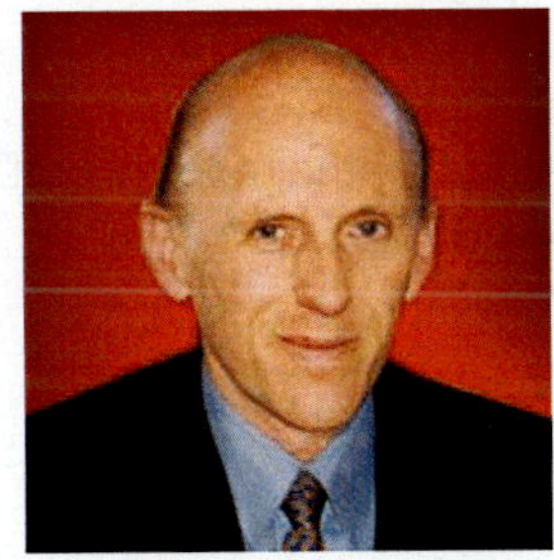

Jorge L Alió MD PhD
Professor and Chairman of Ophthalmology
Medical Director
VISSUM, Instituto Oftalmologico De Alicante
Avda de Denia S/n 03016
Alicante, Spain

Foreword

Laura Elena Campos-Campos (Mexico)

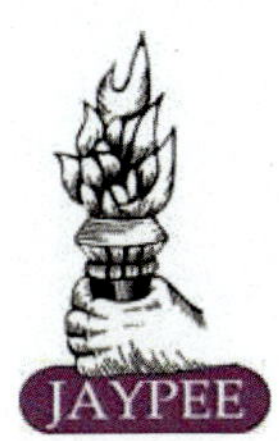

The Health Sciences Publisher

New Delhi | London | Philadelphia | Panama

Editors

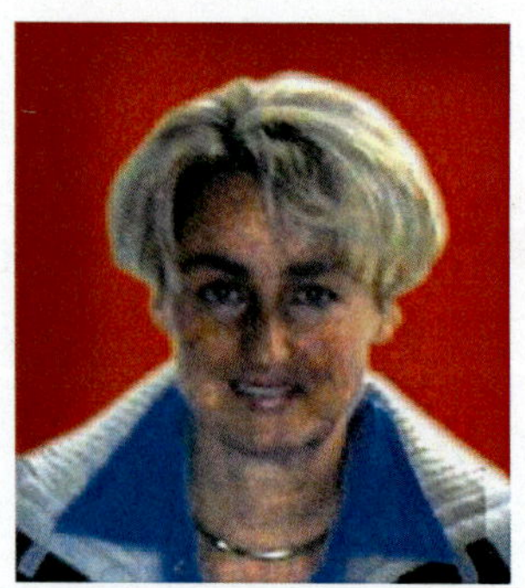

Ewa Oleszczynska Prost MD PhD
Director
Center for Pediatric Ophthalmology
Hertza 9, 04-603, Warsaw
Poland

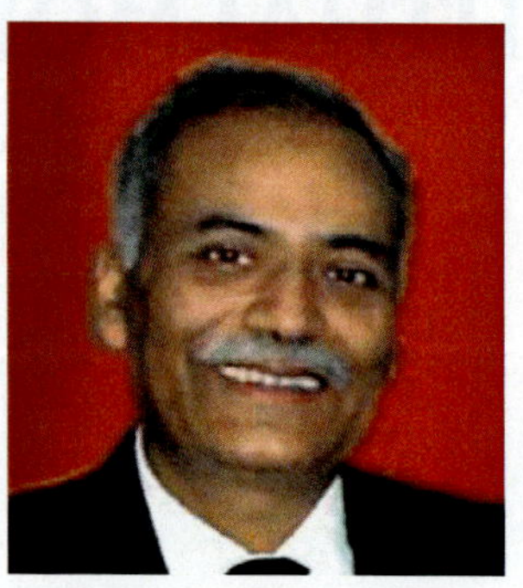

Pradeep Sharma MD
Professor of Ophthalmology
Dr RP Centre for Ophthalmic Sciences
AIIMS, Ansari Nagar
New Delhi-110029
India

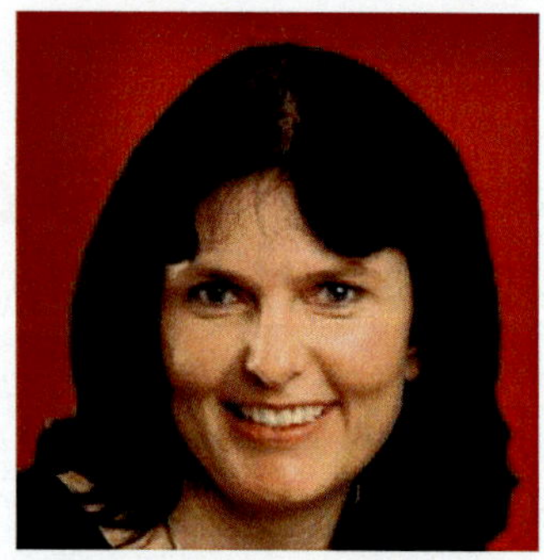

Brigitte Pajic-Eggspuehler MD
Chairman
Swiss Eye Research Foundation
Eye Clinic ORASIS
Titlisstrasse 44
5734 Reinach AG
Switzerland

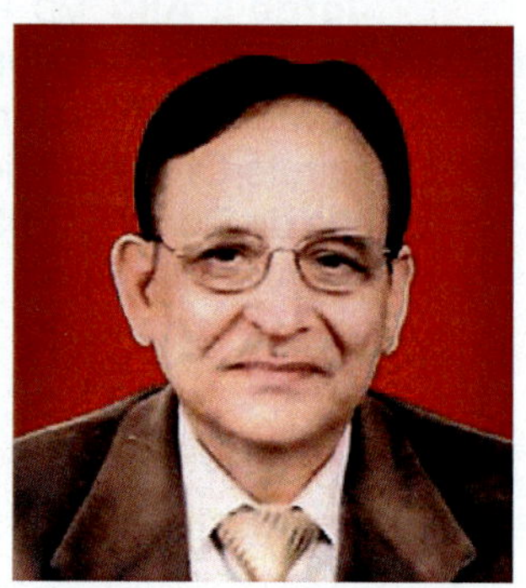

CS Dhull MS PhD FIAO
Sr Professor and Head
Regional Institute of Ophthalmology
Director, PGIMS
Rohtak-124001
India

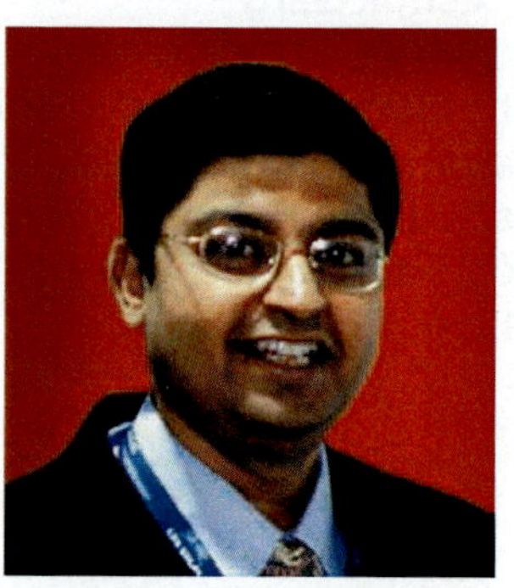

Rohit Saxena MD
Associate Professor of Ophthalmology
Dr RP Centre for Ophthalmic Sciences
AIIMS, Ansari Nagar
New Delhi-110029
India

Dedicated to

- My Respected Param Pujya Guru Sant Gurmeet Ram Rahim Singh Ji for his blessings and motivation.
- My Respected Parents, teachers, my wife Aruna Garg, son Abhishek and daughter Anshul for their constant support and patience during all these days of hard work.
- My dear friend Dr Amar Agarwal, a renowned International Ophthalmologist for his constant support, guidance and expertise.

– Ashok Garg

- To Mayca, Jorge, Fernando and Maria Lucia and most especially to my beloved wife Maria, for the hours that were taken from our family life to make this book possible.

– Jorge L Alió

- My parents, husband and son for patience and understanding.

– Ewa Oleszczynska Prost

- I dedicate this book to my spiritual master Saint Gurmeet Ram Rahim Singh Insaan of Dera Sacha Sauda, Sirsa for teaching the true meaning of human life of the love for one and all.

– Pradeep Sharma Insaan

- To my wonderful husband Bojan, the light of my life.

– Brigitte Pajic-Eggspuehler

- My dear wife Indira Dhull and my children Tushar and Chirag.

– CS Dhull

- My wife and son for helping me appreciate life in full stereoscopy.

– Rohit Saxena

Contributors

Amar Agarwal MS, FRCS, FRC Ophth
Consultant
Agarwal's Eye Hospital
19, Cathedral Road
Chennai-600086, India

Ankur Sinha MD
Senior Registrar
Strabismology, Glaucoma and Neurophthalmology Services
Dr RP Centre for Ophthalmic Sciences
AIIMS, New Delhi-110029, India

Arturo Perez-Arteaga MD
Medical Director
Centro Oftalmologico Tlanlnepantla
Dr Perez-Arteaga Vallarta No 42
Tlalnepantla, Centro
Estado de Mexico 54000, Mexico

Ashok Garg
MS PhD FIAO FRSM ADM FAIMS FICA
Chairman and Medical Director
Garg Eye Institute and Research Centre
235-Model Town, Dabra Chowk
Hisar-125005, India

Ashish Kakkar MD
Dr RP Centre for Ophthalmic Sciences
AIIMS, New Delhi-110029, India

Belquiz A Nassaralla MD PhD
Goiania Eye Institute
Department of Cornea and Refractive Surgery
Goiania, GO, Brazil

Berdine M Burger MD
Department of Ophthalmology
Storm Eye Institute
Medical University of South Carolina
167, Ashley Avenue
Charleston SC 29425, USA

Brigitte Pajic-Eggspuehler MD
Chairman
Swiss Eye Research Foundation
Eye Clinic ORASIS
Titlisstrasse 44,
5734 Reinach/AG
Switzerland

B Shukla MS PhD MAMS FICS
Director of Research
RJN Institute of Ophthalmology
Chandra Bhawan, 1, Jhansi Road
Gwalior-474002, India

BV Ventura MD
Medical Doctor
University of Pernambuco
Pernambuco, Brazil

Carlos Laria MD
VISSUM, Instituto Oftalmologico De Alicante
Avda de Denia, S/n, 03016
Alicante, Spain

CS Dhull MS PhD FIAO
Professor and Head
Regional Institute of Ophthalmology
Director
PGIMS
Rohtak-124001, India

Cyres K Mehta MS FSVH FAGE
Director and Consultant
Mehta International Eye Institute
Seaside, 147, Colaba Road
Mumbai-400005, India

Ewa Oleszczynska Prost MD PhD
Director
Center for Pediatric Ophthalmology
Hertza 9, 04-603
Warsaw, Poland

Fabrizio Gabas MD
Instituto Laser Microchirurgia Oculare
Crystal Palace
Via Cefalonia, 70
25124 Brescia, Italy

Harinder Singh Sethi MS
Dr RP Centre for Ophthalmic Sciences
AIIMS, Ansari Nagar
New Delhi-110029, India

HC Almeida MD PhD
Department of Ophthalmology
Federal University of Minas Gerais Belo Horizonte, Brazil

Ilaria Sireno OD
Instituto Laser Microchirurgia Oculare
Crystal Palace, Via Cefalonia, 70
25124 Brescia, Italy

JL Goyal MD DNB
Professor of Ophthalmology
Guru Nanak Eye Center
Maulana Azad Medical College
New Delhi-1100002, India

João J Nassaralla Jr MD PhD
Faculty of Health Sciences
University of Brasilia, DF
Goiania Eye Institute
Department of Retina and Vitreous
Goiania, GO, Brazil

Jorge L Alió MD PhD
Medical Director
VISSUM, Instituto Oftalmologico De Alicante
Avda de Denia, S/n, 03016
Alicante, Spain

Keiki R Mehta MS DO FIOS
Chairman and Medical Director
Mehta International Eye Institute
147, Shahid Bhagat Singh Road
Colaba Road, Mumbai-400005, India

Kumar J Doctor MS
Director
Doctor Eye Institute Pvt Ltd
Spenta Mansion, 1st Floor
SV Road, Andheri (W)
Mumbai-400058, India

LO Ventura MD PhD
Department of Pediatric
Ophthalmology and Strabismus
Altino Ventura Foundation and
Pernambuco Eye-Hospital (HOPE)
Pernambuco, Brazil

Marcel PM Ten Tusscher MD PhD
Consultant in Neuro-ophthalmology
University Hospital Antwerp, Belgium

Mayur Moreker MS
Surya Eye Hospital
Mulund, Mumbai, India

M Edward Wilson MD
Pierre Gautier Jenkins
Professor and Chairman
Department of Ophthalmology
Director
Albert Florens Storm Eye Institute
Medical University of South Carolina
Charleston, SC, USA 29425

MT Miller MD
Department of Ophthalmology and
Visual Science, University of Illinois
Chicago, USA

PA Jorge MD
Department of Ophthalmology
Altino Ventural Foundation
Pernambuco, Brazil

Paromita Datta MD
Senior Resident
Dr RP Centre for Ophthalmic Sciences
AIIMS, Ansari Nagar
New Delhi-110029, India

P Bhasin MS
Director
RJN Ophthalmic Institute
Gwalior (MP), India

Pooja Deshmukh MS
Doctor Eye Institute Pvt Ltd
Spenta Mansion, 1st Floor
SV Road, Andheri (W)
Mumbai-400058, India

Pradeep Sharma MD
Professor of Ophthalmology
Dr RP Centre for Ophthalmic Sciences
AIIMS, New Delhi-110029, India

Rashmi Shukla
PD Hinduja National Hospital
Mumbai, India

Reena Sharma MD
Senior Resident
Dr RP Centre for Ophthalmic Sciences
AIIMS, Ansari Nagar
New Delhi-110029, India

Roberto Pinelli MD
Instituto Laser Microchirurgia Oculare
Crystal Palace
Via Cefalonia, 70
25124 Brescia, Italy

Rohit Saxena MD
Associate Professor of
Ophthalmology
Dr RP Centre for Ophthalmic Sciences
AIIMS, Ansari Nagar
New Delhi-110029, India

Sachin Mehta MS
Guru Nanak Eye Centre
Maulana Azad Medical College
(MAMC)
New Delhi-110002, India

SB Travassos MD
Department of Pediatric
Ophthalmology and Strabismus
Altino Ventura Foundation and
Pernambuco Eye-Hospital (HOPE)
Pernambuco, Brazil

Sheetal Kharatmal MS
PD Hinduja National Hospital and
Medical Research Centre
Mumbai, India

Shui H Lee MD FRCS FAAO
Medical Director
Sunay Outpatient Aesthetic
Multispecialty Surgical Center
Medical Director
Central Square Medical Eye Clinic
Unit 255-4231 Hazel Bridge Way
Richmond BC V6X 3L7, Canada

Sneha Kataria MD
OD Class 2012
New England College of Optometry
Boston, USA

Sumit Sachdeva MS
Assistant Professor
Regional Institute of Ophthalmology
PGIMS, Rohtak-124001, India

Sunil Moreker MD
Consultant Ophthalmologist
PD, Hinduja National Hospital and
Medical Research Centre
Veer Savarkar Marg, Mahim
Mumbai-400016, India

Swati Phuljhele MS
Registrar
Dr RP Centre for Ophthalmic Sciences
AIIMS, Ansari Nagar
New Delhi-110029, India

Foreword

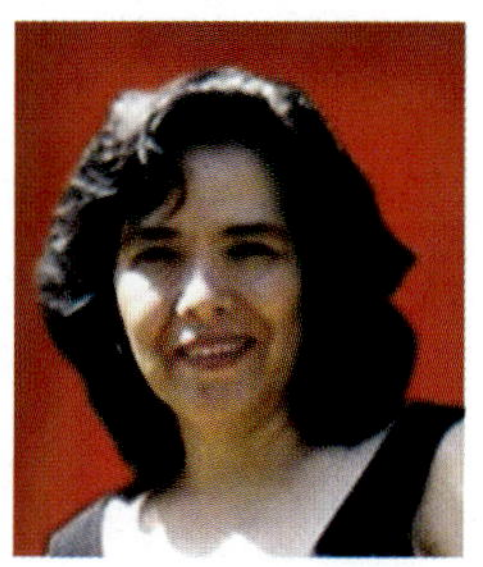

To start with a book project is always a tremendous challenge for someone who has decided this particular duty. To write the foreword is a glad distinction and also a great opportunity to show my feelings about it and make it visible to all the readers; I sincerely thank Dr Ashok Garg for this particular and personal distinctive.

To talk about strabismus is to see an image of thousands of people with "eye deviation", due to many different causes and because of this with many different treatment modalities. The focus of this book is the study of the patient with strabismus; it has a very nice clinical approach, and make us travel since the specific basic topics of the disease until the surgical techniques and its innovations.

Very important for me, was to see, when reading the content of this book, the particular approach to the pediatric patient. It is during this age when most of the strabismus become manifest. During the pediatric years the diagnosis and treatment based upon a complete knowledge of the disease, are of prime importance. Terrible complications can occur, like the development of amblyopia, if a misdiagnosis is done or if a delayed treatment happens. The physician must also think that the cosmetic appearance of the patient at the pediatric age, can lead to adverse psychological effects that can produce a landmark for the patient at very long term.

This textbook is the result of the tremendous effort of worldwide recognized ophthalmologists, who have dedicated their lives to the study of the strabismus. The target audience is the general ophthalmologist who deserves to go deep in the knowledge of this pathology or in some particular cases when a doubt arises or when a particular concept must be clear. The physician can be sure that he will find the answers needed. Because of its wide coverage and current data, it is a mandatory reference in the field.

I am sure it will be a complete success.

Prof Laura Elena Campos-Campos

Chairman of the Department of Pediatric Ophthalmology
General Hospital; National Medical Center "La Raza"
National Institute of Social Security
Mexico
Ph. 0044-5554534699, 5557874500
E-mail: dra_compos@yahoo.com.mx

Preface

Ophthalmic Surgery Technology has undergone rapid advancements and innovations in last two decades. From modest and conventional surgical techniques in early eighties, now it has become high-tech surgery with least indoor stay and excellent visual outcomes. Microincision surgery in both anterior and posterior segments, corneal and lenticular refractive surgery, modern keratoplasty techniques, pediatric and strabismus surgery, oculoplastic and reconstructive surgery and stem cell transplantation have entirely changed the scenario in ophthalmic surgery today.

Modern ophthalmic surgery is a vast subject. It is important for ophthalmologists to master various surgical steps in the ophthalmic surgery procedures of their interest. There are very few quality international Surgical Techniques in Ophthalmology books which can teach and guide the ophthalmologists to master various surgical techniques properly. Keeping in view of this factor we have conceptualized the present series *Surgical Techniques in Ophthalmology* which shall contain 8 volumes. These volumes shall cover all aspects of ophthalmic surgery in a comprehensive and easy to read format. These volumes shall focus specially on Cataract surgery, Corneal and Lenticular Refractive surgery, Glaucoma surgery, Corneal surgery, Retinal surgery, Pediatric surgery, Oculoplastic and Reconstructive surgery, Strabismus and Neuro-ophthalmic surgery. A panel of International eminent ophthalmologists are contributing chapters in these volumes for the benefit of ophthalmologists worldwide.

This volume is dedicated to strabismus surgery, an important branch of ophthalmology. Section-I of this volume deals with various neurophysiological aspects, surgical anatomy, instrumentation and various surgical techniques of strabismus surgery. Section-II includes all new and innovative techniques of strabismus surgery developed in recent times specially related to pediatric strabismus, 3D video oculography, sutureless strabismus surgery and amblyopia management and rehabilitation by corneal wavefront lasik surgery and orthoptics.

Our gratitudes are due to Shri Jitendar P Vij (Chairman and Managing Director), Mr Tarun Duneja (Director–Publishing) and all staff members of our publisher M/s Jaypee Brothers Medical Publishers (P) Ltd. who took keen interest in this project and for speedy completion of this mega task.

We expect that present series of *Surgical Techniques in Ophthalmology* books shall serve as Quick look reference books for ophthalmologists worldwide to sharpen their surgical skills.

Editors

Contents

Section I: Clinical Strabismus

Section II: Recent Advances and Innovative Techniques in Strabismus Surgery

Section I: Clinical Strabismus

Binocular Vision

Belquiz A Nassaralla, João J Nassaralla Jr (Brazil)

Binocular vision is the integration of the sensation produced by the light stimulus in each eye into a unified perception. It is an acquired, conditioned reflex, which has some requisites for its development:

1. There must be proper fixation with each eye. The muscles controlling the movements of each eye must function normally and turn both eyes in such a manner that the object of regard is fixated by corresponding retinal areas, e.g. the two foveas.
2. The visual fields of the two eyes must overlap to a large extent.
3. Approximately similar images must be formed on each retina. The images, therefore, must be approximately of the same size, shape, color, and intensity.
4. The retinas must possess physiologically corresponding points, i.e. retinal receptors which are so related that they have a common visual direction.
5. The eyes must be coordinated by the reflex activities which produce the fusional movements at all times so that retinal receptors which have a common visual direction will receive the same image at all times.

Based on the classic teaching of Claude Worth around the turn of the century, binocular vision has traditionally been broken down into three levels or grades:

1. Simultaneous binocular perception,
2. Fusion, and
3. Stereopsis.

SIMULTANEOUS BINOCULAR PERCEPTION

Simultaneous binocular perception in the context of Worth's scheme refers to the subjective visual superimposition of dissimilar objects viewed by the two eyes. An example of this lowest grade of binocularity is the ability to perceive a lion in a cage (Fig. 1) when viewing the cage with one eye and the lion with the other through a synoptophore (Fig. 2).

Simultaneous perception of differing binocular images is limited by the phenomenon of *rivalry*, which may exclude from visual awareness part of the input from one fovea or the other when the two differ sufficiently.

If a person looks into a stereoscope at two dissimilar targets with overlapping nonfusible contours, first one contour, then the other will be seen, or mosaics of one and the other, but not both contours simultaneously. In Figure 3, taken from Panum, each eye sees a set of oblique lines, one going from above right to below left, seen by the left eye (Fig. 3A), and another set going from above left to below right, seen by the right eye (Fig. 3B). When observed in a stereoscope, these lines are not seen as crossing lines but as a changing pattern of patches of oblique lines going in one or the other direction (Fig. 3C).

It is of interest that it takes a certain buildup of time (150 m) before dissimilar visual input to the eyes causes binocular rivalry. Dichoptic stimuli were perceived as "fused" when presented for shorter periods.

The phenomenon of retinal rivalry is basic to binocular vision and may be explained as follows. Simultaneous excitation of corresponding retinal areas by dissimilar stimuli does not permit fusion; but since such excitations are localized in the same visual direction and since two objects localized in the same place give rise to conflict and confusion, one or the other is temporarily suppressed.

Which of the two is suppressed more depends on the greater or lesser dominance of one eye rather than on the attention value of the visual object seen by each eye. In other words, it is the eye and not the stimulus that competes for dominance under a wide range of conditions. Stimulus rivalry occurs only within a limited range of spatial and temporal parameters.

It is at once clear that rivalry phenomena, or rather their absence, must in some fashion be related to what is known as suppression in strabismic patients. Constant foveal suppression of one eye with cessation of rivalry leads to complete sensory dominance of the other eye, which is a major obstacle to binocular vision. Return of retinal rivalry is a requisite for re-establishment of binocular vision.

The retinal rivalry phenomenon has been explained in neurophysiologic terms by the presence of separate channels for the right and left eyes that compete for access to the visual cortex. A third binocular channel is activated only by fusible input. Because of this competition and the inhibition elicited, only fragments of the image seen by each eye are transmitted to the striate cortex in the case of nonfusible binocular input. Competitive interaction occurs not only in the primary visual cortex but continues at several afferent levels of the visual pathway, well after the inputs to the two eyes have converged.

In the clinical setting, normal rivalry can be evaluated by looking closely at the white spot in the worth four-dot display through the red-green viewing glasses (Fig. 4). A shifting combination of red and green areas is seen within the spot, rather than the uniform (yellow) color that would result if the red and green images were physically superimposed on the retina.

When rivalry is in effect, input from the involved foveal region is excluded from conscious perception regardless of whether it is part of the disparate image that is responsible for the rivalry. In particular, the images of small test spots that are briefly projected onto the same retinal area are excluded. A rivalry *scotoma* can therefore be demonstrated using binocular perimetry, in which the visual field of one eye only is probed with conventional targets during binocular viewing with a dichoptic device. If the intensity of the stimulus within the rivalry scotoma is increased beyond a threshold level, it suddenly breaks through into visibility. Because the rivalry scotoma is present only under certain viewing conditions, it is described as *facultative*.

SENSORY FUSION

A retinal element is a small retinal patch that has an associated directional value. The fovea's directional value is defined subjectively as straight ahead; peripheral retinal elements possess directional values in other orientations. Corresponding retinal points are a pair of retinal elements, one in each eye, that have the same directional value. Comfortable single binocular vision occurs when objects in the binocular field (Fig. 5) stimulate corresponding retinal points and the higher cortical function (termed sensory fusion) occurs.

The locus in space that represents the intersection of all points in space that stimulate corresponding retinal points is termed the horopter (Fig. 6). Interestingly, sensory fusion still occurs if the object that projects upon a retinal element in one eye projects upon a range of elements that surrounds the corresponding retinal element in the second eye. The area in space that projects from this range of elements in the second eye that intersects with the projection from the retinal element in the first eye is termed the Panum fusional areas (Fig. 6). This Panum fusional area surrounds the horopter anteriorly and posteriorly; it permits fusion to take place when exact retinal correspondence does not occur. The binocularly perceived object imaged on noncorres-ponding retinal loci, but fused within the Panum fusional area, is perceived to have one subjective visual direction. The foveal Panum area is circular, of diameter about 14 min of arc; thus, an object projected upon the fovea of one eye may be displaced by this amount and the patient still maintains bifoveal vision. The size of the Panum fusional area increases toward the retinal periphery, but the ultimate size and shape depend upon the temporal and spatial frequency of the patient's alignment drift when fixing upon a stationary target (Fig. 6).

Objects in front of or behind the Panum fusional areas stimulate physiologic diplopia, which is not usually noted but may in turn stimulate fusional vergence eye movements. The horopter shape may be defined in a pair of perfectly spherical eyes that have refractive seats at the nodal points of each eye as the locus of points of zero vertical disparity relative to the fixation point. In a horizontal plane, the horopter, which includes the fovea, is the Vieth-Müller circle (Fig. 7). In a living animal visual system, the horopter is flatter (the Hering-Hellebrand horopter deviation). The vertical horopter tilts away from the observer, who stands on the horopter; the inclination is a function of fixation distance.

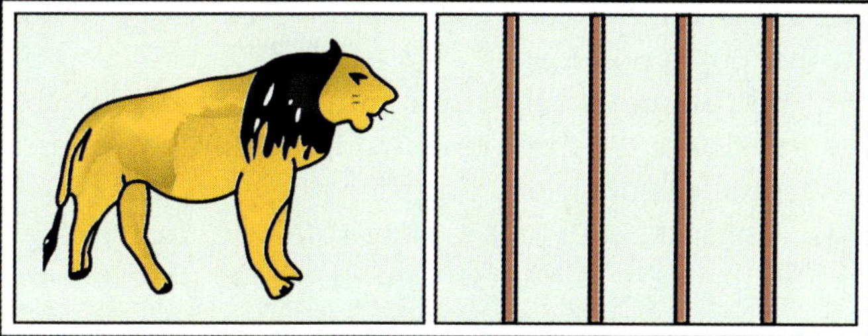

Fig. 1: Simultaneous perception slides – Lion and Cage (Haag-Streit-UK)

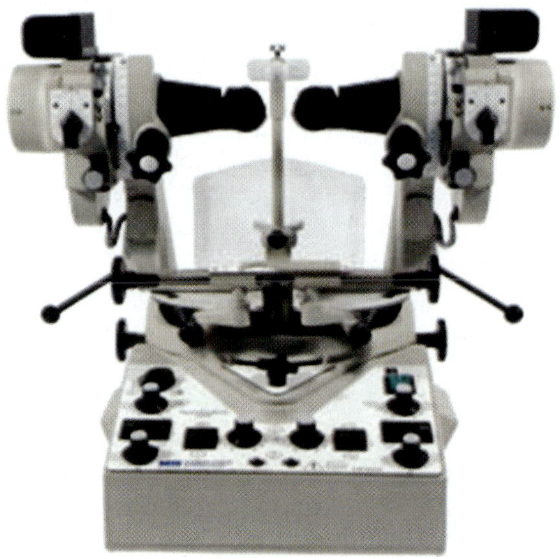

Fig. 2: Synoptophore—This instrument permits assessment of the angle alpha, the objective angle, abnormal retina correspondence, cyclophoria, hyperphoria and horizontal vertical vergences (Haag-Streit-UK)

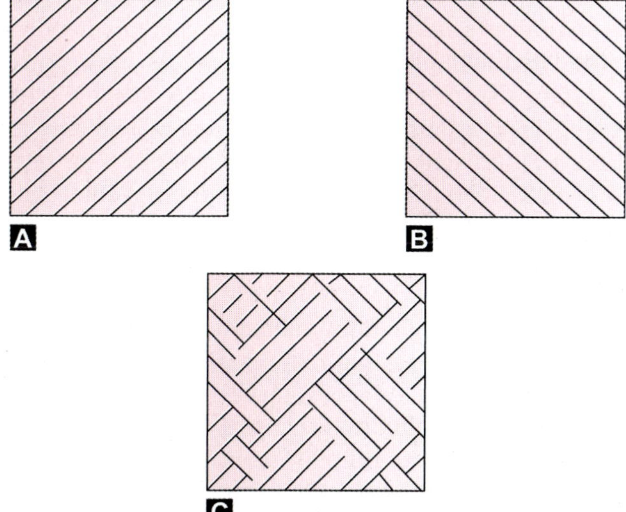

Figs 3A to C: Rivalry Pattern (A) Pattern seen by the left eye (B) Pattern seen by the right eye (C) Binocular impression. (Millodot: Dictionary of Optometry and Visual Science, 2009)

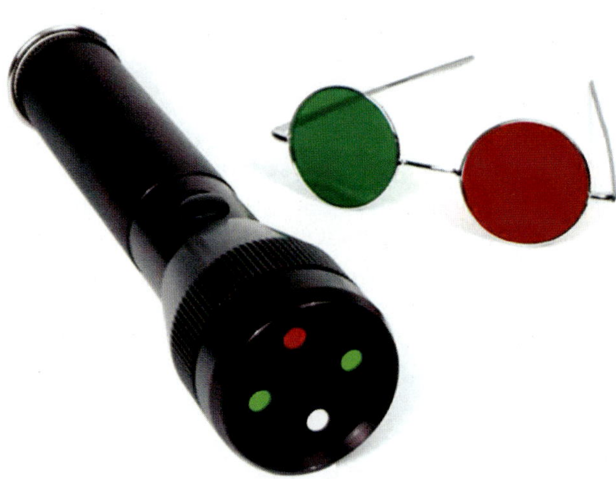

Fig. 4: Worth four-dot test consists of a black background and four illuminated disks: two green, one red and one white. Patient wears red/green glasses which makes each eye cancel the complimentary color (Gulden Ophthalmics)

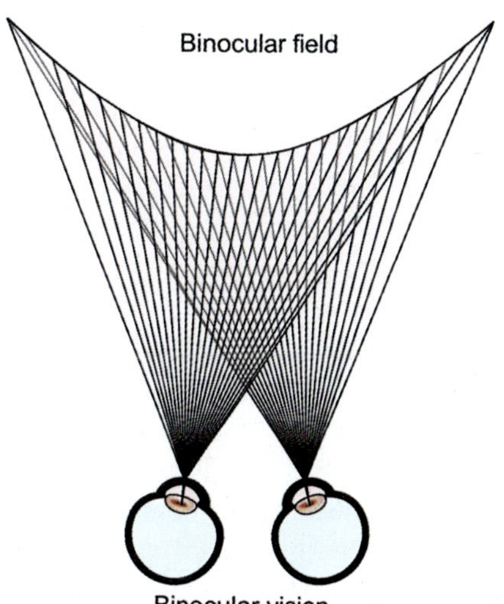

Fig. 5: Single binocular vision occurs when objects in the binocular field stimulate corresponding retinal points and sensory fusion occurs

STEREOPSIS

Stereopsis is the perception of the third dimension (relative nearness and farness of object points within Panum's area) obtained from fusible but disparate retinal images. It is possible to appreciate the relative location of objects using one eye (monocular cues).

Some monocular cues allow relative distance and depth to be judged. These monocular cues include:

1. *Relative size:* Retinal image size allow us to judge distance based on our past and present experience and familiarity with similar objects. As the car drives away, the retinal image becomes smaller and smaller. We interpret this as the car getting further and further away. This is referred to as size constancy. A retinal image of a small car is also interpreted as a distant car.
2. *Interposition*: Interposition cues occur when there is overlapping of objects. The overlapped object is considered further away.
3. *Linear perspective*: When objects of known distance subtend a smaller and smaller angle, it is interpreted as being further away. Parallel lines converge with increasing distance such as roads, railway lines, electric wires, etc.
4. *Aerial perspective*: Relative color of objects gives us some clues to their distance. Because of the scattering of blue light in the atmosphere, creating a "wall" of blue light, distance objects appear bluer. Thus, distant mountains appear blue. Contrast of objects also provides clues to their distance. When the scattering of light blurs the outlines of objects, the object is perceived as distant. Mountains are perceived to be closer when the atmosphere is clear.
5. *Light and shade*: Highlights and shadows can provide information about an object's dimensions and depth. Because our visual system assumes that the light comes from above, a totally different perception is obtained if the image is viewed upside down.
6. *Monocular movement parallax*: When our heads move from side to side, objects at different distances move at a different relative velocity. Closer objects move "against" the direction of head movement and farther objects move "with" the direction of head movement.

However, it is the lateral displacement of the eyes that provides two slightly different views of the same object (disparate images) and allows acute stereoscopic depth discrimination. The stereopsis determination hence is made on the basis of differences in interretinal distances of the fusible images within Panum's area: the greater interretinal image distances are projected by nearer object points, and the lesser interretinal image distances are projected by further object points.

Simultaneous binocular perception, fusion, and stereopsis are the three essential but distinctly different perceptual phenomena comprising single binocular vision. All three usually are capable of functioning simultaneously, although simultaneous perception is usually suppressed unless voluntarily recognized. There are some congenitally esotropic patients who, after their eyes have been straightened by surgery, only develop the simultaneous perception and fusion components of single binocular vision and never develop stereopsis. Binocular vision is a cortical function, and there are separate specialized cortical cells for each component. The cortical cells serving simultaneous perception, fusion, and stereopsis are conjectured to be completely individualized in their morphology, physiology, and distribution frequency throughout the cortex. They are indeed considered to be three separate neurophysiologic phenomena, sharing only the fact that they function only during the cortical processing of the images projected simultaneously on each retina.

There are two groups of clinical tests used to measure stereopsis. These are the contour stereotests and the random-dot stereotest.

Random-dot stereograms are pairs of images of random-dots which when viewed with the aid of a stereoscope, or with the eyes focused on a point behind the images, produce a sensation of depth, with objects appearing to be in front of or behind the actual images. The random-dot stereogram technique was first used by Dr Béla Julesz (1960) to eliminate monocular cues. As there are no contours, depth perception (stereopsis) can only be appreciated when binocular fusion occurs. Two process of stereopsis are used and these are local and global stereopsis. Local stereopsis exists to evaluate the two horizontally disparate stimuli. This process is sufficient for contour stereotests. Global stereopsis is required in random-dot stereogram when the evaluation and correlation of corresponding points and disparate points are needed over a large retinal area.

An example of a contour stereotest used in the clinic is the Titmus stereotest (Fig. 8). Vectograph cards dissociate the eyes optically. A vectograph consists of Polaroid material on which the two targets are imprinted so that each target is polarized at 90° with respect to the other. When the patient is provided with properly oriented Polaroid spectacles, each target is seen separately with the two eyes. This principle is used in the Titmus stereotest (Fig. 8). In this test a gross stereoscopic pattern representing

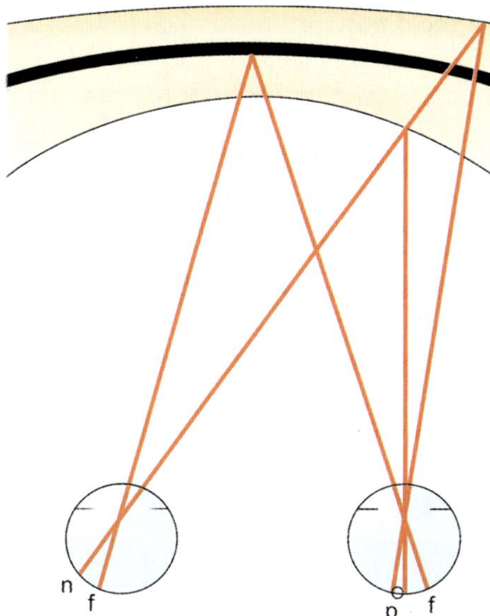

Fig. 6: Panum fusional area—The eyes are fixating "*x*" on the horopter "*h*". Stimulation of point "*n*" in the left retina and of any point within Panum's area "*p*" of the right retina gives rise to a perception of singleness and stereopsis

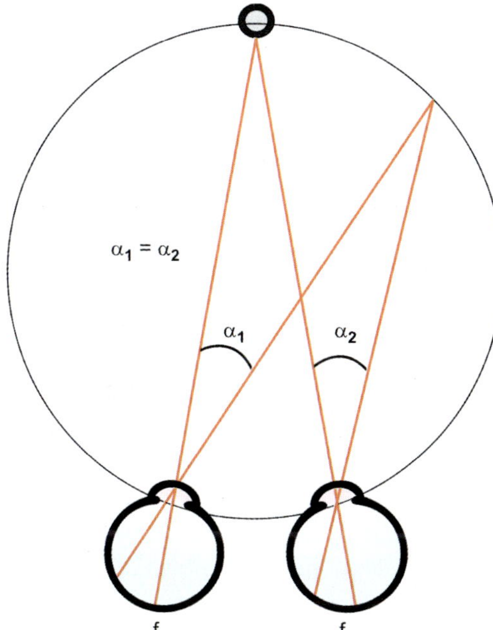

Fig. 7: Vieth-Müller Circle. This represents the theoretical location of points in space that will produce corresponding retinal points. Notice that the locations form a circle. If the eyes are assumed to be spherical with rotational centers at the nodal points, all points in space that have a zero disparity fall on this circle. Angle α_1 = angle α_2; thus, equal retinal distances map into equal angles in space in this idealized system

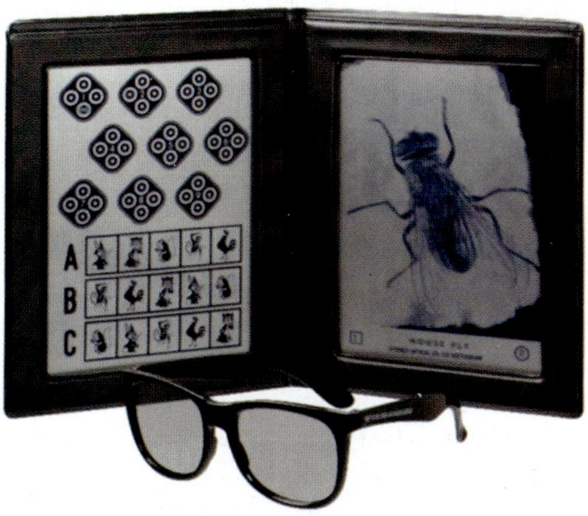

Fig. 8: Titmus stereotest. The standard for stereodepth perception testing. Evaluate both gross stereopsis (2500 to 1200 seconds of arc) and fine depth perception

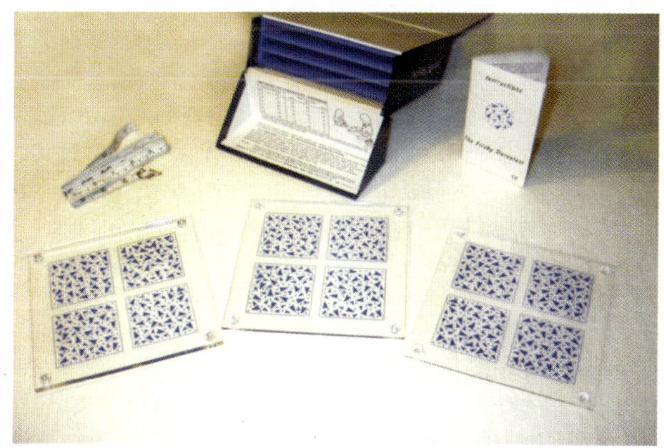

Fig. 9: Frisby stereotest. This test consists of three test plates (6 mm, 3 mm, and 1.5 mm thick), which permit stereoacuity measurements in a range of 600 - 15 sec of arc. No special glasses are required. The hidden shape can only be detected if stereopsis is present. Suitable for a wide age range, even young pre-schoolers

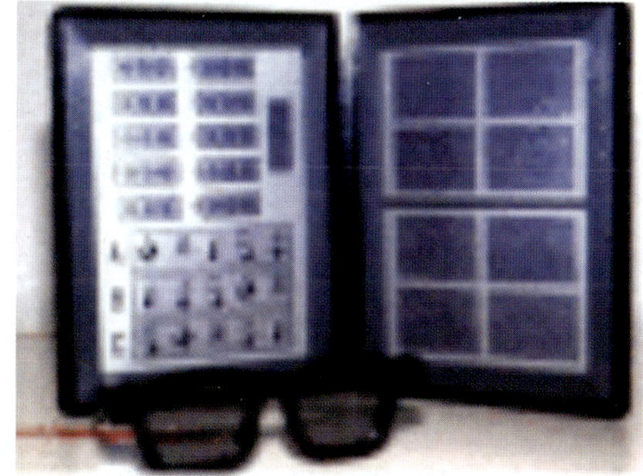

Fig. 10: Randot stereotest with Polaroid glasses. Tests the ability to identify six geometric forms from random-dot backgrounds. Figures cannot be identified without glasses to discourage guessing. 500 to 20 seconds of arc

a housefly is provided to orient the patient and to establish whether there is gross stereopsis (threshold: 3000 seconds of arc). In testing young children, one must ask questions the child will understand. For example, one may ask the child to take hold of the wings of the fly. If the child sees them stereoscopically, the child will reach above the plate. The Polaroid test also contains three rows of animals, one animal in each row imaged disparately (thresholds: 100, 200, and 400 seconds of arc, respectively). The child is asked which one of the animals stands out. The animal Figures contain a misleading clue. In each row one of the animals, correspondingly imaged in two eyes, is printed heavily black. A child without stereopsis will name this animal as the one that stands out. Last, the Titmus test (Fig. 8) contains nine sets of four circles arranged in the form of a lozenge. In this sequence the upper, lower, left, or right circle is disparately imaged at random with thresholds ranging from 800 to 40 seconds of arc. If the child has passed the other tests, he or she is now asked to "push down" the circle that stands out, beginning with the first set. When the child makes mistakes or finds no circle to push down, the limits of stereopsis are presumably reached.

Examples of random-dot stereotests used in the clinic are the Frisby stereotest (Fig. 9), the Randot stereotest (Fig. 10), the Random-dot E stereotest (Fig. 11) and the Lang stereotest (Fig. 12).

The Frisby stereotest has three transparent plates (Fig. 9). One of these is shown on each presentation to the subject. The target that the patient has to detect is printed on one side of each plate. This target is a cluster of randomly arranged arrowheads of differing sizes. On the other side of each plate is printed a background of similar texture. An observer with normal binocular stereovision can readily detect the target because it appears to stand out from the background (or to recede from the background, depending on which way round the plate is shown). Such an observer is essentially seeing the thickness of the plate by virtue of the texture elements printed on the two sides. An observer lacking normal binocular stereovision (or a normal observer viewing with one eye only) fails to be able to detect the target as it can be distinguished only on the basis of binocular disparity cues to depth.

Both the Randot (Fig. 10) and the Random-dot E stereotests (Fig. 11) use crossed polarized filters. Disparity is also constructed vectographically. The Randot stereotest uses modified animals and ring designs with random-dot backgrounds to eliminate monocular cues. The Lang stereotest uses a panographic technique (Fricke and Siderov, 1997) to present disparity; therefore, no filters are required. Patients are required to identify pictures on the Lang stereotest. The Lang II stereotest has a monocularly visible shape on it (Fig. 12).

All the tests provide a measure of stereoacuity by asking the patient to identify the correct target that has stereoscopic depth (target with disparity). The working distance and interpupillary distance will need to be taken into consideration when calculating stereoacuity. Patients with disturbed binocular vision or different refractive error in one eye will perform poorly on depth discrimination tests.

Patients with a large manifest deviation do not have useful stereopsis in casual seeing. Nevertheless, they can function quite well in space, making use of nonstereoscopic clues to depth perception, especially if the strabismus is of early origin. They may have trouble with fast-moving objects, such as flying balls, and this experience may be frustrating to young children. However, when the strabismus is acquired later in life the loss of stereopsis is felt acutely and may present a real handicap. It appears as if stereopsis is useful in the comprehension of complex visual presentations and those requiring good hand-eye coordination.

Although the importance of stereopsis is often stressed, studies addressing the functional effects of stereoscopic deficits are sparse. It is always interesting and useful to determine whether a patient with strabismus has stereopsis or the potential for such.

Fig. 11: Random-dot E test set. (From Simons K, Reinecke RD: Amblyopia screening and stereopsis. In Symposium on strabismus: Transactions of the New Orleans Academy of Ophthalmology. St. Louis, Mosby–Year Book, 1978, p 15.)

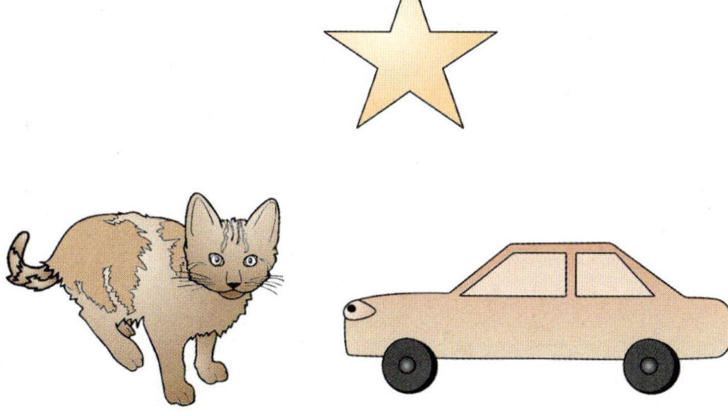

Fig. 12: The Lang II stereotest. It measures disparities: Moon and Star are 200, car 400 and elephant 600 seconds of arc plus monocularly visible star. In this test, the random dots are smaller and less dense. This disparity is finer, namely 200 seconds of arc for the moon and the star, 400 for the car, and 600 for the elephant when viewed at a distance of 40 cm.

Surgical Anatomy

Ewa Oleszczynska Prost (Poland)

ANATOMY OF THE EXTRAOCULAR MUSCLES

Six muscles are responsible for eye movements. These are:

- Four rectus muscles: medial, lateral, inferior and superior rectus.
- Two oblique muscles: superior and inferior.

All these muscles originate from the common ring tendon (annulus of Zinn) at the posterior segment of the orbit. The inferior oblique muscle originates from the lesser wing of the sphenoid bone, above the common ring tendon, whereas inferior oblique muscle arises from the lacrimal groove in the part of the inferior orbital wall (Fig. 1).

Then, all these muscles run divergently forward and insert in sclera with their tendinous part. Rectus muscle insert in sclera above the equator of the eyeball, whereas oblique muscles below it. Points of rectus muscles insertion gradually remove from the limbus, starting from medial rectus through inferior, lateral, and superior rectus muscle. The line of insertion is called spiral of Tillaux (Fig. 2).

RECTUS MUSCLES

Medial Rectus Muscle

It is the thickest and strongest ocular muscle. Its tendinous part is short, of about 4 mm, and width at the insertion in sclera is about 10 mm. Its insertion in sclera is 5.5 mm from the limbus. Check ligament of this muscle is well developed. Contraction of the medial rectus muscle produces:

- Adduction of the eyeball (vertical axis) (Fig. 3).

This muscle has no fascial attachments to other muscles and can retract to the orbital apex, if severed from the globe. Faden procedure is effective because of the short arc of contact. The muscle penetrates Tenon's capsule 12 mm behind its insertion.

Lateral Rectus Muscle

It has long and thin tendinous part of about 8 mm. Its insertion in sclera is about 9 mm and is located about 7 mm from limbus contraction of this muscle produces:

- Abduction of the eyeball (Fig. 3).

The ligament connect both inferior oblique and lateral rectus. During weakening of the rectus, accurate section of the intermuscular septum and separation of muscle are necessary. It prevents shift of the inferior oblique muscle toward lateral rectus muscle.

The lateral rectus has the longest arc of contact, making Faden procedure on this muscle ineffective.

Surgery of both inferior and superior recti may be associated with changes of the palpebral opening.

Superior Rectus Muscle

Runs forward above the eyeball together with levator palpebrae muscle with which is closely connected by fascial capsules. This muscle is about 41.8 mm long. Its tendinous part is about 5 mm long, and insertion – 10.6 mm. It inserts in sclera about 7.7 mm from the limbus. Contraction of superior rectus muscle produces:

- Elevation of the eyeball (frontal axis = X-axis of Fick), most prominent at abduction by 23°.
- Sligth adduction (vertical axis = Z-axis of Fick).
- Intorsion (sagittal axis = Y-axis of Fick).

Superior rectus muscle shares a common tendon of origin with the superior levator palpebrae muscle. Weakening of the superior rectus muscle (resection) may narrow palpebrae, a recession may cause retraction.These attachments must be removed, being careful to stay close to the muscle to avoid penetration of Tenon's capsule and manipulation of orbital fat. Pseudoptosis may occur as

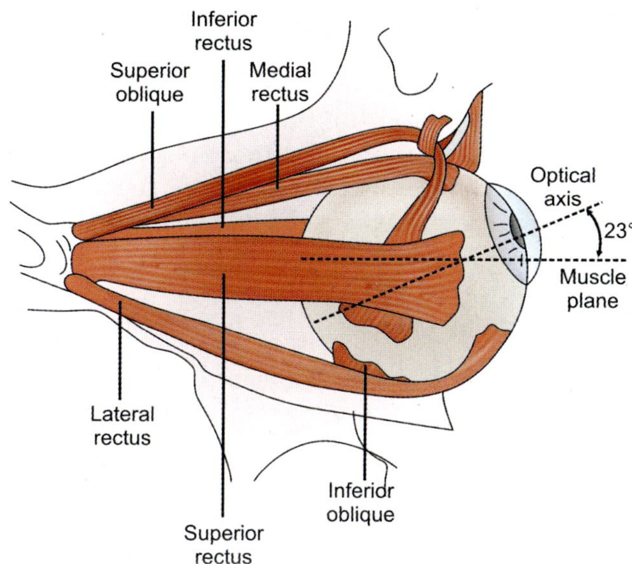

Fig. 1: Extraocular muscles of the right eyeball in the primary position, seen from above

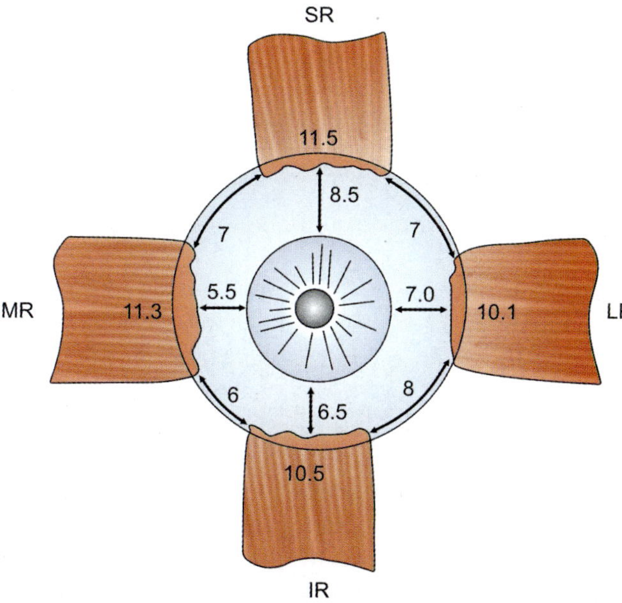

Fig. 2: Spiral of Tillaux. Distance of the rectus muscles from the limbus (mm)

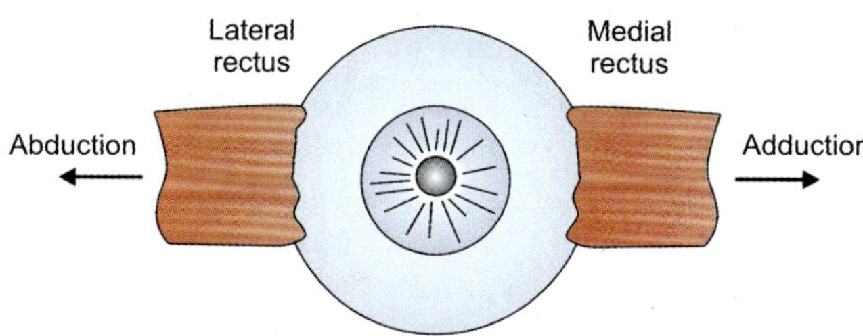

Fig. 3: Action of the medial and lateral rectus muscles

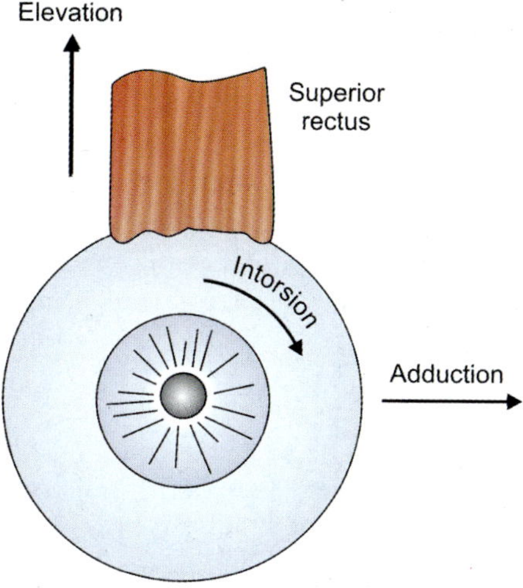

Fig. 4: The action of the superior rectus muscle

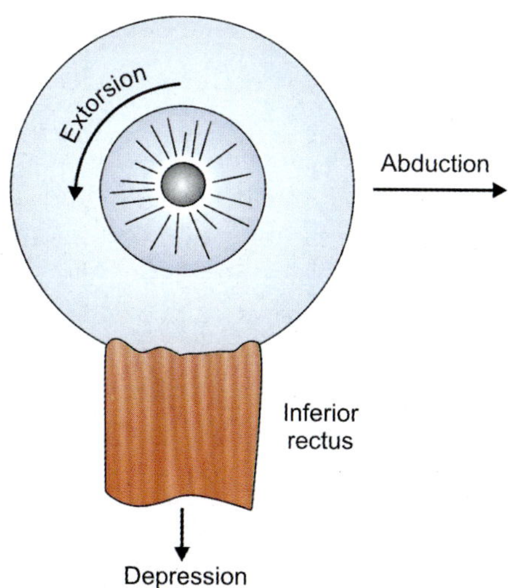

Fig. 5: The action of the inferior rectus muscle

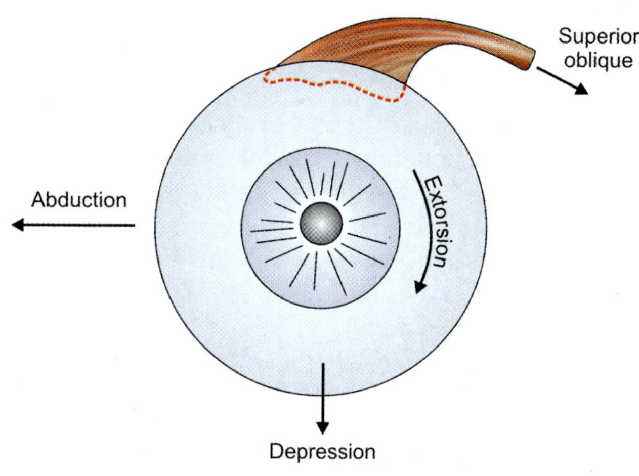

Fig. 6: Superior oblique muscle action

the upper lid movement follows superior rectus muscle action. Secondary ptosis may also occur in case of excessively large range of surgery and less delicate manipulations which may lead to the levator palpebrae muscle damage. Particular attention should be payed during removal of intermuscular septum because of adjacent of the anterior part of the superior oblique muscle.

Actions of the superior rectus muscle is shown in Figure 4.

Inferior Rectus Muscle

Its tendinous part is about 5.6 mm long and insertion about 10 mm wide. The insertion is located about 6.5 mm from the limbus. Contraction of inferior rectus muscle produces:

- Depression of the eyeball (X-axis of Fick), most prominent at abduction by 23°.
- Adduction (Z- axis of Fick).
- Extorsion (Y-axis of Fick).

Actions of the inferior rectus muscle is shown in Figure 5.

Inferior rectus muscle is connected with inferior oblique and the lower eyelid retractors called the Lockwood's ligament. Retraction of the inferior rectus muscle leads to widening of palpebral fissure and depression of the lower eyelid. Its shortening narrows palpebral fissure through elevation of the lower eyelid. The fascial connections beetwen the inferior rectus and inferior oblique work to the surgeon's advantage in looking for a lost inferior rectus muscle.

Eyeball wall is the thinnest at insertion of recti into the sclera and slightly backward. Therefore, operations of rectus muscle retraction or weakening may be complicated by perforation of sclera.

OBLIQUE MUSCLES

Superior Oblique Muscle

It is the longest ocular muscle. It arises from the lesser wing of the sphenoid bone, passing cartilaginous pulley (trochlea) attached to the nasal side of the superior orbital rim. Then, it passes under under the superior rectus muscle and inserts into sclera just below the equator. It is about 60 mm long and size of its insertion is variable. Contraction of this muscle produces:

- Depression of the eyeball (frontal axis), most prominent at abduction by 51°.
- Abduction of the eyeball (vertical axis).
- Intorsion (peroneal axis).

Actions of the superior oblique muscles are shown in Figure 6.

At 1/3 between the beginning of rectus muscle and trochlea, nerves insert into the muscles. It should be considered during surgery. The broad posterior insertion extends to 6.5 mm of optic nerve. So during sugery extreme care must be taken not to inadvertently disturb the optic nerve.

Inferior Oblique Muscle

It runs from lacrimal fossa in the lower part of the orbit, passes backward and to the temple under the inferior rectus muscle and inserts in sclera below this muscle. Posterior end of its insertion is adjacent to the macula, about 2 mm in the front and 1 mm below it. Optical nerve is only 4 mm distant from it while arteries and ciliary nerves run near posterior end of the insertion. Inferior oblique muscle is 37 mm long and its insertion into sclera is 5 to 13 mm wide. This muscle has the longest and one of the best developed check ligaments (suspensory Lockwood's ligament). Contraction of the inferior oblique muscle produces:

- Eyeball elevation, most prominent at abduction by 51°.
- Abduction (vertical axis)
- Extorsion (sagittal axis).

Actions of the inferior oblique muscle are shown in Figure 7.

Inferior oblique muscle travels together with parasympathetic nerves of pupillary sphincter and ciliary muscle at the point of transversing the inferior rectus muscle. Lesion to this area may disturb the size of pupils. Vorticose vein runs about 10 to 12 mm below the posterior insertion near ciliary nerves and arteries. The posterior end of insertion is near macula: 1 to 2 mm in the front and 1 mm below it, and optic nerve is about 4 mm further. Removal of the muscle from the globe or passage of suture through the muscle still attached to the globe must be done with extreme care to avoid scleral perforation and damage to the macula. The inferotemporal vortex vein is in close proximity to the inferior oblique muscle so sometimes it is inadvertently damaged. Nerve enters the muscle about 15 mm nasal to the insertion.

Detailed anatomical relationships of the extraorbital muscles insertions into sclera at corneal limbus area are shown in Figure 1. Proper globe straight position is named prime globe position. All ocular muscles participate in such a positioning and it is muscle prime function (different for each muscle: abduction, adduction, elevation,

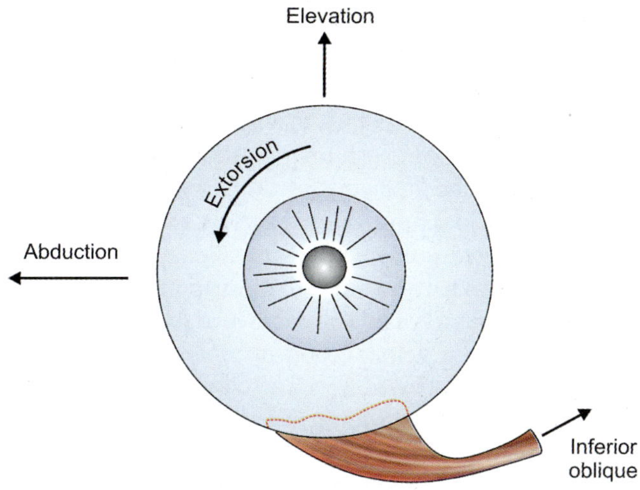

Fig. 7: Inferior oblique muscle action

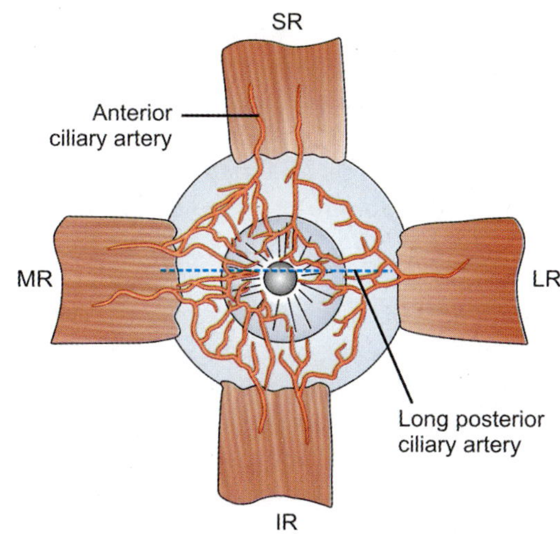

Fig. 9: Vascularization of the anterior part of the globe

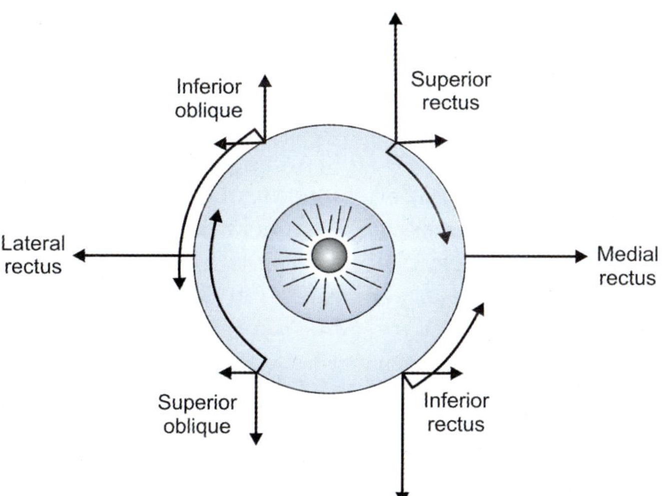

Fig. 8: The action of the extraocular muscles: Right eye

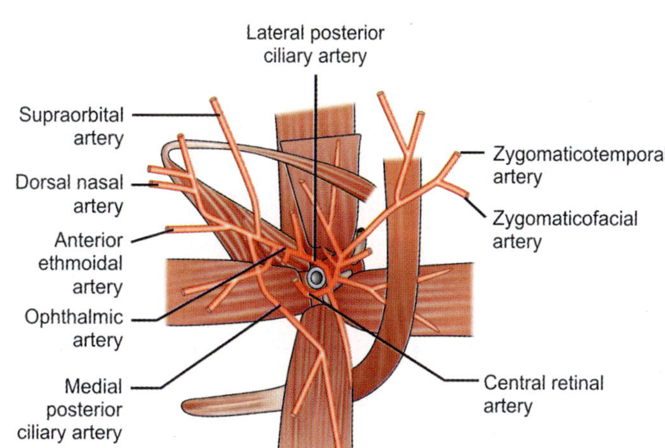

Fig. 10: Arterial supply to the orbit—coronal view

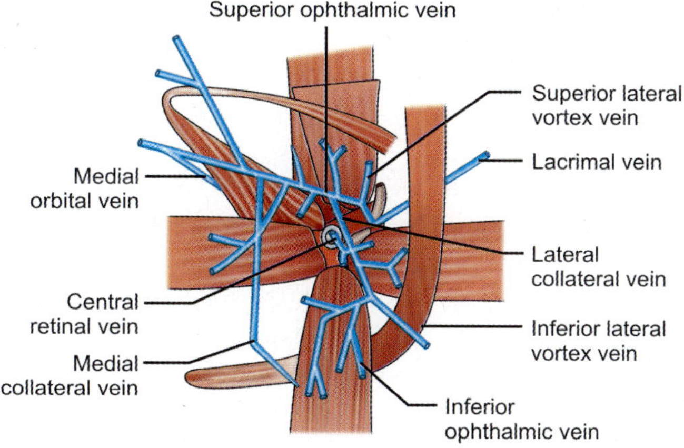

Fig. 11: Venous supply to the orbit—coronal view

depression, intorsion, extorsion) and their muscular planes form appropriate angle with optic axis.

Actions of extraocular muscles are shown in Figure 8.

Muscular plane runs parallelly to the long axis of the muscle and is shared by each pair of muscles.

There are three pairs of muscles, forming muscular planes:

1. Medial and lateral rectus muscles giving an angle of 90° with optic axis at prime position.
2. Inferior and superior rectus muscles giving an angle of 23° with optic axis at prime position.
3. Inferior and superior oblique muscles giving an angle of 51° with optic axis at prime position.

The secondary and tertiary functions of the muscles exert an extra effect on the globe position, when it is in the prime position. Detailed characteristics of the extraocular muscles is shown in Table 1.

VASCULARIZATION OF THE EXTRAOCULAR MUSCLES

Muscles are mainly supplied by the ophthalmic artery. Lateral muscular branch supplies blood to the medial and inferior rectus muscle and oblique inferior muscles as well as lateral and superior rectus muscle and inferior oblique muscles. Medial muscular branch supplies blood to the medial and inferior rectus muscles and inferior oblique muscle. Additionally inferior rectus muscle and inferior oblique muscle are partially supplied by infraorbital artery, whereas lateral rectus muscle by lacrimal artery. Anterior ciliary arteries (seven) being branches of muscular arteries run along rectus muscles. They enter episclera and supply blood to the anterior part of the globe. Most blood flows through the anterior ciliary arteries of the inferior and superior recti. Long posterior ciliary arteries (two) penetrates into the globe posteriorly. Beneath the equator at 3 and 9 o'clock and running forward, joining with anterior ciliary circulus arteriosus.

Ocular veins run similarly to the arteries. Near inferior and superior rectus muscles, backward from the equator, are four vorticose veins. Blood outflows to the superior and inferior orbital vein.

Vessels supplying blood to extraocular muscles run along the rectus muscles. They also enter to episclera and supply anterior part of the globe. Therefore, surgery on all recti may produce ischemia of this area.

Vascularization of the extraocular muscles and the globe is shown in Figures 9 to 11.

INNERVATION OF EXTRAOCULAR MUSCLES

Ocular muscles are innervated by three cranial nerves:

1. Oculomotor nerve (n. III) – inferior division innervates medial rectus, inferior rectus, and inferior oblique muscles; superior division innervates superior rectus muscle. Superior division innervates also levator muscle of the upper eyelid. Inferior division sends branches to ciliary ganglion, innervating ciliary muscles and papillary sphincter. Nucleus of the nerve

Table 1: Characteristics of the ocular muscles

Muscle	*Nerves*	*Origin*	*Anatomic insertion*	*Length of muscle (mm)*	*Length of tendon (mm)*	*Width of tendon (mm)*	*Angle of prime position (°)*	*Arc of contact (mm)*	*Muscle actions: *P **S ***T*
Medial rectus	III	Zinn annulus	5.5	41	4	10.3	90	6	*Adduction
Lateral rectus	VI	Zinn annulus	7.0	41	8	9.2	90	10	*Abduction
Superior rectus	III	Zinn annulus	7.7	41.8	5	10.6	23	6.5	* Elevation **Intorsion *** Adduction
Inferior rectus	III	Zinn annulus	6.51	40	5.6	10	23	7	* Depression **Extorsion *** Adduction
Superior oblique	IV	Above orbit apex Zinn annulus	Posterior, lateral Upper quadrant	32	26	10.8	51	12	*Intorsion ** Depression
Inferior oblique	III	Lacrimal fossa	Lower quadrant	35	1	9.6	51	15	*Extorsion ** Elevation *** Abduction

Muscle actions: *Primary; **Secondary, *** Tertiary.

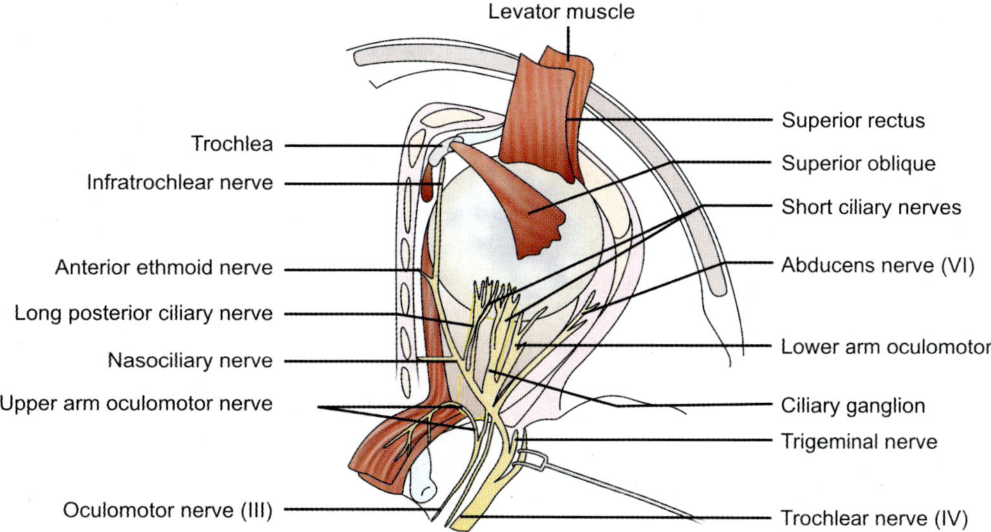

Fig. 12: Ocular course of the cranial nerves III, IV and VI – cross-section from the temporal side

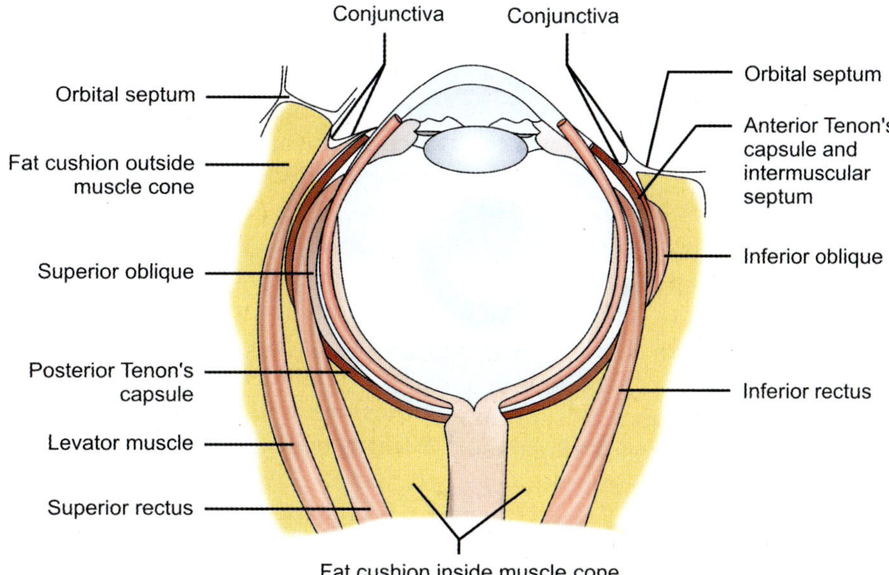

Fig. 13: Sagittal section of orbital tissues through the vertical recti

is located beneath cerebral aqueduct at the level of superior colliculus of the lamina quadrigemina. It consists of four nuclei:

- Dorsolateral and ventromedial nuclei innervate oculomotor muscles and levator of the upper eyelid.
- Accessory nucleus, autonomic (Edinger-Westphal), innervates pupillary sphincter.
- Single central caudal nucleus (Perla) innervates ciliary muscle. Fibers leaving the nucleus are partially crossed.

2. Abducent nerve (n. VI) – innervates lateral rectus muscle. Its nucleus is located on the floor of rhomboid fossa, beneath facial colliculus in the pons. It is surrounded by geniculum of the facial nerve. Fibers leaving the nucleus run to the lateral rectus muscle on the same side.
3. Trochlear nerve (n. IV) – innervates superior oblique muscle. Its nucleus is located beneth cerebral aqueduct at the level of inferior colliculus of the lamina quadrigemina, near the nucleus of the oculomotor nerve. Fibers leaving the nucleus are crossed and reach the superior oblique muscle on the other side (48, 50).

Innervation of extraocular muscles and the globe is shown in Figure 12.

ORBIT: FACIAE, TENDONS AND SURROUNDING TISSUES

In the orbit, eyeball together with extraocular muscles is supported by a complex of fibroelastic structures with fatty lining. Each muscle is surrounded by **sheath** of the connective tissue. At muscle insertion in sclera, forward from the equator, only thin basal laminae of the connective tissue are present. It is called **intramuscular septum,** extending between four rectus muscles, connecting them with each other and with the globe. Due to septum, muscles smoothly slide on the globe surface.

At the equator, the sheaths, crossing Tenon's capsule sheath, thicken gradually. Surrounding the whole body of the muscle, run with it, exending several fascicles attaching the muscle to the orbital wall and forming functional end of the muscle, i.e. check ligaments. Check ligaments fix the globe in a permanent position and prevent its retraction in depth of the orbit during recti contraction or its expulsion during oblique muscles contraction. The longest and strongest is Lockwood's ligament covering the inferior rectus and inferior oblique muscles from the point of crossing. Muscles, their sheaths, and intramuscular septum form **muscular cone**, extending backward from the equator up to the orbital apex. At the distance of about 10 mm from limbus, muscular cone is surrounded by a large amount of fatty tissue. It is also present inside the cone and separated by Tenon's capsule from the sclera. Fatty tissue helps to absorb shocks and keep the eye in the orbit.

Main ocular fascia, forming socket in which the globe moves, is named **Tenon's capsule**. This elastic connective tissue originates from the intramuscular septum, about 3 mm from the limbus. Passing backward, it fuses with optic nerve sheath. Tenon's capsule is thick and strong at the equator and beneath it. Forward equator—it is pierced by oblique muscles while rectus muscles pierce it about 10 mm backward from their insertions. From this point, Tenon's capsule encapsulates all muscles, separating them from orbital fat and structures outside muscular cone. It also forms sheaths of the connective tissue around the muscles. Its posterior part encapsulates optic nerve as well as vessels and ciliary nerves, is thin and elastic. It enables free eyeball. Tenon's capsule connecting with orbital tissues suspends the globe in springboard-like manner.

Precise understanding and respecting anatomical relationships between extraocular muscles and connective tissue orbital structures together with blood vessels and nerves is crucial for the success of surgery.

Rectus muscles retraction does not require extensive preparation of the intramuscular septum contrary to their weakening, which requires precise cutting the septum and muscle.

Discontinuation of Tenon's capsule, especially more than 9 mm backward from the limbus, should be avoided at the first instance. Fatty tissue may fall out from the capsule, leading to the adhesions between the muscles, sclera, conjunctiva, and intramuscular septum. Such adhesions will reduce eyeball motility. Maintaining integrity of the muscular sheaths reduces also hemorrhage during surgery and protects smooth surface of the muscle.

Section of orbital tissues is shown in Figure 13.

BIBLIOGRAPHY

1. Agarwal S, Agarwal A, Agarwal A, Garg A. Supranuclear pathways for eye movements. w Garg A, Prost M (red.): Surgical and medical management of pediatric ophthalmology. Jaypee Brothers, New Dehli, 2007.
2. Bron AJ, Tripathi RC, Tripathi BJ. (red). Wolff's anatomy of the eye and the orbit. 8th ed London: Chapman and Hall, 1997.
3. Diamond GR: Evaluating vision in preverbal and preliterate infants and children., in: Ophthalmology, Mosby St. Louis, 2004; 549-634.
4. Diamond GR. Strabismus. In: Ophthalmology, Mosby, St. Louis 2004;550-556.

5. Fells P, Lee IP. Strabismus. In: Spalton DJ, Hitchings RA, Hunter PA (Eds): Atlas of Clinical Ophthalmology. London, New York: Gower Medical Publishing 1984; 6-7.
6. Friendly DS, Parelhoff ES, McKeown CA. Effect of severing the check ligaments and intermuscular membranes on medial rectus recession in infantile esotropia.Ophthalmology 1993; 100:945-8.
7. Helveston EM, Merriam WW, Ellis FD, et al. The trochlea. A study of the anatomy and physiology. Ophthalmology 1982; 89:124-33.
8. Helveston, EM. The influence of superior oblique anatomy on function and treatment. The 1998 Bielschowsky Lecture. Binoc Vis Strabismus Q 1999;14:16-21.
9. Krzystkowa K. Narząd ruchu gałki ocznej i jego zaburzenia. Okulistyka współczesna, PZWL Warszawa 1986;2(15):179-223.
10. Krzystkowa K, Kubatko-Zielińska A, Pająkowa J, Nowak-Brygowa H. Choroba zezowa-rozpoznawanie i leczenie. PZWL, Warszawa, 1997.
11. Kushner BJ. A surgical procedure to minimize lower-eyelid retraction with inferior rectus recession. Arch Ophthalmol, 1992;110:1011-4.
12. MacEwen C, Gregson R. Manual of Strabismus Surgery. Elsevier Limited, 2003.
13. Parks MM: Ocularmotility and strabismus. in: Duane's clinical ophthalmology. Philadelphia, Lippincott, 1993; 1:1-20.
14. Pediatric Ophthalmology and Strabismus. American Academy of Ophthalmology, Basic and Clinical Science Course 2002;6 (II):13-29.
15. Scott AB: Ocular motility. in: TasmanT,Jaeger EA(red): Bio-medical foundations of ophthalmology. vol.2 Philadelphia: Lippincott 1997.
16. Wright KW. Color Atlas of Ophthalmic Surgery: Strabismus. JB Lippincott Comp, Philadelphia, 1991.

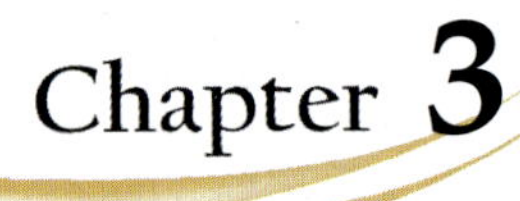

Chapter 3

The Neuroanatomical Basis of Accommodation and Vergence

Marcel PM Ten Tusscher (Belgium)

The near synkinesis triad consists of accommodation of the lenses, convergence of the eyes, and miosis of the pupils. Central cortical and brainstem pathways as well as the accommodative final pathway through the autonomic nerves and ciliary ganglion are discussed. At the end accommodative and vergence dysfunctions are described.

ACCOMMODATION

Human accommodation is largely realized by changes in power of the crystalline lens. About the way in which these changes in shape and power of the lens are achieved there still are controversies. Although corneal curvature and anteroposterior displacement of the crystalline lens may theoretically influence accommodation, most authors agree that changes in the shape of the lens are the most important for the realization of accommodation. The balance between elastic forces of both the lens and its capsule give the lens its accommodated, most powerful form. Zonular fibers are attached near the equator of the lens and along the ciliary processes. The ciliary body contains meridional, radial and circular muscle fibers. Contraction of these muscle fibers reduces the diameter of the concentric ciliary body circumference. Subsequently the zonular fibers are relaxed and the lens takes on its accommodated form. This, however, is the classical description of Hermann von Helmholtz.[9] Schachar,[18] among others, believes that torsional forces on the lens equator increase during accommodation. This would, in their view, cause the lens to become flatter at its periphery while the central curvature would become steeper.

Accommodation is linked to convergence. The near response is often described as a near triad: when attention is brought to bear on a near object, three reactions occur simultaneously: the eyes adduct, the ciliary muscles contract and the pupils become smaller. Stakenburg,[20] however, showed that pupil constriction is under independent control. It appeared that the pupil is very sensitive to alignment. With perfect alignment he was able to show that blur induced accommodation may occur without corresponding papillary reaction.

Accommodation only occurs, if luminance levels allow cone activity. If the luminance level is progressively lowered the accommodation response to a stimulus diminishes.[1]

The true synkinetic relationship between accommodation of the lens and accommodative convergence is often expressed as a ratio AC/A (prism diopters/sphere diopters).

The peripheral nervous system is classically separated into a somatic division containing both afferent and efferent pathways and an autonomic division composed of efferents only. The somatic afferent division is divided in A- and B-neurons. The B-neurons are supposed to be autonomic afferents as part of a reflex system involved in homeostasis. Data obtained by neuronal tracing and immunohistochemical experiments concerning the eye related peripheral nervous system endorse the existence of these peripheral reflex systems.[21,22]

Somatic afferents of trigeminal origin synaptically innervate parasympathetic neurons in the pterygopalatine ganglion. This probably represents a pathway mediating autonomically regulated ocular activity in response to sensory stimulation. In addition, it has been hypothesized that trigeminal sensory nerve fibers have an efferent function in response to noxious stimuli, e.g. the ocular injury response. Sympathetic nerve fibers originating in the superior cervical ganglion course through the trigeminal and pterygopalatine ganglion without forming direct synaptic contacts. These fibers, however, contain clusters of vesicles suggesting some kind

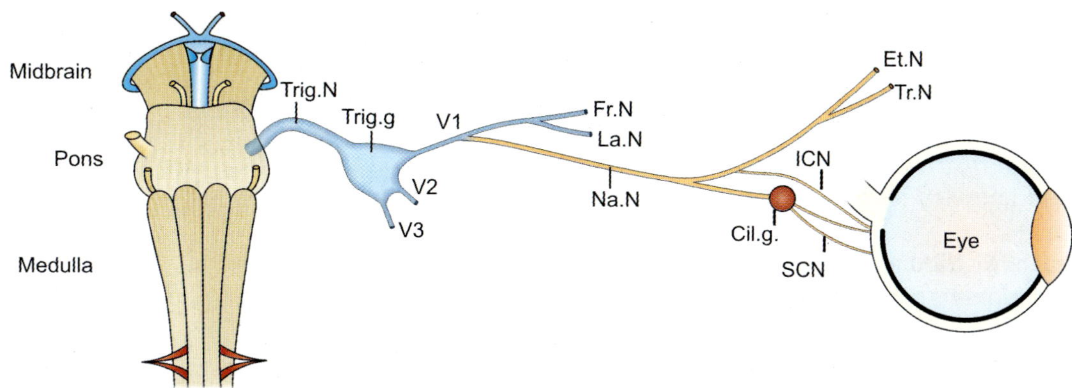

Fig. 1A: Outline of the main branches of the nerves that supply the anterior eye. A: The sensory trigeminal nerve (Trig. N) courses to the trigeminal ganglion (Trig.G.) and gives rise to the ophthalmic nerve (V1), the maxillary nerve (V2), the mandibulary nerve (V3), the lacrimal nerve (La.N.), the frontal nerve (Fr.N), the nasociliary nerve (Na.N), the posterior ethmoid nerve (Et.N), the infratrochlear nerve (Tr.N), the short ciliary nerves (SCN) and the long ciliary nerve (ICN). Cil.g.: ciliary ganglion

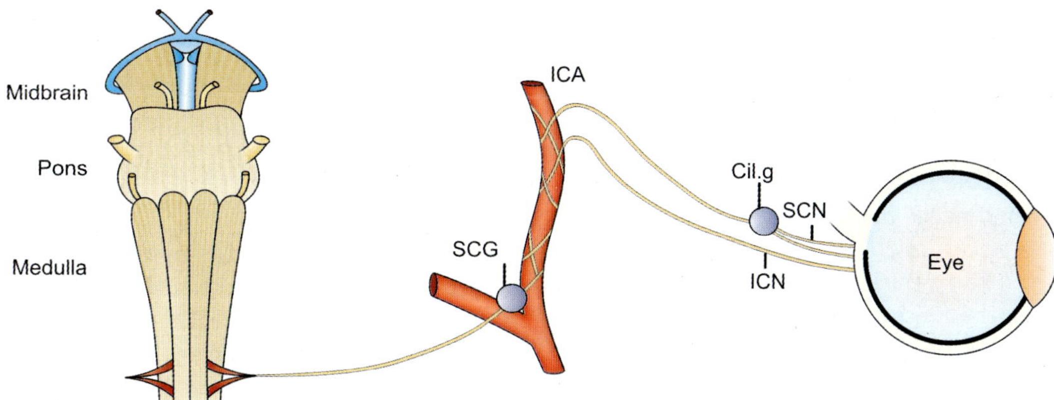

Fig. 1B: The sympathetic nerve branches run to the superior cervical ganglion (SCG) and from a plexus around the internal carotid artery (ICA). The sympathetic nerve fibers reach the eye along with arteries and nerves through the short ciliary nerves and long ciliary nerve

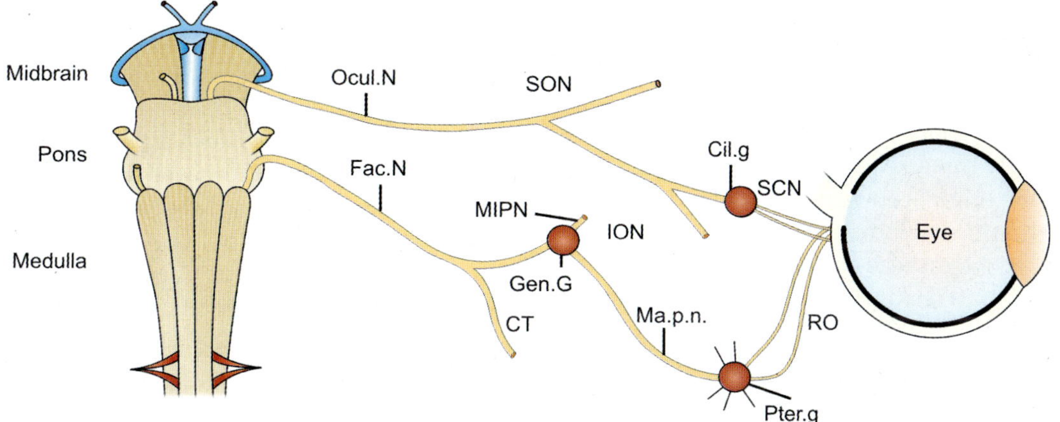

Fig. 1C: The parasympathetic nerve fibers run to the eye along with motor fibers in the oculomotor nerve (Ocul.N.) and the facial nerve (Fac.N.). The motor fibers in the oculomotor nerve branch into the superior oculomotor nerve (SON) and the inferior oculomotor nerve (ION). The parasympathetic nerve fibers run to the ciliary ganglion and reach the eye through the short ciliary nerves. The facial nerve gives rise to the chorda tympani (CT), the geniculate ganglion (Gen G.), the minor petrosal nerve (MIPN), the major petrosal nerve (Ma.p.n.), the pterygopalatine ganglion (Pter.g.) and the rami oculars.

of interneural communication. Parasympathetic nerve fibers of pterygopalatine origin course through the ciliary ganglion. These nerve fiber terminals also contain clusters of vesicles without direct synaptic contacts. Experimental data concerning the distribution of neuropeptides revealed a more detailed knowledge of the anterior eye segment innervation.

We studied the distribution of sensory trigeminal nerve fibers in the anterior eye segment and the autonomic eye related ganglia,[24] i.e. the parasympathetic ciliary and pterygopalatine ganglia and the sympathetic superior cervical ganglion in rats. For this the trigeminal ganglion was injected with tritiated leucine and wheat germ agglutinin coupled to horseradish peroxidase (WGA-HRP). After injection of WGA-HRP into the trigeminal ganglion, ganglion cell somata in the superior cervical and the pterygopalatine ganglion were labeled. As labeling of these cell bodies with WGA-HRP is the result of retrograde transport it must be assumed that cell bodies in these ganglia project to the trigeminal ganglion. [3H]Leucine injection into the trigeminal ganglion revealed the presence of labeled nerve fibers in the pterygopalatine ganglion. Labeled nerve fibers were absent in the ciliary and superior cervical ganglion. As [3H]leucine labeling of nerve fibers is the result of anterograde transport exclusively, it can be concluded that trigeminal nerve fibers project to the pterygopalatine ganglion, but not to the ciliary and superior cervical ganglion. In the retrobulbar structures, sensory nerve fibers occurred between the inferior oblique and the lateral rectus muscle and were present medial to the medial rectus muscle. Within the anterior eye segment, sensory nerve fibers were found in the cornea epithelium, stroma and adjacent to the endothelium. In addition, labeled fibers were found in the anterior stroma of the ciliary body, throughout the iris up to the pupillary border and in the conjunctiva. Most sensory nerve fibers which innervate the cornea, the iris and the ciliary body traverse the ciliary cleft.

In addition the origin, course and distribution of pre- and postganglionic neurons of the pterygopalatine ganglion (PPG) in the rat was studied using acetylcholinesterase staining,[26] wheat germ agglutinin coupled to horseradish peroxidase (WGA-HRP) histochemistry and autoradiography. These methods were used in a selected and planned fashion to reveal details concerning the innervation of the lacrimal gland and portions of the eye. The PPG in rats consists of a rostral triangular portion and additional perikarya surrounding the distal part of the major petrosal nerve. Fibers from the superior cervical ganglion (SCG) reach the PPG via the inferior petrosal sinus. Application of WGA-HRP was made after transections:

1. Rostral to the PPG; and
2. Caudal to the PPG.

The first of these applications labeled mainly fibers in the PPG; the second application labeled preganglionic parasympathetic brainstem neurons dorsolateral to the facial nucleus (i.e. the lacrimal nucleus), rostral cells in the SCG and trigeminal sensory fibers. WGA-HRP injections of the lacrimal gland, the conjunctiva and the anterior chamber of the eye all labeled cells in different parts of the PPG. This means that the PPG contains sensory and sympathetic nerve fibers and that the PPG has a topographical organization along the rostrocaudal axis. Isotope injections of the PPG anterogradely labeled fibers passing through the ciliary ganglion that innervated the conjunctiva, the limbus and parts of the choroid.

Our research in peripheral ganglia showed that satellite cells in autonomic ganglia comprise an effective barrier for WGA-HRP and HRP and probably large molecules in general. This barrier appears to be absent in sensory ganglia.[23]

Selective labeling of sympathetic nerves was obtained by means of injection of [3H]leucine into the superior cervical ganglion.[25] Bundles of sympathetic nerve fibers were found in the trigeminal ganglion and the pterygopalatine ganglion but were absent in the ciliary ganglion. In addition individual sympathetic nerve fibers, which may have contacts with trigeminal ganglion cells, were found between the ganglion cell bodies all over the trigeminal ganglion indicating a sympathetic innervation of this ganglion. In the anterior eye segment, there appeared to be a sympathetic innervation of the ciliary cleft, the ciliary body and the iris. Within the ciliary body sympathetic nerve fibers innervate the central stroma and the stroma of the ciliary processes. Labeled sympathetic nerve fibers were also observed in the stroma of the iris and were most abundant in its periphery. Most sympathetic fibers reach the iris and ciliary body by way of the base of the ciliary body. Only few sympathetic fibers are present in the ciliary cleft. No sympathetic innervation of the cornea was found.

VERGENCE

During vergence the eyes move in opposite directions at the same time. These movements are triggered by either the locations of an image on the two retinas, causing diplopia which induces fusion movements, or blur due to defocus which leads to accommodation.

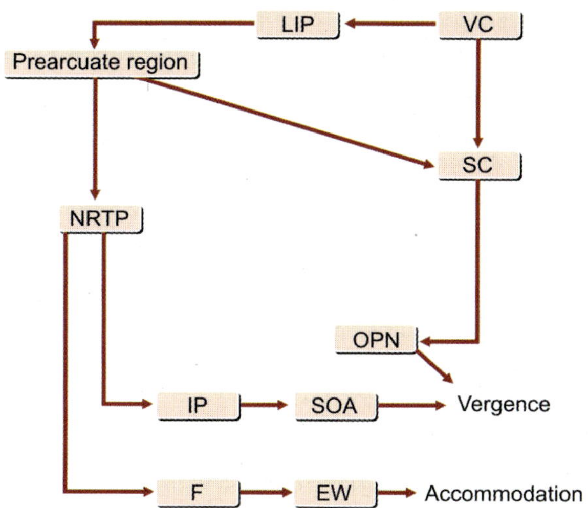

Fig. 2: Pathways involved in vergence. Fast vergence is realized through the striate en extrastriate cortex (VC) via the superior colliculus (SC) to the omnipause neurons (OPN). Slow vergence and accommodation are part of the near reflex in which from the visual cortex,lateral intraparietal area in the parietal cortex (LIP), the prearcuate region near the frontal eye fields and the medial nucleus reticulari stegmenti pontis (NRTP) project to the cerebellar nucleus interpositus (IP)and the fastigial nucleus (F). These cerebellar nuclei give rise to accommodation and vergence via the supraoculomotor area (SOA) and the Edinger Westphal nucleus (EW)

Eye movements are controlled by a variety of neural circuits. The vestibulo-ocular reflex and the optokinetic reflex, which reside in the brainstem, are controlled by circuits that are phylogenetically older than the circuits mediating vergence. Vergence is a phylogenetically new system that fascilitates binocular vision, resides in the cortex and is weaker in cats than in primates.[30]

Recently much research focused on identifying the neural substrates for vergence eye movements.[4-7,12-14,27-29] The supraoculomotor area and adjacent reticular formation around the oculomotor nucleus contain premotor neurons for vergence and accommodation. Connection tracing studies showed that the posterior interposed nucleus (IP) of the cerebellum projects to the supraoculomotor area (vergence) and that the fastigial nucleus projects also to the Edinger-Westphal nucleus (accommodation). Single-unit recording identified the nucleus reticularis tegmenti pontis (NRTP) as the precerebellar nucleus which receives input from the cerebral cortex. Physiological evidence suggests five areas involved in blur or disparity: prestriate cortex, posterior parietal cortex, the prearcuate cortex, cerebellum and superior colliculus. Both the superior colliculus and the prearcuate cortex (near the frontal eye fields) project to the paraoculomotor area.

All models of the vergence system include cross-coupling between blur-induced vergence and disparity-induced vergence. In these models the supraoculomotor area is connected to the posterior interposed nucleus (IP) of the cerebellum and the fastigial nucleus. Cerebral connections relay through the medial nucleus reticularis tegmenti pontis (NRTP) to these cerebellar nuclei. It appeared that the firing response of the IP neurons and the NRTP neurons is modulated both during disparity vergence and during accommodative vergence. Therefore, these areas are expected to be located after the cross-coupling between vergence and accommodation.

VERGENCE PATHWAYS

Retinal image disparity is the most important depth cue. Depth discrimination is essential for correct foveation of visual stimuli. Neurons showing disparity sensitivity have been found in the primary visual area (V1)[15] and in many other extrastriate visual areas, e.g. the middle temporal (MT) area[11] and the medial superior temporal (MST) area.[3] In addition, in the lateral intraparietal area LIP[8] and in the FEF, anatomically connected with MT, MST, and LIP,[16,19] disparity sensitive neurons have been demonstrated.

Stimulation of neurons in a prearcuate area of the frontal lobe could elicit both saccadic and vergence eye movements. Anatomically the prearcuate area, the lateral intraparietal area and the superior colliculus are connected. Gnadt and Mays[8] suggest that these two major cortical areas (FEF and LIP) involved in saccade production probably have a role in the guidance of disconjugate eye movements as well. LIP, FEF, and SC probably form a network for the control of both disconjugate and conjugate eye movements.

With functional imaging the striate cortex has been shown to react to blur cues.[16,19]

Vergence eye movements are separated into two different components: fast vergence, which is best elicited by stimuli with large retinal disparity errors, and slow vergence, elicited by small disparity velocities of less than $3^0/s$. In patients with acute cerebellar lesions it showed that slow vergence is impaired while fast vergence is unaffected.[17] So, the pathway from the caudal FEF via the nucleus reticularis tegmenti pontis to the cerebellum (the corticopontocerebellar circuit) may only be involved in slow vergence.

Zhou and King[10] suggested that fast vergence may be due to the ability of the saccadic system to generate unequal saccades in the two eyes. Both the rostral cap of the superior colliculus and omnidirectional pause neurons may be involved in fast vergence control.[2] Probably saccades and fast vergence have a shared gating system for movement initiation.

The effect of a change in accommodation on convergence is expressed as the ratio between accommodation in diopters and the associated change in convergence in prism diopters. (AC/A). One prism diopter is defined as the prism power needed to deviate a ray of light 1 centimeter at a distance of one meter. Therefore, theoretically the convergence requirement in prism diopters is the interpupillary distance divided by the fixation distance in meters or multiplied by the fixation distance in dioptres. So, a person with an interpupillary distance of 6 cm should converge 6 diopters for every diopter of accommodation. This ratio is usually far smaller than the amount needed to fixate binocularly. This means that both blur-induced vergence (accommodative vergence) and disparity induced vergence together align the eyes during near vision.

In clinical practice the AC/A is measured with the heterophoria method. The latent deviation of the eyes, determined with the alternate cover test, at distant and near fixations are compared. Clinically, however, the calculation method suffers from the influence of proximal accommodation and convergence.

The gradient method determines the AC/A by measuring the difference between the deviation of the eyes for a given distance after changing the accommodation with lenses in front of the eyes.

The AC/A tends to decrease with age. This decrease is most marked in the period when presbyopia develops.

Accommodative and vergence dysfunctions are diverse visual anomalies that are easily overlooked by the clinician. Symptoms possibly related to accommodative and vergence anomalies include blurred vision, headache, ocular discomfort, eyestrain, diplopia, motion sickness, and loss of concentration during visual tasks. In patients with a marked difference in eye alignment between far and near fixation, analysis of the AC/A may be useful. The patient may suffer from convergence insufficiency, convergence excess, divergence insufficiency or divergence excess.

Spasm of the near reflex has been characterized as the variable appearance of pseudomyopia, convergent strabismus and miosis. It may erroneously be diagnosed as a bilateral sixth nerve palsy. In patients with significant hypermetropia it may become manifest if the patient is unable to relax accommodation. Spasm of the near reflex is characterized by transient attacks of convergence, accommodation, and miosis. It is usually observed in young individuals and may be functional. Spasm of the near reflex was also diagnosed in patients who had associated neurologic disorders, e.g. posterior fossa abnormalities (cerebellar tumor, Arnold-Chiari malformation), thalamic esotropia (thalamic hemorrhage, pineal tumors), pituitary tumors, vestibulopathy, and a history of antecedent head trauma.

Vergence deficits may also be associated with acquired neurological disorders. Cerebellar vermis lesions, drug intoxication, progressive supranuclear palsy, pontine lesions as well as cerebral pathology may all lead to impairment of fast or slow vergence.

REFERENCES

1. Campbell FW. The minimum quantity of light required top elicit the accommodation reflex in man. J. Physiol 1954;123: 357-66.
2. Chaturvedi V, Gisbergen van JAM. Perturbation of combined saccade-vergence movements by microstimulation in monkey superior colliculus. J Neurophysiol 1999;81:2279-96.
3. Eifuku S, Wurtz RH. Response to motion in extrastriate area MSTl: Disparity sensitivity. J Neurophysiol 1999;82:2462-75.
4. Gamlin PDR, Clarke RJ. Single-unit activity in the primate nucleus reticularis tegmenti pontis related to vergence and ocular accommodations. Journal of Neurophysiol 1995;73: 2115-19.
5. Gamlin PDR, Yoon K, Zhnagh H. The role of cerebroponto-cerebrellar pathways in the control of vergence eye movements. Eye 1996;10:167-71.
6. Gamlin PDR, Yoon K. An area for vergence eye movements in primate frontal cortex. Nature 2000;407:1003-07.
7. Gamlin PDR. Neural mechanisms for the control of vergence eye movements. Annals of the New York Academy of Sciences 2002; 956:264-72.
8. Gnadt JW, Mays LE. Neurons in monkey parietal LIP are tuned for eye-movement parameters in three-dimensional space. J Neurophysiol 1995;73:280-97.
9. Helmholtz von H. Handbuch der physiologischen Optik, 2. umgearb Aufl, Hamburg: Voss 1886.
10. King WM, Zhou W. New ideas about binocular coordination of eye movements: Is there a chameleon in the primate family tree? The anatomical record 2000;261:153-61.
11. Maunsell HR, van Essen DC. Functional properties of neurons in middle temporal visual area of the macaque monkey. II. Binocular interactions and sensitivity to binocular disparity. J Neurophysiol 1983;49:1148-67.
12. Mays LE. Neural control of vergence eye movements: Convergence and divergence neurons in the midbrain. J Neurophysiol 1984;51:1091-1108.
13. Mays LE, Gamlin PDR. Neuronal circuitry controlling the near response. Current Opinion in Neurobiology 1995;5:763-8.
14. Mays LE, Porter JD, Gamlin PDR, Tello CA. Neural control of vergence eye movements: Neurons encoding vergence velocity. Journal of Neurophysiology 1986;56:1007-21.
15. Poggio GF, Fisher B. Binocular interaction and depth sensitivity in striate and prestriate cortex of behaving rhesus monkey. J Neurophysiol 1977;40:1392-1405.

16. Richter HO, Costello P, Sponheim SR, Lee JT, Pardo JV. Functional neuroanatomy of the human near/far response to blur cues. Eur J Neurosci 2004;20:2722-32.
17. Sander T, Sprenger A, Neumann G, Machner B, Gottschalk S, Rambold H, Helmchen C. Vergence deficits in patients with cerebellar lesions. Brain 2009;132:103-15.
18. Schachar RA. Qualitative effect of zonular tension on freshly extracted intact human crystalline lenses: Implications for the mechanism of accommodation. Invest. Ophthalmol. Vis Sci 2004; 45:2691-5
19. Schall JD, Morel A, King DJ, Bullier J. Topography of visual cortex connections with frontal eye field in macaque: Convergence and segregation of processing streams. J Neurosci 1995;15:4464-87.
20. Stakenburg M. Accommodation without pupillary constriction. Vision Res 1991;31:267-73.
21. Tusscher MPM ten. Peripheral ganglia and the eye - a connection tracing study. PhD thesis, Maastricht, the Netherlands 1989.
22. Tusscher MPM ten, Klooster J, Vrensen GFJM. The innervation of the rabbit's anterior eye segment: A retrograde tracing study. Exp Eye Res 1988;46:717-30.
23. Tusscher MPM ten, Klooster J, Vrensen GFJM. Satellite celles as blood ganglion cell barrier in autonomic ganglia. Brain Res 1989;490:95-102.
24. Tusscher MPM ten, Klooster J, Want JJL van der, Lamers WPMA Vrensen GFJM. The allocation of nerve fibers to the anterior eye segment and peripheral ganglia of rats. I The sensory innervation. Brain Res 1989;494:95-104.
25. Tusscher MPM ten, Klooster J, Want JJL van der, Lamers WPMA, Vrensen GFJM. The allocation of nerve fibers to the anterior eye segment and peripheral ganglia of rats. II The sympathetic innervation. Brain Res 1989;494:105-13.
26. Tusscher MPM ten, Klooster J, Baljet B, Werf F van der, Vrensen GFJM. Pre- and post-ganglionic nerve fibers of the pterygopalatine ganglion and their allocation to the eyeball of rats. Brain Res 1990;517:315-23.
27. Zee DS, Levi L. Neurological aspects of vergence eye movements. Review of Neurology (Paris) 1989;145:613-20.
28. Zhang Y, Mays LE, Gamlin PDR. Characteristics of near-response cells projecting to the oculomotor nucleus. Journal of Neurophysiology 1992;76:944-60.
29. Zhang HY, Gamlin PDR. Neurons in the posterior interposed nucleus of the cerebellum related to vergence and accommodation I. Steady-state characteristics. Journal of Neurophysiology 1998;79:1255-69.
30. Zuidam I, Collewijn H.Vergence eye movements of the rabbit in visuomotor behavior. Vision Res 1979;19:185-94.

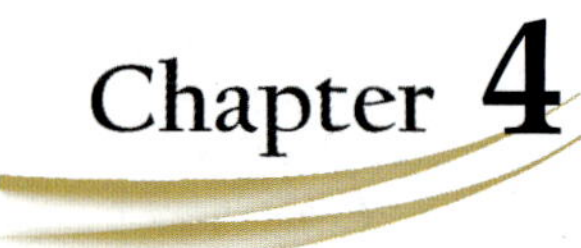

Chapter 4

Strabismus Examination: An Overview

Amar Agarwal, Ashok Garg (India)

INTRODUCTION

The pediatric strabismus examination should be done meticulously and carefully. One can divide the examination into three groups:
(i) Preliminaries, (ii) motor tests, and (iii) sensory tests.

HISTORY

One should take a good history of the patient. If it is an adult case, the patient can be asked and if a child, the parents. One should try to find out:

- If the patient has more of tropia than being orthophoric (as in intermittent tropia) and if the tropia increases on the patient being tired
- Family history
- Mother's pregnancy and other details
- Age at which the patient's eyes became abnormal
- Diplopia and questions on it
- Any associated epilepsy or other neurological problems.

VISUAL ACUITY AND REFRACTION

One should check the visual acuity of the child or adult. It is difficult in small children. In our hospital we use the video vision analyzer which is a type of pediatric autorefractor. In this, infrared light is passed into the child's eyes. The child sits at 1 meter distance from the instrument. The child can sit on the mother's lap also. Then the reflection is captured onto a video camera and the data analyzed by a computer, which tells us the refractive power of the eye.

Optokinetic nystagmus and the Allen preschool vision test can also be done. The cards using illiterate E can be used in children. One should preferably dilate the child with atropine and perform retinoscopy to rule out any high hypermetropia. Cycloplegic refraction is quite important in assessing the child's refraction.

EXAMINATION OF THE EYE

One should check the eye thoroughly on a slit lamp. Check the intraocular pressure (IOP).

Fundus examination should be done with the indirect ophthalmoscope.

CHECK FOR PSEUDOSTRABISMUS

One should check for angle kappa or for any epicanthal folds, which might give a pseudostrabismus appearance.

OCULAR MOVEMENTS

One should test for uniocular and binocular movements.

Uniocular Movements

All uniocular movements are termed ductions. There are six ductions.

- Adduction—in which the eye is moved medially
- Abduction—in which the eye is moved laterally
- Supraduction or sursumduction—the eye moves up
- Infraduction or deorsumduction—the eye moves down
- Incycloduction or intorsion—the eye rotates inwards
- Excycloduction or extorsion—the eye rotates outwards.

The normal limit of abduction is the limbus of the lateral part of the eye touching the outer canthus and the limit of adduction is the junction of the inner one-third and outer two-third of the cornea reaching an imaginary line drawn between the upper and lower punctum.

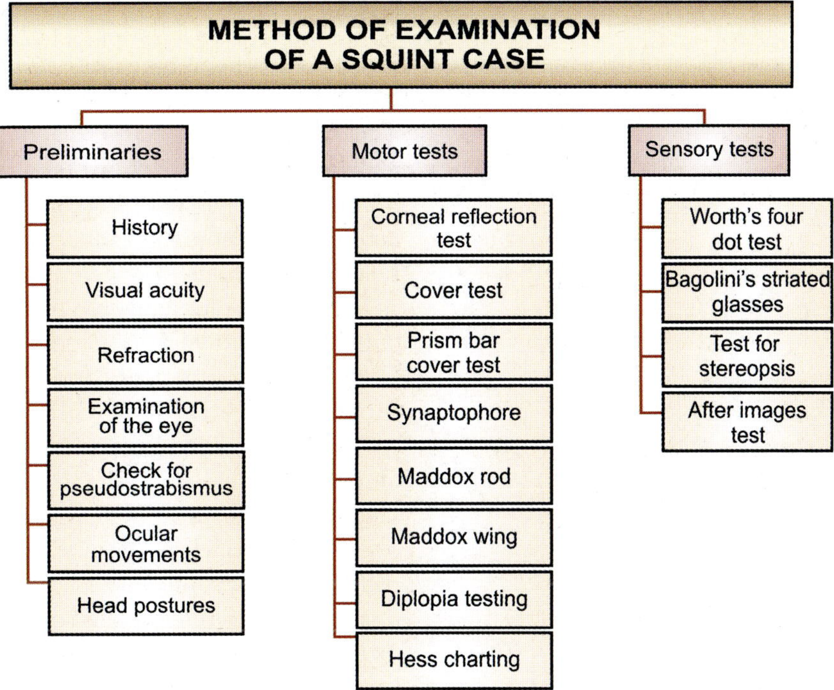

Fig. 1: Methods of examination of a squint case

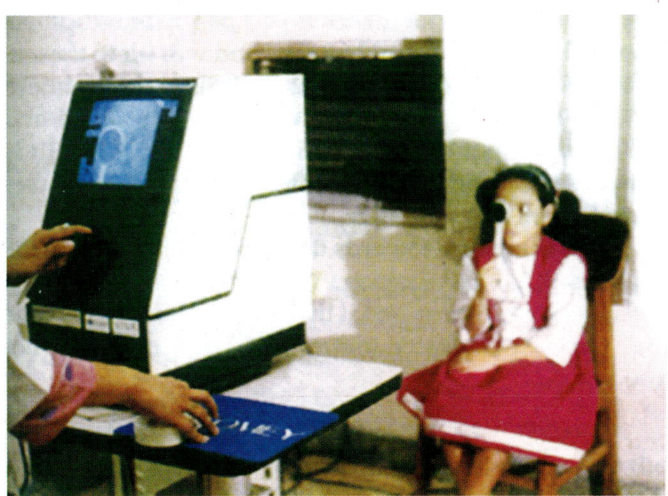

Fig. 2: Video vision analyzer

Binocular Movements

- Synchronous simultaneous movement of the two eyes in the same direction is called versions.
- Synchronous simultaneous movement of the two eyes in opposite directions is called vergence.

Versions

Basically, the actions of each muscle is shown as:

LR—Abductor
MR—Adductor
SR—Adductor, elevator and intorter
IR—Adductor, depressor and extorter.
SO—Abductor, depressor and intorter
IO—Abductor, elevator and extorter

Remember

RAD—recti are adductors, and
SAI—superiors are intorters.

The muscles involved in versions are:

Dextroversion—RE LR and LE MR,
Levoversion—RE MR and LE LR,
Dextroelevation—RE SR and LE IO,
Levoelevation—RE IO and LE SR,
Dextrodepression—RE IR and LE SO and
Levodepression—RE SO and LE IR.

Vergences

There is only one vergence that is normally possible and that is convergence, in which both eyes move medially.

We should remember two important laws concerning ocular movements. They are: Hering's law, and Sherrington's law.

Hering's Law

Hering's law states that the movement of the two eyes is equal and symmetrical.

Sherrington's Law

Sherrington's law states that whenever an agonist receives an impulse to contract, an equivalent inhibitory impulse is sent to its antagonist, which relaxes and actually lengthens.

HEAD POSTURES

Introduction

Head postures develop in a paralytic squint and depending on the muscle involved the head posture is typical.

Basics

Head postures can take three different forms:

- Head turn to the right or left
- Chin elevation or depression
- Head tilt to either shoulder.

Head turn will take place in the direction of the field of action of the paralyzed muscle to avoid diplopia in that field and maintain single binocular vision.

The chin will be elevated or depressed in the direction of the paralyzed vertical muscle. For instance, if the case is of SR palsy, the patient cannot look up, so to solve the problem the head posture will be with the chin elevated up.

Head tilt will be depending on whether the muscle is an intorter or extorter. The idea of the head posture is to keep the head tilt in such a position where the muscle does not work. This is mainly for the obliques. Remember the superiors are intorters. So, if the SO or SR are involved, the head will be tilted to the opposite side of the paralyzed muscle. This is because if right SO is paralyzed then tilting the head to the right will make the right eye intort and the left eye extort. If the right eye intorts the right eye SO will be working and as it is paralyzed, diplopia occurs. To solve this problem the head will tilt to the left. In this position the left eye will intort and the right eye will extort. So, the right SO will not be utilized and diplopia will not be present. **So remember head tilt is towards the opposite side of the eye involved in cases of superiors (SO and SR).**

Head tilt will be towards the same side in cases of the inferiors (IO and IR) getting involved. This is because the inferiors are extorters and if the head is tilted to the same side the eye of that side intorts and the extorters are not used.

Individual Muscles Involved

Table 1 shows the head postures of each muscle.

Table 1: Head postures

Paralyzed muscle	*Head (Face) turn (Important for horizontal recti)*	*Chin (Important for vertical recti)*	*Head tilt (Important for obliques)*
Right LR	Right	Nil	Nil
Right MR	Left	Nil	Nil
Right SR	Right	Elevated	Left shoulder
Right IR	Right	Depressed	Right shoulder
Right SO	Left	Depressed	Left shoulder
Right IO	Left	Elevated	Right shoulder

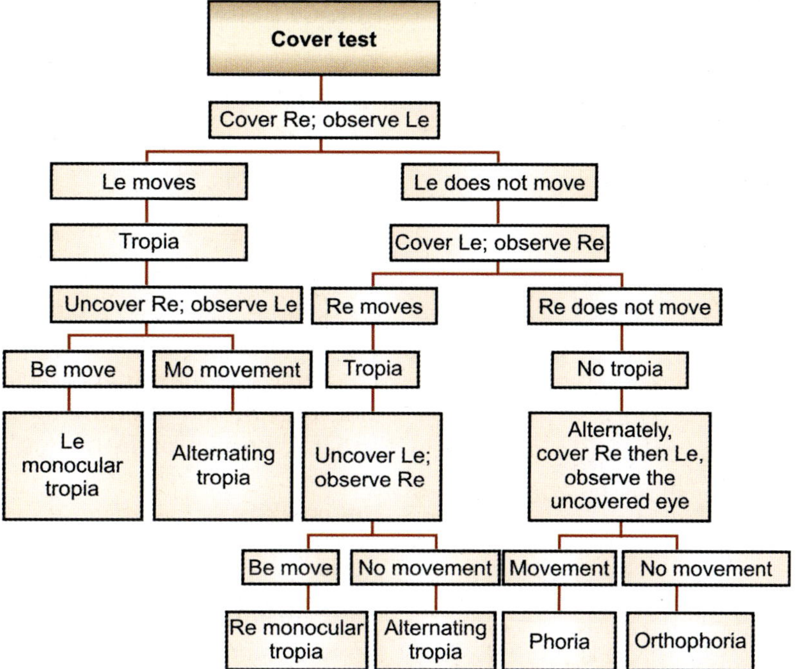

Fig. 3: Cover test

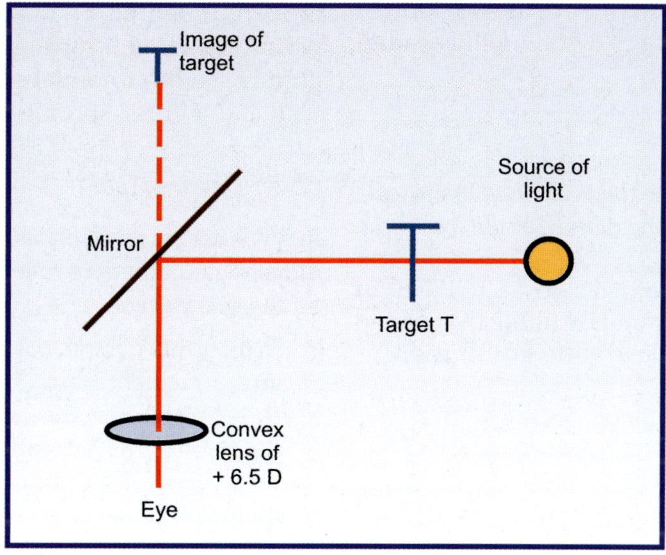

Fig. 4: Synaptophore

Right LR Palsy

The patient will move the head (face) towards the right side, i.e. towards the diseased side. This is because in this position, the right LR is not working at all and only the right MR is working.

Right MR Palsy

The patient will move the head (face) towards the left side, i.e. towards the normal side. This is because in this position the right MR is not working and only the right LR is working.

Right SR Palsy

In all vertical muscle palsies three things have to be noted: (i) Chin, (ii) face turn, and (iii) head tilt.

In SR palsy,

- The chin will be elevated to overcome the decrease in the upward movement.
- The face will be turned towards the diseased side, i.e. in this case to the right. This is because the SR works in abduction, and so by turning the face to the right will adduct the eye and the SR will not work.
- The head is tilted to the left side, i.e. to the normal side because SR is an intorter and so the eye tries to extort to prevent diplopia. Thus, it does by tilting the head to the normal side.

Right IR Palsy

- The chin is depressed, as the depression effect is lost.
- The face is turned towards the diseased side, i.e. to the right.
- The head is tilted to the diseased side, i.e. to the right because the IR is an extorter and by tilting the head to the right side the eye is made to undergo intorsion.

Right IO Palsy

- The chin is elevated
- The face is turned toward the normal side, i.e. to the left side
- The head is tilted to the diseased side, i.e. toward the right side.

Right SO Palsy

- The chin is depressed
- The face is turned towards the normal side, i.e. towards the left side
- The head is tilted to the normal side, i.e. left side.

HIRSCHBERG'S CORNEAL REFLECTION TEST

Test

Hirschberg found that each 1 mm of decentration of the corneal reflex corresponded to 7 degrees of deviation of the visual axis. Thus,

1 mm = 7 degrees.

In this test, the examiner stands in front of the patient and shines a light in the patient's eyes and observes the position of the reflection of the light on the cornea. It should normally be at the center of the pupil. If it is at the edge of a normal pupil, it is approximately 15 degrees of squint and if at the edge of the limbus, it is 45 degrees.

COVER TEST

Parts

There are three parts in the cover test: (i) simple cover test, (ii) cover-uncover test, and (iii) alternate cover test.

Simple Cover Test

In this, first of all observe both the eyes. Then just cover one eye after the patient has fixated a target. Note the behavior of the uncovered eye. Each eye should be tested in turn. It should be done for near and distance and performed in all 9 cardinal positions of gaze. The head posture should be normal and the test should be performed with and without spectacles.

Cover-Uncover Test

In this, after covering one eye, the cover is removed and the movements of the eyes noted. The findings vary depending on the diagnosis.

- In a normal person, covering one eye will not produce any movement of the other eye.
- In heterophoria, the covered eye will deviate in the direction of the heterophoric position. When the eye is uncovered, it will move in the direction opposite to that while under cover to re-establish binocular fixation. The opposite eye maintains fixation and makes no movement. **Thus, if only one eye moves it is a phoria.**
- In heterotropia, if the fixating eye is covered, the opposite eye, provided it is able to do so, will make a movement from the heterotropic position and the covered eye will make a corresponding movement in accordance with Hering's law. On uncovering the formerly fixating eye, it will either resume fixation and the other eye will again deviate or the previously

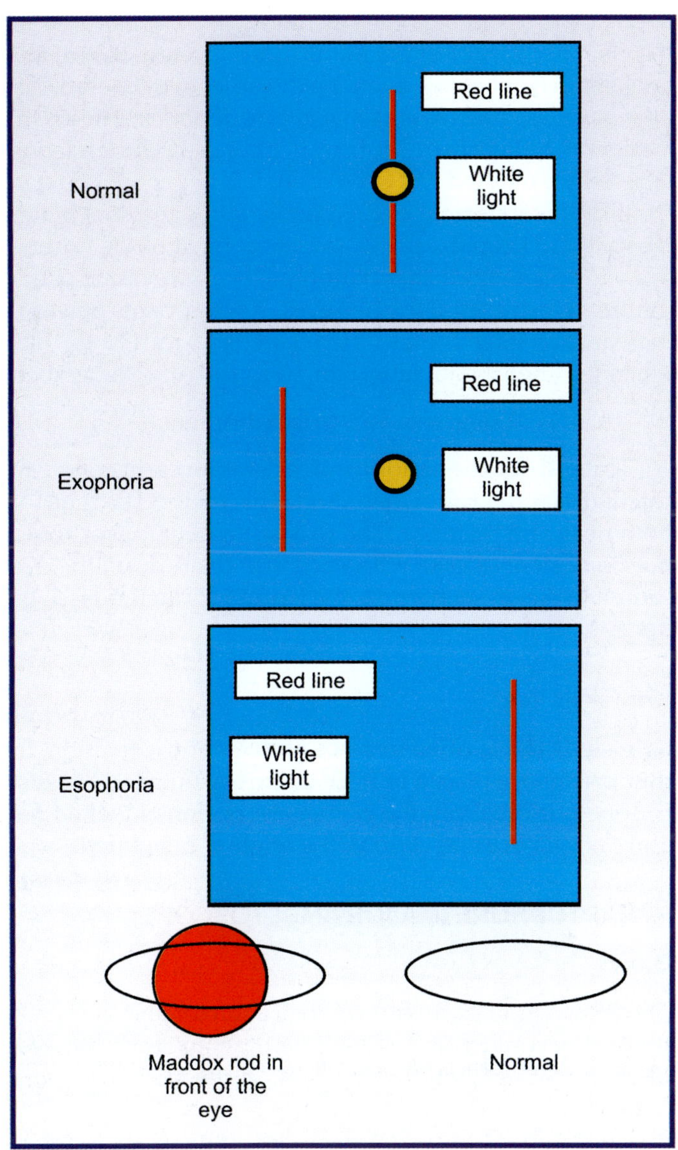

Fig. 5: Maddox rod

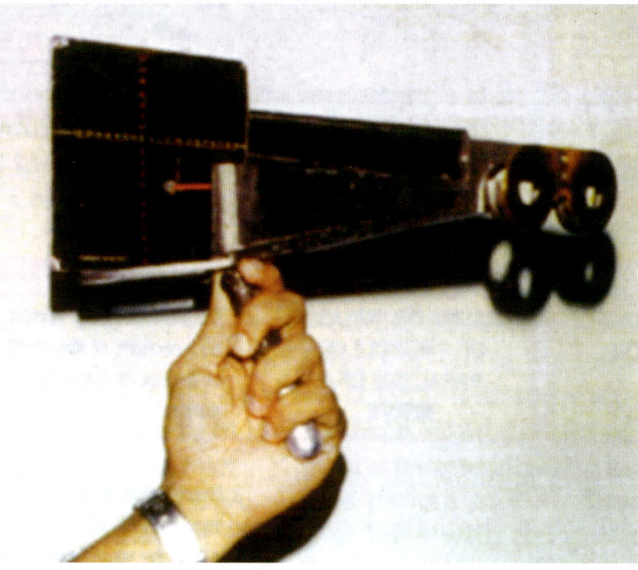

Fig. 6: Maddox wing

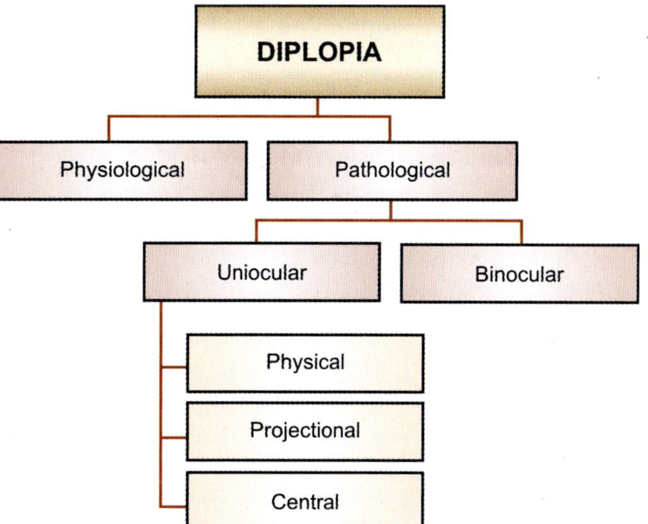

Fig. 7: Classification of diplopia

deviated eye will maintain fixation and the newly uncovered eye will remain deviated, depending on whether one is dealing with a unilateral or an alternate heterotropia. *Thus, if both eyes or none move, it is a tropia.*

Alternate Cover Test

In this, the patient looks at the fixation target with both eyes open and each eye is alternately covered and uncovered several times. This prevents fusion of the two eyes and thus reveals a latent squint. It is used to diagnose a latent squint of even 2 degrees and small degrees of tropia.

Primary and Secondary Deviation

The deviation of the squinting eye behind the screen when the non-squinting eye is fixing is called the *primary deviation*. Its direction and extent is revealed when the non-squinting eye is covered and the squinting eye takes up fixation. The deviation of the non-squinting eye behind the screen when the squinting eye is fixing is called the *secondary deviation*. Its deviation and extent is revealed when the squinting eye is covered so that the non-squinting eye resumes fixation. Now,

- If both deviations are equal, the squint is comitant. The reason why the primary and secondary deviation is equal because of Hering's law, which means that the movement of the two eyes is equal and symmetrical.
- If the secondary deviation is greater than the primary, the squint is incomitant and paretic. This is because the attempt to get the paralyzed eye into line creates an abnormal effort of innervation and since this energy is involuntarily shared between the two eyes, the movement of the sound eye in the direction of the paralyzed muscle [secondary deviation] will be excessive.
- If the primary deviation is greater than the secondary, the squint is spastic and fibrotic (incomitant). In this, due to contractures, a slight innervation will produce a lot of movement of the affected eye and so the primary deviation is greater than the secondary deviation.

Fallacies of the Cover Test

The cover test produces fallacies in:

- Eccentric fixation
- Uncooperative or mentally retarded patient
- If the vision is very much decreased and
- Nystagmus.

PRISM BAR COVER TEST

Test

In prism bar cover test or Duane's parallax test, the prisms are kept in front of one eye with the other eye covered. *The prisms are kept with the apex towards the deviation*. The prism ladder can be kept in front of any eye but in eccentric fixation [Krimsky's method has to be used, it is better to keep it in front of the abnormal eye. Actually some feel it is better normally to keep the prism ladder in front of the normal eye. Now, one should alternately cover each eye and check for the movements of the two eyes. As the prisms power is increased, a stage comes when there is no movement, i.e. when the angle of deviation can be found out. Remember,

1 degree = 1.75 prism diopters

Thus, from the amount of prisms present, one can calculate the degree of deviation. This method is done for both near and distance. The prism bar cover test should not be done in a case with eccentric fixation, as the eye cannot fixate. In such a case, the Krimsky's method is to be done.

Krimsky's Test

Krimsky's test is done in cases with eccentric fixation. In this, prisms are placed in front of the eye but no cover test is done with it. Only the corneal reflection is looked for and once it becomes central, the angle is calculated.

SYNAPTOPHORE (MAJOR AMBLYOSCOPE)

Basics

The rays of light from the target hit a mirror and then pass through a convex lens of +6.5 diopters to reach the eye. Thus, the image will be seen behind the mirror, i.e. at a distance of 6 m which will be equal to the focal length of the lens. Thus, the synaptophore images are seen at distance and not near. This is because we do not want the patient to use his or her accommodation. If we want to use the synaptophore for near, then we keep a – 3 diopter lens in front of the eye.

Usage of the Instrument

Interpupillary Distance (IPD)

First of all the IPD is checked.

Simultaneous Macular Perception

Now, we use the simultaneous paramacular perception slides.

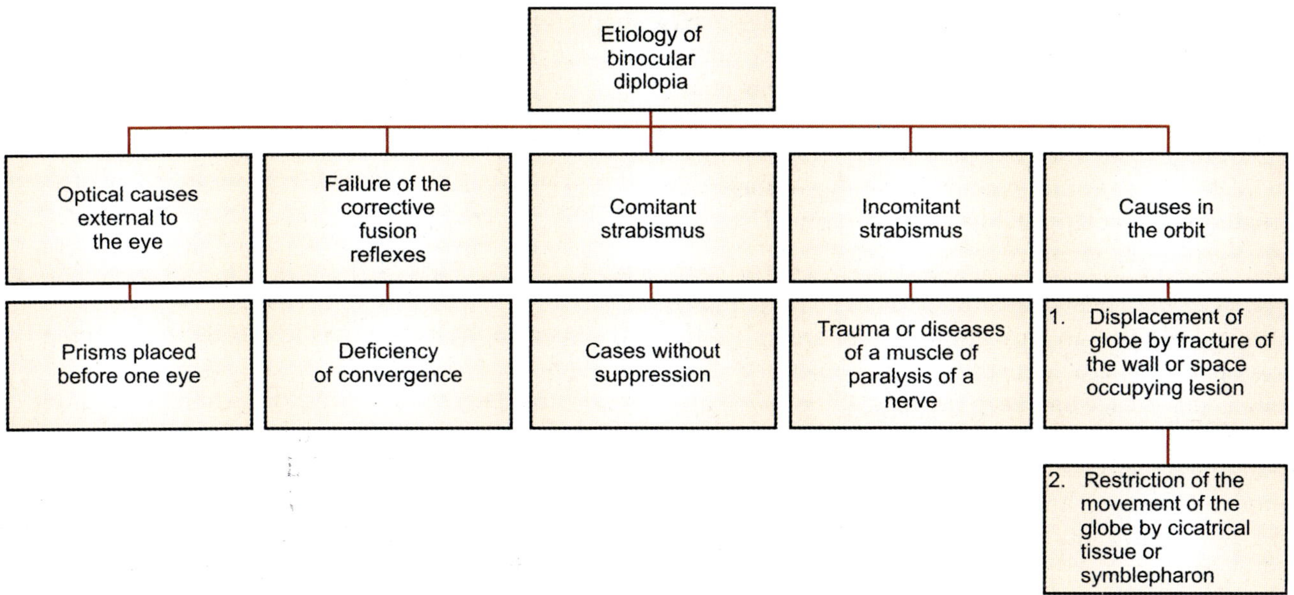

Fig. 8: Etiology of binocular diplopia

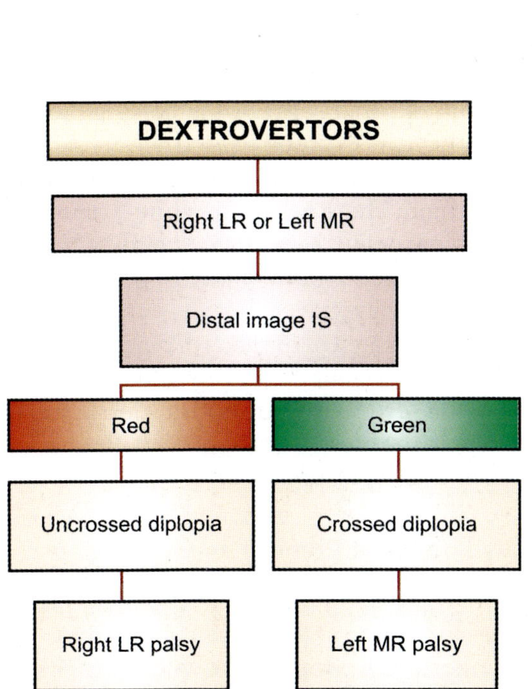

Fig. 9: Dextrovertors

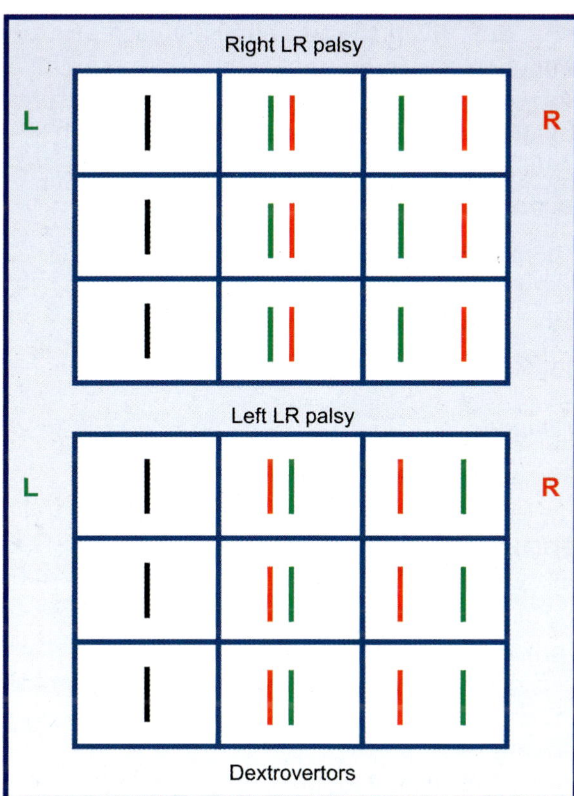

Fig. 10: Diplopia testing of dextrovertors

Objective angle: The objective angle of squint is checked in all 9 cardinal positions of gaze. In these, one is the primary position and the other 8 are 15 degrees from the primary position. To test the objective angle, keep one arm of the synaptophore fixed at zero degree. Now, move the other arm till there is no movement of the eyes when you alternately on and off the lights of the two arms. The point where the eyes do not move is the objective angle.

Subjective angle: Then check the subjective angle in all 9 positions of gaze. In this again, fix one arm of the synaptophore at zero degree. Show the patient the slides of a lion and its cage and keep the cage in the arm that is fixed. Now, ask the patient to move the other arm [containing the slide of the lion] and ask the patient to put the lion in the cage. The angle at which this is done is the subjective angle of squint.

Fusion

Now check for fusion. In this, two slides are used. One is that of a rabbit without a tail and the other of a rabbit without ears. Keep the two slides in each arm of the synaptophore and fix the arms at the angle of squint. If the patient sees both the ears and the tail, then fusion is present. If the patient sees either the tail or the ears, fusion is absent.

Stereopsis

Test stereopsis with slides containing paratroopers with a plane in the background. The patient should be able to tell if the paratroopers are in front of the plane or not which indicates good stereopsis.

After Images

After images can also be done.

MADDOX ROD

Principle

Maddox rod depends on the effect of a cylindrical lens in converting the image of a point object into a linear form.

Apparatus

Apparatus consists of one or several cylinders of red glass placed side by side in a frame. When a spot of light is passed through it, the image is formed as a focal line running perpendicular to the axis of the cylinders. With the rod before one eye that eye sees a red line running perpendicularly to the direction of the cylinders while the other eye sees the spot of light.

Distance

The Maddox rod is the only test done at a distance of 5 metres.

Results

- In orthophoria, the red line runs through the white light.
- With a latent or manifest deviation, the red line does not pass through the white light. With the cylinders running in a horizontal direction, a deviation to the right or left indicates a lateral deviation. With the cylinders vertical, a deviation above or below indicates a vertical deviation. The degree of deviation can be read off on a tangent scale [This is a scale at which the patient can fixate]. If the rod is in front of the RE, and there is an uncrossed diplopia, then it indicates an esodeviation. If there is a crossed diplopia, it indicates an exodeviation.

MADDOX WING TEST

Instrument

In this instrument, there are two slit holes in the eyepiece. The fields which are exposed to each eye are separated by a diaphragm in such a way that they glide tangentially into each other. The RE sees a white arrow pointing vertically upwards and a red arrow pointing horizontally to the left. The LE sees a horizontal row of Figures in white and a vertical row in red.

These are calibrated in diopters of deviation. The arrow pointing to the horizontal row of Figures and the arrow pointing to the vertical row are both at zero in the absence of a squint or in the presence of a squint with a harmonious abnormal retinal correspondence.

Clinically Important Points

- The Maddox wing should be held pointing at 15 degrees inferiorly, as you hold it for reading
- It is important to do the test with and without correction for refractive errors. If there is a high degree of hypermetropia and/or presbyopia, it may not be possible to carry out the Maddox wing test with vision unaided owing to the patient being unable to read the numbers on the scale

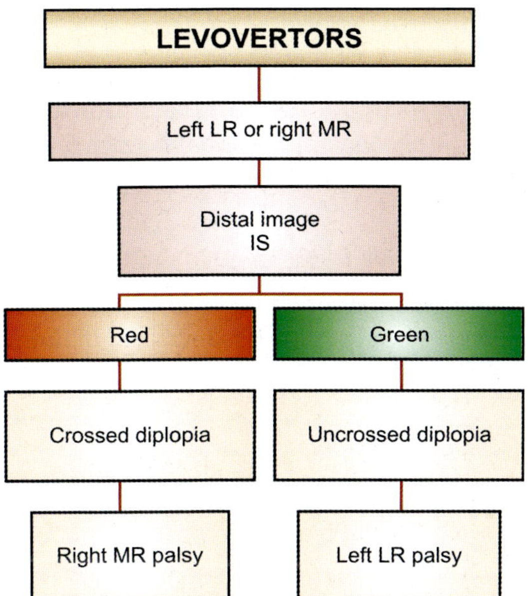

Fig. 11: Levovertors

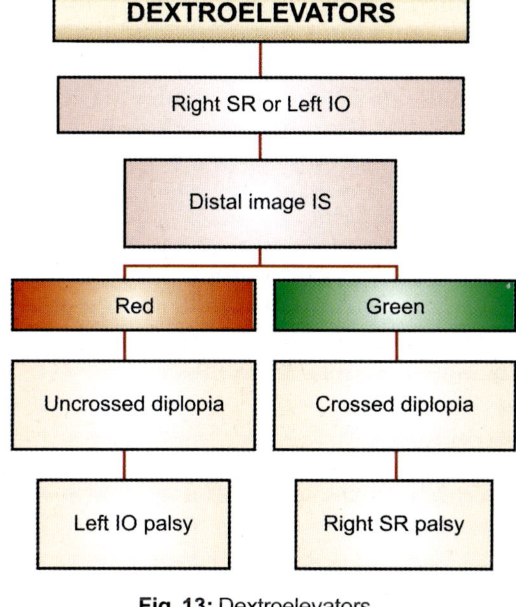

Fig. 13: Dextroelevators

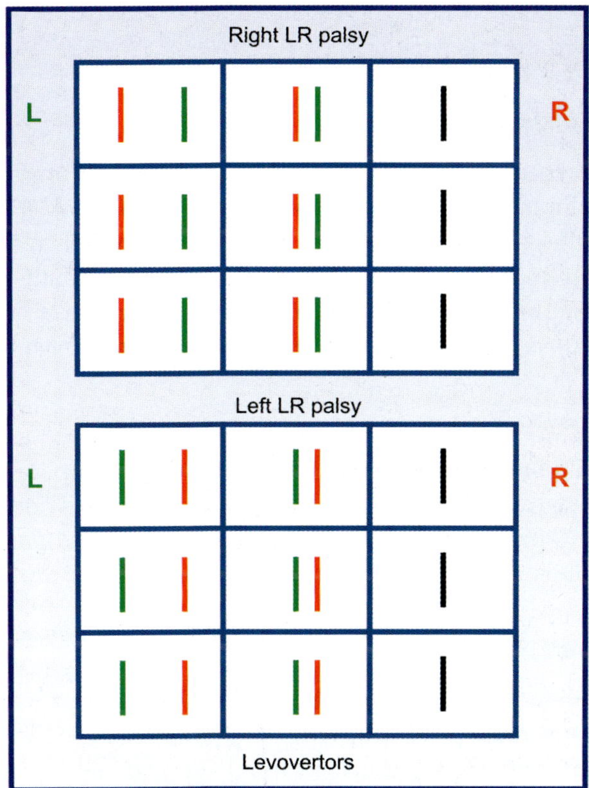

Fig. 12: Diplopia testing of levovertors

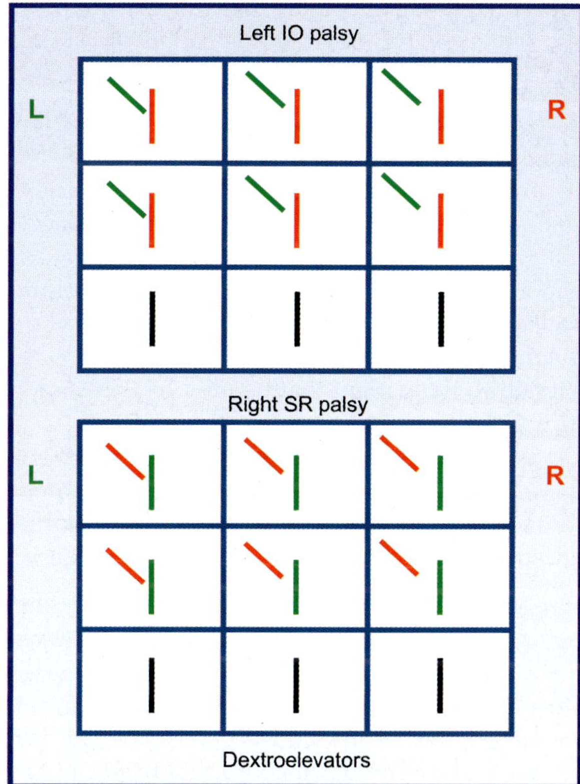

Fig. 14: Diplopia testing of dextroelevators. Remember, RAD- recti are adductors; so SR works like MR and so paralysis for SR produces an uncrossed squint and so crossed diplopia

- The ability of the patient to give an answer on the Maddox wing does not mean that the patient has normal binocular vision for the patient can have abnormal retinal correspondence (ARC) or rapid alteration.

DIPLOPIA

Diplopia Definition

Diplopia is due to identical objects imaged on disparate retinal areas and therefore seen in different visual directions and thus seen as double.

Types of Diplopia

Diplopia can be physiological or pathological.

Physiological Diplopia (Fixation Disparity)

Explanation: When two images of an object fall on corresponding retinal points, single vision is attained. Fusion is still possible for a certain margin of disparity, but if the images fall on widely disparate points, diplopia results which being inevitable is called physiological diplopia.

Clinical significance: Fixation disparity is a variant of normal binocular vision. The disparity is usually –5 to +3 min of arc. It has a two-fold clinical significance.

- *Undesirable:* Occasionally, a person becomes accidentally aware of physiological diplopia. Since double vision must appear as an abnormal situation, the patient seeks the help of an ophthalmologist, who after diagnosing physiological diplopia may not be able to explain to the patient that he only has physiological diplopia.
- *Desirable:* In the diagnosis of binocular cooperation, the presence of physiological diplopia indicates that the patient is capable of using both eyes in casual seeing and presumably does so.

Normal: Physiological diplopia is a phenomenon inherent in the organization of the sensory apparatus for vision. The question arises, "Why are we not always aware of diplopia?" From the first moment in which binocular vision is established, we become accustomed or conditioned to the arrangements provided for binocular seeing and hence to physiological diplopia. We learn how to disregard it and unless some abnormal process interferes we never become aware of diplopia.

Physical Uniocular Diplopia

Physical uniocular diplopia is due to optical causes in the eye like keratoconus, iridodialysis, double pupils, subluxation of the lens, spherophakia, incipient cataract and retinal detachment.

Projectional Uniocular Diplopia

Projectional uniocular diplopia is seen in eccentric fixation when a single visual stimulus is localized in normal and abnormal directions.

Central Uniocular Diplopia

Central uniocular diplopia is seen in calcarine lesions, multiple sclerosis and basal meningitis.

Binocular Diplopia

The causes of binocular diplopia are many.

Images: In diplopia, one image is distinct and is called the true image, whereas the other image is indistinct and is called the false image.

Uncrossed Diplopia

Uncrossed diplopia is also known as homonymous diplopia. In convergent squint, the image of the object falls on the nasal side of the fovea. But this point usually receives light from the temporal fields and so, it results in the false image on the outer side of the true image. *Thus, a convergent squint or crossed squint produces an uncrossed diplopia.*

Crossed Diplopia

In a divergent squint, the image falls on the temporal side of the fovea. But this is perceived from the nasal field. So, the term is heteronymous diplopia. Thus, a divergent squint or uncrossed squint gives rise to a crossed diplopia.

Paradoxical Diplopia

In this, the type of diplopia is opposite to that usually found in the particular type of squint present, so that an uncrossed diplopia occurs in a divergent squint and a crossed diplopia in a convergent squint. It may occur after surgical correction of a squint with abnormal retinal correspondence.

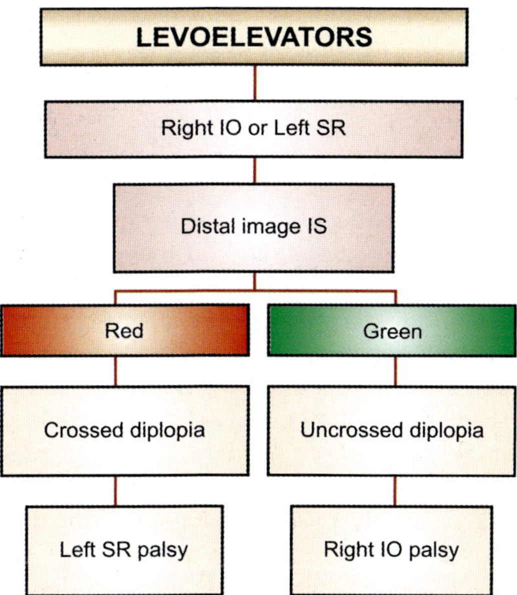

Fig. 15: Levoelevators

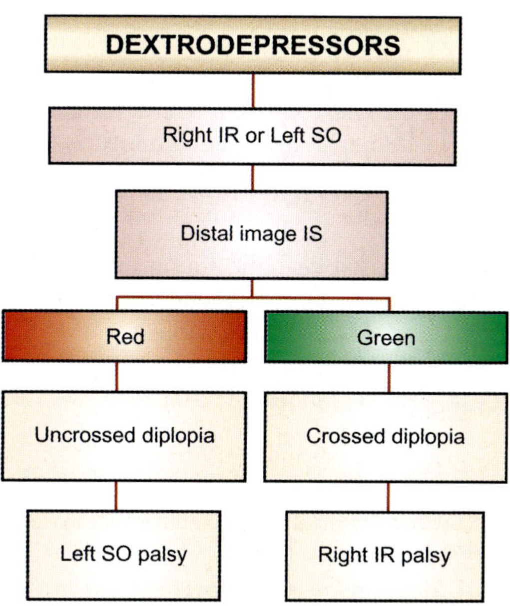

Fig. 17: Dextrodepressors

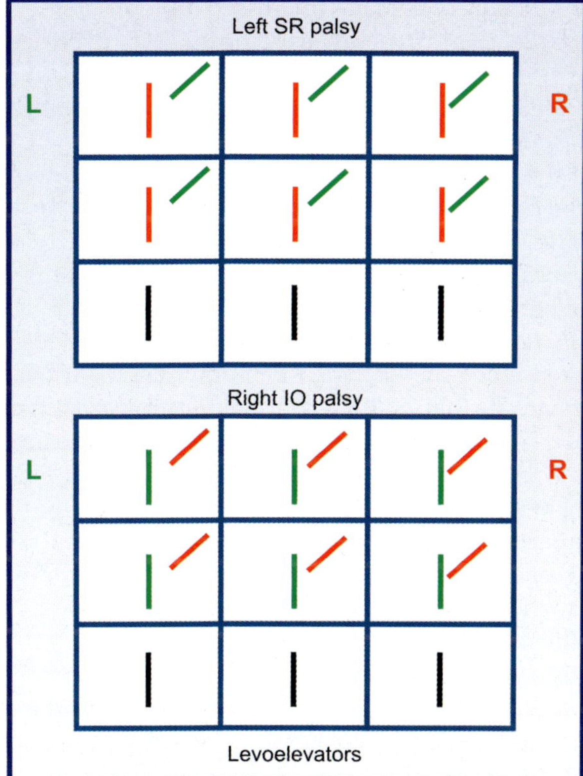

Fig. 16: Diplopia testing of levoelevators. Remember, RAD- recti are adductors; so SR works like MR and so paralysis for SR produces an uncrossed squint and so crossed diplopia

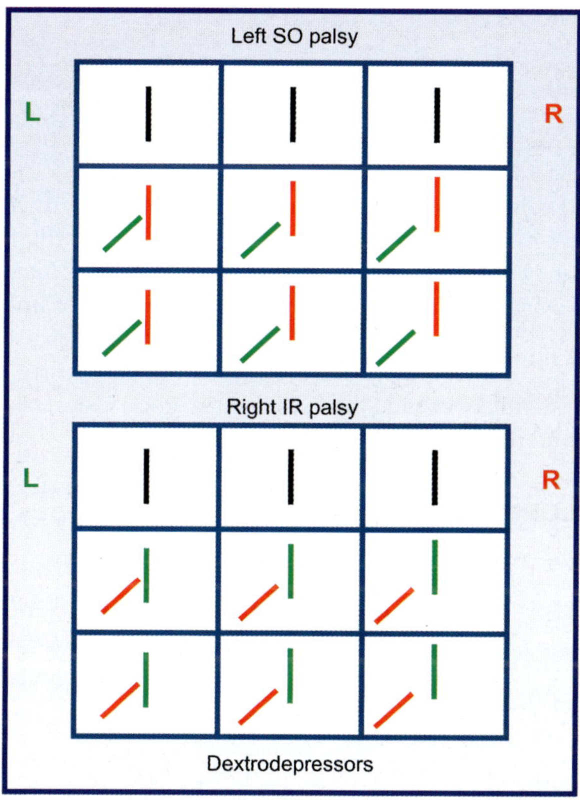

Fig. 18: Diplopia testing of dextrodepressors. Remember, RAD- recti are adductors; so SR works like MR and so paralysis for IR produces an uncrossed squint and so crossed diplopia

Congruous Diplopia

When the distance between the double images (measured in degrees of arc) corresponds to the deviation of the deviating eye, then it is said to be a congruous diplopia.

Incongruous Diplopia

When the distance between the double images [measured in degrees of arc] does not correspond to the angle of squint, the diplopia is said to be incongruous.

Overcoming Diplopia

When a patient develops diplopia, the body tries to overcome it by certain ways. They are:

- A direct muscular effort by corrective fusion movements as in heterophoria
- Closure of one eye—*monoblepsia*
- Suppression of one image
- The development of abnormal retinal correspondence
- The adoption of abnormal head postures
- The development of amblyopia and eccentric fixation
- The development of Swan's syndrome.

Swan's Syndrome

Swan described a mechanism in which some patients with an esotropia of 30 to 40 prism diopters make use of the blind spot to overcome diplopia. In other words, the false image is made to fall on the optic disk so that the false image is not noticed. This is also known as the *blind spot mechanism*. Occasional diplopia and confusion of images characterize this syndrome. Other features are—esotropia of 12 to 18 degrees, blind spot of the deviating eye consistently overlying the fixation area, good vision of each eye and normal correspondence.

DIPLOPIA TESTING

Introduction

Diplopia testing is a very important test in diagnosing the muscle paralyzed in a paralytic squint. Further, it is a very inexpensive test, as it requires only a source of light and a red green goggles.

Procedure

Put on a red green goggles on the patient with red in front of the right eye and green in front of the left eye. Hold a torch in your hand and cover it with some tape so that only a slit of light is seen. Then stand in front of the patient (about 1 meter). Make the patient sit, keep his or her head straight and ask the patient to look directly forward so that the light is at level with the patient's eyes. Now ask the patient the *first question—"Do you see one light or two?"* If the patient confirms seeing two lights he or she has diplopia.

Then ask the patient the *second question—"Is one above the other or are they side by side?"* If the answer is side by side, we are dealing with a horizontal muscle palsy but if they are one above the other, a vertical muscle is involved. *If the diplopia is horizontal*, then move the torch slowly to the patient's left, the patient being instructed to watch the lights. The patient is then asked the *third question—"Do the two lights get further apart or not?"* The same question is asked by moving the torch to the patient's right. If the two lights become further apart when looking to the right, there is paresis of the dextrovertors, i.e. *right LR* or *left MR* and if it happens when looking to the left there is paresis of *the levoovertors*, i.e. *left LR* and *right MR*. Now, to find out which of these muscles is at fault, ask the *fourth question—"Is the outer image red or green in color?"* If the dextrovertors are involved and the distal image or outer image is red then it means that the patient has uncrossed diplopia. Remember a crossed squint (or an esotropia) will produce an uncrossed diplopia and a crossed squint will occur only by a lateral rectus palsy so the diagnosis would be a *right LR paresis*.

If the levovertors are involved, the muscles involved are the right medial rectus and the left lateral rectus.

If the diplopia is vertical, then the torch is moved slowly upwards and the patient is asked to follow the lights with his or her eyes. He or she is then asked the *third question—"Do the two lights get further apart or not?"* The same question is asked when moving the torch downwards. If the two lights are further apart when looking upwards there is paralysis of one of the elevators, i.e. SR or IO. The torch is moved up and to the right and then up and to the left and the patient asked in which of these two positions the lights are apart more vertically. If the answer is up and to the right, one of the dextroelevators are involved and if up and to the left one of the levoelevators are involved. Now ask the *fourth question—"Is the outer image red or green in color?"*

Similarly, one can work for the depressor muscles.

HESS CHARTING

Instrument

Hess charting consists of a black cloth, three and a half feet long, marked out by a series of red lines subtending

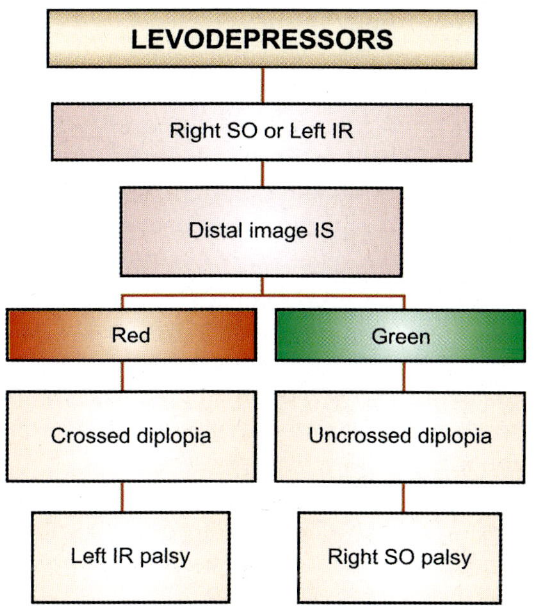

Fig. 19: Levodepressors

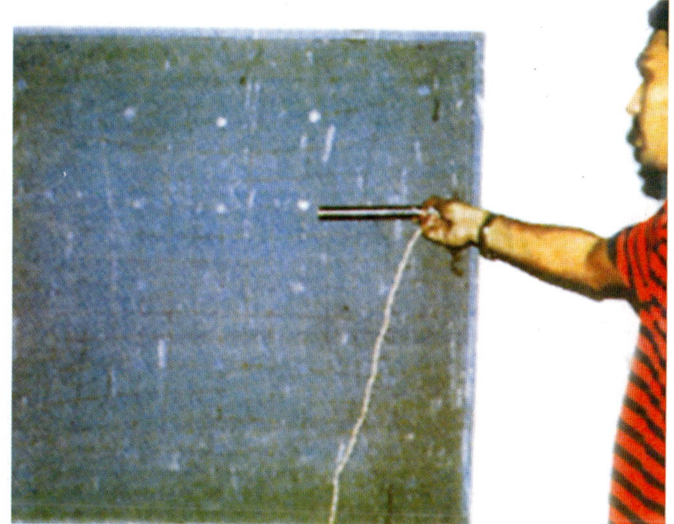

Fig. 21: Hess chart

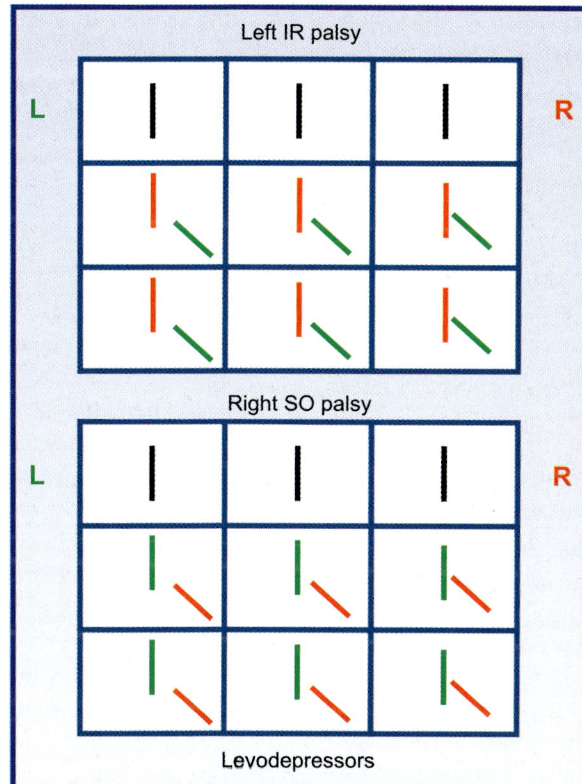

Fig. 20: Diplopia testing of levodepressors. Remember, RAD- recti are adductors; so SR works like MR and so paralysis for IR produces an uncrossed squint and so crossed diplopia

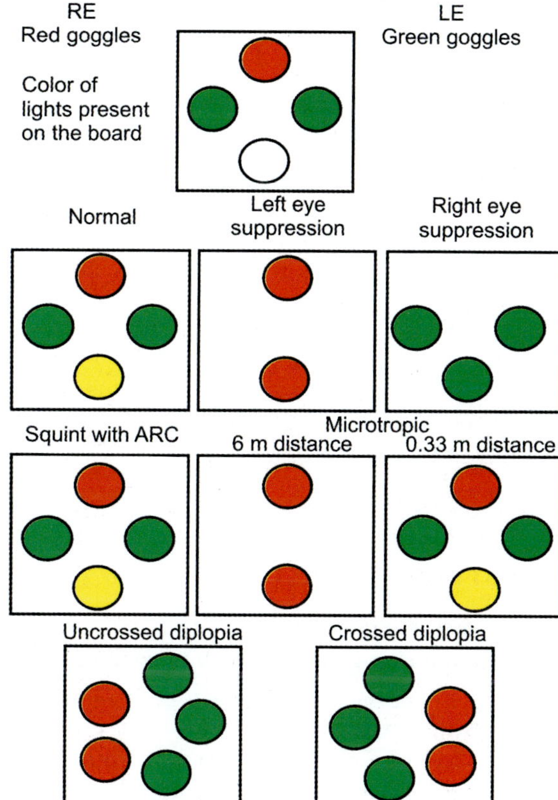

Fig. 22: Worth's four dot test

between them an angle of 5 degrees. At the zero point of this coordinate system and at each of the points of intersection of the 15 and 30 degree lines with one another and with corresponding vertical and horizontal lines, there is a red dot. These dots form an inner square of 8 dots and an outer square of 16 dots. An indicator is provided with a green light.

Test

The patient wears red green goggles and is seated 50 cm from the screen. The patient thus sees the red dots with one eye and the green light with the other eye. The patient is asked to place the green light over each of the red dots in turn. The examiner marks the positions indicated by the patient on a small card with a reduced copy of the screen. Straight lines connect the points found by the patient. The red green goggles are now reversed with the red filter in front of the LE. This gives us the final Hess chart from which we can detect which muscle is paralyzed.

Results

- After charting, the eye in which smaller squares are made is the diseased eye.
- In any muscle palsy, there will be an overaction of the ipsilateral antagonist and contralateral synergist with underaction of the antagonist of the contralateral synergist.
- If you get a straight line on the Hess chart it means a mechanical restriction as in blow-out fractures, Duane's syndrome or Brown's syndrome.
- If you get underaction of a muscle without overaction of the ipsilateral antagonist, it is due to mechanical restriction.
- If you have a line that is not straight and there is no overaction, then it is due to combination of a palsy and mechanical restriction.

WORTH'S FOUR DOT TEST

The apparatus consists of an illuminated box with 4 apertures of colored glass one red, two greens and one white. The patient at 6 meters wears a red-green goggles with the red in front of the right eye and green in front of the left eye. **To check if the goggles are alright, combine the red with the green and look through them. If one is not able to see anything, that means that the goggles are good. This is because the red goggles will allow only red light through and as the green allows only green light, nothing will be seen. Before starting the test, check if the patient is colorblind.** The reason we use red and green is because they are complimentary colors. Now, ask the patient to see and tell how many dots are there.

- *If the patient sees four*—one red, two green and the fourth yellow, pink or light green (depending on whether he or she has no dominant eye, right eye dominant or left eye dominant respectively) he or she is normal.
- *If the patient sees only two red lights*—the right eye is dominant and left eye suppressed.
- *If the patient sees three green lights*—the left eye is dominant and right eye suppressed.
- *If the patient sees 5 lights*—the patient has diplopia.
- *If the patient sees 4 lights and has a squint*—the diagnosis is abnormal retinal correspondence.
- *If the patient sees 2 or 3 lights at 6 meters and 4 lights at 0.33 m*—the diagnosis is microtropia. When the Worth's four dot test is done at 6 meters, it projects approximately 1.25 degrees on the retinal area and so when the patient stands at a distance of 6 meters, the dots fall on his or her foveal scotoma and the patient sees either two red dots or three green dots depending on the eye involved. Now, as the patient is brought closer to the dots at a distance of 0.33 meters, the dots project at approximately 6 degrees—in other words, the retinal projection area of the image exceeds the size of the scotoma and the patient sees four dots.

BAGOLINI'S STRIATED GLASSES TEST

In this test, the patient fixates a small light, after having been provided with plano lenses with a narrow fine striation across one meridian. These glasses do not affect the vision or the accommodation of the patient but cause the fixation light to appear as an elongated streak, since the glasses are *micro-Maddox cylinders*. In these glasses, the lines are made oblique and not vertical as scotomas generally occur vertically so abnormal retinal correspondence (ARC) might be missed if the lines were made vertical.

In NRC (normal retinal correspondence,) the lines cross in the center, whereas in ARC they do not. In microtropia, the lines are not seen in the center and this indicates foveal suppression. The Bagolini's striated glasses are the best test for ARC as it takes the most physiological position of the patient. When the patient is walking on the streets, he or she does not see after images but he or she would see something like in Bagolini's striated glasses. The difference between the Bagolini's test, and the after images test is that in the after image test, the fovea of both eyes is being stimulated, whereas in the Bagolini's, the fovea of one eye and an abnormal point of the other eye is being stimulated.

If a patient has a squint, then if the lines cross in the center, it is a case of ARC and if the lines do not cross in the center, it is a case of NRC. In cases of RE or LE suppression, one of the lines will not be seen.

TESTS FOR STEREOPSIS

Definition of Stereopsis

It is the perception of the third dimension, i.e. relative nearness and farness of objects.

Difference Between Stereopsis and Fusion

Fusion has a motor component whereas stereopsis does not. Further fusion of only one object point in an otherwise formless field can occur, but this is inadequate as a stimulus for stereopsis. For stereopsis to occur, the retina has to be stimulated by at least two object points having a different proximaldistal relationship with each other. Lastly, fusion localizes points in a two-dimensional plane for the observer, whereas stereopsis localizes in the third dimension of depth.

Tests

Synaptophore: The slides used are that of paratroopers jumping from a plane. This is described under synaptophore.

Titmus fly test: This is a test containing vectograph cards. The patient puts on special glasses and is shown the book. The patient is asked if the fly can be caught. Further quantification of the test can also be done thus telling the exact amount of stereopsis present.

AFTER IMAGES TEST

After images test demonstrates the visual direction of the two foveae. The right fovea is stimulated by a vertical bright flash of light and the left by a horizontal flash. The patient then draws the relative positions of the after images. If the two after images are seen as a cross, the patient has normal retinal correspondence. If there is ARC, the two images will not cross. In the case of an esotropia with ARC, the vertical after image (belonging to the RE) will be seen to the left of the horizontal after image (belonging to the LE). These findings are reversed in exotropia.

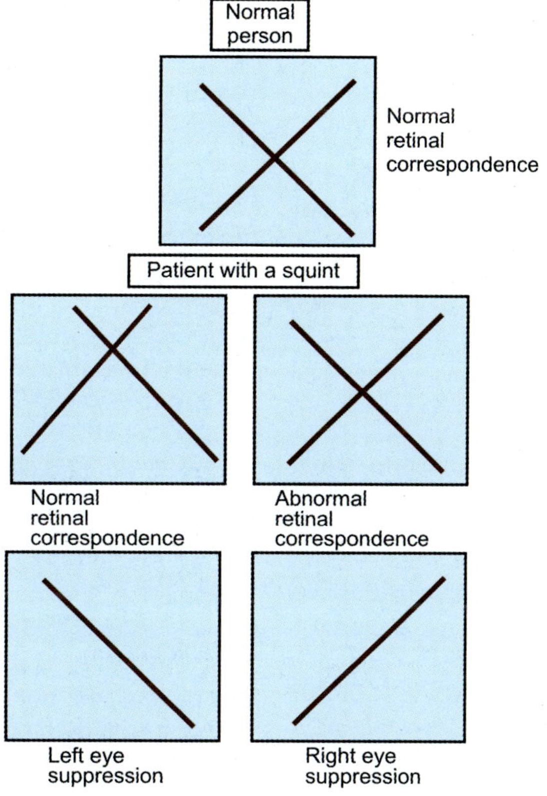

Fig. 23: Bagolini's striated glasses test

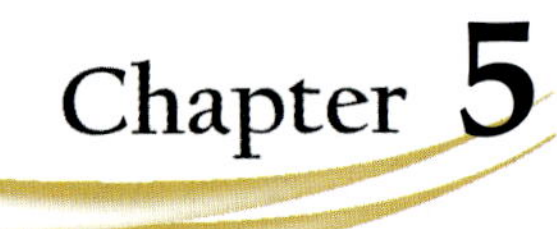

Chapter 5

Clinical Features and Adaptations in Strabismus

Amar Agarwal, Ashok Garg (India)

INTRODUCTION

Certain signs, symptoms and adaptations are seen in strabismus, which one should understand. They are: (i) confusion, (ii) diplopia, (iii) suppression, (iv) amblyopia, (v) eccentric fixation, and (vi) abnormal retinal correspondence.

CONFUSION

Definition

Visual confusion results when dissimilar images project unto corresponding retinal points.

Introduction

Confusion is caused by different images falling on corresponding points (particularly the two fovea) so that the images of two different objects arise together into consciousness with the result that a second dissimilar image may be projected as if superimposed upon the fixation object.

Comparison with Diplopia

In diplopia, the same object is imaged on desperate retinal areas. In other words, the same object falls on the fovea of one eye and some point other than the fovea in the other eye. This leads to the patient seeing double.

DIPLOPIA

Diplopia is discussed separately.

SUPPRESSION

Definition

Suppression is a positive inhibitory reflex occurring within the framework of single binocular vision permitting the cortex to ignore the visual sensations despatched from the retina of the non-fixing eye.

Difference from Amblyopia

Suppression and amblyopia are two different phenomena. In amblyopia there exists decreased vision in uniocular and binocular states whereas in suppression there is good vision in the uniocular state.

Tests to Detect Suppression

Worth's Four Dot Test

Worth's four dot test is discussed separately in Pediatric Strabismus Examination.

FRIEND Test

FRIEND test has the same principle as the Worth's four dot test. In this FIN is colored green and RED in red. The patient wears red green goggles with red in front of the right eye. A normal person reads FRIEND, whereas a patient with right eye suppression reads FIN and with left eye suppression RED.

Bagolini's Striated Glasses

In this (refer under Bagolini's glasses), only one line is seen either of the right or left eye depending on which eye is suppressed.

Synaptophore

The patient will not see one image from one eye when testing fusion (Refer under synaptophore). This is discussed separately.

AMBLYOPIA

Amblyos means dull and ops means vision.

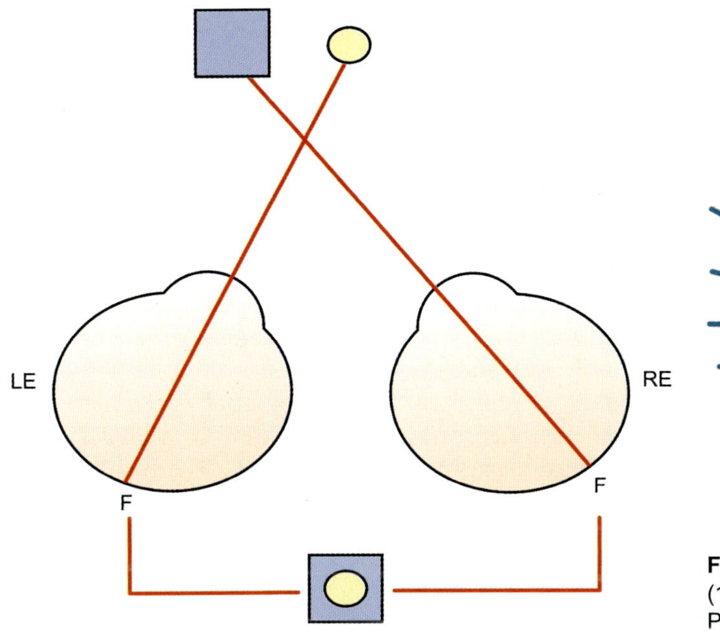

Fig. 1: Confusion

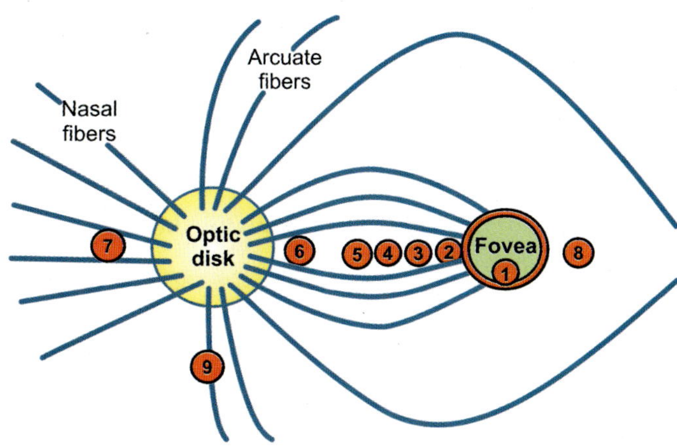

Fig. 3: Eccentric fixation. 1. Unsteady foveal fixation. 2. Perifoveal (1 degree from fovea). 3. Parafoveal (1-3 degrees from fovea). 4. Paramacular (3-5 degrees from fovea). 5. Centrocecal. 6. Juxtacecal. 7. Nasal to the disk. 8. Temporal to the fovea. 9. Nonfixation

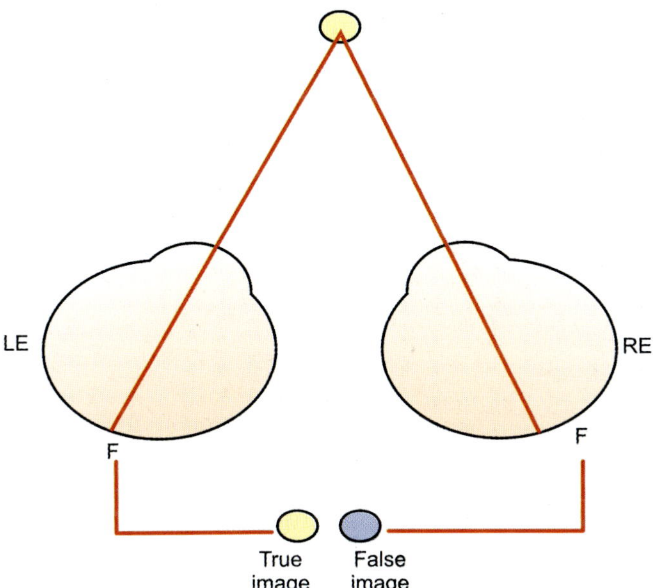

Fig. 2: Diplopia

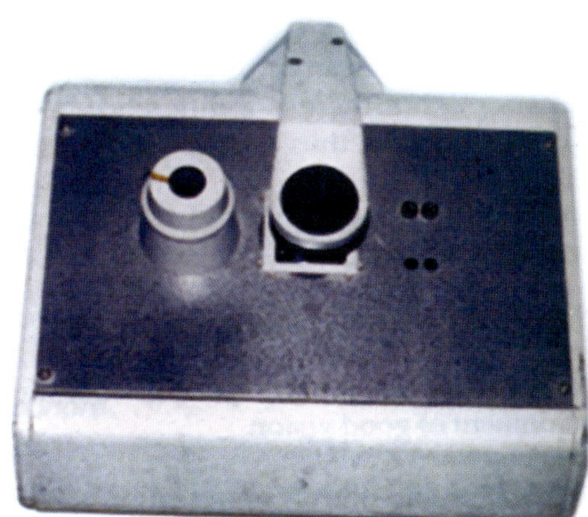

Fig. 4: The coordinator

Definition

Amblyopia is a unilateral or bilateral decrease of vision for which no obvious cause can be detected by the physical examination of the eye and which in appropriate cases is correctable by therapeutic measures.

Incidence

2 to 2.5 percent of the general population has functional amblyopia.

Types

Amblyopia Ex Anopsia

Amblyopia ex anopsia is used to denote diminution of vision in early life due to disuse of the eye. This is due to lack of formation of retinal images in early life—stimulation deprivation amblyopia—by such pathological lesions such as a complete congenital cataract or total congenital ptosis.

Organic (Congenital) Amblyopia

Organic amblyopia refers to that type of amblyopia, which occurs from birth in the apparent absence of retinal or central nervous system (CNS) lesion.

Anisometropic Amblyopia

Anisometropic amblyopia is due to a failure in fusion because of anisometropia.

Aniseikonic Amblyopia

Aniseikonic amblyopia can occur when there is absence of anisometropia but there is a difference in the axial lengths of the two eyes, thus producing an optical form of aniseikonia.

Ametropic Amblyopia

Ametropic amblyopia occurs in one or both eyes in the presence of a significant error of refraction when the adequate provision of correcting spectacles does not result in the attainment of good vision.

Strabismic Amblyopia

Strabismic amblyopia occurs after an interval in a uniocular squint. It is functional in type and occurs as the result of a squint and is due to an active inhibition or suppression adopted as a means of eliminating the adverse effects of diplopia and visual confusion.

CLINICAL FEATURES

- There is a fall in visual acuity. The visual acuity of such an eye is better when used alone. A difference in vision of two lines on a visual acuity chart is a diagnostic criterion for amblyopia. *With neutral density filters the visual acuity in amblyopia does not change or it can slightly improve, but in central retinal lesions, the visual acuity decreases. A normal person shows a fall by two lines with a neutral density filter.*
- The *crowding phenomenon* can be seen. In patients with amblyopia it is always of interest to compare the vision obtained with visual acuity symbols presented in a row to that obtained with isolated symbols on a uniform background. Many patients with amblyopia are capable of discriminating rather small visual acuity symbols when they are presented singly against a uniform background, whereas when these symbols are presented in a row as on a visual acuity chart, the symbols must be larger. In other words, in amblyopia there is an inability to discriminate symbols that are crowded closely together. Thus, amblyopic eyes have two visual acuities—one is called line or Snellen acuity and the other single E acuity. It is the single E acuity, which represents the true potential functional ability of the eye.
- Visual acuity is better in near fixation than distance fixation in amblyopia due to an improvement in the fixation pattern of the amblyopic eye in downward gaze.
- The amblyopic eyes are better in dark adaptation and the eccentric fixation even might become central fixation. The amblyopic eye is worse in photopic conditions.

Treatment

- *Orthoptics* This is discussed separately in the on Non-surgical Treatment of Squint.
- Treatment of the cause
- Surgical treatment of the squint.

ECCENTRIC FIXATION

Introduction

Eccentric fixation is a uniocular condition in which some part of the retina other than the fovea is used for fixation and in which reorientation of sensory and motor functions may eventually occur so that the new area assumes a foveal type of visual direction. There is another term used, which is called eccentric viewing. This is a uniocular

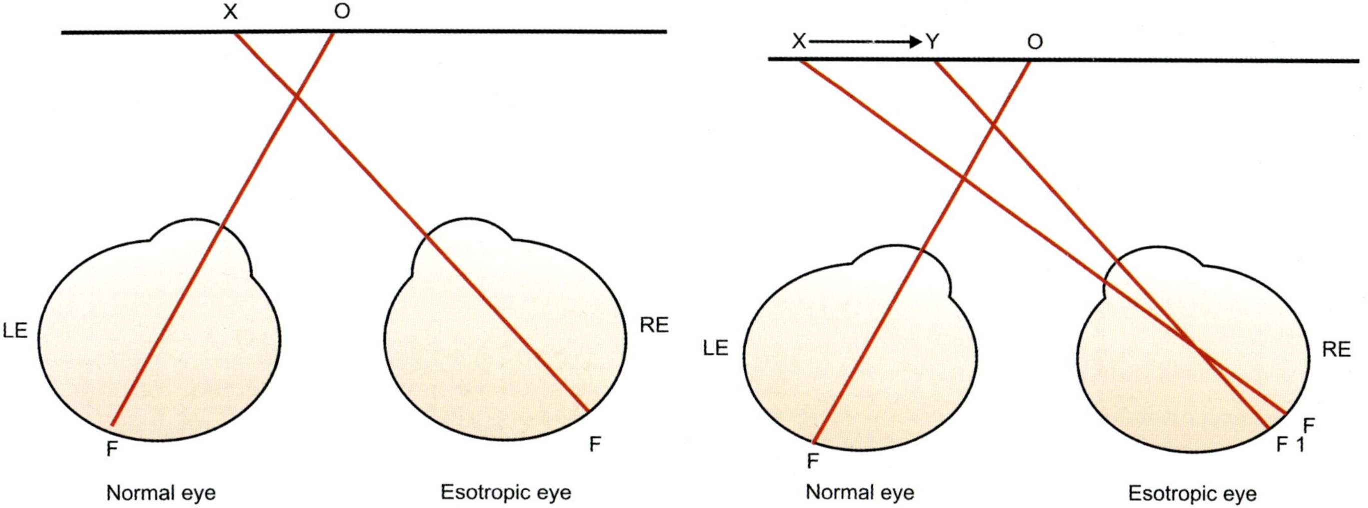

Fig. 5: Normal retinal correspondence

Fig. 6: Non-harmonious abnormal retinal correspondence (ARC)

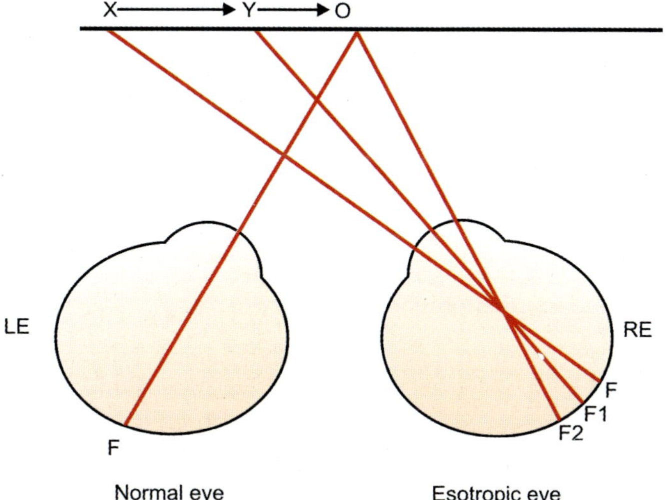

Fig. 7: Harmonious abnormal retinal correspondence (ARC)

condition in which some part of the retina other than the fovea is used for fixation but in which the fovea retains its normal straight ahead projection.

Types

Unsteady foveal fixation In this the patient fixates on the foveola sometimes and sometimes moves away from it.

Perifoveal: In this the fixation is 1 degree away from the foveola.

Parafoveal: This is 1 to 3 degrees away.

Paramacular: This is 3 to 5 degrees away.

Centrocecal: In this the fixation is between the disk and foveola.

Juxtacecal: In this the fixation is next to the disk

Nasal to the disk: The fixation is nasal to the disk

Temporal to the disk: The fixation is temporal to the disk

Nonfixation: In this no definite point is used for fixation.

Paradoxical Fixation

Eccentric fixation corresponds generally to the direction of squint. In an esotropia, the eccentric fixation is situated on the nasal side of the fovea, whereas in exotropia it is on the temporal side. Sometimes, this does not occur and in an esotropia the eccentric fixation may be on the temporal side of the fovea. If this occurs it is known as paradoxical fixation. It can occur as a primary event in cases, which have developed an early infancy and have been untreated. But it develops more usually as a secondary phenomenon in two circumstances.

- After occlusion of the sound eye in the search for an area of improved vision
- In cases wherein the direction of squint has changed either spontaneously or by surgical overcorrection.

Remember

The highest visual acuity in an eccentric fixation patient is the eccentric point and not the fovea.

Investigations

Corneal Reflection Test

By shining a torch on the patient's eyes and occluding the sound eye, one will see that the squinting eye on trying to look at the light will not be able to focus and the reflex of the light on the cornea will not be central.

Ophthalmoscope

Take a direct ophthalmoscope, which has a star in it. Ask the patient to close the sound eye and look with the ophthalmoscope into the squinting eye. Ask the patient to look at the light and judge how far the point of the ophthalmoscope is from the macula. This gives us an indication of the eccentric fixation.

Others

Other instruments that can be used are the Visuoscope of Cupper's, coordinator and the synaptophore with Haidenger's brushes.

Treatment

- *Orthoptics* This is discussed separately in the on Non-surgical Treatment of Squint.
- Surgical treatment of the squint.

ABNORMAL RETINAL CORRESPONDENCE

Definition

Abnormal retinal correspondence, false projection or false macula is said to exist when the fovea of the fixing eye is used simultaneously with a retinal point other than the fovea of the other eye.

Angles

The angles involved in the determination of ARC are as follows:

Angle of deviation: This is the objective angle of the squint.

Subjective angle: This is the angle determined when the patient subjectively merges the two images of the synaptophore.

Angle of anomaly: This is the difference between the objective and subjective angles.

Perversion Quotient

This is *angle of anomaly/angle of squint.*

Explanation

Let us take a patient in whom the LE is normal and the right eye is esotropic. Now, at this stage the left eye looks at a point O with the fovea F. This is normal for that eye. As the right eye is esotropic, the fovea F of the RE looks at another point X as it cannot look at O. At this stage, the patient is having normal retinal correspondence.

Now, to solve this problem of diplopia, the right eye can go in for suppression. Alternately, the eye can go in for the phenomenon called abnormal retinal correspondence. The idea is that both the eyes should focus on one point O. As the LE is looking at O and the right eye looking at X, the right eye decides to change its position to Y. Now some point other than the fovea F1 looks at Y. This point F1 of the RE corresponds with the fovea F of the LE. But still the goal is not achieved as both eyes are still not looking at O. This patient now has a non-harmonious retinal correspondence. The LE looks at O and the right eye has moved its fixation from X to Y.

Again, the RE changes its point of fixation so that yet another point other than the fovea F2 now fixates onto O. Thus, at this stage the fovea F of the LE corresponds with some point (F2) other than the fovea of the RE. At this stage the LE is looking at O. The RE has now changed its position from X to O. This patient now has harmonious abnormal retinal correspondence. The advantage of this is that the patient neither has diplopia nor suppression.

Factors which Favor the Development of Arc

- Convergent squint of early onset, i.e. upto the age of 3 years
- Convergent squint of relatively small and constant angle of deviation.

Cases of Squint in which Arc is Unlikely to Occur

- Cases of convergent squint of late onset, i.e. after the age of 4 years. In these cases, there has been full development and grounding of normal binocular reflexes and there is therefore less likelihood of replacement by abnormal reflexes
- Cases of convergent squint of large degrees example +30 degrees or more
- Cases of squint with variable angle of deviation. The variability causes stimulation over a wide retinal area of the non-fixating eye, hence no one area can be stabilized as a pseudo-fovea
- *Primary divergent squint* This is because of two reasons. One is that in most cases the deviation is initially intermittent and only becomes constant much later when normal binocular function has developed and two due to the lack of visual regard from ARC in divergent squint.

Advantages of Arc

- If the condition is harmonious, it avoids the necessity for dense amblyopia
- It provides a perverted form of binocular function, often permitting an anomalous fusion range to develop and in most cases permitting also some degree of stereoscopic vision
- Its presence prevents consecutive divergence since it provides a stimulus to maintain the eyes in a slightly divergent position
- It allows a form of binocular convergence to take place.

Disadvantage of Arc

Abnormal retinal correspondence is not normal and hence normal binocular function does not occur.

Tests to Detect Arc

Worth's Four Dot Test

If the patient sees four dots and has squint, the diagnosis is harmonious ARC, as if the patient has a squint how can four dots be seen? The patient should see either two reds or three green dots. So by seeing four dots, it means the foveal point of one eye is corresponding with an extrafoveal point of the other eye.

Synaptophore

To detect ARC with the synaptophore determine first the objective angle of squint. This can be done by using slides like a lion and its cage and after fixing one arm of the synaptophore, moving the other arm till there is no movement of the two eyes. This is done by flashing on and off the lights alternately between the two eyes. Once there is no movement of the eyes, we get the objective angle.

Then determine the subjective angle of squint. To detect this, ask the patient to put the lion in the cage (or sentry in the sentry house) and note the angle of the squint at which this is done.

If the patient has NRC then the subjective angle (SA) will be equal to the objective angle (OA). The angle of anomaly (AOA) which is

$$AOA = OA - SA$$

Will show zero. This is because the OA is equal to the SA. Thus, the patient has normal retinal correspondence (NRC).

If the patient has *unharmonious ARC,* then the subjective angle will be less than the objective angle. The difference between the two should be at least 5 degrees or more. Thus, for example if the

OA = 20 degrees

and

SA = 10 degrees

Then

$$AOA = OA - SA = 20 - 10 = 10 \text{ Degrees}$$

Thus, the patient has non-harmonious abnormal retinal correspondence.

If the patient has *harmonious ARC*, then the subjective angle will be zero (which means the patient will put the lion in the cage at zero degrees). Thus, the angle of anomaly (objective angle minus subjective angle) in a harmonious ARC will be equal to the objective angle and in NRC will be zero as in NRC the objective angle will be equal to the subjective angle.

Bagolini's Striated Glasses

Using these glasses, one can detect ARC.

After-images Test

In this after images are produced and ARC detected.

Others

Other tests that can be used to detect ARC are the Maddox rod, Maddox wing and the Haidenger's brushes.

Treatment

- Orthoptics
- Surgical treatment of squint.

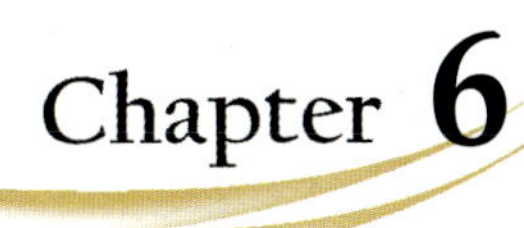

Instrumentation in Orthoptic Setup

Kumar J Doctor, Pooja Deshmukh (India)

In any orthoptic setup or squint clinic, the instrumentation for measurement of strabismus and associated parameters plays a vital role in the diagnosis and management of the squint patient, be it pre- or post-operative. Their usage and the tests associated with these instruments are confusing and require proper interpretation.

This chapter encompasses the varied tests and the usage of vital generic instruments to diagnose particular parameters in evaluation and treatment of squint.

VISUAL ACUITY ASSESSMENT

1. Preverbal Children Less Than 2 Years

Optokinetic Drum (Fig. 1)

Visual angle subtended by smallest strip width which elicits an eye movement is a measure of the visual acuity. Normal values: 6/120 in newborn, 6/6 by 20-30 months.

Checkerboard Pattern Visual Evoked Potential (Fig. 2)

EEG recordings are made from occipital lobe in response to visual stimuli. Normally Expected Values: 6/120 at 1 month of age , 6/6 at 1 year of age.

Hundreds and Thousands Sweet Test (Fig. 3)

Child able to pick up sweets at 33 cm is said to have a visual acuity of 6/24.

Preferential Looking Test (Fig. 4)

Infants with good visual acuity will tend to look at a striped pattern. Grating acuity in infants is better than recognition acuity Normal: 6/120 at 1month, 6/6 at 24-36 month.

Cardiff Acuity Cards (Fig. 5)

2. Verbal Children 2-5 Years

HOTV and Tumbling E Chart (Fig. 6)

Allens Picture Chart (Fig. 7)

Keeler Log MAR Crowded Test (Fig. 8)

Teller Acuity Test (Fig. 9)

Kay Pictures: At 2 years of age to name pictures (Fig. 10)

3. Visual Acuity in Age Group 5 Years to Adults (Fig. 11)

- Visual acuity is the reciprocal of minimum resolvable visual angle.
- 2 points can be seen clearly when they subtend a minimum visual angle of 1min at the nodal point of the eye.
- The letters comprising a visual acuity chart subtend an angle of 5 min of arc. Whereas each stroke of the letter subtends an angle of 1 min of arc.

Stereopsis Assessment

Random Dot E Test (RDT) (Fig. 12)

To detect an E at 50 cm, with polaroids.

Frisby Test (Fig. 13)

To detect a circle pattern in the plastic plates . Without polaroid glasses.

TNO Test (Fig. 14)

It is a Truer measure of stereoacuity.

It consists of 7 plates, red green glasses are worn by patient and the plates read.

First 3 establish stereopsis. Next four to quantify it.

Test Stereo Acuity in a range of 480- 15 secs.

Titmus Test (Fig. 15)

Performed at 16 inches , With polaroids.

Fly: On this plate, try to pick wings , Checks gross Stereo acuity upto 3000 secs.

Circles: On this plate, press the circle which stands out. Checks Fine Stereo Acuity from 800 – 40 secs.

Animals: On this plate point out the animal which stands out.

Checks Fine Stereo Acuity 400 – 100 secs .

Lang Stereo Test (Fig. 16)

PBCT: Prism Bar Cover Test

Instrument (Fig. 17)

Procedure (Fig. 18)

Aim: To quantify objectively the angle of deviation for near and distance.

- Performed for distance and near targets separately. And also in 9 gazes.
- Prism bar is placed with apex towards deviation in front of squinting eye.
- Normal eye fixes the target .
- Alternate cover test is performed with a spielman occluder.
- If the angle of squint is large, i.e. > 35-40°, loose prisms are used.
- The eye which is not undercover will show refixational movements.
- The prism bar is moved with increasing powers in front of the squinting eye till there are no refixational movments. noted anymore → this power of the prism gives the angle of deviation.

Uses: Heterophoria and Heterotropia both are measured $1^o = 1.8\Delta$

Limits: Cannot be performed in blind eye/gross eccentric fixation/Nystagmic eye.

Krimsky's Corneal Reflex (Fig. 20)

- To measure angle of deviation in a blind or deeply amblyopic eye with or without eccentric fixation.
- The patient is asked to fixate on a point light, prisms of increasing strength (with apex towards the direction of manifest squint) are placed in front of the normal fixating eye till the corneal reflex is centred in the squinting eye.
- The power of prism required is equal to the amount of squint in prism diopters.

Advantages

- Useful in testing small children.
- Quicker than prism cover test.
- Can be used in patients in whom deviating eye has low visual acuity and has lost central fixation.

Limitations

- Since the angle kappa is included in measurement, test is inaccurate.
- Not possible to perform the test for distance fixation.

20D Base Out Prism (Fig. 21)

- It detects Binocular Single Vision (BSV) in children who cannot perform stereo tests.
- 20 D BO prism in front of RE causes diplopia and to relieve this RE shifts to left LE looks to left too (Hering's law).
- LE then makes refixational movment to right.
- Removal of prism then causes both eyes to look to right. And then LE makes an outward fusional movement, Confirming good BSV.

Maddox Rod Test (Fig. 22)

Aim : To measure Heterophoria and Heterotropia .

Instrument (Fig. 23): Consists of series of parallel red glass cylinders of higher power set together in metallic disk. Produces a linear image of a point light which is perpendicular to the axis of the cylinder.

Procedure:

- Maddox rod is placed before the squinting eye with the axis of cylinder parallel to deviation-horizontal or vertical.
- The patient fixes on the point of light at the center of the Tangent scale/or any point source of light at 6 m distance.

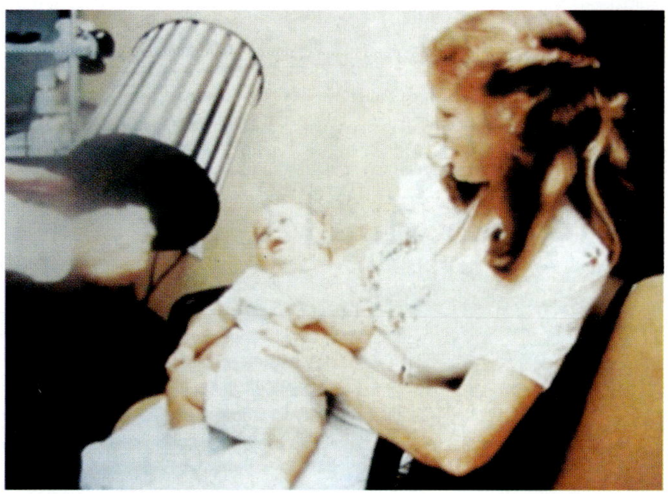

Fig. 1: Optokinetic drum

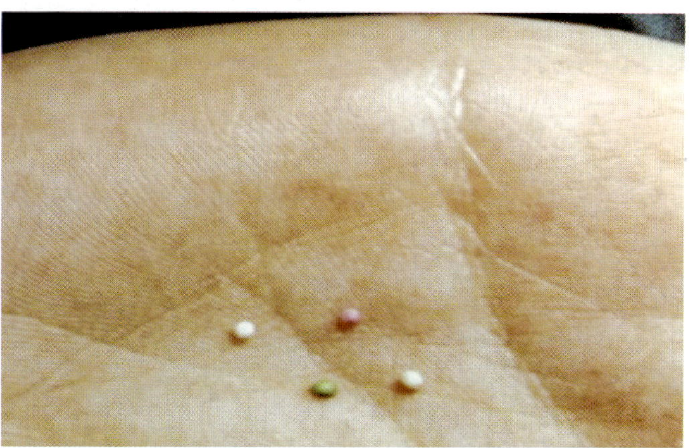

Fig. 3: Hundreds and thousands sweet test

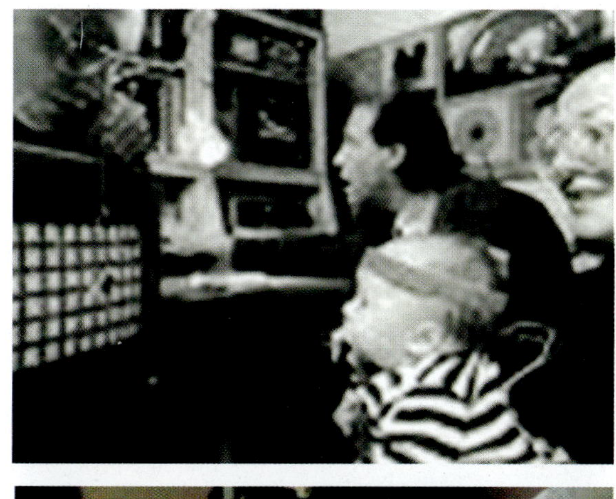

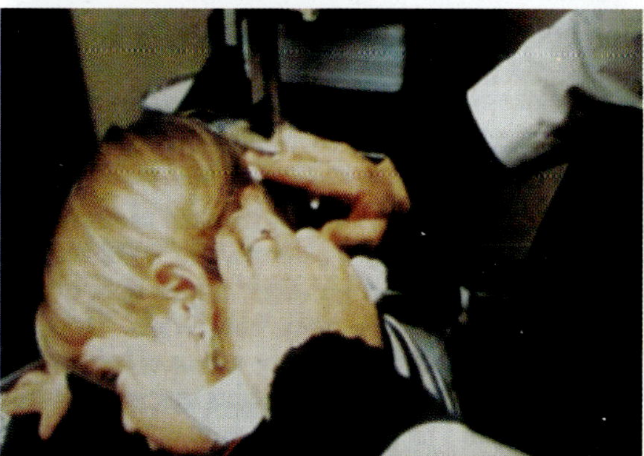

Fig. 2: Checkerboard pattern visual evoked potential

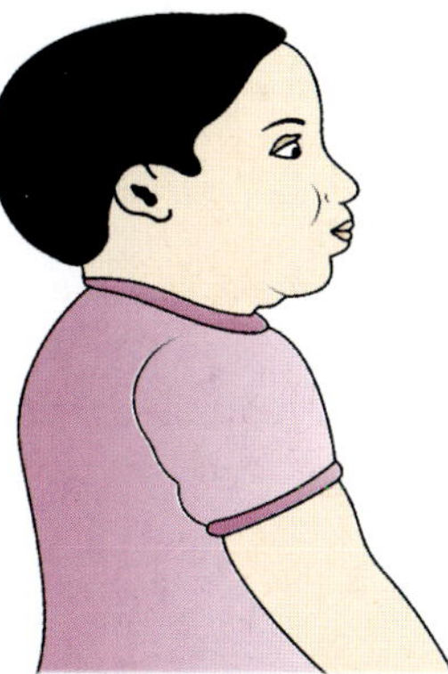

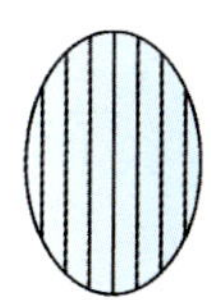

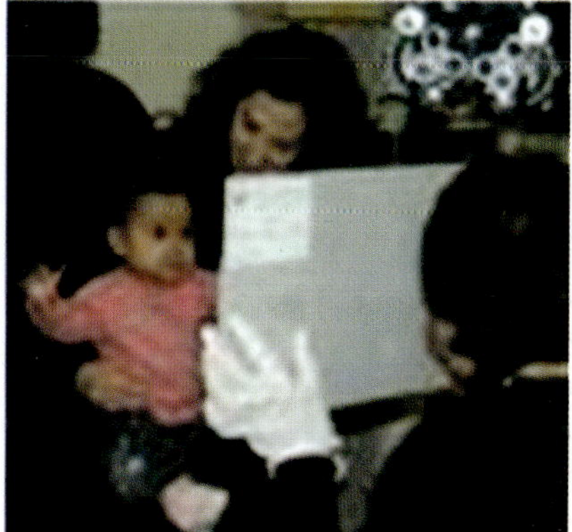

Fig. 4: Preferential looking test

- This gives a red linear image with its axis ⊥ to axis of maddox rod.
- The other eye sees just a point light.
- The red line is seen to either right or left side of the point light in center of tangent scale.
- Where the red line falls on the scale is the degree of deviation.
- Tip: To measure Phorias an occluder is placed before maddox rod, then the patient Fixates and occluder is removed for 1 sec, then patient is asked where the red line falls.
- *Limitations*
  - Can be performed only if there is no suppression .
  - Deviation measured only if patient has NRC.
  - It is useful only to measure small deviations.

Interpretation

For Horizontal Deviations (Fig. 25)
For Vertical Deviations (Fig. 26)

Maddox Wing Test (Fig. 27)

Aim

- Amount of heterophoria for near can be measured subjectively (33 cm).
- Principle : Dissociation of fusion by dissimilar objects.

Procedure (Fig. 28)

- RE sees: white and red arrows
- LE sees : vertical and horizontal line of numbers.
- Patient tells which number on horizontal line does the white arrow touch , this is the angle of the *Horizontal Phoria* . TIP: Even nos. EXO, Odd nos. ESO.
- Patient also tells which number on the vertical line does the red arrow touch, this is the angle of the *Vertical Phoria.*
- Patient tells us which arrow in horizontal line does red arrow touch, this is the detected *Cyclophoria* .

Disadvantages

- IPD not adjustable so cannot be used in kids.
- Subjective test.

MADDOX DOUBLE PRISM

Aim : Test to detect cyclodeviations.

Instrument: They are two 4 D Prisms

Procedure (Fig. 29):

- With both eyes open Patient looks at horizontal line with a blank background.
- They are two 4 D Prisms placed base to base kept in front of the RE.
- With both eyes open patient looks at black horizontal line with a blank background.
- RE sees 2 red split lines.
- LE sees one black line.

Interpretation (Fig. 30)

Disadvantages

- Qualitative test
- Cannot differentiate between a cyclophoria and a cyclotropia.

JAMPOLSKY 4 D BASE OUT PRISM

Aim: To detect central suppression scotoma and small angle tropias (Fig. 31).

- 4 D BO prism is placed in front of the normal eye, this causes the image to stimulate a point 2° (4D) temporal to the fovea. This causes an inward movement of that eye with a versional outward movment of the other (suspect) eye.
- Following this the image now falls on the temporal side of the fovea of the suspect eye, which if normal, makes a refixational corrective movement to primary position.

Procedure

- But if a suppression scotoma is present in the suspect eye, then the fovea will not attempt a refixational movment in that eye and the suspect eye will hence remain deviated showing no corrective movements.

RED FILTER LADDER (FIG. 32)

- To measure the depth of suppression.
- It consists of a series of red gelatinous filters of increasing density.
- With both eyes open patient is asked to fixate a point light and the ladder is run in front of the eye to be tested. Till the patient sees double lights.
- The darker the red filter needed to produce this effect, the deeper the suppression.

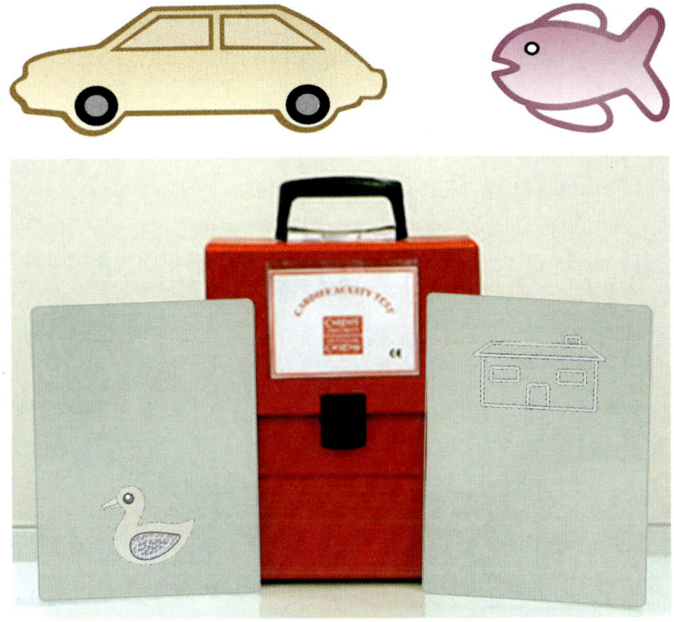

Fig. 5: Cardiff acuity cards

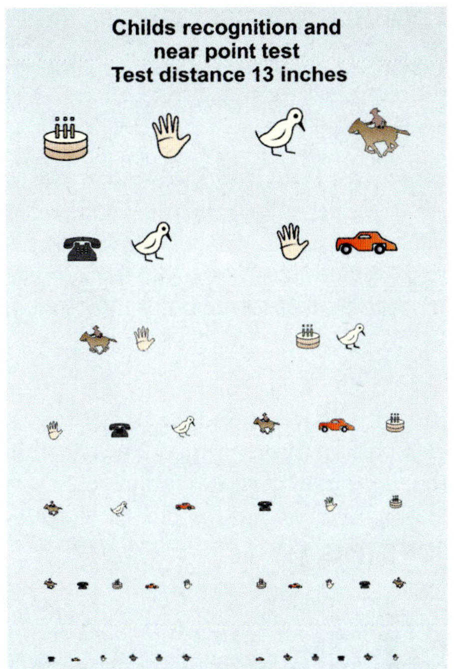

Fig. 7: Allens picture chart

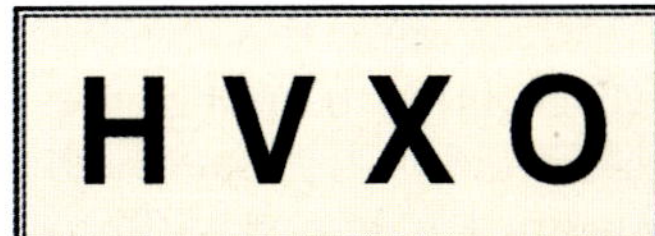

Fig. 8: Keeler log MAR crowded test

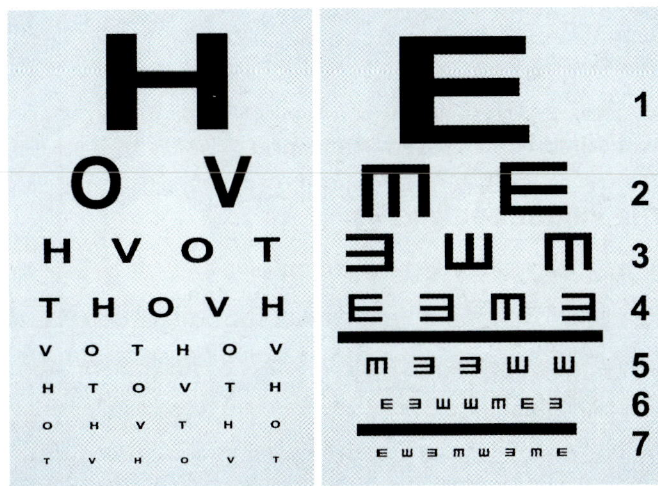

Fig. 6: HOTV and Tumbling E chart

Fig. 9: Teller acuity test

MADDOX DOUBLE ROD (FIG. 33)

Aim : To measure a cyclophoria and a cyclotropia.

Instrument and Procedure

- In Suspect eye put : Red Maddox Rod in trial frame at 90°
- In Normal eye put : Black/White Maddox Rod in trial frame at 90°, with a 6D prism behind it (only in case of horizontal cyclodev.- to separate the 2 images).
- Patient has to fixate a white point light in a dark room.

Interpretation (Fig. 34)

- The red rod is then rotated such that both lines seen parallel to patient this reading on the trial frame, which gives the degrees of cyclodeviation.

DIPLOSCOPE (FIG. 35)

- To detect suppression.
- To detect lack of Binocular Single Vision (BSV).
- With normal retinal correspondence (NRC) and BSV the patient will see 3 holes with the word DOG in them.

BAGOLINI STRIATED GLASS TEST

Aim: To detect suppression/Retinal correspondence.

Instrument: Consists of transparent glasses with Striations on RE and LE at 45 and 135 degrees which converts a light point to 2 oblique lines intersecting each other.

Procedure: With both eyes open point light target could be for near 33 cm as well as distance 6 m.

Interpretation

- Normal Retinal Correspondence (NRC)/ Harmonious Anomalous Retinal Correspondence (ARC) (cover test will show tropia) (Fig. 36)
- Constant tropia, ARC, Diplopia no suppression (Fig. 37)
- Suppression (Fig. 38)
- Suppression area with NRC/Unharmonious ARC (Fig. 39)

Advantages

- Physiological.
- Simple and easy.

Disadvantages

- Very subjective.
- Small tropias can be missed.

WORTH'S 4 DOT TEST (W4DT) (FIG. 40)

Aim: To detect suppression/Retinal correspondence.

Procedure

- Patient wears Red-Green goggles.
- The box has 1 red 2 green 1 white bulb.
- Patient looks at it and draws how many lights and which colored lights are seen by him/her.

Interpretation

- All 4 seen with no manifest squint = Normal BSV
- All 4 seen with manifest squint = ARC
- 2 red lights = LE suppression
- 3 green lights = RE suppression
- 2 red lights and 3 green lights alternately = Alternating Suppression
- 5 lights = Diplopia

W4DT for near (Fig. 41)

Disadvantages

- It is very subjective.

BIELSCHOWSKY AFTER IMAGE TEST (FIG. 42)

Aim: It demonstrates the visual direction of foveae.

Procedure

- Bright light stimulates both eyes for 15 secs each.
- Patient draws what he sees when light is shut off.

Disadvantages

- Subjective test.
- Difficult for children to interpret.

THE VISUSCOPE (FIG. 43)

Aim : To detect Eccentric Fixation

Procedure: To examine monocular fixation pattern : close one eye

- A disk with concentric rings ½ degree away with a central green star is thrown onto the patient's fundus.
- Normally the star lies on fovea if fixation is central.

Interpretation (Fig. 44): The position of the star to foveola is noted to arrive to conclusion of fixation.

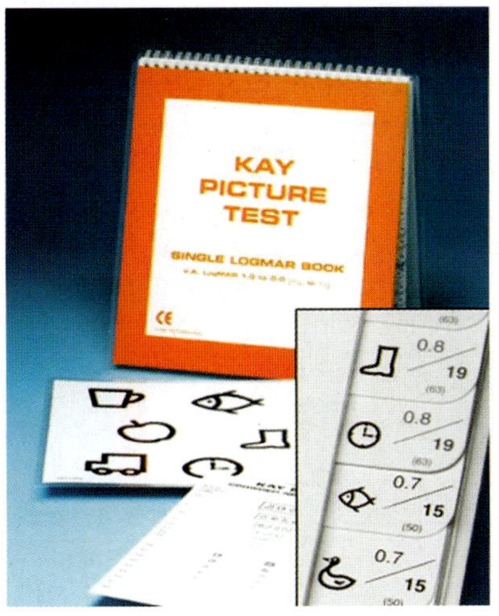

Fig. 10: Kay picture test

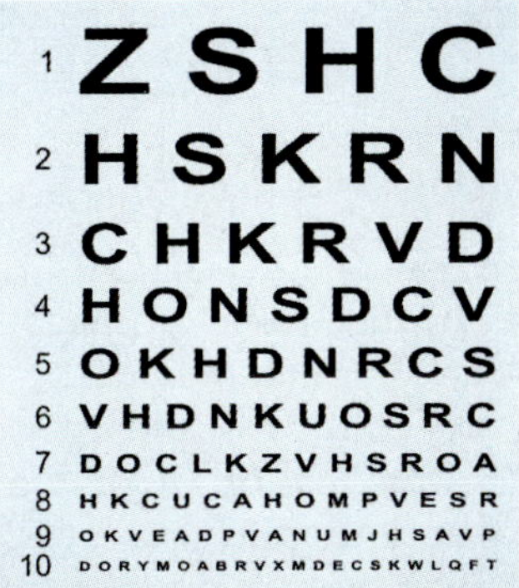

Fig. 11: Visual acuity in age group 5 years to adults

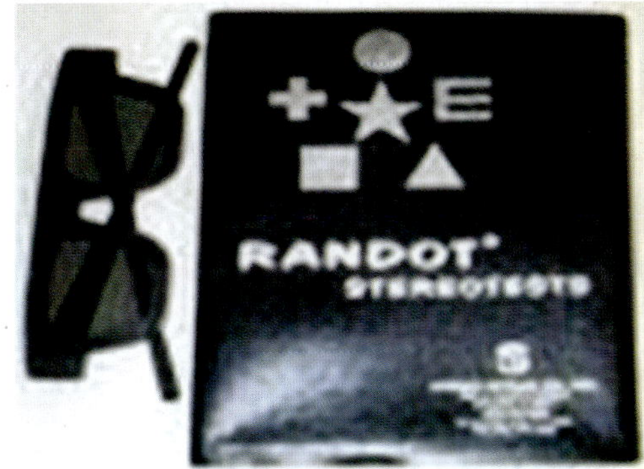

Fig. 12: Random dot E Test

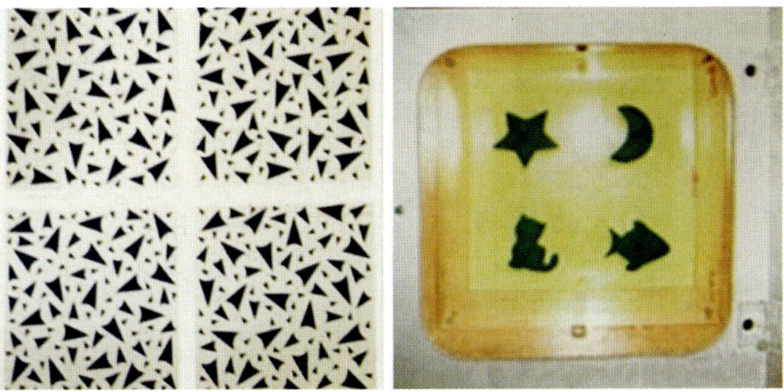

Fig. 13: Frisby test

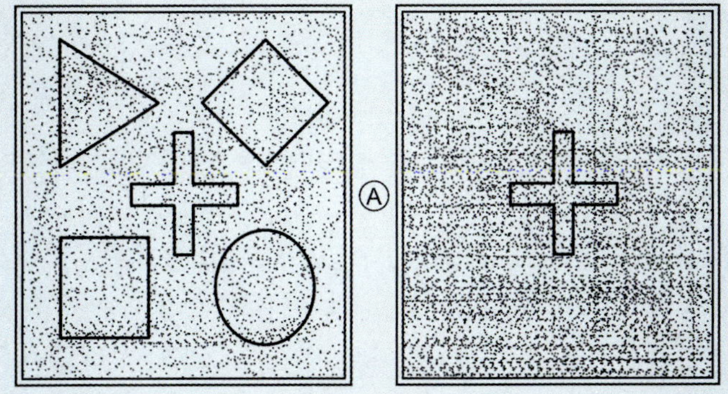

Fig. 14: TNO test

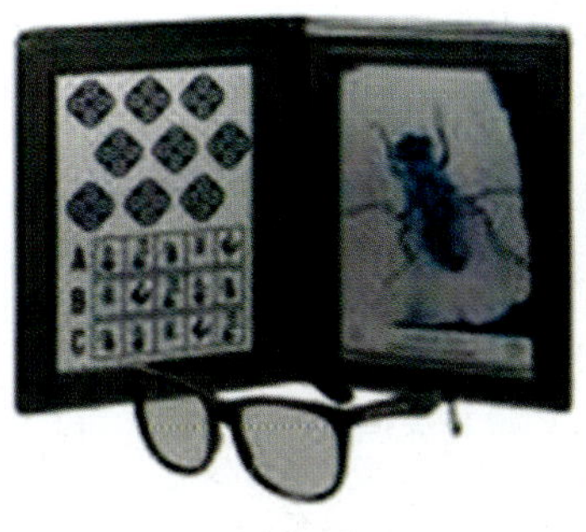

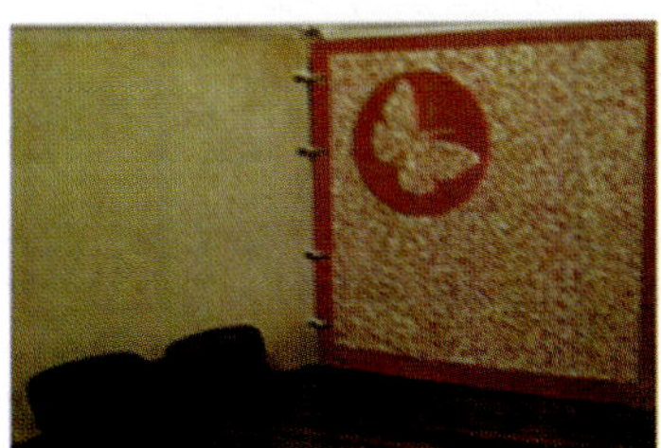

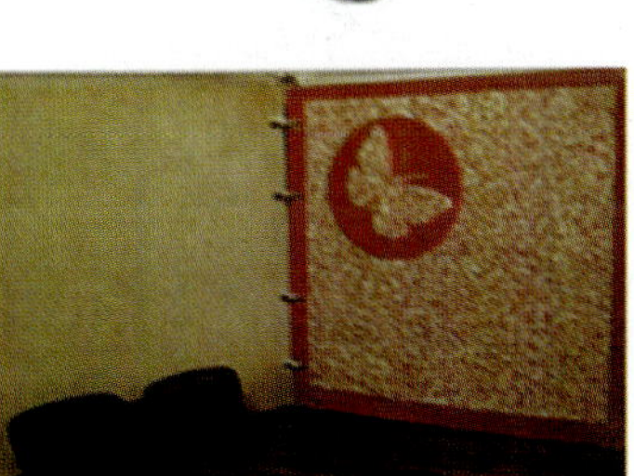

Fig. 15: Titmus test

RAF RULE (ROYAL AIR FORCE RULE) (FIG. 45)

Aim: To measure Near Point Convergence (NPC) /Near point of Accommodation (NPA).

Instrument:

- Rule Bar/Rod. Each side of bar will measure marks in centimeters, inches, diopters and age.
- A wing like cheek rest on one end which sits snugly on patients lower orbital margins.
- A sliding target mover towards the patient which contains :
  - Print for NPA.
  - Single target for NPC.

Procedure

NPA (Near point of Accommodation):

- It is the nearest point at which eyes can maintain clear focus.
- Wear full optical correction.
- RAF print 6/9 letter moving towards patient.
- Patient tries to read till print is blurred. (Clarity is the criteria).
- First uniocular then binocular
- + / - lenses added to counter act too low or too high amplitude of accommodation.
- Normal NPA: 8-10 cm/Depends on age of patient.

NPC (Near point of convergence)

- It is the nearest point at which the eyes can maintain binocular **single** vision.
- Patient fixates a single vertical line target which moves closer to patient.
- When patient's eye loses fixation and drifts laterally → Objective NPC.
- When patient says that he has diplopia → Subjective NPC.
- Normal **NPC**
  - Average value = 7 cm
  - Average range = 5-10 cm
  - Excessive in children = <5 cm
  - Defective/remote = 10 cm
  - Convergence insufficiency=25-30 cm

LIVINGSTON BINOCULAR GAUGE (FIG. 46)

Aim : To measure Point Convergence (NPC) /Near point of Accommodation (NPA).

Procedure

- Black section of rod is to be seen singly till eye diverges to gauge the Objective convergence N = 6-10 cm.
- Vertical part of cross on card is to be seen singly till diplopia to obtain Subjective convergence. N = <20 cm
- Horizontal limb of cross on card has ALT printed alongside which are to be read clearly till blurring to obtain Subjective Accommodation values.

DIPLOPIA CHARTING (FIG. 47)

Aim : To Assess extraocular muscle Paresis in a patient of incomitance with diplopia.

Procedure

- In front of RE : Red filter.
- In front of LE: Green filter.
- A Linear streak of light shone to patient.
- Working distance : 4 feet.
- Show target in all 9 gazes.
- Patient has diplopia and gives clues which help the surgeon find the culprit paretic muscle.

Interpretation and Questions to ask

- Is the diplopia crossed/uncrossed? If Crossed: Culprit muscle is MR or other Recti. If image is uncrossed: Culprit muscle is LR or other obliques.
- Quadrants involved? If superior quadrant has diplopia: culprit muscle is SR/IO if inferior quadrant has diplopia : culprit muscle is IR/SO.
- Quadrant with maximum image separation?
- The yolk muscles acting in that quadrant?
- The peripheral image in that quadrant belongs to the eye with the paralyzed muscle.
- In case of Recti/Obliques- Inturning /Outturning of deviating Image? If Inturn: SR/SO, If Outturn: IR/IO.

Disadvantages

- Qualitative.
- Requires cooperative and intelligent patient.
- Cant test in color blind patients.
- Not useful in congenital palsies and long standing cases , because in deep suppression diplopia cannot be elicited.

HESS CHARTING (FIG. 49)

Aim: To assess extra ocular muscle paresis or restriction in a patient with incomitance.

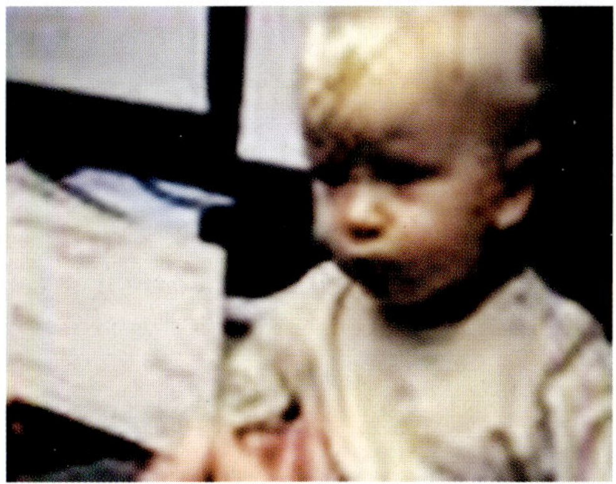

Fig. 16: Long stereo test

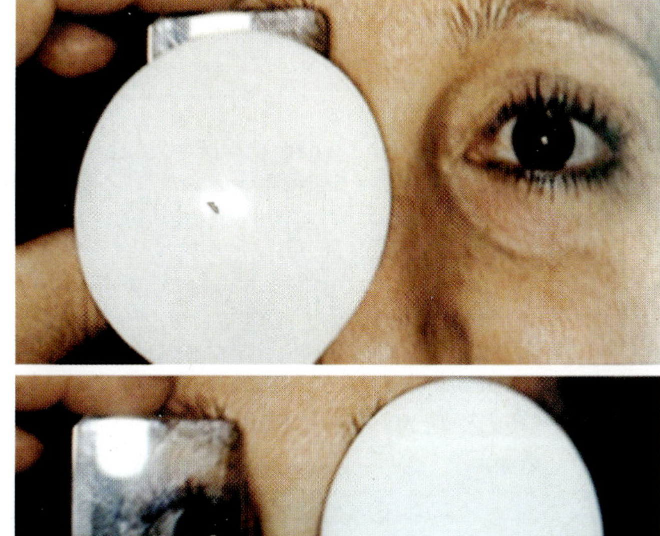

Fig. 19

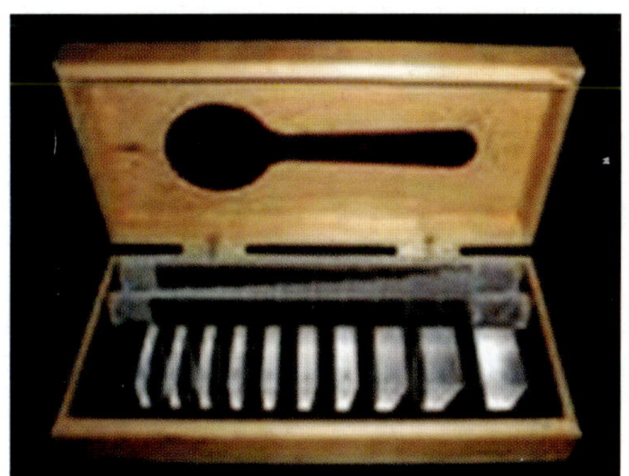

Fig. 17: Instrument of PBCT

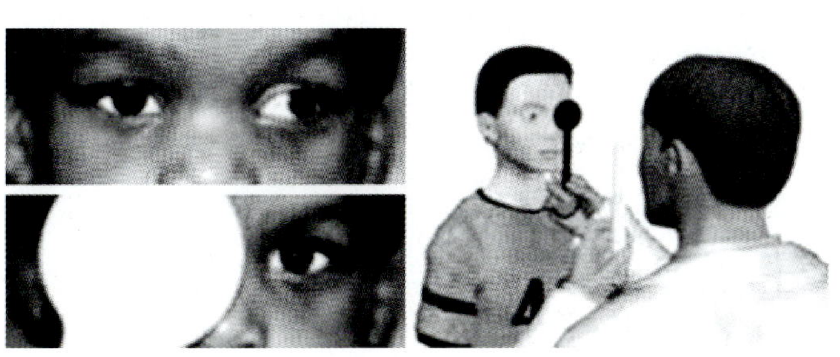

Fig. 18: Procedure of PBCT

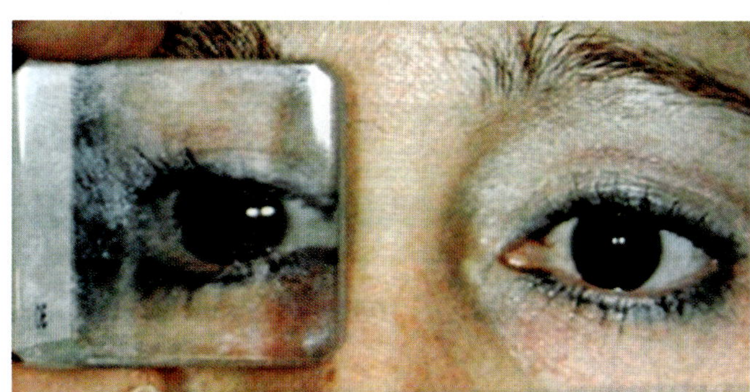

Fig. 20: Krimsky's corneal reflex

Instrument (See Figure 49)

Procedure

- Patient sits at 50 cm and wears diplopia goggles with Green in front of the eye being tested.
- Patient is given a horizontal slit green laser pointer. Patient sees the red lights (from eye which has red filter in front of it), he superimposes these red dots which light up with the green laser pointer.
- The positions that patient points out are connected with straight lines to draw a chart.
- Repeat same with green in front of other eye.

Interpretation

The two charts are compared (Fig. 50).

- The smaller chart indicates the eye with the paretic muscle.
- The larger chart indicates the eye with the overacting muscle.
- The smaller chart shows restriction in the field of paretic muscle.
- The larger chart shows expansion in the field of the paretic yoke muscle.
- Fields of similar shape and size are suggestive of concomitant deviation.

LEES SCREEN (FIG. 51)

Aim: To assess extraocular muscle paresis or restriction.

Instrument and Procedure

while examining **RE**:

- Patient faces non illuminated Left screen at 50 cm.
- Both eyes are dissociated by the rim of the central mirror
- Patients RE sees the mirror in which he sees the illuminated Right Screen.
- while LE directly sees the non-illuminated left screen.
- Examiner projects dots on the illuminated screen, which the patient has to superimpose on the non-illuminated screen.
- Procedure is repeated with LE now facing the non illuminated screen.

Interpretation

- Compression = underaction
- Expansion = overaction
- Smaller field= eye with paretic muscle.
- Larger field = other eye with contralateral synergist.

THE SYNOPTOPHORE (FIG. 52)

Instrument

- Consists of an instrument with two right angled tubes, with mirrors at the angles, mounted on a base having a chin rest and a forehead rest.
- Each eyepiece has a +6.5 D lens which optically sets testing distance to 6 meters.
- Each arm has at distal ends a slide carrier.
- Each arm can be rotated vertically/horizontally/ torsionally with knobs rading off scales.
- Each arm can be illuminated together or alternately to carry out the cover tests.
- Readings from 0 mark in represent BO prisms or Degrees of convergence (+) and vice versa.

Diagnostic Uses

- To measure IPD.
- To measure Objective and Subjective angle of Deviation in phorias and tropias .
- To measure primary and secondary Deviation.
- To detect state of retinal correspondence.
- To estimate grades of BSV.
- To detect type of suppression.
- To measure angle kappa.
- To measure range of fusion or vergence.
- To measure deviation in cardinal positions of gaze.

1. To measure deviations in heterophorias and heterotropias both subjectively and objectively

Objective Method

- Simultaneous macular perception (SMP) slides are put in.
- Arm adjusted by examiner till there is no deviation of either eye on alternate cover test done by flashing the lights alternately.
- Horizontal and vertical both components are measured.
- For near put –3D lenses.
- Patient has to accommodate 3D for each lens diopter, i.e. 9 D for 1 eye or 18 for both eyes.
- for Esodeviation subtract 18.
- for Exodeviation add 18.

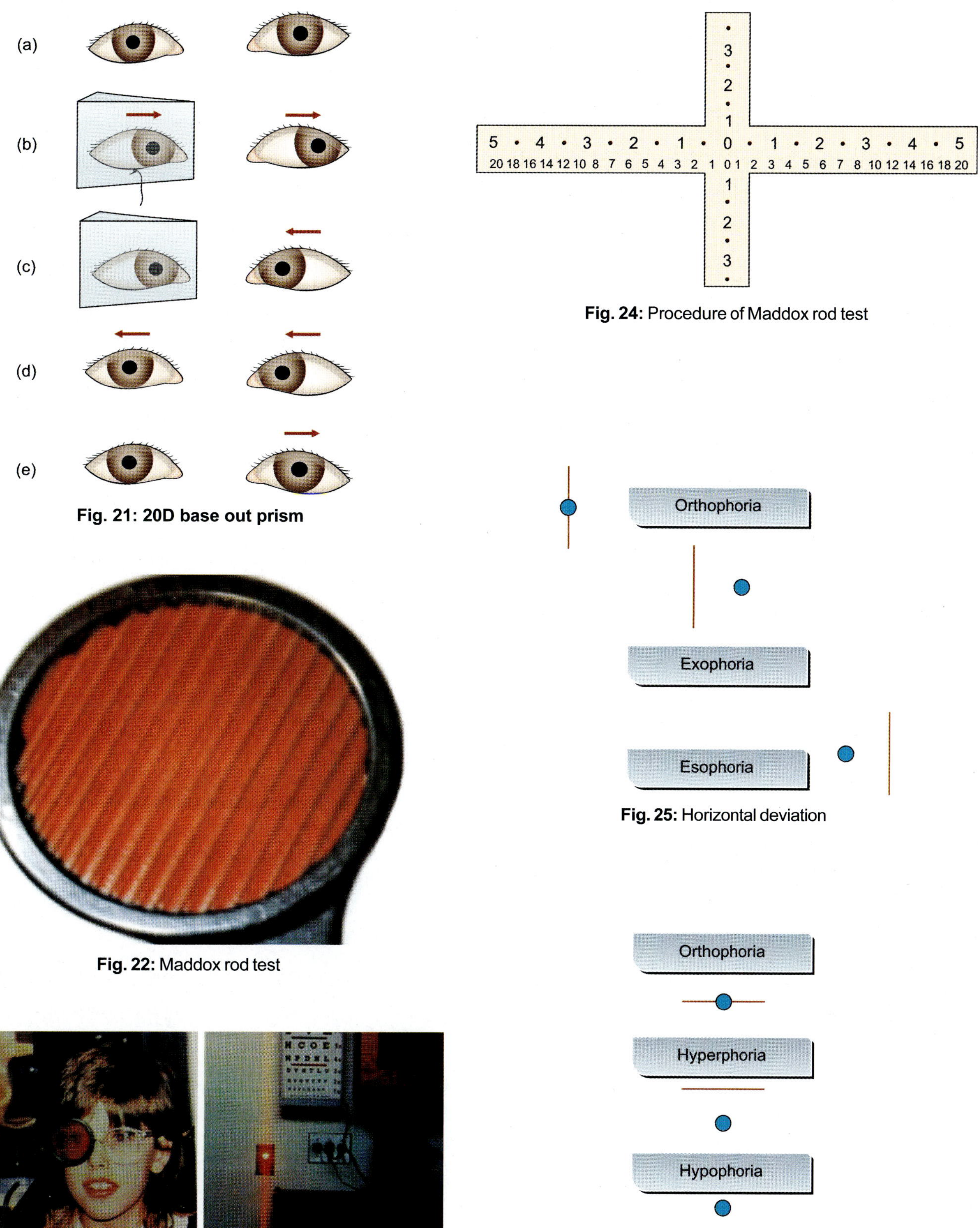

Fig. 21: 20D base out prism

Fig. 22: Maddox rod test

Fig. 23: Instrument of maddox rod test

Fig. 24: Procedure of Maddox rod test

Fig. 25: Horizontal deviation

Fig. 26: Vertical deviation

Subjective Method

- Arms are at 0.
- Ask the patient to superimpose lion in cage SMP slides by moving the tube which is in front of the non-fixating eye.
- Record readings.
- Cyclodeviation can be measured only by subjective method.

Limitations

- Suppression may prevent superimposition; use paramacular slides.
- May never succeed in superimposition, point of crossing is subjective angle.

2. **To estimate grades of binocular single vision (BSV) (Fig. 53):**
3. **To detect state of retinal correspondence**

- Obtain the objective and subjective angles of deviation from the above method.
- OA= Objective Angle, SA = Subjective Angle.
- NRC=Normal retinal correspondence.
- ARC= Anomalous retinal correspondence.
  - If OA=SA → NRC present .
  - IF OA>SA → ARC present.
  - OA – SA = AA (angle of anomaly).
  - If SA is zero.
  - Then OA = AA → Harmonious ARC.
  - If OA > AA → Unharmonious ARC.

4. **To measure and detect type of suppression:**

a. Normally patients would see both lion and cage on SMP slides.
b. If patient sees only lion or only cage , then suppression present.
c. Begin with Simultaneous Foveal Perception (SFP), if not appreciated go to larger slides:
   i. SFP: simultaneous foveal perception slides
   ii. SMP : simultaneous macular perception slides
   iii. SPP: simultaneous paramacular perception slides.
d. Suppression scotoma can be mapped out in the horizontal meridian:
   i. One arm of S is rotated and points read off the scale when the target disappears and then reappears.

5. **To measure range of fusion or vergences:**

- Obtain Subjective Angle and objective Angle with 1st and 2nd grade SMP slides.
- To measure divergence:
  - Arms are diverged till patient reports diplopia or dissappearance of control mark of rabbit slide → Break point.
  - Arms are then converged till patient reports fusion → Recovery point.
  - Repeat vice versa for convergence.
- For vergences at Near, repeat same procedure with -3D lens in front of both eyes.

6. **To measure interpupillary distance:**

- The patient is asked to fixate a picture with his RE (to be tested), in the right tube of synoptophore.
- The examiner with his RE closed, aligns the reflection of a vertical white line in the center of the patient's pupil.
- Similar procedure is repeated for patient's LE.
- The IPD is then read off the scale in mm.

7. **To measure angle kappa:**

- A special slide consists of
  4 3 2 1 0 A B C D
  at intervals of 1°
- Patient sees the 0 mark on this slide with the eye to be tested while examiner looks for the corneal reflex.
- If the reflex is on the nasal side of the pupil the angle is positive
- If the reflex is on the temporal side of the pupil, the Angle is negative.
- The patient is then asked to look at one number at a time till examiner notices that the patient's corneal reflex is centered → this gives the angle kappa in degrees .

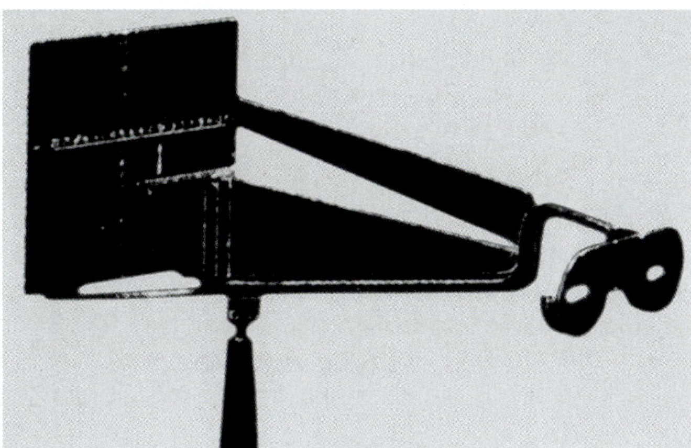

Fig. 27: Maddox wing test

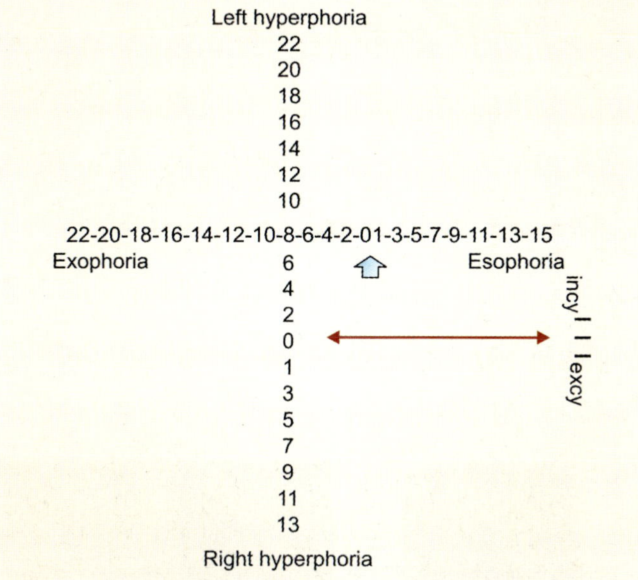

Fig. 28: Procedure of Maddox wing test

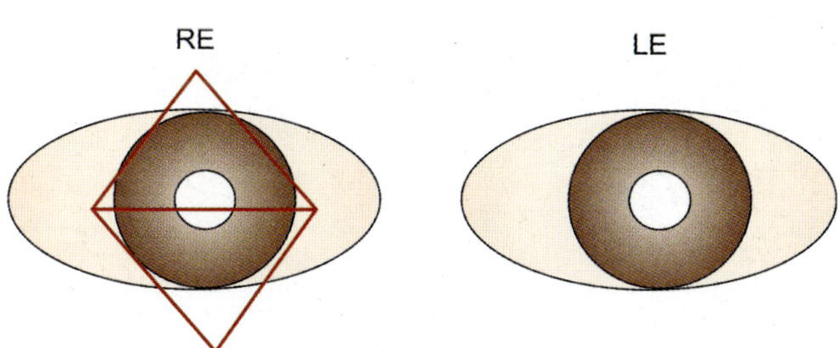

Fig. 29: Maddox double prism

Absence of Cyclophoria

Incyclophoria (tilt to the same side)

RE Incycloph: (RE line tilts to right)

LE Incycloph: (LE line tilts to left)

Excyclophoria (tilt to the opp. side)

RE Excycloph: (RE line tilts to left)

LE Excycloph: (LE line tilt to right)

Fig. 30: Interpretation of Maddox double prism

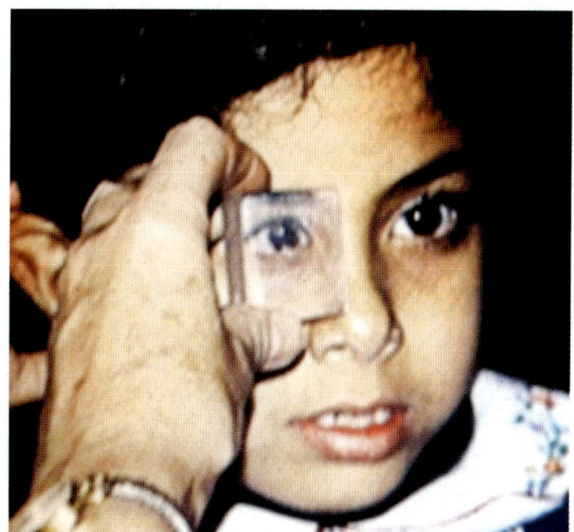

Fig. 31: Jampolsky 4D base out prism

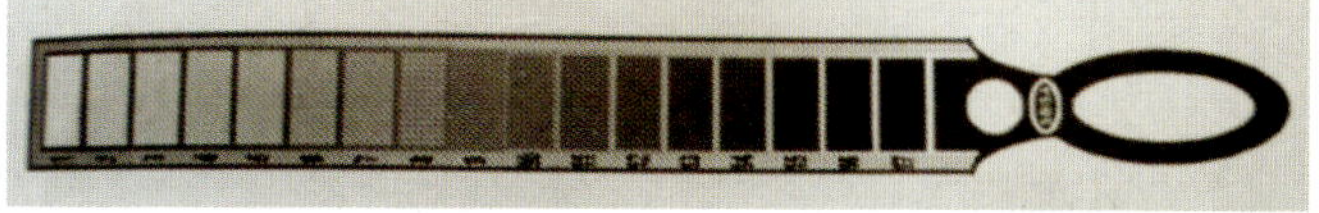

Fig. 32: Red filter ladder

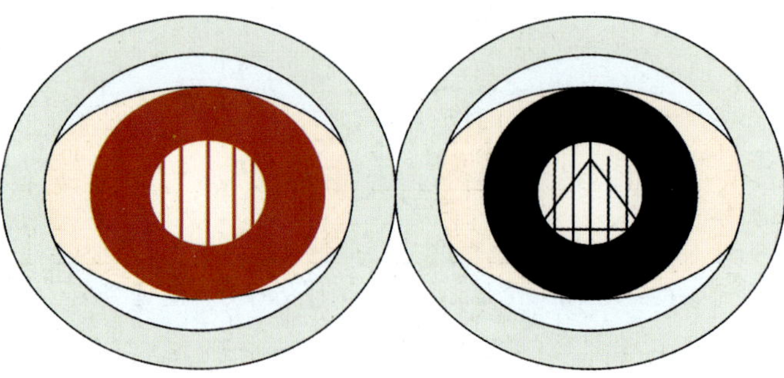

Fig. 33: Maddox double rod

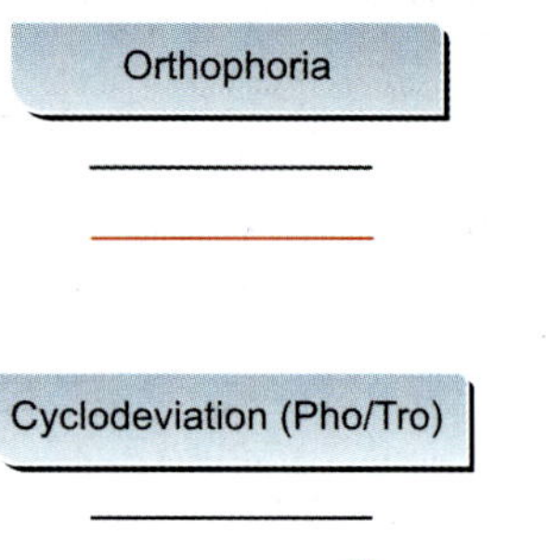

Fig. 34: Interpretation of Maddox double rod

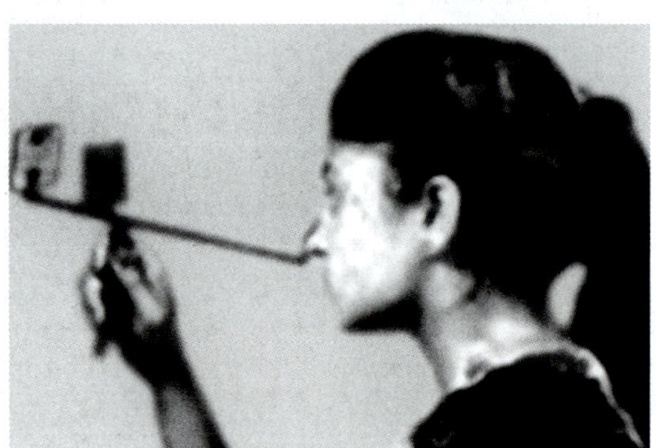

Fig. 35: Diploscope

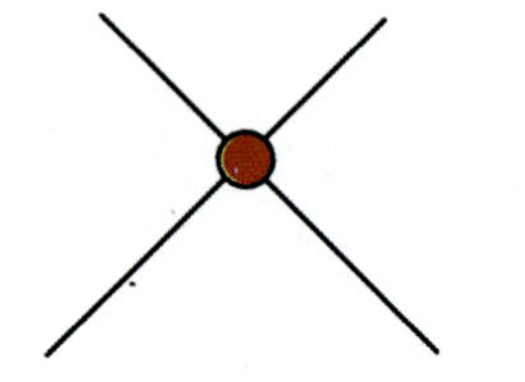

Fig. 36: NRC/Harmonious ARC

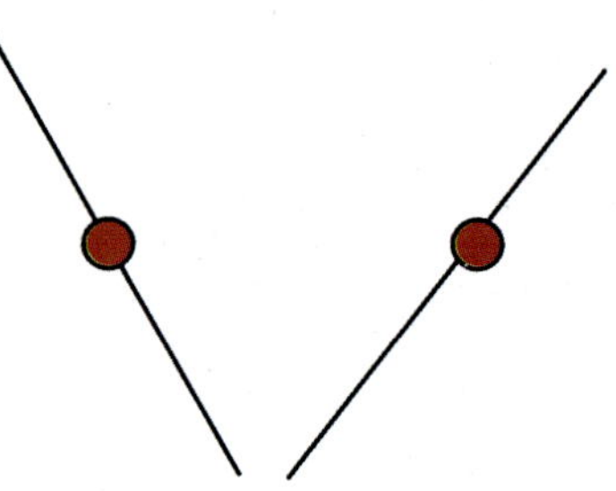

Fig. 37: Diplopia no suppression

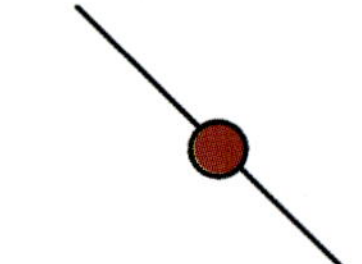

Fig. 38: Suppression

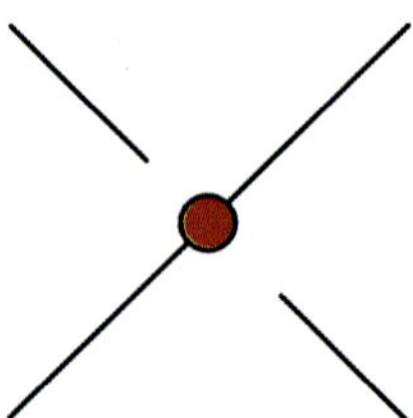

Fig. 39: Suppression area with NRC/unharmonious ARC

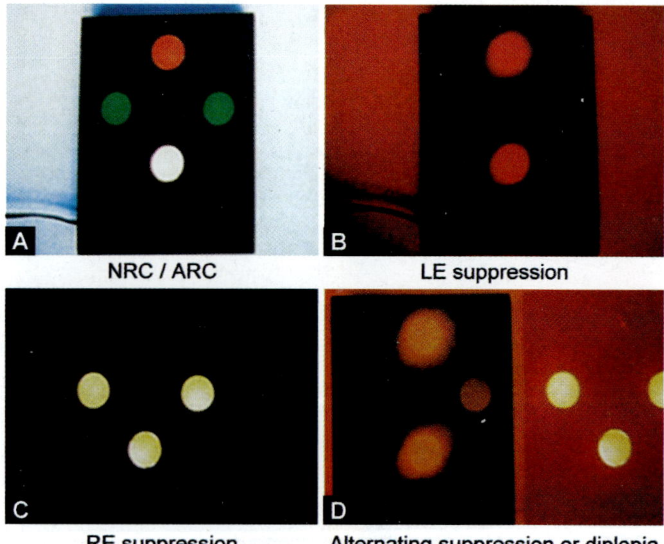

Figs 40A to D: Worth's 4 dot test (W4 DT)

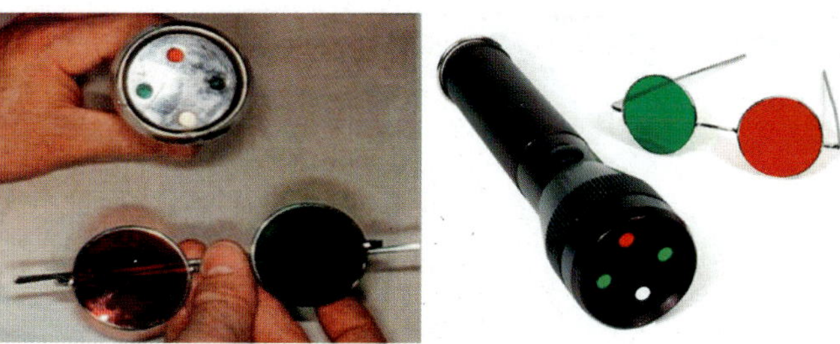

Fig. 41: W4DT for near

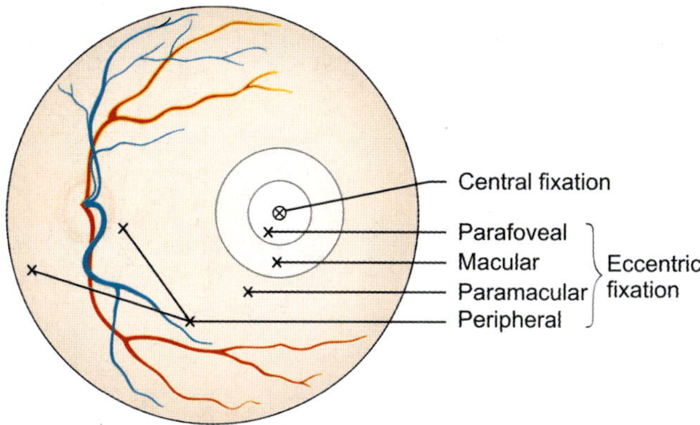

Fig. 44: Interpretation of Visuscope

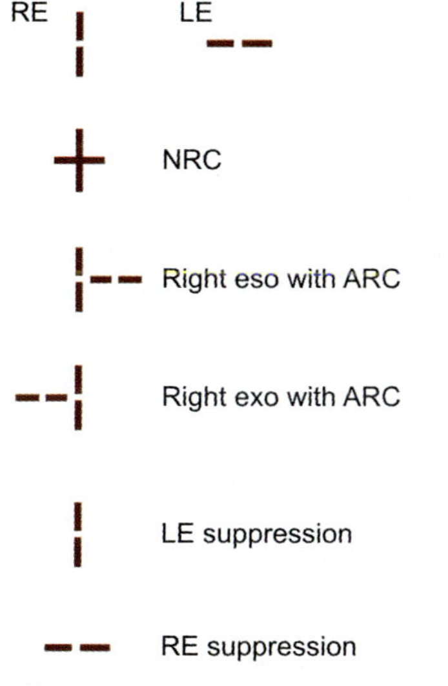

Fig. 42: Bielschowsky after image test

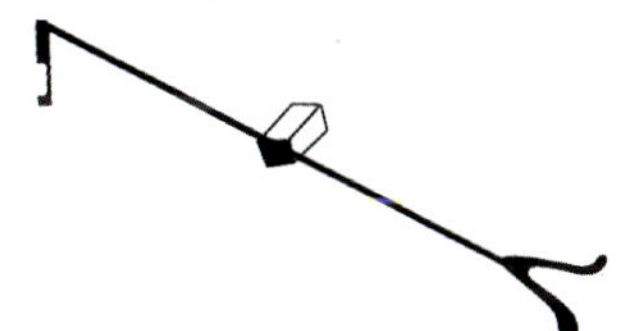

Fig. 45: RAF rule

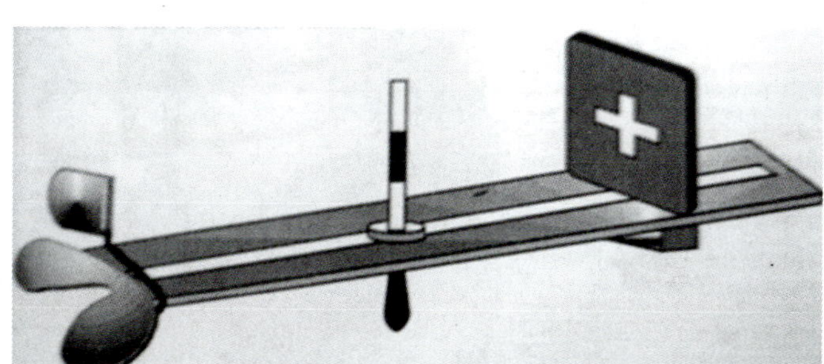

Fig. 46: Livingston binocular gauge

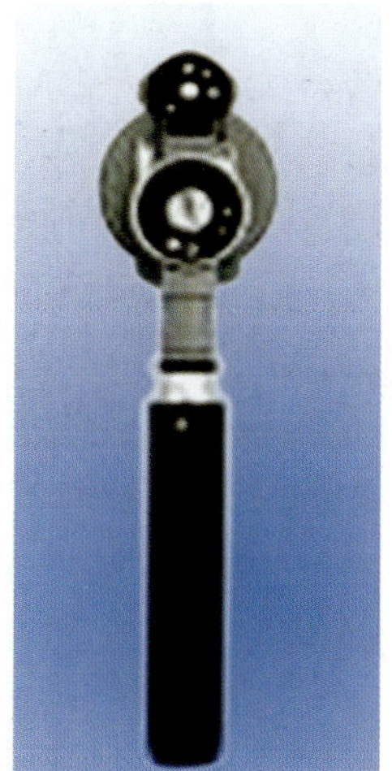

Fig. 43: Visuscope

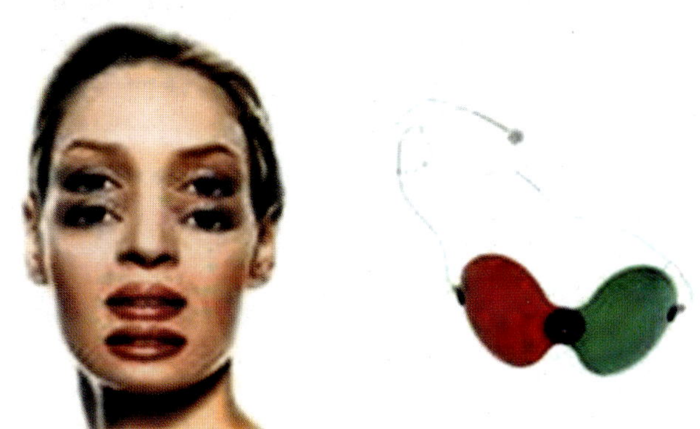

Fig. 47: Diplopia charting

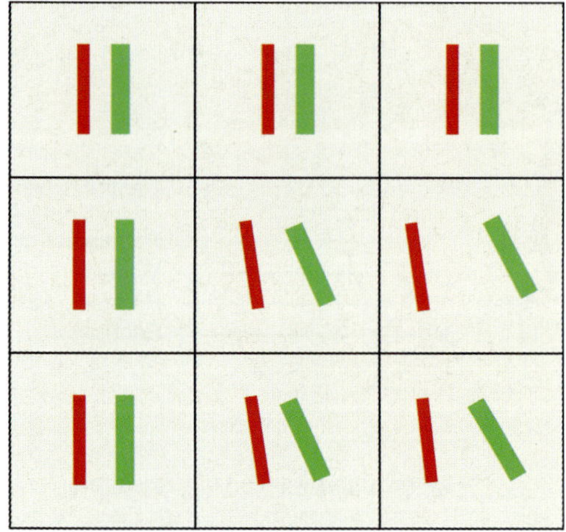

Fig. 48: Diplopia Charting

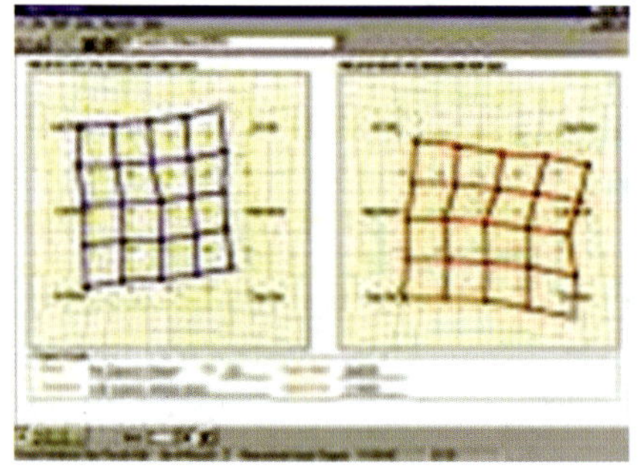

Fig. 49: Hess Charting

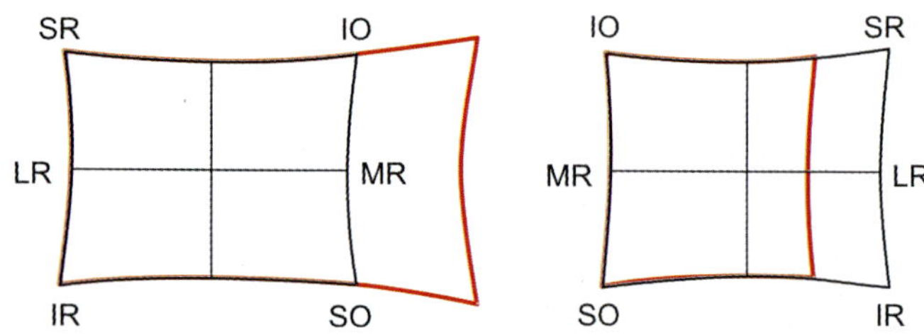

Fig. 50: Comparing two charts (with smaller and longer)

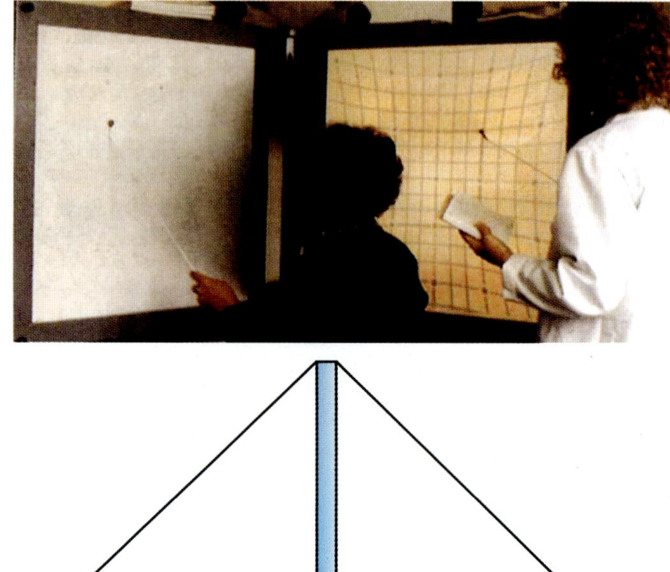

Fig. 51: Lees screen

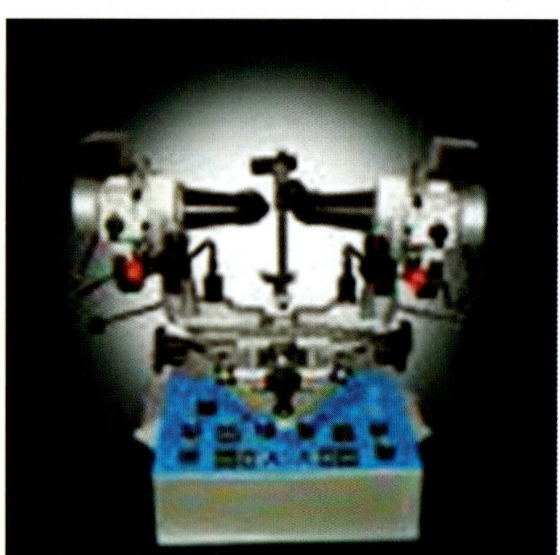

Fig. 52: Synoptophore

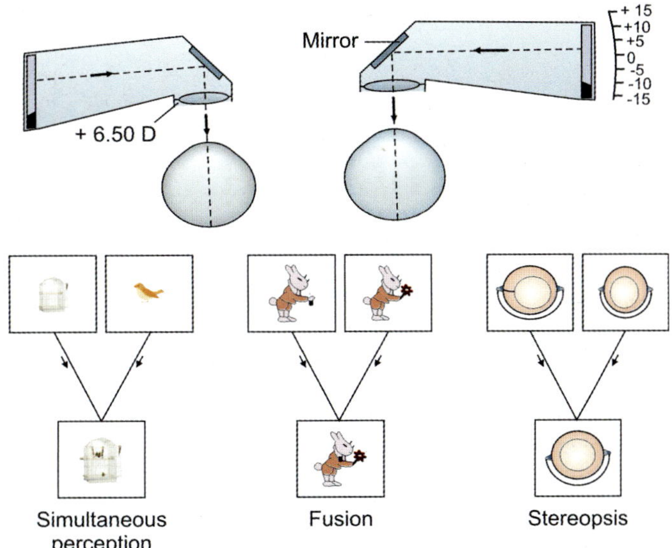

Fig. 53: Estimate grades of binocular single vision

BIBLIOGRAPHY

1. Bielschowsky A. Lectures on motor anomalies. Hanover NH, 1943 (Reprinted 1956), Dartmouth College Publications.
2. Duke Elder S, Wybar K. System of Ophthalmology. In Duke Elder S (ed) Ocular Motility and Strabismus, Vol 6. St.Louis, Mosby, 1973.
3. Khurana AK. Evaluation of a case of strabismus and orthoptic Instruments. In: Theory and Practice of Squint and Orthoptics, CBS Publications 1999.
4. Mukherjee. Case of squint. In: Clinical Ophthalmology 2006.
5. Noorden, GK Von. Infantile Esotropia: A continuing riddle. Am.Orthopt. J 34;52:1984.
6. Rubin ML. Optics for Clinicians, Gainesville, Fl, Triad,1974.

Amblyopia

Shui H Lee (Canada)

INTRODUCTION

Amblyopia, otherwise known as lazy eye, is a disorder of the visual system that is characterized by poor vision in an eye that is otherwise physically normal, or out of proportion to associated structural abnormalities. The problem is caused by either no transmission or poor transmission of the visual image to the brain for a sustained period of dysfunction or during early childhood.

Amblyopia normally only affects one eye, but it is possible to be amblyopic in both eyes if both are similarly deprived of a good, clear visual image. Detecting the condition in early childhood increases the chance of successful treatment.

The term functional amblyopia often is used to describe amblyopia, which is potentially reversible by occlusion therapy. Organic amblyopia refers to irreversible amblyopia.

Most vision loss from amblyopia is preventable or reversible with the right kind of intervention. The recovery of vision depends on how mature the visual connections are, the length of deprivation, and at what age the therapy is begun. It is important to rule out any organic cause of decreased vision because many diseases may not be detectable on routine examination.

Pathological Consideration

Amblyopia is a developmental problem in the brain, not an organic problem in the eye (although organic problems can induce amblyopia which persist after the organic problem has resolved). The part of the brain corresponding to the visual system from the affected eye is not stimulated properly, and develops abnormally. This has been confirmed via direct brain examination. Researchers David H Hubel and Torsten Wiesel had won the Nobel Prize in Physiology or Medicine in 1981 for their work demonstrating the irreversible damage to ocular dominance columns produced in kittens by sufficient visual deprivation during the so-called "critical period". The maximum critical period in humans is from birth to two years old.

Although many types of amblyopia exist, it is believed that their basic mechanisms are the same even though each factor may contribute different amounts to each specific type of amblyopia. In general, amblyopia is believed to result from disuse from inadequate foveal or peripheral retinal stimulation and/or abnormal binocular interaction that causes different visual input from the foveae.

Other Important Features of Amblyopia

Prevalence of amblyopia is difficult to assess and varies in the literature, ranging from 1.0-3.5% in healthy children to 4.0-5.3% in children with ophthalmic problems. Most data show that about 2% of the general population has amblyopia.

Amblyopia is an important socioeconomic problem. Studies have shown that it is the number one cause of monocular vision loss in adults. Furthermore, persons with amblyopia have a higher risk of becoming blind because of potential loss to the sound eye from other causes. No racial preference is known. No gender preference is known.

Amblyopia occurs during the critical periods of visual development. An increased risk exists in those children who are developmentally delayed, were premature, and/or have a positive family history.

Symptoms and Signs

Symptoms and signs of amblyopia are variable. Many people with amblyopia, especially those who are only mildly so, are not even aware they have the condition until

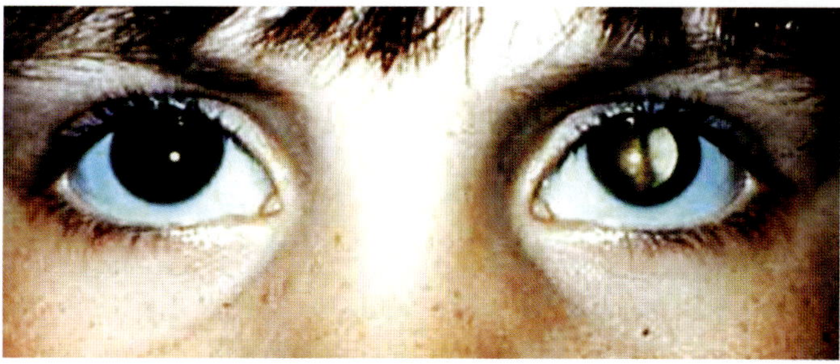

Fig. 1: Child with left retinoblastoma – left organic or form deprivation amblyopia

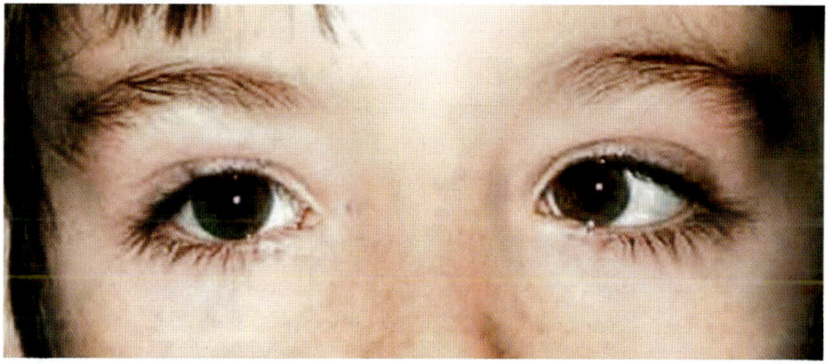

Fig. 2: Child with left esotropia, left strabismic amblyopia

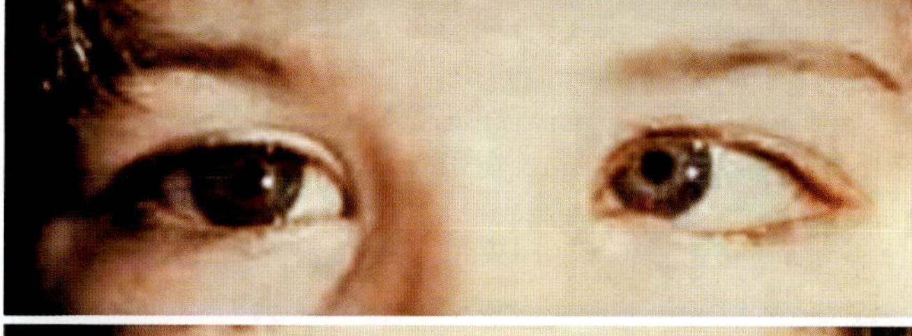

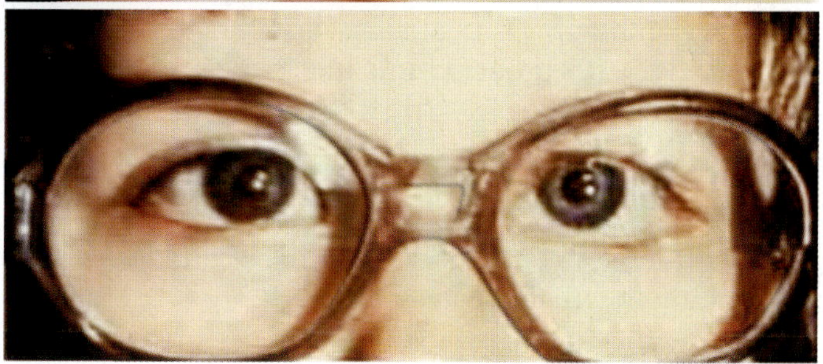

Fig. 3: Child with left accommodative esotropia secondary to left eye with high hyperopia refractive error, and after optical correction, the left eye is normally aligned with the right eye, and the amblyopia is resolved.

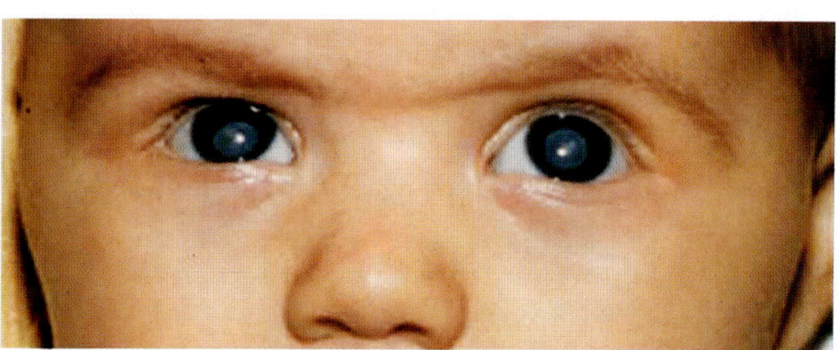

Fig. 4: Child with bilateral congenital cataracts, bilateral form deprivation amblyopia

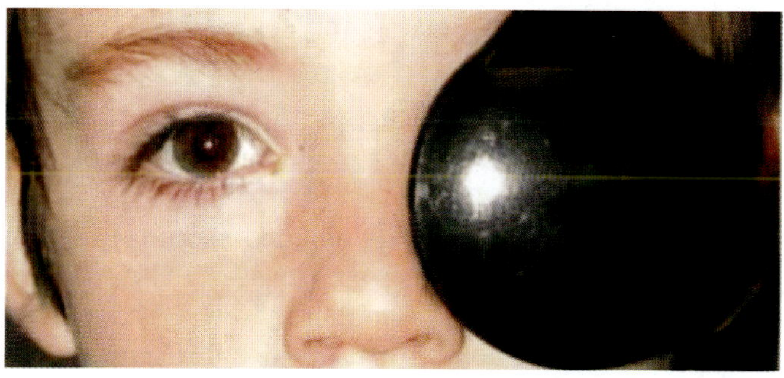

Fig. 5A: Cover test—Tropia-manifest

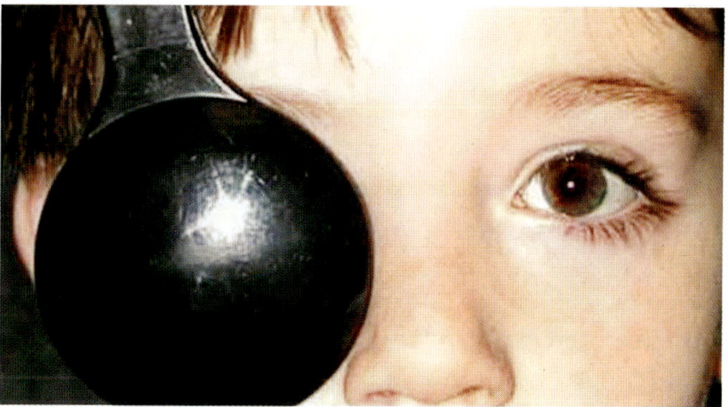

Fig. 5B: Alternate cover test—phoria-latent

tested at older ages, since the vision in their stronger eye is normal. However, people who have *severe* amblyopia may experience associated visual disorders, most notably poor depth perception.

Usually, symptoms and signs are depending upon the types of amblyopia.

In general , there are three types of amblyopia:

1. Strabismic amblyopia - squinting or closing one eye while reading or watching television, crossed or turned eye and turning or tilting the head when looking at an object.
2. Refractive or anisometropic amblyopia.
3. Form-deprivation or visual pathway obstruction amblyopia, such as poor vision in one or both eyes.

INVESTIGATION

For Refractive or Anisometropic Amblyopia

Check Visual Acuity

Diagnosis of amblyopia usually requires a 2-line difference of visual acuity between the eyes; however, this definition is somewhat arbitrary and a smaller difference is common. *Crowding phenomenon:* A common characteristic of amblyopic eyes is difficulty in distinguishing optotypes that are close together. Visual acuity often is better when the patient is presented with single letters rather than a line of letters.

Diagnosis is not an issue in children old enough to read or with use of the tumbling E. Testing in preverbal children.

If the child protests with covering of the sound eye, amblyopia can be diagnosed if it is dense.

Fixation preference may be assessed, especially when strabismus is present.

Induced tropia test may be performed by holding a 10-prism diopter before one eye in cases of an orthophoria or a microtropia.

In infants who cross-fixate, pay attention to when the fixation switch occurs; if it occurs near primary position, then visual acuity is equal in both eyes.

Contrast sensitivity: Strabismic and anisometropic amblyopic eyes have marked losses of threshold contrast sensitivity, especially at higher spatial frequencies; this loss increases with the severity of amblyopia.

Neutral density filters: Patients with strabismic amblyopia may have better visual acuity or less of a decline of visual acuity when tested with neutral density filters compared to the normal eye. This was not found to be true in patients with anisometropic amblyopia or organic disease.

Binocular function: Amblyopia usually is associated with changes in binocular function or stereopsis.

Eccentric fixation: Some patients with amblyopia may consistently fixate with a nonfoveal area of the retina under monocular use of the amblyopic eye, the mechanism of which is unknown. This can be diagnosed by holding a fixation light in the midline in front of the patient and asking them to fixate on it while the normal eye is covered. The reflection of the light will not be centered.

Refraction: Cycloplegic refraction must be performed on all patients, using retinoscopy to obtain an objective refraction. In most cases, the more hyperopic eye or the eye with more astigmatism will be the amblyopic eye. If this is not true, one needs to investigate further for ocular pathology.

Rest of examination: Perform a full eye examination to rule out ocular pathology.

In summary, refractive amblyopia may result from anisometropia (unequal refractive indices between the two eyes).

Anisometropia exists when there is a difference in the refraction between the two eyes. The eye which provides the brain with a clearer image (closer to 20/20) typically becomes the dominant eye. The image in the other eye is blurred, which results in abnormal development of one half of the visual system.

Refractive amblyopia is usually less severe than strabismic amblyopia. Frequently, amblyopia is associated with a combination of anisometropia and strabismus. Pure refractive amblyopia is treated by correcting the refractive error early with prescription lenses and patching or penalizing the good eye.

For Strabismic Amblyopia

Strabismus, sometimes erroneously also called *lazy eye*, is a condition in which the eyes are misaligned. Strabismus usually results in normal vision in the preferred sighting (or "fellow") eye, but may cause abnormal vision in the deviating or strabismic eye due to the discrepancy between the images projecting to the brain from the two eyes. Adult-onset strabismus usually causes double vision (diplopia), since the two eyes are not fixated on the same object. Children's brains, however, are more neuroplastic, and therefore can more easily adapt by suppressing images from one of the eyes, eliminating the double vision. This plastic response of the brain, however, interrupts the brain's normal development, resulting in the amblyopia.

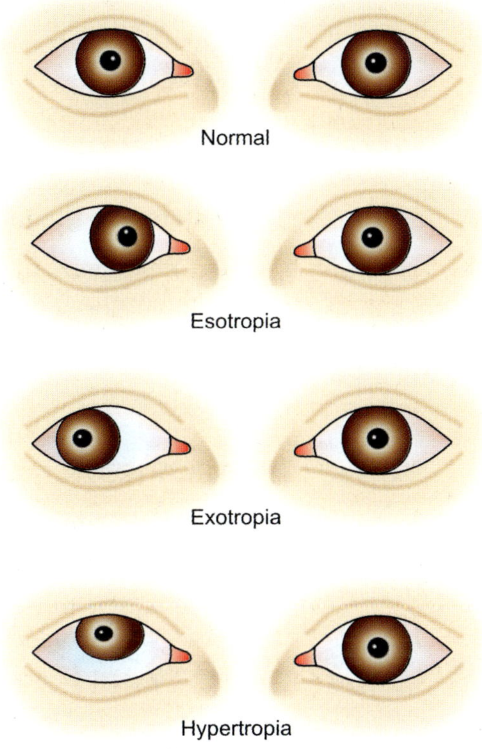

Fig. 6: Types of tropia

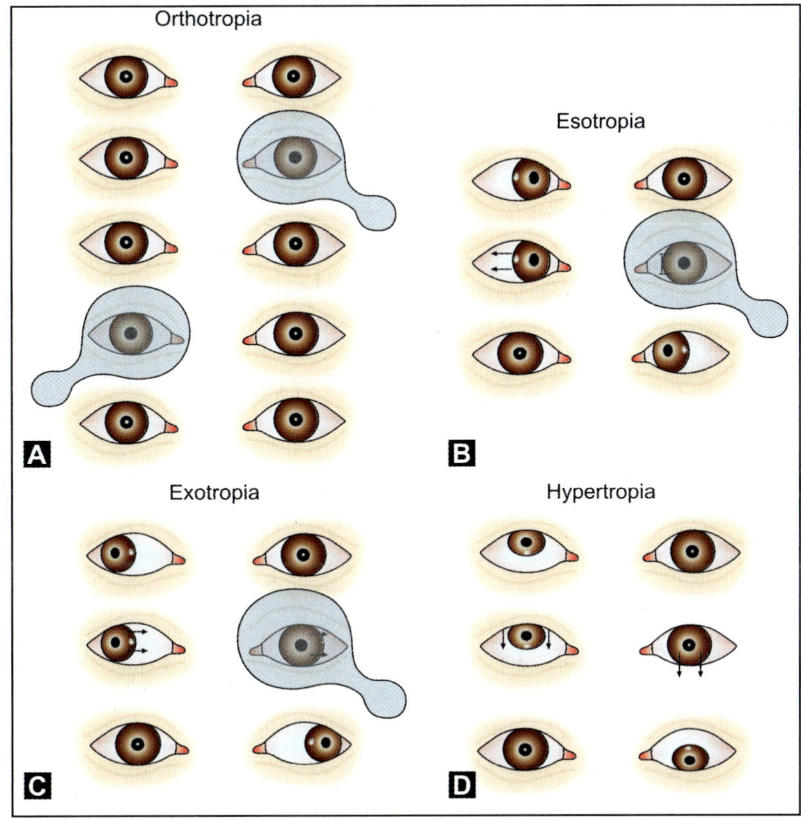

Figs 7A to D: Cover test to detect the type of tropia

Types of Strabismus

Esotropia and Exotropia, A-patterns
Esotropia and Exotropia, V-patterns
Esotropia, Accommodative
Esotropia, Acquired
Esotropia, Infantile
Esotropia, with High AC/A Ratio
Exotropia, Acquired
Exotropia, Congenital
Monofixation Syndrome
Any type of the above strabismus will lead to strabismus amblyopia if not treated in children after the critical time of visual pathway development.

Testing for Strabismus

Alternate cover test-phoria-latent
Cover test to detect the type of tropia alternate cover test to detect latent strabismus-phoria-strabismus.

Other tests for screening strabismus can be done in a large clinical center with aide of orthoptic technician at Children hospital.

Form-deprivation and Visual Pathway Obstruction Amblyopia

Form-deprivation amblyopia (*Amblyopia ex anopsia*) results when the ocular media become opaque, such as is the case with cataracts or corneal scarring from forceps injuries during birth. These opacities prevent adequate visual input from reaching the eye, and therefore disrupt development. If not treated in a timely fashion, amblyopia may persist even after the cause of the opacity is removed. Sometimes, drooping of the eyelid (ptosis) or some other problem causes the upper eyelid to physically occlude a child's vision, which may cause amblyopia quickly. Visual pathway obstruction amblyopia may be a complication of a hemangioma that blocks some or all of the eye.

Other Problems to be Considered

Consider organic problems that may be subtle or difficult to diagnose such as optic nerve hypoplasia.

Imaging Studies

If suspicion exists of an organic cause for decreased vision and the ocular examination is normal, then further investigations into retinal or optic nerve causes should be initiated. Studies to perform include imaging of the visual system through CT scan, MRI, and fluorescein angiography to assess the retina.

Other Tests

Although differences in the electrophysiologic responses of normal versus amblyopic eyes have been reported, these techniques remain investigational and the differences are controversial.

Differential Diagnosis of Amblyopia

It is important to differentiate the three main different types of amblyopia, i.e. strabismus, refractive-anisometropia, and form deprivation amblyopia with the above chart. The treatment of amblyopia depends upon the etiology of the amblyopia.

TREATMENTS— MEDICAL AND SURGICAL

Medical Care

The clinician must first rule out an organic cause and treat any obstacle to vision (e.g. cataract, occlusion of the eye from other etiologies).

Remove cataracts in the first 2 months of life, and aphakic correction must occur quickly.

Treatment of anisometropia and refractive errors must occur next.

The amblyopic eye must have the most accurate optical correction possible. This should occur prior to any occlusion therapy because vision may improve with spectacles alone.

Full cycloplegic refraction should be given to patients with accommodative esotropia and amblyopia. In other patients, a prescription less than the full plus measurement that was refracted may be prescribed given that the decrease in plus is symmetric between the two eyes. Because accommodative amplitude is believed to be decreased in amblyopic eyes, one needs to be cautious about cutting back too much on the amount of plus. Refractive correction alone can improve amblyopia in about one third of children.

The next step is forcing the use of the amblyopic eye by occlusion therapy. Occlusion therapy has been the mainstay of treatment since the 18th century. The following are general guidelines for occlusion therapy:

Patching may be full-time or part-time. Standard teaching has been that children need to be observed at intervals of 1 week per year of age, if undergoing full-time occlusion to avoid occlusion amblyopia in the sound eye. The recent and ongoing Amblyopia Treatment Studies (ATS) have helped to provide new information on the effect of various amounts of patching.

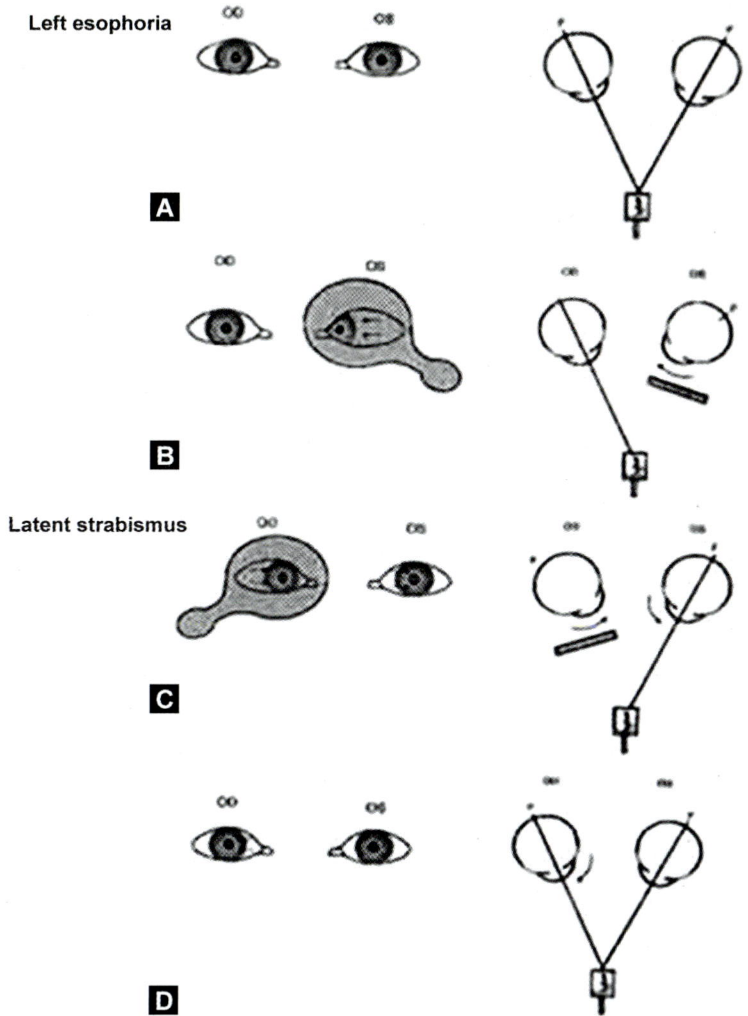

Figs 8A to D: Alternate cover test to detect latent strabismus—phoria-strabismus

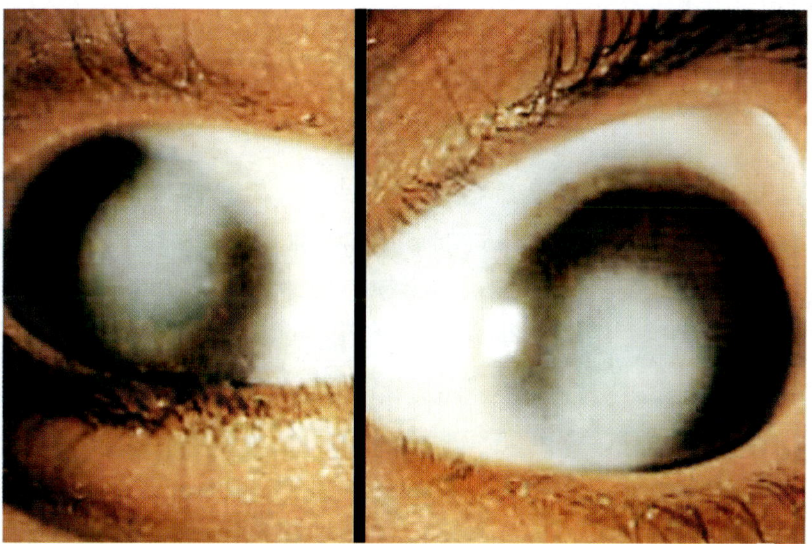

Fig. 9: Peter's abnormality—Bilateral corneal scarring

Always consider lack of compliance in a child where visual acuity is not improving. Compliance is difficult to measure but is an important factor in determining the success of this therapy.

In addition to adhesive patches, opaque contact lenses, occluders mounted on spectacles, and adhesive tape on glasses have been used.

Establishing the fact that the vision of the better eye has been degraded sufficiently with the chosen therapy is important.

The Amblyopia Treatment Studies have helped to define the role of full-time patching versus part-time patching in patients with amblyopia. The studies have demonstrated that, in patients aged 3-7 years with severe amblyopia (visual acuity between 20/100 and 20/400), full-time patching produced a similar effect to that of 6 hours of patching per day. In a separate study, 2 hours of daily patching produced an improvement in visual acuity similar to that of 6 hours of daily patching when treating moderate amblyopia (visual acuity better than 20/100) in children aged 3-7 years. In this study, patching was prescribed in combination with 1 hour of near visual activities.

Data from the Amblyopia Treatment Studies are also available for older patients. For patients aged from 7 years to younger than 13 years, the Amblyopia Treatment Studies have suggested that prescribing 2-6 hours a day of patching can improve visual acuity even if the amblyopia has been previously treated. For patients aged from 13 years to younger than 18 years, prescribing 2-6 hours a day of patching might improve visual acuity when amblyopia has not been previously treated; however, this is likely to be of little benefit if amblyopia was previously treated with patching. Long-term results from these studies are still pending.

The Amblyopia Treatment Studies have also found that about one fourth of children with amblyopia who were successfully treated experience a recurrence within the first year after discontinuation of treatment. Data from these studies suggest that patients treated with 6 or more hours a day of patching have a greater risk of recurrence when patching is stopped abruptly rather than when it is reduced to 2 hours a day prior to cessation of patching. Randomized studies have still yet to be performed.

Penalization Therapy

In the past, penalization therapy was reserved for children who would not wear a patch or in whom compliance was an issue. The Amblyopia Treatment Studies, however, have demonstrated that atropine penalization in patients with moderate amblyopia (defined by the study as visual acuity better than 20/100) is as effective as patching. The Amblyopia Treatment Studies were performed in children aged 3-7 years.

The Amblyopia Treatment Studies have also demonstrated that weekend atropine provided an improvement in visual acuity similar to that of daily atropine when treating moderate amblyopia in children aged 3-7 years.

Atropine drops or ointment (Atropine sulfate 0.5% to 2.0%) is instilled in the nonamblyopic eye. This therapy is sometimes used in conjunction with patching or occlusion of the glasses (eg, adhesive tape, nail polish) by individual practitioners. In the Amblyopia Treatment Studies that evaluated patching versus atropine penalization, atropine penalization and patching were used in conjunction with 1 hour of near visual activities.

This technique may also be used for maintenance therapy, which is useful especially in patients with mild amblyopia.

Other options include optical blurring through contact lenses or elevated bifocal segments.

The endpoint of therapy is spontaneous alternation of fixation or equal visual acuity in both eyes.

When visual acuity is stable, patching may be decreased slowly, depending on the child's tendency for the amblyopia to recur.

Because amblyopia recurs in a large number of patients (Prognosis), maintenance therapy or tapering of therapy should be strongly considered. This tapering is controversial, so individual physicians vary in their approaches.

Treatment of strabismus generally occurs last. The endpoint of strabismic amblyopia is freely alternating fixation with equal vision. Surgery generally is performed after this endpoint has been reached.

Surgical Care

Surgical therapy for strabismus generally should occur after amblyopia is reversed. Disadvantages to surgical therapy prior to correction of amblyopia include difficulty in telling if amblyopia is present because there is no longer a strabismus to assess fixation preference and higher potential to being lost to follow-up, as the child cosmetically looks better. The improved cosmesis gives the parents a false sense of security about the vision improving.

Other surgical therapy for form deprivation amblyopia include cataract surgery for congenital cataracts, corneal transplants for bilateral corneal scarring, retinoblastoma etc.

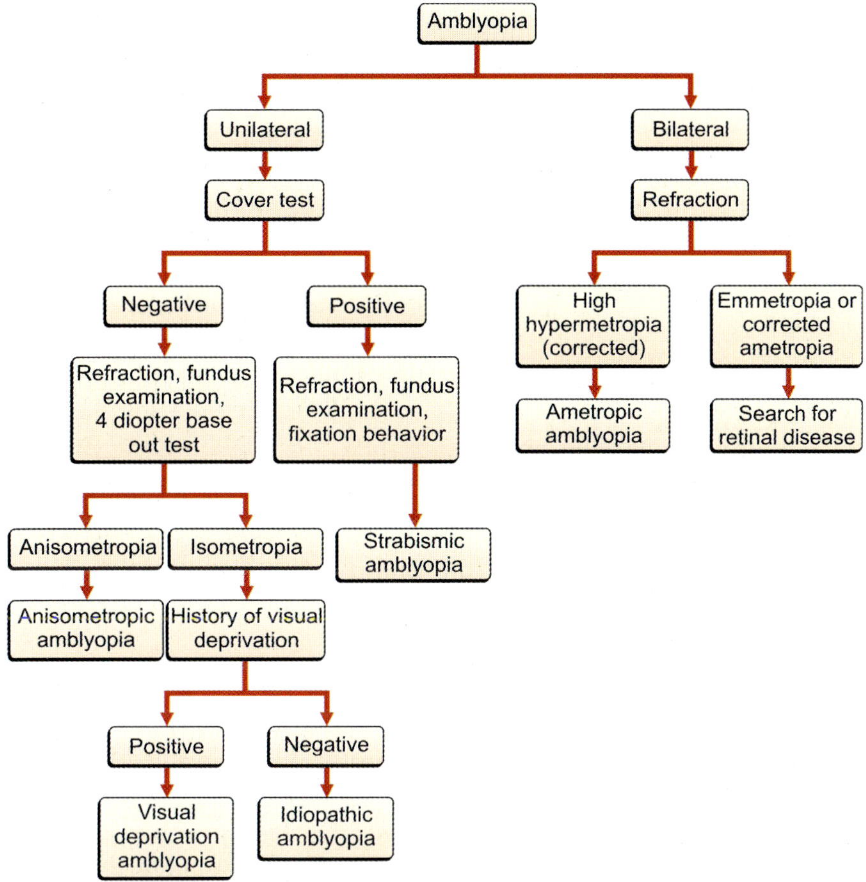

Fig. 10: Flow chart of determination of differential diagnosis of amblyopia

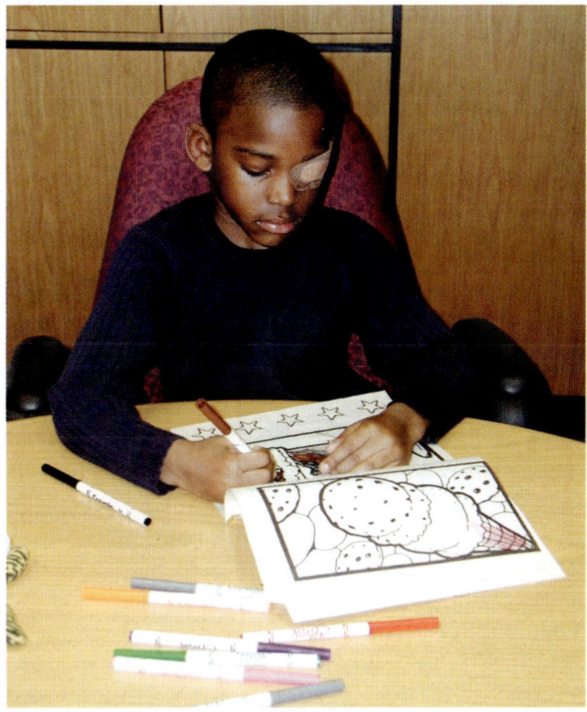

Fig. 11: Child with left patching to treat the right amblyopia

Activity after Treatment

Close supervision during occlusion therapy is necessary to make sure children do not peek. Various methods of preventing children from removing patches have been considered, from a reward system for older children to arm splints and mittens for infants.

Atropine penalization–Atropine sulfate 0.5–2.0 % (with either ointment or drops) is an alternative method of blurring vision in the sound eye of patients who refuse patching. It may be applied once a day to patients in the preferred eye only.

Further Follow-up Care

Outpatient follow-up care needs to continue beyond the primary completion of amblyopia treatment because visual deterioration occurs in many children. In a multicenter study conducted as part of the Amblyopia Treatment Studies, one-fourth of patients experienced recurrence of amblyopia within the first year after treatment, with the risk of recurrence greater if the treatment was stopped abruptly rather than tapered. One study by Levartovsky et al showed deterioration in 75% of children with anisometropia of 1.75 diopters or more after occlusion therapy. Recidivism can occur even several years after the initial treatment period and is as high as 53% after 3 years.

Deterrence/Prevention

Vision screening programs: Studies have shown these programs to be technically easy and that they help reduce cost as well as incidence of amblyopia because of early treatment and detection. Current programs include use of the photorefractor and school vision screening programs.

Amblyopia after Trauma

Young patients who have trauma to their eyes often are at risk for occlusion amblyopia. Possible reasons include lid edema, hyphema, occlusive dressing, vitreous hemorrhage, and traumatic cataract.

This amblyopia often is superimposed on a visual deficit caused by any structural abnormality and needs to be taken into account when treating these children.

Vision needs to be monitored closely in children after ocular trauma, especially up to 6 years and in nonverbal children. Occlusive therapy needs to be instituted if there is any suggestion of decrease vision in the injured eye.

Complications

Most cases of amblyopia are reversible if detected and treated early, so this vision loss is preventable. The main complication of not treating amblyopia is long-term irreversible vision loss.

Clinical Trials and Experiments

A recent study, widely reported in the popular press, has suggested that repetitive transcranial magnetic stimulation may temporarily improve contrast sensitivity and spatial resolution in the bad eye of amblyopic adults. These results await verification by other researchers.

Virtual reality computer games where each eye receives different signals of the virtual world that the player's brain must combine in order to successfully play the game have shown some promise in improving both monocularity in the affected eye as well as binocularity.

In another recent clinical trial conducted in a hospital in China and coordinated with a research program at University of Southern California, 28 of 30 patients being treated for amblyopia showed dramatic gains with some developing 20/20 vision. The treatment involved only the use of basic computer desktop software and vision training exercises.

Prognosis

After 1 year, about 73% of patients show success after their first trial of occlusion therapy. Studies have shown that the number of patients who retain their level of visual acuity decreases over time to 53% after 3 years.

Risk factors for failure in amblyopia treatment include the following:

Type of amblyopia: Patients with high anisometropia and patients with organic pathology have the worse prognosis. Patients with strabismic amblyopia have the best outcome.

Age at which therapy began: Younger patients seem to do better.

Depth of amblyopia at start of therapy: The better the initial visual acuity in the amblyopic eye, the better the prognosis.

Parents need to be educated about the importance of treatment and compliance as well as the visual implications because the treatment of amblyopia often lies in the hands of the parents.

The clinician must educate parents and patients of the implications of not treating amblyopia. Delay in treatment beyond the critical period results in irreversibility of amblyopia and could result in liability claims against the physician.

CONCLUSION

Early treatment and detection is the key to visual rehabilitation in amblyopic patients. Methods of identifying children at risk or who have amblyopia are needed. Further research into the mechanism of amblyopia is needed to be able to address and treat the direct etiology.

BIBLIOGRAPHY

1. Hess RF, Mansouri B, Dakin SC, and Allen HA. "Integration of local motion is normal in amblyopia." J Opt Soc Am A Opt Image Sci Vis 2006;23(5):986-92.
2. Holmes, Repka, Kraker and Clarke. "The treatment of amblyopia." Strabismus 2006;14(1):37-42.
3. "Information from your family doctor. Amblyopia ("lazy eye") in your child." American family physician 2007;75(3):368.
4. Jeffrey Cooper and Rachel Cooper. "All About Strabismus". Optometrists Network. Retrieved on 2008-03-09.
5. Levi DM. "Visual processing in amblyopia: Human studies." Strabismus 2006;14(1):11-19.
6. McKee SP, Levi DM, Movshon JA. "The pattern of visual deficits in amblyopia." J Vision 2003;3(5):380-405.
7. Tyler CW. Binocular Vision In, Duane's Foundations of Clinical Ophthalmology. Tasman W, Jaeger EA (Eds), JB Lippincott Co: Philadelphia 2004;2.
8. Weber JL, Wood Joanne. "Amblyopia: Prevalence, Natural History, Functional Effects and Treatment 2005.

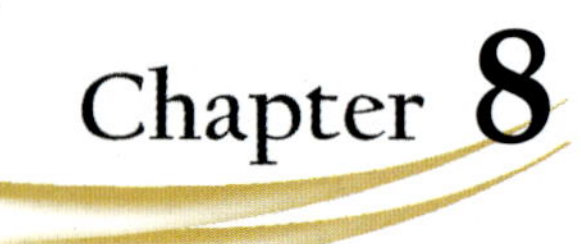

Rectus Muscles Strengthening Surgery

Ewa Oleszczynska Prost (Poland)

Procedures that strengthen muscle actions involve:

- Rectus muscle resection (Fig. 1)
- Anteposition (Fig. 2)
- Muscle-scleral tuck (Fig. 3)

In case of exotropia – medial rectus muscle and esotropia – lateral rectus muscle, surgery to the horizontal recti is frequent procedure, leading to their strengthening. In hypertropia or hypotropia, surgery to the vertical recti is performed less frequently. Its technique is basically similar to the procedure on horizontal recti.

Incision of conjunctiva is made in the limbus (See Fig. 1 in chapter 2) or deflection (See Fig. 2 in chapter 2), similarly other procedures on the rectus muscles.

RECTUS MUSCLE RESECTION

Resection increases the action of the muscle reflected in the length-tension curve (Figs 1A to G).

INDICATIONS

- Strengthning lateral rectus muscle action for esotropia, unilateral or bilateral.
- Strengthning medial rectus muscle action for exotropia, unilateral or bilateral.
- Not used in restrictive strabismus.

SURGICAL TECHNIQUE

Figures 1A to G.

ANTEPOSITION

This procedure aims at strengthening muscle actions. It comprises of placing muscle insertion forward from its normal position, so that the length of the contact arch with the globe surface is elongated with subsequent increase in the torque of contracting muscle (Figs 2A to E).

INDICATIONS

- Additional procedure to increase shortening of the muscle.
- Sometimes in paretic squint.

SURGICAL TECHNIQUE

Figures 2A to G.

MUSCLE-SCLERAL TUCK

This procedure produces a leash effect by tightening the muscle. This leash can cause a restriction of ocular rotation in the direction away from the muscle (Figs 3A and B).

INDICATIONS

- Strengthening of rectus muscle actions, especially in case of muscular atrophy and significant thinning of the muscle:
  - congenital anomalies
  - prolonged muscular paralysis.
- Actually, this procedure is rarely performed because of a possibility of plane adhesions with the globe as well as mutilation of muscle and its blood vessels.

SURGICAL TECHNIQUE

Figures 3A and B.

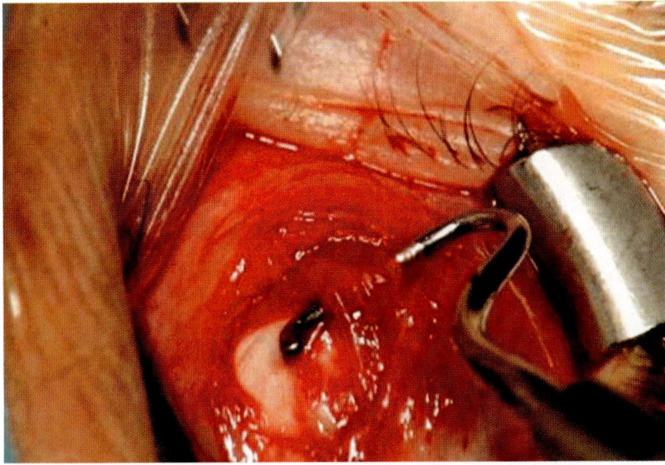

Fig. 1A: The muscle is identified and the hook placed beneath it

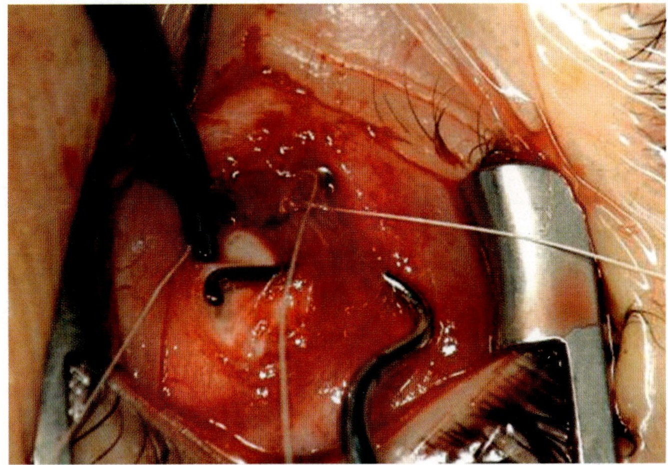

Fig. 1D: The sutures are tightened and tied

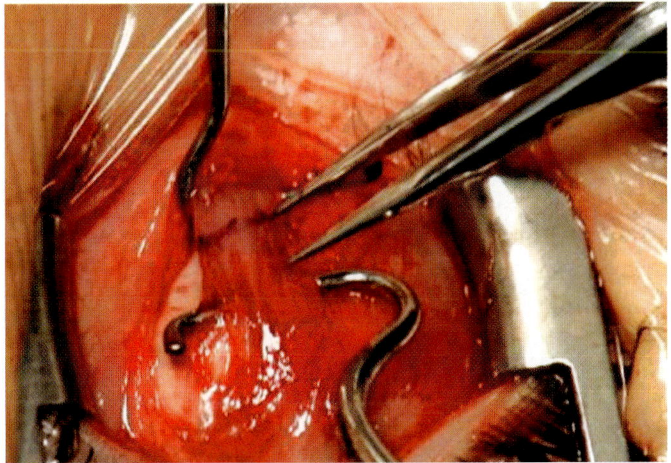

Fig. 1B: The exact amount of resection is measured by the calipers

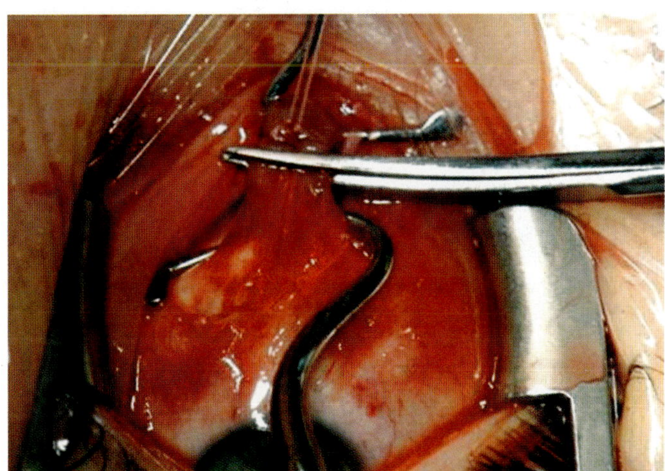

Fig. 1E: Muscle is divided between sutures and insertion

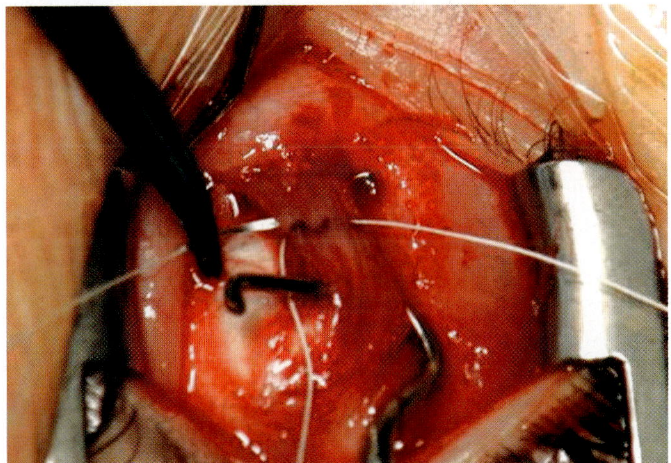

Fig. 1C: Sutures are placed at measured distance from insertion

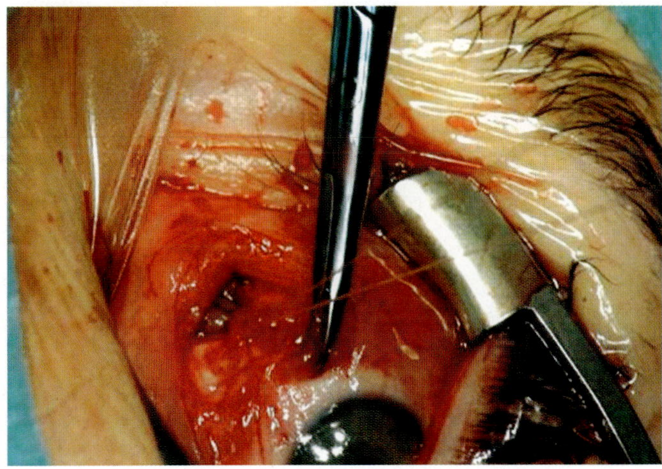

Fig. 1F: Muscle is re-sutured to the original insertion

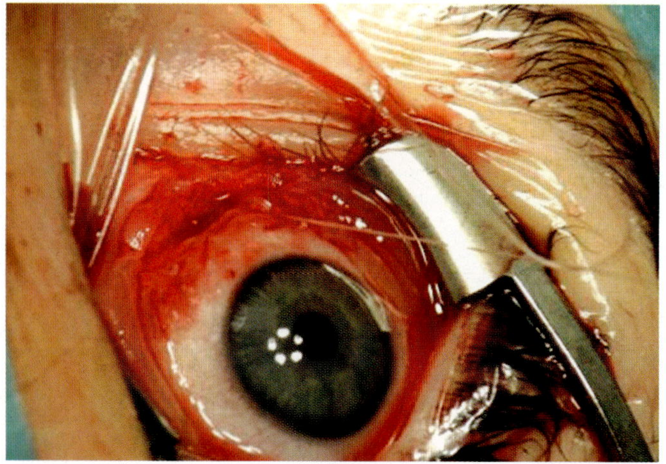

Fig. 1G: Tenon's capsule is repositioned over the incision site and conjunctiva closed with one continuous 8/0 suture

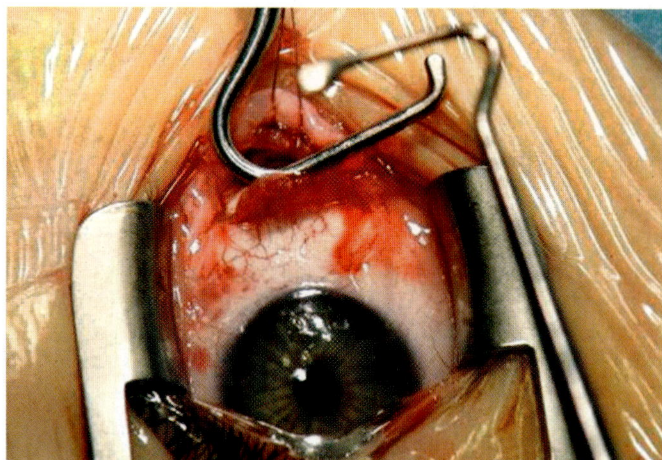

Fig. 2C: Muscle tendon is disinserted from the globe

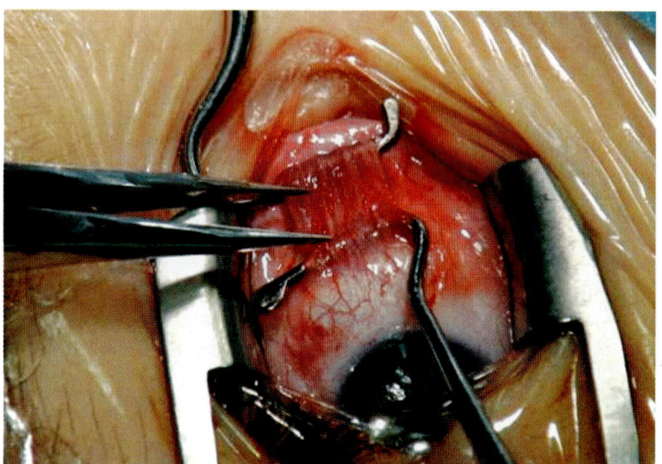

Fig. 2A: The calipers measuring the exact distance for the muscle resection

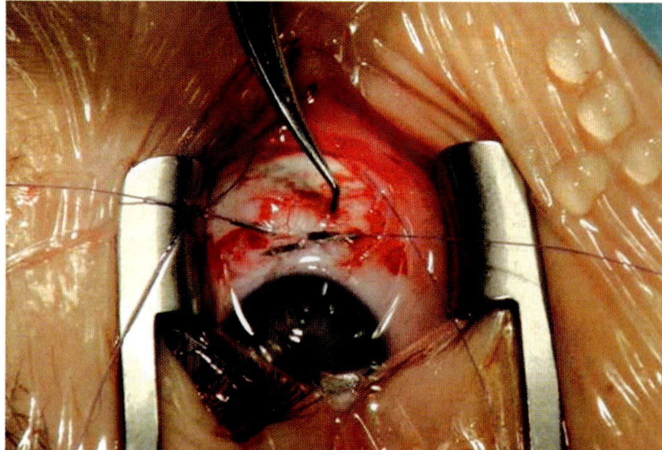

Fig. 2D: Both needles of double-armed suture are placed through the sclera anterior to the first insertion

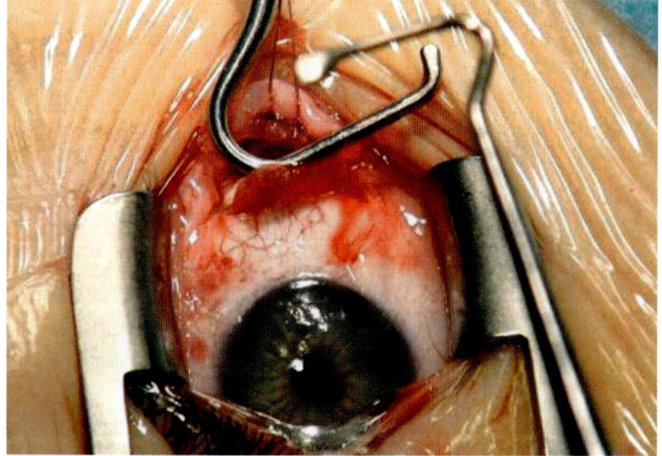

Fig. 2B: Two sutures are passed through the peripheral 1/3rd of the muscle width

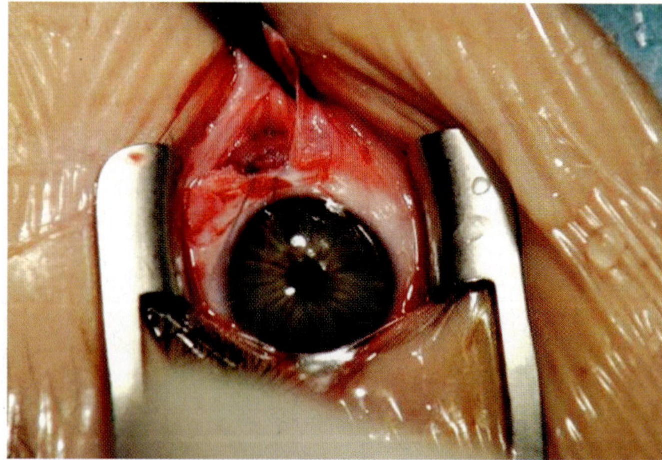

Fig. 2E: The muscle is pulled completely to the desired recession site

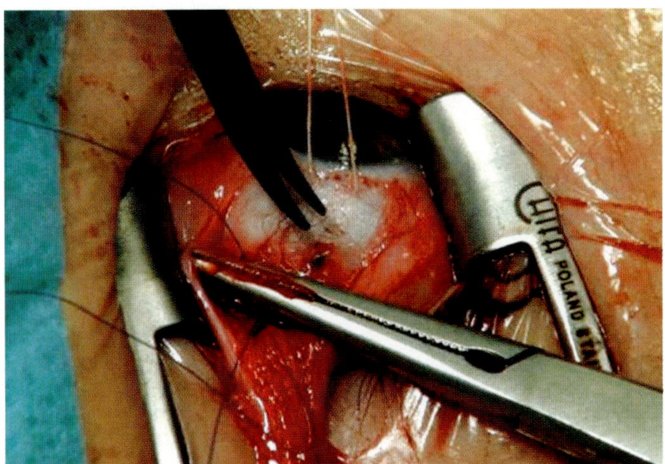

Fig. 3A: Needles are passed through half-thickness of muscle, starting in its center, aiming perpendicular to the muscle fibers toward the muscle edge. Identical pass is performed on both sides of the muscle

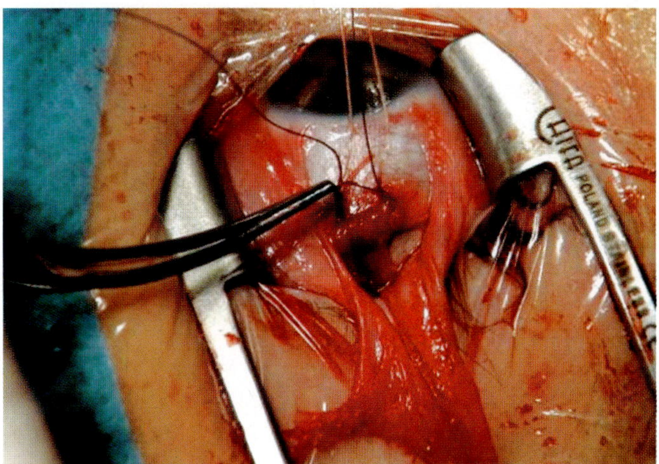

Fig. 3B: Needles are passed through the sclera just anterior to the muscle insertion.Posterior muscle is advanced by pulling on the double-armed sutures.The double-throw overhand knot is secured

BIBLIOGRAPHY

1. Biglan AW. Early surgery of infantile exotropia. Trans Pa Acad Ophthalmol Otolaryngol 1983;36:161-8.
2. Fells P, Lee IP. Strabismus, in: Spalton DJ, Hitchings RA, Hunter PA, eds.: Atlas of clinical ophthalmology. London, New York: Gower Medical Publishing 1984;6-7.
3. Hardesty H: Management of intermittent exotropia. BinocVis Quart, 1990;5:145.
4. Hermann JS: Surgical therapy for convergence insufficiency. J Pediatr Ophthalmol Strabismus , 1981;18:28.
5. Krzystkowa K. The surgery of oculomotor muscles. in: Orłowski W (ed.): Modern ophthalmology. PZWL, 1992;3:550-80.
6. Pratt-Johnson JA, Barlow JM, and Tillson G: Early surgery in intermittent exotropia. Am J Ophthalmol 1977;84:689.
7. Scott WE, Keech R, and Mash J: The postoperative results and stability of exodeviations. Arch Ophthalmol 1981;99: 1814.
8. von Noorden GK. Exodeviations. In: von Noorden GK, Campos EC, (Eds): Binocular Vision and Ocular Motility: Theory and Management of Strabismus. 6th ed. St Louis: Mosby; 2002; 356-76.
9. von Noorden GK: Resection of both medial rectus muscles in organic convergence insufficiency. Am J Ophthalmol 1976; 81:223.
10. Wright KW. Exotropia. In: Wright KW, (Ed): Pediatric Ophthalmology and Strabismus. St. Louis: Mosby; 1995;39: 195-202.
11. Wright KW, Bruce-Lyle L. Augmented surgery for esotropia associated with high hypermetropia. J Pediatr Ophthalmol Strabismus, 1993;30:167-70.
12. Wright KW, Edelman PM, Terry A, et al: High grade stereo acuity after early surgery for congenital esotropia. Arch Ophthalmol, 1994;112:913-19.

Rectus Muscles Weakening Surgery

Ewa Oleszczynska Prost (Poland)

Surgery to the horizontal rectus muscles, in the form of weakening, is commonly performed for esotropia – medial rectus muscle and exotropia – lateral rectus muscle. Surgery to the vertical rectus muscles in hypetropia or hypotropia is less commonly performed, but is basically similar to horizontal rectus muscle surgery.

The operation begins with the incision of the conjunctiva. There are two types of incisions:

1. Limbal incision (Figs 1A and 1B).
2. Fornix incision (Figs 2A and 2B).

Procedures that weaken muscle actions involve:

- Rectus muscle recession (Figs 3A to 3G).
- Hang-Back technique recession (Figs 4A to 4H)
- Elongation of the muscle
  1. Incision of the muscle part (myotomy) (Fig. 5A).
  2. Excision of the muscle part (myectomy) (Fig. 5B).

Each patient requires an individual surgical approach to the management of their squint.

RECTUS MUSCLES RECESSION

Indications

- Standard procedure for weakening medial rectus in esotropia unilateral or bilateral.
- Standard procedure for weakening lateral rectus in exotropia unilateral or bilateral.

SURGICAL TECHNIQUE

See Figures 3A to 3G.

HANG-BACK TECHNIQUE OF RECESSION

Indications

- Weakening rectus muscle in case of the difficult access:
  - in the young baby
  - if very large recession is required.
- High risk of perforation during suturing:
  - very thin sclera
  - inexperienced surgeon.
- Use of adjustable sutures.

SURGICAL TECHNIQUE

See Figures 4A to 4H

ELONGATION OF THE MUSCLE

Elongation of the rectus muscle comprises cutting tendinous part or muscle body to elongate it and in consequence weaken muscle actions. There are two ways of performing surgery:

1. Incision of the muscle part (myotomia) (Fig. 5A).
2. Excision of the muscle part (myectomy) (Fig. 5B).

Indications

- Additional weakening of the rectus muscle:
  - reoperation after recession of the rectus muscle
  - weakening of secondary contracted muscle in paretic squint
  - minimal surgical intervention is required on previously operated globe, following retinal ablation, ocular trauma, high myopia or other weakening of eyeball walls.
- Surgery to the rectus muscles is infrequent, whereas elongation of both superior and inferior oblique muscles is made frequently.

SURGICAL TECHNIQUE

See Figures 5A and 5B

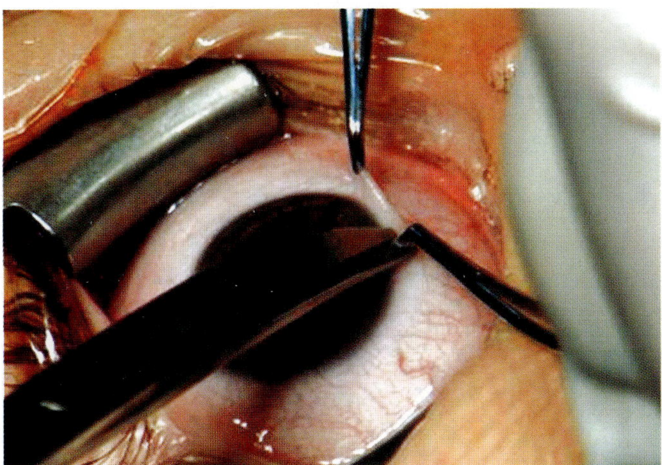

Fig. 1A: The conjunctiva is incised. Approach to medial rectus with relieving incision radially and 100° limbal peritomy

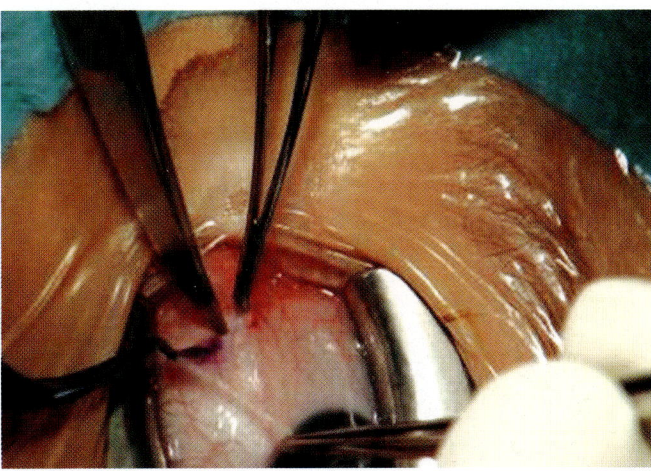

Fig. 2B: The fornix incision made by cutting straight down through the conjunctiva in the white zone

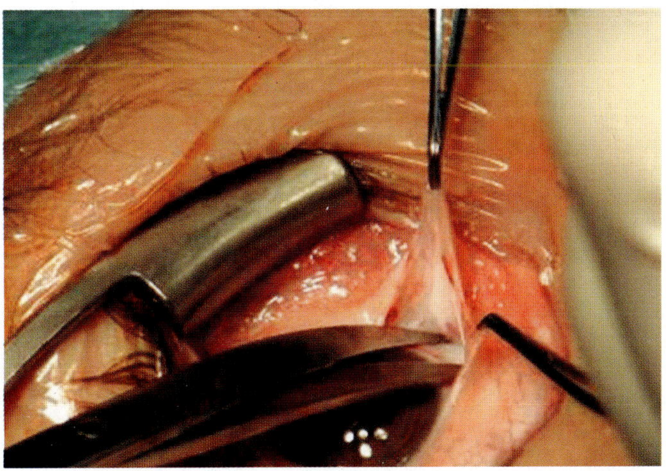

Fig. 1B: The subconjunctival space is dissected down on either side of the muscle.Tenon's capsule is cleaned from the muscle

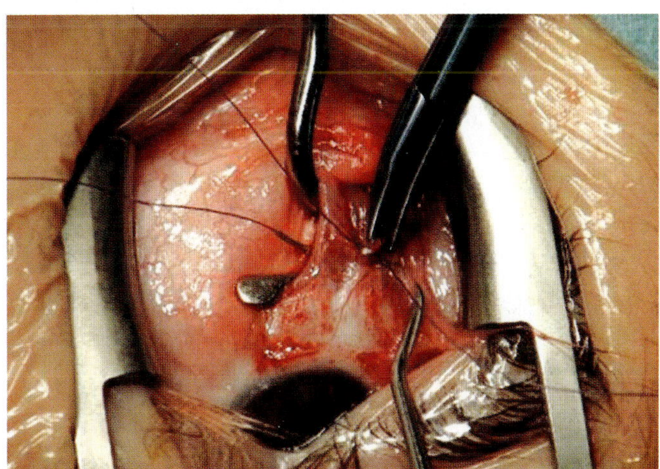

Fig. 3A: The squint hook lifts the muscle away from the globe

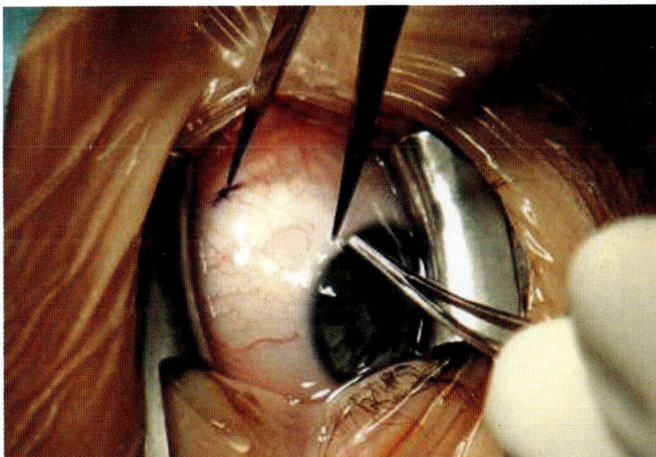

Fig. 2A: The fornix incision after measurement approximately 8 mm posterior to the limbus

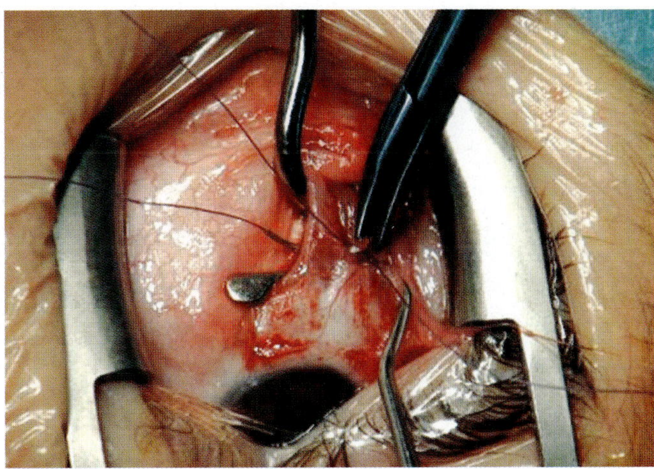

Fig. 3B: Two sutures are passed peripheral 1/3rds of the muscle width

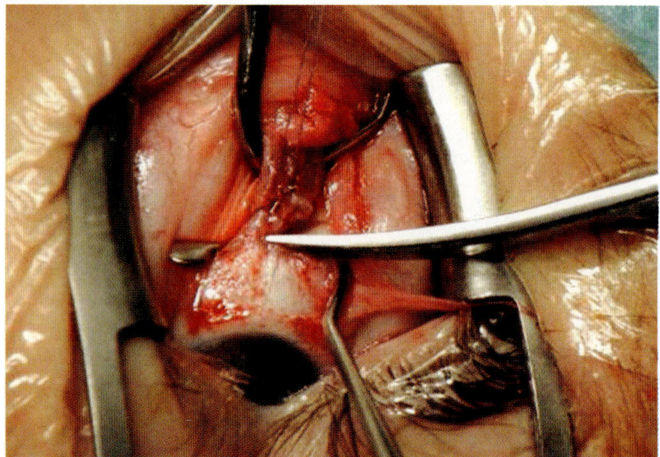

Fig. 3C: Removal of rectus muscle from the globe

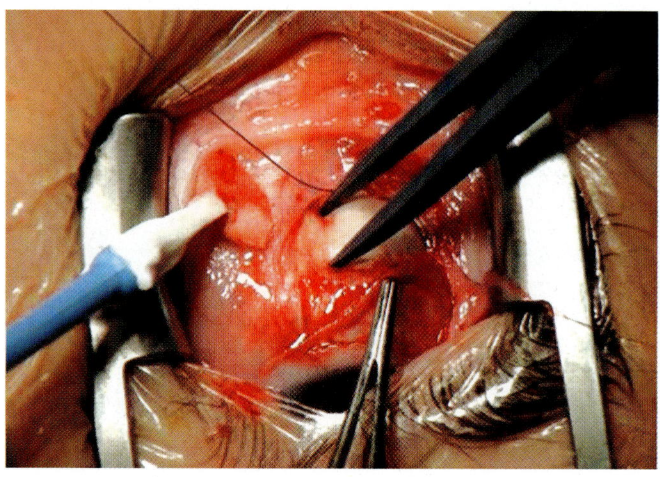

Fig. 3D: The distance of the muscle has to be recessed is measured by calipers

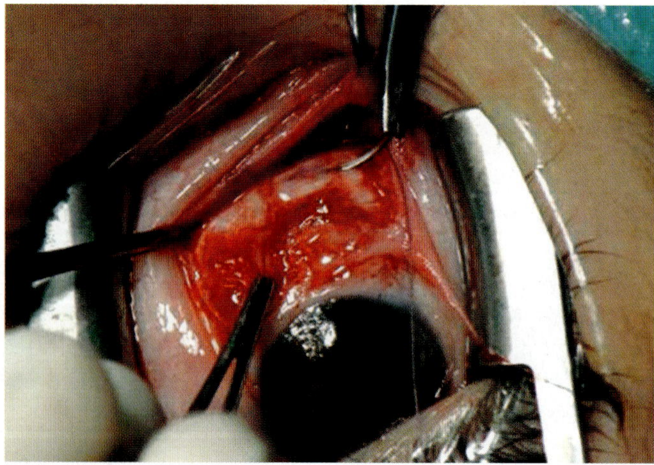

Fig. 3E: The first needle of the double-armed suture is placed through the sclera, parallel to the orginal insertion

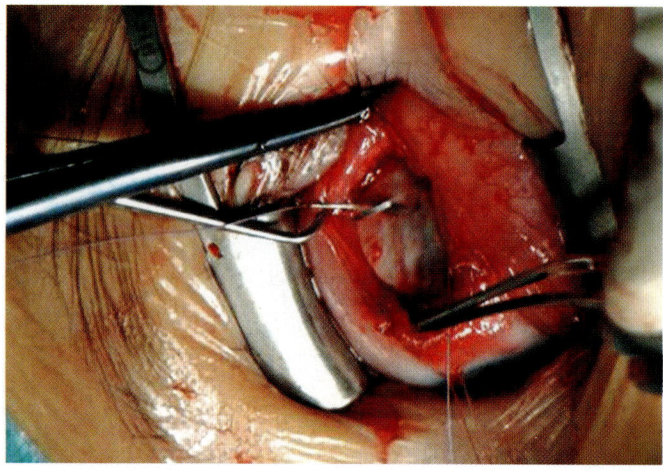

Fig. 3F: The second arm of double-armed suture is placed in similar fashion

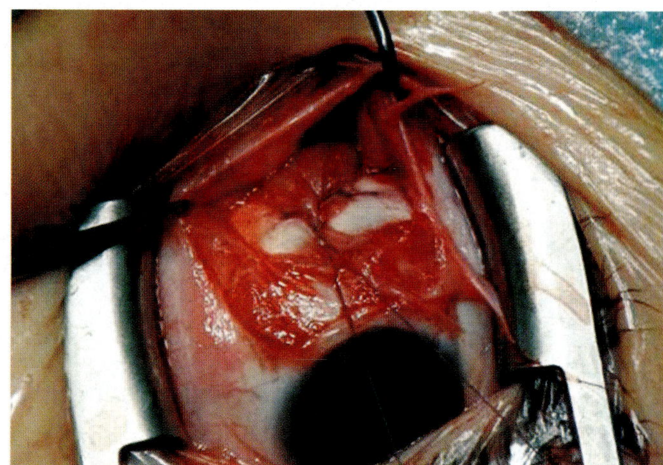

Fig. 3G: The muscle is pulled fully to the desired recession site and sutures are tightened, tied, and cut

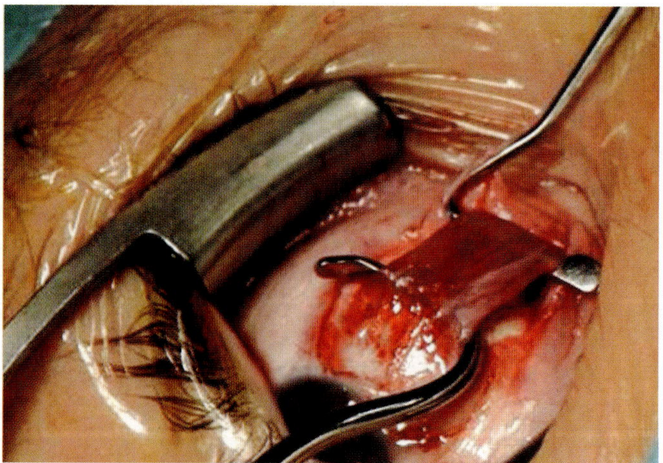

Fig. 4A: Two hooks are placed to spread the muscle

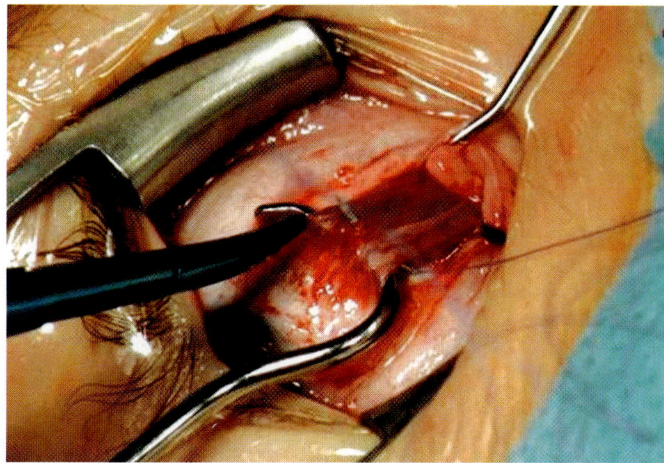

Fig. 4B: A 6/0 absorbable suture is placed in the middle of the tendon to the margin, parallel to the insertion

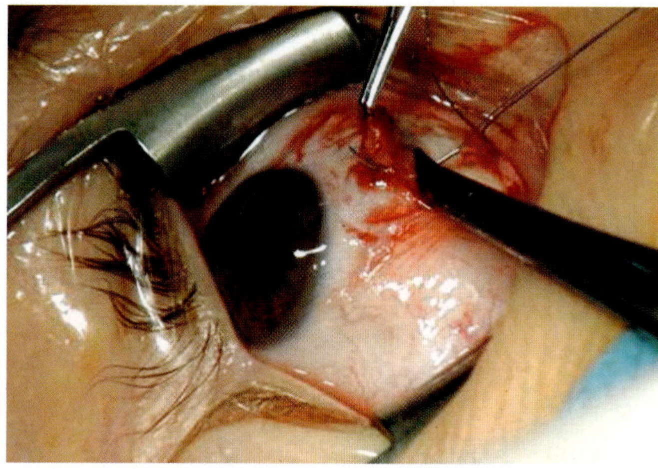

Fig. 4E: After disinserting the muscle from the sclera, suture should be passed from posterior to anterior through center of the insertion

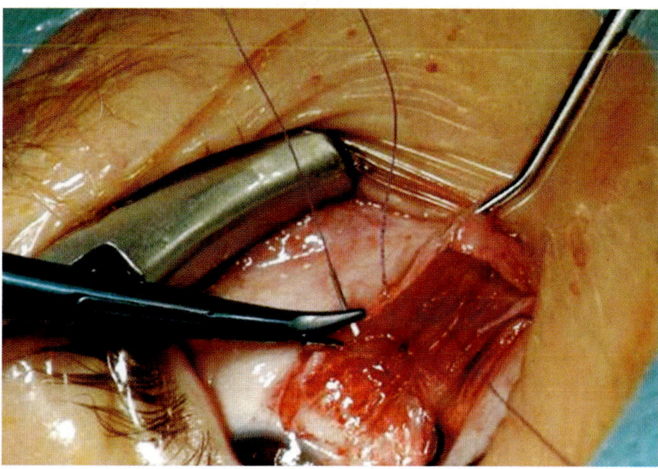

Fig. 4C: A lock bite is performed at the margin of the muscle

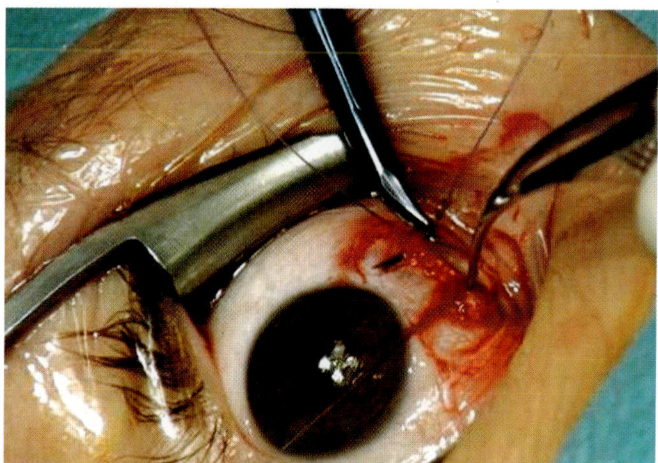

Fig. 4F: The second suture is placed similarly to the first one

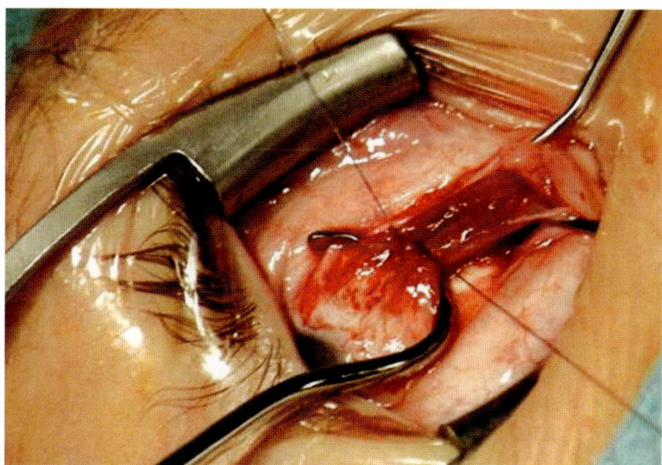

Fig. 4D: Following a double bite, this suture should be locked with one throw.

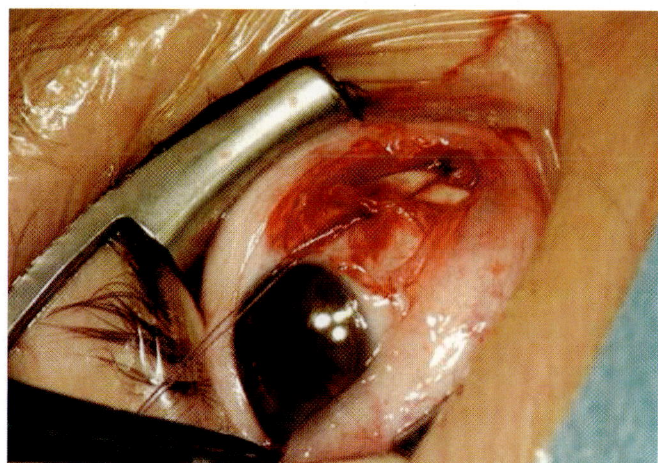

Fig. 4G: The muscle is advanced to the required recession and the suture is tied

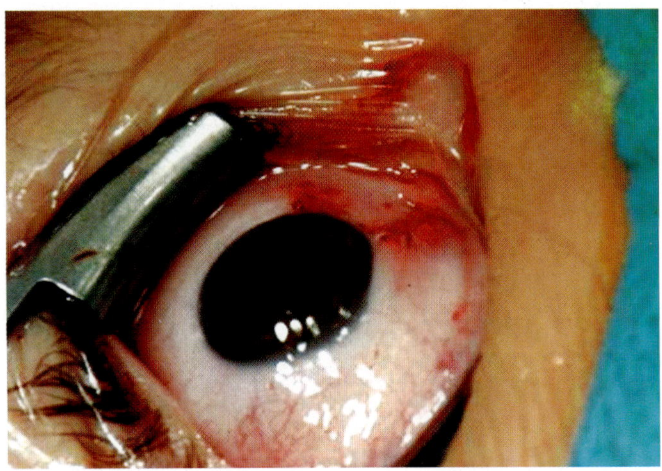

Fig. 4H: The conjunctiva is closed with single 8/0 sutures

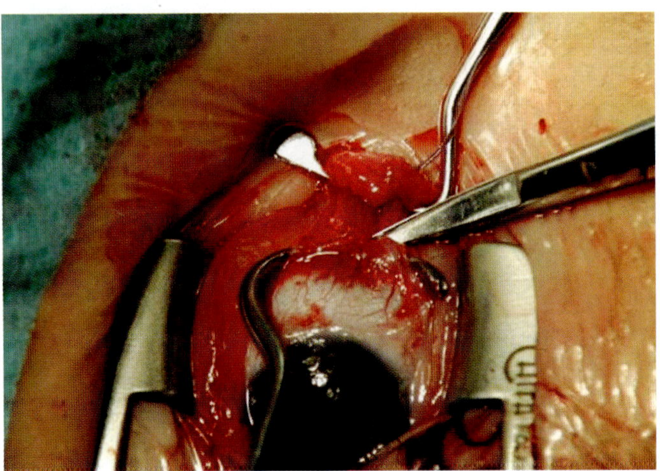

Fig. 5A: Myotomy of medial rectus muscle in the left eye

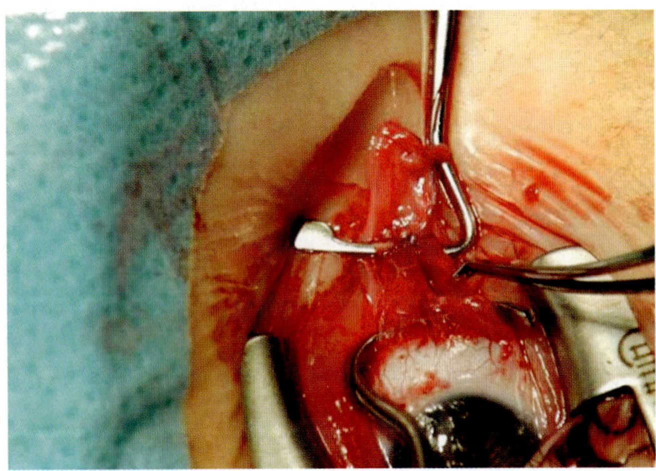

Fig. 5B: Myectomy of the medial rectus muscle

BIBLIOGRAPHY

1. Biedner B, Marcus M, David R, Yassur Y. Congenital con-stant exotropia: surgical results in six patients. Binocul Vis Eye Muscle Surg Q 1993;8:137-40.
2. Biglan AW, Davis JS, Cheng KP, Pettapiece MC. Infantile exotropia. J Pediatr Ophthalmol Strabismus 1996;33(2):79-84.
3. Biglan AW. Early surgery of infantile exotropia. Trans Pac Acad Ophthalmol Otolaryngol 1983;36:161.
4. Diamond GR. Strabismus. In: Ophthalmology, Mosby St.Louis 2004:549-634.
5. Gunter K, Von Noorden GK, Wong SY. Surgical results in nystagmus blockage syndrome. Ophthalmology 1986;93: 1028-32.
6. Hardesty H. Management of intermittent exotropia. BinocVis Quart 1990,5:145.
7. Hermann JS. Surgical therapy for convergence insufficiency. J Pediatr Ophthalmol Strabismus 1981;18:28.
8. Hiles DA, Watson A, Biglan AW. Characteristics of infantile esotropia following early bimedial rectus recession. Arch Ophthalmol 1980;98:697-703.
9. Jampolsky A. Ocular Deviations. Int Ophthalmol Clin 1964; 4:567-701.
10. Krzystkowa K. The surgery of oculomotor muscles. In: Or»owski W (Ed.): Modern Ophthalmology, PZWL, Warsaw 1992;3:550-80.
11. MacEwen C, Gregson R. Manual of etrabismus surgery. Blutterworth - Heinemann, Edinburg 2003.
12. Oleszczyñska-Prost E. Concomitant strabismus. In: Garg A, Prost M. (Eds:) Surgical and Medical Management of Pediatric ophthalmology. Jaypee Brothers Medical Publishers, New Delhi 2007:753-91.
13. Oleszczyñska-Prost E. Concomitant strabismus. In: Pediatric ophthalmology PZWL,Warsaw 1998:31-56.
14. Pickering IB, Simon JW, Ratliff CD, et al. Alignment success following medial rectus recessions in normal and delayed children. Pediatr Ophthalmol Strabismus 1995;32:225-7.
15. Prieto-Diaz J. Large bilateral medial rectus recession in early esotropia with bilateral limitation of abduction. J Pediatr Ophthalmol Strabismus 1980,17:101-5.
16. Raab EL, Parks MM: Recession of the lateral recti: Early and late postoperative alignments. Arch Ophthalmol 1969;82:203.
17. von Noorden GK. Divergence excess and simulated divergence excess. Diagnosis and surgical management. Ophthalmologica 1969;26:719.
18. von Noorden GK. Resection of both medial rectus muscles in organic convergence insufficiency. Am J Ophthalmol 1976;81:223-5.
19. Williams F, Beneish R, Polomeno RC, Little JM. Congenital exotropia. Am Orthopt J 1984;34:92-4.
20. Wright KW, Bruce-Lyle L. Augmented surgery for esotropia associated with high hypermetropia. J Pediatr Ophthalmol Strabismus 1993;30:167-70.
21. Wright KW:Strabismus and amblyopia In: Wright KW: (Ed): Pediatric Ophthalmology and Strabismus, Mosby, St. louis 1995;89-209.
22. Zak TA , Morin JD. Early surgery for infantile esotropia: Results and influence of age upon results. Can J Ophthalmol 1982; 17:213-8.

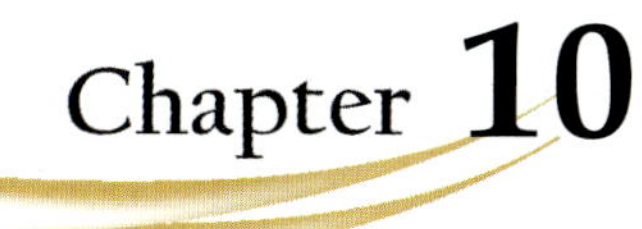

Chapter 10

Concomitant Strabismus

Ewa Oleszczynska Prost (Poland)

Strabismus is a disease characterized by the eyes misalignment. It may be present constantly or intermittently, and may appear at near or distant vision. Strabismus is present in 2 to 5% of children, being an important cause of both visual and psychological problems. Strabismus may be congenital or acquired abnormality. One should remember that:

- Children do not outgrow strabismus.
- Treatment should be started immediately after detection of this abnormality as child's age plays crucial role in the development of the normal binocular vision.
- Alignment of the eyes is possible in any age of the child and contributes to vision improvement.
- Treatment of strabismus is both non-surgical and surgical.

ANATOMY AND PHYSIOLOGY

Anatomy of the Extraocular Muscles

Movement of each eye is controlled by six extraocular muscles. Four of them are rectus muscles: medial, lateral, inferior, and superior muscles. Two muscles are oblique: inferior and superior muscles. All these muscles originate at the posterior segment of the orbit, i.e. common ring tendon, except inferior oblique muscle, which originates from the nasolacrimal groove in the anterior segment of the orbital inferior wall, run divergently forward, and insert onto the eyeball, becoming tendinous. Rectus muscles insert in the front of eyeball equator, whereas oblique muscle insert behind it (Fig. 1).

Extraocular muscles are built from the stratial muscular fibers, similarly to skeletal muscles. However, they contain large amounts of connective tissue, are rich in blood vessels and both nervous fibers, and endings.

Extraocular muscles are innervated by three cranial nerves:

1. Oculomotor nerve (III cranial nerve) innervating the medial, superior, and inferior rectus muscles, and the inferior oblique muscle.
2. Abducens nerve (VI cranial nerve) innervating the lateral rectus muscle.
3. Trochlear nerve (IV cranial nerve) innervating the superior oblique muscle.

Ocular artery branches (anterior ciliary arteries) and lacrimal artery are supplying the blood. Blood outflows through the superior and inferior ophthalmic veins.

Rectus Muscles

Medial Rectus Muscle

It is the thickest and strongest extraocular muscle. Its tendon is short, about 4 mm long and 10.9 mm wide at the point of insertion onto the eyeball. Contraction of this muscle produces rotation of the eyeball medially, i.e. its adduction.

Lateral Rectus Muscle

It has long and thin tendon: about 8 mm long and about 9, 8 mm at the point of insertion onto the eyeball. Its contraction produces lateral rotation of the eyeball, i.e. its abduction.

Superior Rectus Muscle

It runs above the eyeball together with the levator muscle of upper eyelid and is tightly connected with this muscle by fascia. The superior rectus muscle is about 41.8 mm long, its tendon is about 5 mm long and about 11 mm wide at the point of insertion onto the eyeball. This muscle is the major elevator of the eye, therefore, its actions are: supraduction, adduction and intortion. Maximum elevation is seen when the eyeball is adducted by 23° (Fig. 2).

Inferior Rectus Muscle

Its tendon is about 5.6 mm long and about 10 mm wide at the point of insertion onto the eyeball. This muscle depresses, adducts, and excyclotorts the eyeball. Maximum depression of the globe is seen, when the eyeball is abducted by 23°.

Oblique Muscles

Superior Oblique Muscle

It is the longest extraocular muscle. It originates on the body of sphenoid bone and runs forward, passing to the trochlea attached to the nasal side of the superior orbital rim. Next it passes under the superior rectus muscle and inserts into the sclera behind the equator of the eyeball. It is about 60 mm long. Its insertion is of variable wideness. The major action of the superior oblique muscle is incycloduction but also depression, and abduction of the eyeball. Maximum action is seen, when the eyeball is adducted by 51°.

Inferior Oblique Muscle

It runs from the nasolacrimal groove in the inferior segment of the orbit backwards and toward the temple under the inferior rectus muscle and inserts onto the eyeball below the oblique rectus muscle. Its posterior insertion is adjacent to the macula: about 2 mm towards and 1 mm below the macula. It is 37 mm long and its insertion is 5 mm to 13 mm wide. This muscle has the longest and best developed suspensory ligament of the eyeball (Lockwood suspensory ligament). Contraction of the inferior oblique muscle excycloducts, elevates, and abducts the eyeball.

Detailed anatomy of the extraocular muscles insertions onto the eyeball surface around the corneal limbus is shown in Figure 3. Relationship between rectus muscles, obliques muscles, vortex veins and macula is seen in Figure 4.

LAWS OF THE EYEBALLS MOTILITY

The eyeball supported by the fascia and ligaments moves around three axes, called Fick axes (Fig. 5).These are the axes passing through the eyeball rotation point:

- vertical axis (Z): around it abduction and adduction are realized;
- horizontal axis (X): around it sursumduction and deorsumduction are realized;
- anterior-posterior axis (Y): determining rotational movements: intorsion and extorsion.

All position of gaze can be achieved by rotations around axes that lie on Listing's plane: O-axis is present between z-axis and x-axis of Fick, which allows oblique eye rotation. (Fig. 6)

Monocular movements are called ductions.

Binocular movements are called:

- versions, when both eyes rotate in the same direction at the same time
- vergence, when both eyes rotate in the opposite direction.

Each extraocular muscle has its synergistic muscle (acting in the same direction) and antagonist (acting in the opposite direction). It concerns the muscles of one eye (homolateral synergistic or antagonistic muscle) or both eyes (heterolateral synergistic or antagonistic muscle).

Extraocular muscles responsible for the eyeballs movements are subject of two laws.

Sherrington's Law

Contraction of one muscle produces relaxation of its antagonistic muscle.

Hering's Law

For movements of both eyes in any direction, the same and simultaneous nervous stimuli are transferred from the oculomotor centers to the corresponding muscles of both eyes participating in the rotation of the eyeballs to the said direction. Level of the impulse is the same for the right and left eye. Therefore, appropriate synergistic and antagonistic muscles of one eye (homolateral) and fellow eye (heterolateral) are cooperating. Six pairs of muscles responsible for the eyeballs movements during binocular vision are formed (Fig. 7)

BINOCULAR ROTATIONS

Versions

Binocular versions may be divided into the primary sight position and the secondary, tertiary, and torsional rotations. During the binocular movement from the primary to the secondary position the following muscles are involved:

- dextroversion: the right lateral rectus and the left medial rectus muscles;
- levoversion: the right medial rectus and the left lateral rectus muscles;
- supraversion: the right superior rectus and the left superior rectus muscles;

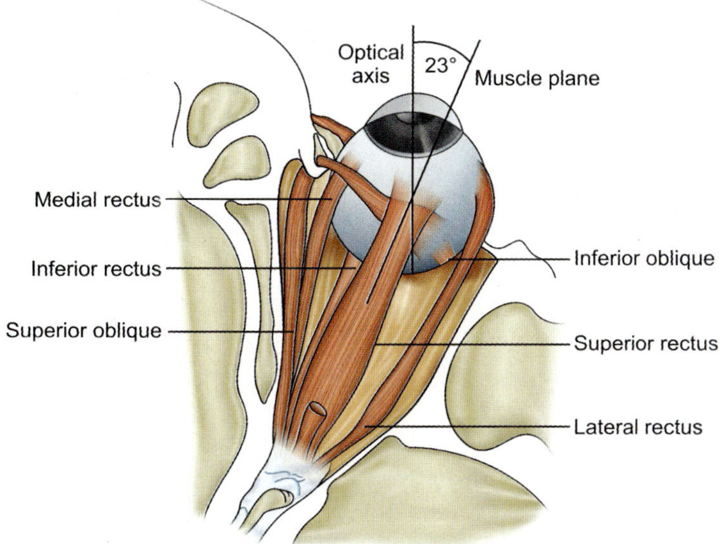

Fig. 1: Top view of the eye and muscles in primary position

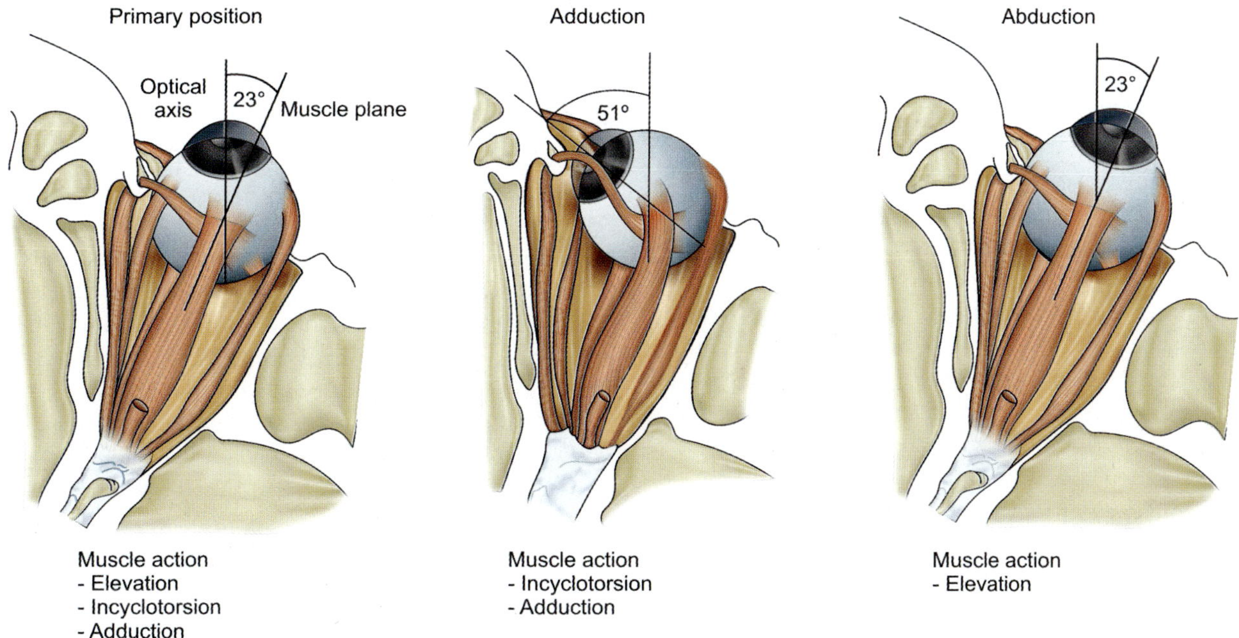

Fig. 2: The actions of the superior rectus muscle

- infraversion: the right inferior and the left inferior rectus muscles.

During the movement of both eyes from the primary to the tertiary position the following synergistic muscles are involved:

- dextrasupraversion: the right superior rectus and the left inferior oblique muscles;
- levosupraversion: the right inferior oblique and the left superior rectus muscles;
- dextroinfraversion: the right inferior rectus and the left superior oblique muscles;
- levoinfraversion: the right superior oblique and the left inferior rectus muscles.

Binocular torsional rotation is called: cycloversions, when both eyes rotate excyclotorsionally or incyclotorsionally in regard to Y Fick's axis. Torsional rotation may be assessed during the cornea observation.

Vergences

Convergence is a symmetrical, horizontal convergent movement of the eyeballs, leading to the binocular fixation on the viewing subject. Convergence movement may be conditioned reflex, but in fact it is a reflex related to accommodation and pupillary stenosis.

Strength of the total convergence is measured by the determination of the proximal convergence point. Normal value of this point is about 4 cm to 6 cm in children. In this case the crucial role is played by accommodation. Normal rate between accommodation and convergence is quantitatively determined by the accommodation convergence (AC) to accommodation (A) ratio, called AC/A ratio. High AC/A ratio means excessive convergence, predisposing the patient to near sight esotropy development. Low AC/A ratio produces convergence insufficiency, causing near sight exotropy. The normal AC/A ratio is between 4PD to 6PD of convergence for every diopter accommodation.

The range of the total convergence includes:

1. Tonic convergence, dependent on the rest ocular muscle tone at distant sight.
2. Accommodative convergence responsible for binocular fixation of the viewed object.
3. Fusional convergence, i.e. optometric reflex leading to the fusion of the binocular images, due to the bitemporal disparation of the retinal images.
4. Psychological convergence determined by the cognition of near fixation point.
5. Spontaneous convergence stimulated by the near-positioned objects.

Divergence means moving apart anterior poles of both eyes. It depends on the fusion range and is produced by the disparation of the nasal retinal images. Divergence may be caused also by the inhibition of convergence tonus or wide interpupillary distance.

Reflex Eyeballs Movements

Normal position and rotation of the eyes are also dependent on voluntary eyeball rotations. They are modified by the appropriate spatial position of the head assuring proper alignment.

Optometric Reflexes

They develop, when the eyes turn toward the object attracting our attention (tracing reflex). Marked difference between the visual acuity of the macula and peripheral retina is a mechanism, which automatically directs the eye to the fixation object (fixation reflex). Then, fusion reflex starts to act, leading to the single binocular vision. It might be said that it is a factor supervising all other ocular reflexes. Convergence reflex enables combination of both fixation and fusion reflexes, while bringing near the fixed object the eyes converge as long as the image is fixed on the foveas.

Postural Eyeball Reflexes

Postural eyeball reflexes are influenced by several complex factors, in which vision does not play any important role. Reflexes from the labyrinth of the ear and neck muscles have been studied in detail. Magnus divided them into static and static-kinetic reflexes. The former are gravitational body reaction at rest, while the latter are related to the body movements and caused by an acceleration or deceleration. Main role is played by both labyrinths receiving these changes and producing reflex nervous activity, leading to the changes in the whole body musculature. Tonic stimuli are transferred to the ocular muscles. This reflex mechanism aims at maintaining the eyes in the initial position despite head movements (the doll's head maneuver).

Optokinetic Nystagmus

Nystagmus with both rapid and slow phases may be artificially produced, when fixation reflex is developed. It is physiological and reflex phenomenon. There are diseases in which such a nystagmus cannot be evoked. Nystagmus can be assessed with the aid of special cylinder

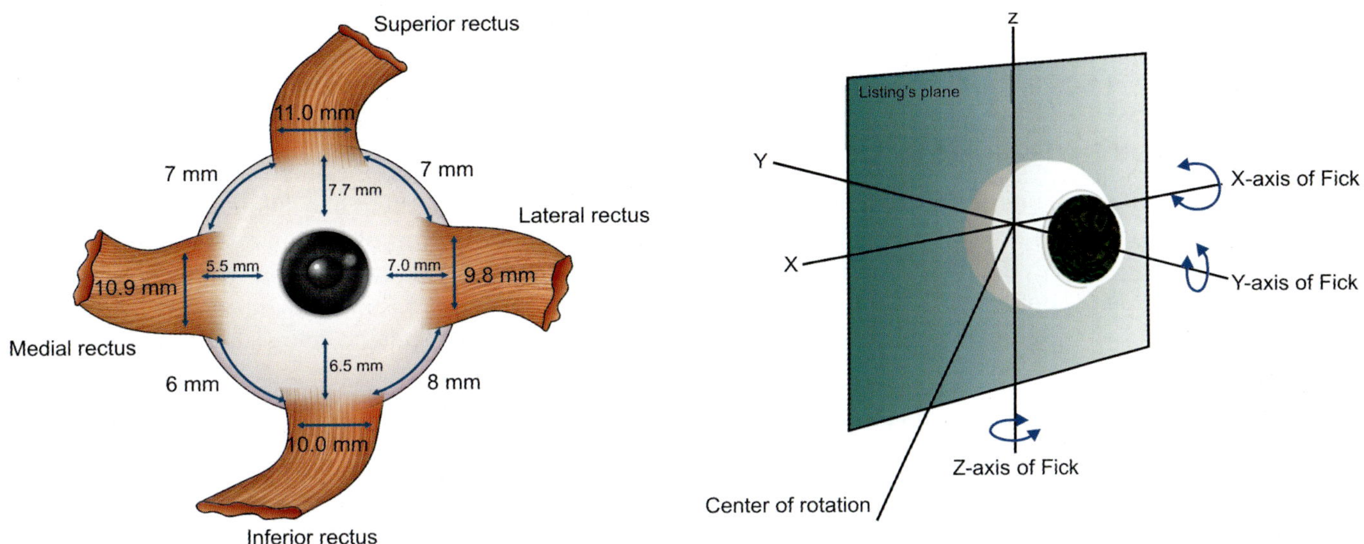

Fig. 3: The rectus muscle insertions around the limbus

Fig. 5: The axes of Fick

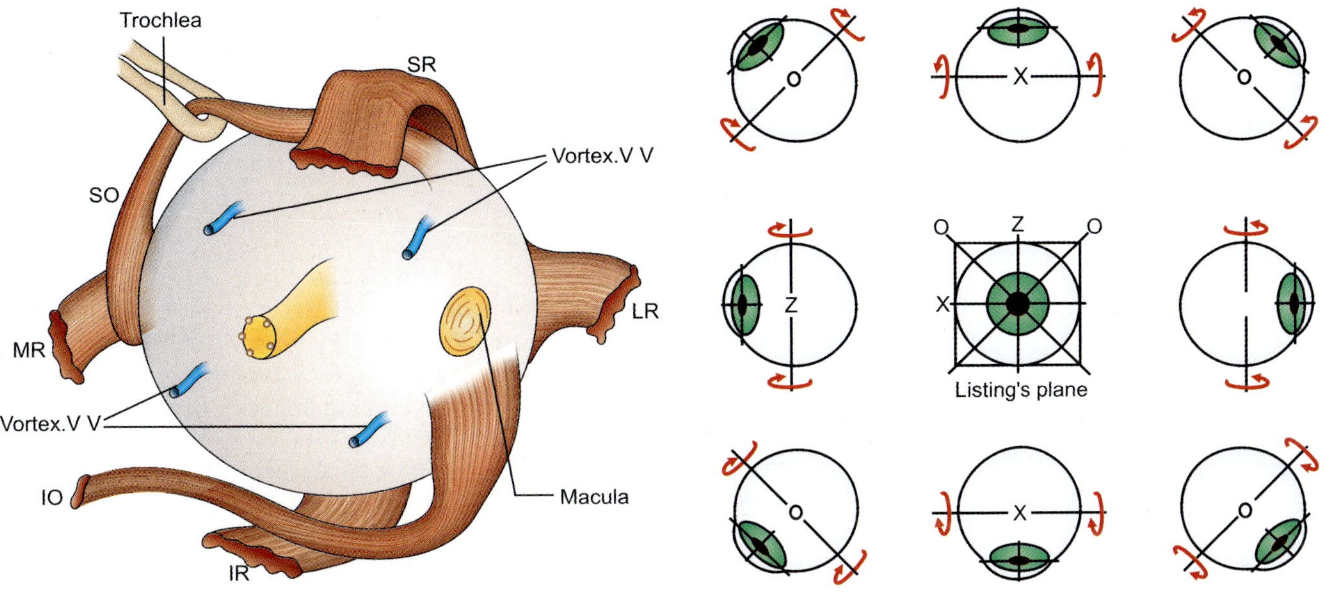

Fig. 4: Posterior anatomy of the eye and muscles

Fig. 6: Listing's plane

covered with black-and-white vertical strips. Under normal viewing condition we may also see accommodative nystagmus (at viewing rapidly moving objects) and latent nystagmus (which may appear with covering one eye).

BINOCULAR VISION PHYSIOLOGY

Binocular vision is the most perfect function of the vision. It is a physiological process involving an integration of retinal image from two eyes into the single three-dimensional visual perception.

Visual Development

Development of binocular vision starts at the child birth. Both photoreceptor organ of the eye and vision are changing. In children, size and shape of the eyeball differ from the adult eye. Retina and its nervous elements, especially cones in the macular area, are not fully developed. Peripheral temporal segments of the retina also develop. Development is very rapid: inner retinal layers are shifted more peripherally and sensory cells (rods and cones) become elongated, thinner, and denser. Myelination of the optic nerve is also not completed. Crossed nervous pathways maturate earlier than non-crossed ones. These time, visual centers in the brain, such as lateral geniculate bodies and striated visual cortex (17 and 18 visual fields of the occipital lobe, according to Brodman) are also differentiating. Development of vision is very rapid during the first week of life.

By 4 to 6 weeks, central foveal fixation is established along with accurate smooth pursuit. By 6 weeks of age, smooth pursuit and reproducible responses to optokinetic stimuli are seen. The first 2 - 3 months of life are the period of very intensive development of vision, when foveal fixation reflex with straight localization are completely developed. It is assumed that the most important time of vision development is the period between 6 and 10 weeks of age, when infant comes to the visual contact with the mother for the first time; responding with smile to the smile. That time, the eyes are in the primary straight position. Many investigators, using visual evoked potential, have found 6/60 visual acuity in term newborns but only 6/120, when optokinetic nystagmus has been used. Visual acuity of 6/6 may be demonstrated by 6 - 12 months of age (visual evoked potential), by 26 - 30 months (optokinetic nystagmus), and by 18 - 24 months (preferential looking). Binocular vision development occurs together with improving vision acuity.Convergence and fusion may be seen by 2-3 months of life. The development of stereopsis improves gradually from 3-6 month of age.

BINOCULAR VISION

Binocular vision is a coordinated action of both eyes, leading to the achievement of a single visual image with depth perception (stereopsis). Light rays, coming from the external objects, after passing through the cornea, lens and vitreous, reach the retina and form the image. The retina is a complex nervous system being able to change light stimulus into the nerve signal and to transfer it by the optic nerve and visual pathways to the cerebral cortex of the occipital lobe (fields 17 and 18, according to Brodman). There, an analysis and acknowledgment of the said object features take place, i.e. proper vision (Fig. 8).

Photosensitive elements (photoreceptors: rods and cones) are not uniformly distributed in the retina. Cones controlling vision at day light and color perception are mostly localized in the macula, mainly in the fovea. Anatomically and functionally the macula significantly prevails over the rest of retina. Stereoscopic model of the visual field examined quantitatively with Goldman perimeter shows these relations (Fig. 9). Foveal vision prevails in the form of the high peak over the rest of the visual field. Visual acuity decreases gradually toward the peripheral retina. Retinal sensitivity is presented in the form of circular isopters, connecting points of equal visual acuity, forming slanting planes.

Fixation reflex is directly connected with the fovea Phylogenetically coded reflex in every healthy individual is the fixation of fovea on the object of the interest. It is called central fixation connected with this object position straight ahead. One or both eyes may fix simultaneously. Binocular vision is created with binocular fixation. Capability to see two different images formed on the retina of one eye is the I degree of the binocular vision, called simultaneous perception. Fusion of one stereoscopic image from the 2 images seen simultaneously by two eyes is the II degree of the binocular vision. It is the central process, dependent on the cerebral cortex. Convergence movement produced by the binocular fixation stimulates the fusion. Its degree depends also on attention, fatigue, and age of the examined individual, accommodation tone, exercises, and fusion images size. Fusion is assessed by the measurement of fusional movements of the eyes, it is so-called fusion vergence amplitudes.

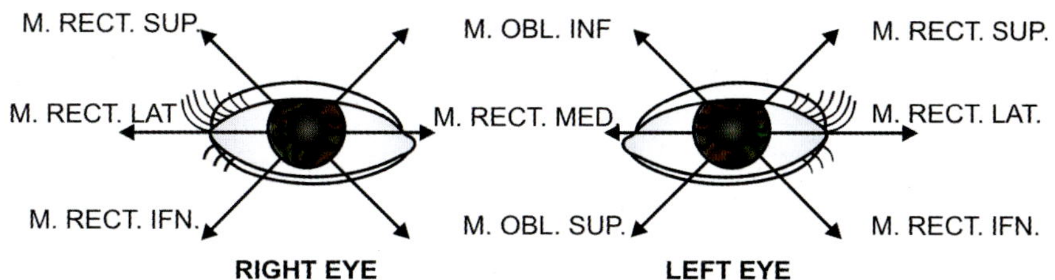

Fig. 7: Movements of six pairs of the eyes muscles. Vector indicates the direction of movement

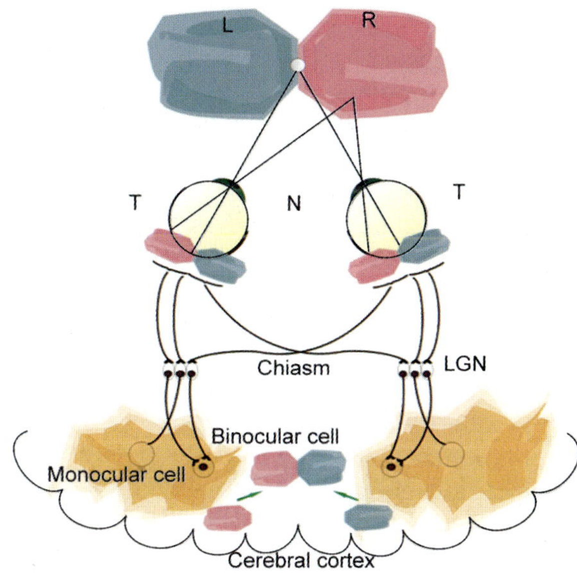

Fig. 8: Demonstration of the afferent visual pathways. Nasal retinal images cross by the chiasm to the contralateral lateral geniculate nucleus (LGN). Temporal retinal images project to the ipsilateral LGN

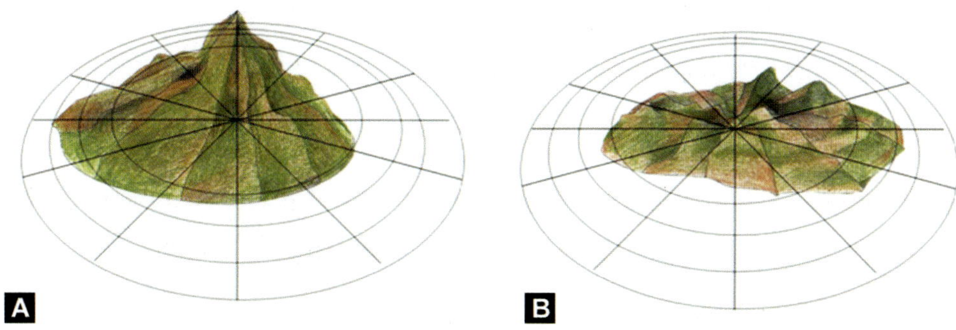

Fig. 9: Stereoscopic models of the visual field. A-normal eye with the high peak on the region of fovea. B-amblyopic eye with the depth depression on the region of fovea

Normal fusion vergence amplitudes is:

	Distance (6 meters)	Near (1/3 meter)
Convergence	18-22 PD	30-38 PD
Divergence	6-8 PD	10-16 PD
Vertical vergence	2-3 PD	2-3 PD

Fusion is possible only when the corresponding retinal points are stimulated. In 2 eyes there are pairs of the similar retinal points distant in the same direction. Stimulation of these corresponding retinal points and the higher cortical cells produces visual impression localized in the same place in the space. Normal retinal correspondence is produced, and these points are called corresponding retinal points. Retinal points of different visual directions are called noncorresponding, or disparat retinal points.

The object with the image produced in these disparate points, is localized in two different visual directions and seen as being in two places. Images received by the corresponding retinal points are seen in one place. Geometric place of all points seen in one place is called empirical horopter. Points adjacent to the horopter are also seen in one place, despite the fact that they are received by the noncorresponding retinal points. The brain can combine and fuse images from corresponding and slightly noncorresponding retinal points. It is possible because in the front of and behind the empirical horopter there is small wedge-shaped area of the permissible tolerance, so-called Panum's fusional area (Fig. 10). If the images are outside empirical horopter but within Panum's fusional area, stereoscopic vision is produced (III degree of the binocular vision). Vision becomes the most precise when the three-dimensional perception is projected to binocular cortical cells in the striate cortex. Stereopsis is related to the binocular parallax. It depends of the fact that 2 eyes are at interpupillary distance and there are subtle differences between two images. Convergence and accommodation are necessary to the depth and distance perception, especially at near vision. Streoscopy is expressed in arc seconds. Under ideal conditions, foveal stereoacuity is 10 arc seconds. Stereoscopic depth perception is associated with foveal vision.

Good binocular vision acquired:
- Normal anatomy of two eyes and their position in the orbits.
- Properly corrected refractive errors
- Good vision in both eyes.
- Normal action of the extraocular muscles.
- Proper activity of the visual pathways responsible for the perceptive and transfer visual images to the visual cerebral cortex.
- Normal functioning of the cerebral cortex to receive, change and interpret visual impressions.

PATHOPHYSIOLOGY OF BINOCULAR VISION

Strabismus is an abnormality in which precise mechanism of the binocular vision, based on the normal retinal correspondence, is disturbed. Light stimuli reach noncorresponding retinal points in two eyes, mainly retinal fovea, producing **diplopia**. Different images are produced in the corresponding retinal points, leads to **visual confusion**. The body defends such a situation as it is completely unable spatial orientation.

Adaptation mechanism is produced which gradually leads to the abnormal forms of the binocular vision:
1. Inhibition of the cortical activity cortical suppression amblyopia.
2. Anomalous retinal correspondence (ARC).

Initially, **inhibition** is present, i.e. psychic exclusion of the visual impressions in the squint eye. If it is of transient character, only during binocular vision, it is called **suppression** (Fig. 11).

Typically it is present in the alternating squints, in the actually squinting eye and disappears, when this eye becomes fixing eye. In the monocular squint a constant suppression is present, which persists even after cessation of the inhibiting stimuli from the fellow eye. There is a status when **amblyopia** developed.

Its other name is **central scotoma**. It develops in the deviating eye foveal area, preventing visual confusion. Central scotoma is always larger during the binocular vision than during monocular vision. This syndrome is called monofixation and is present most frequently in anisometropia, strabismus of the small angle $< 4^{o}$ following earlier surgery of the congenital strabismus, and congenital monocular cataract. Characteristic is peripheral fusion without central fusion. Patients with monofixation syndrome usually have stereo acuity in the range between 3000 arc sec to 70 arc sec. If the viewing foveas alternate freely in the young children, amblyopia does not occur, even in patients who are free of strabismus.

Peripheral scotoma is present in both alternating and monocular squint fixation point, preventing diplopia. It is an area of depressed vision within the retina of the deviating eye corresponding to the fixating eye fovea. It is of suppression character and disappears under monocular viewing conditions. Scotomas are perfectly visualized on the stereoscopic models of the visual field in strabismus, produced by Wilczek on the specially designed scotometer. Significant disorders of the deviating eye visual field are

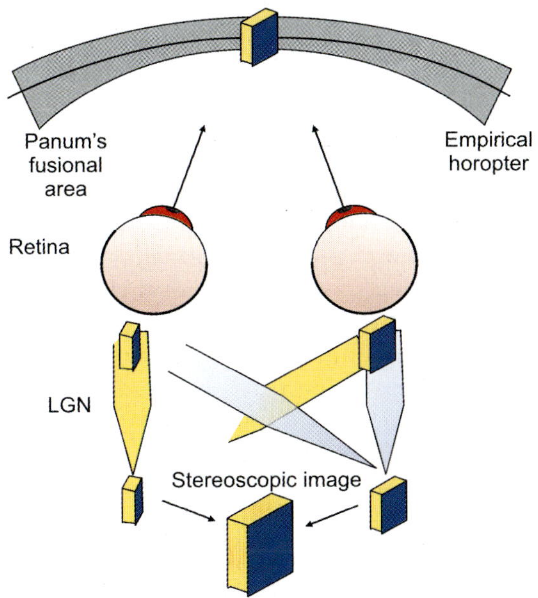

Fig. 10: Panum's fusional area. The target stimulates noncorresponding retinal points that provide stereoscopic vision

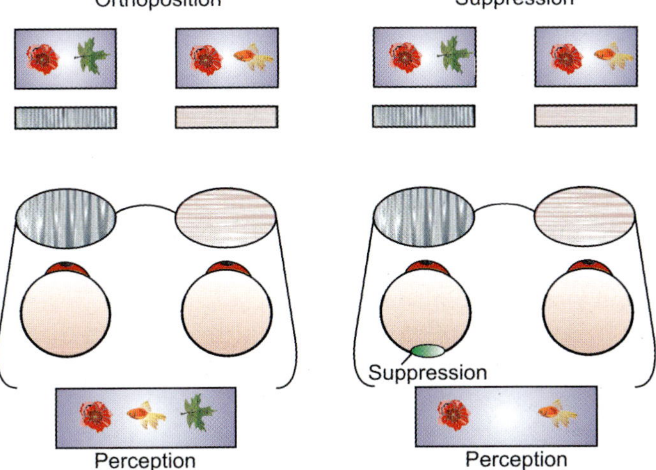

Fig. 11: Suppression test with polaroid glasses and pictures are projected to the two polarized screens oriented 90 degrees to each other

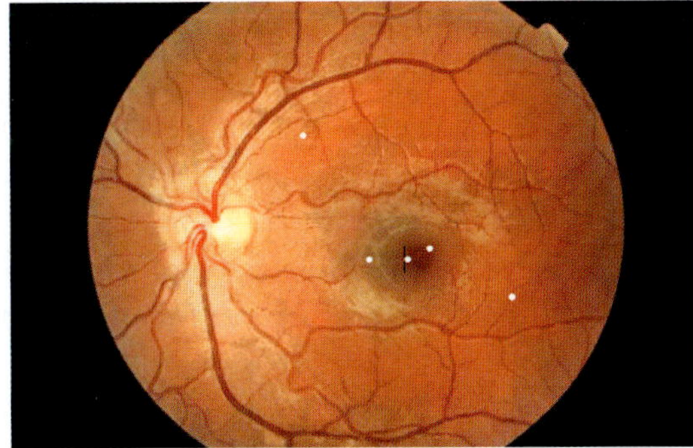

Fig. 12: Examination of one eye fixation. The star of visuscope is seen in the different place on the fundus, depends on type on fixation

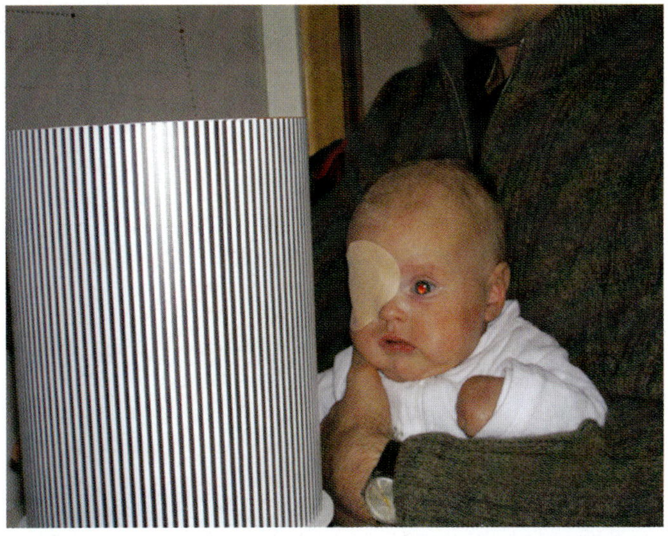

Fig. 13: Optokinetic Nystagmus examination of 3 months child

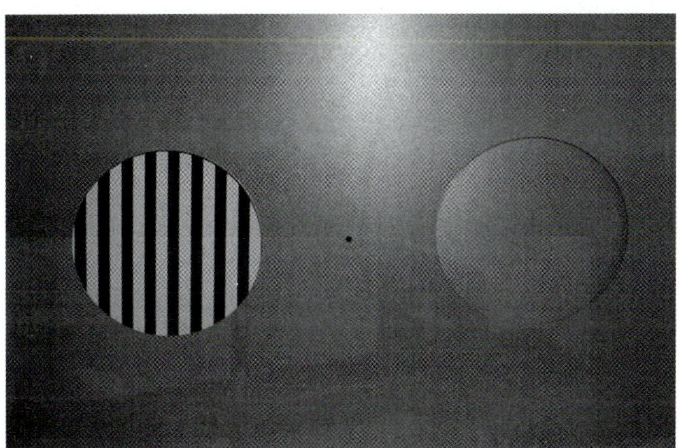

Fig. 14: Test setup for prefential looking using Teller acuity cards

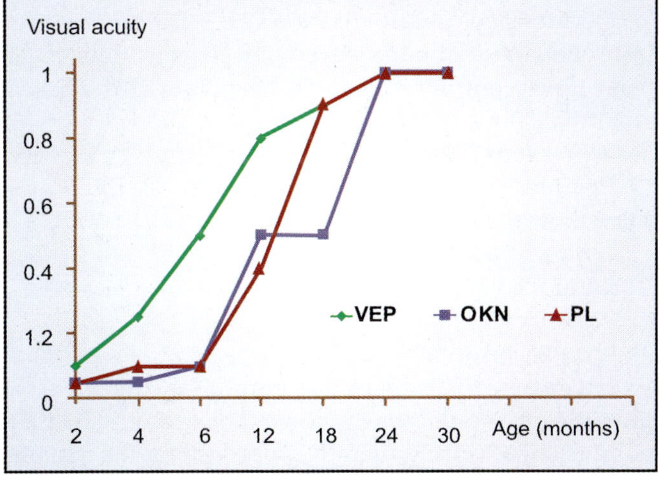

Fig. 15: Visual acuity estimates by test method of infant eyes

seen, mostly in the most valuable central and paracentral retina (Fig. 9).

Amblyopia

Amblyopia may refer to poor vision of any cause. It may be divided into two large groups:
- Functional amblyopia (amblyopia ex anopsia).
- Organic amblyopia.

Amblyopia may involve one or two eyes.
Organic amblyopia may be caused by the structural abnormalities in the eyeballs or the brain and should be distinguished from the functional amblyopia. Differentiation of the organic amblyopia and functional amblyopia is presented in Table I.

Table 1: Causes of functional and organic amblyopia

Functional amblyopia	*Organic amblyopia*
Anisometropia	Corneal opacity (Peter's opacity)
Bilateral high hypermetropia	Monocular and binocular cataract
Bilateral high myopia	Vitreous hemorrhage
Strabismic amblyopia	Vitreous opacity
	Optic nerve atrophy
	Macular scar
	Brain damage

The term amblyopia is generally reserved for the poor vision caused by abnormal visual development, secondary to abnormal visual stimulation. It is a process of image suppression in the deviating eye at the cerebral cortex level. Strabismic amblyopia is caused by the vision suppression in the foveal area in the absence of organic disease. Visual acuity is reduced to the different degree similarly to the contrast sensitivity. It is related to the poor fixation and abnormal localization straight ahead.

Deviating eye uses for fixation an eccentric retinal area instead of fovea. Abnormal eye-hand coordination results from the eccentric fixation. Hand points at the object abnormally localized by the eccentric fixation point. This has been showed in the studies conducted by Starkiewicz.

Retinal fixation is divided into (Bangerter's, Krzystkowa) (Fig. 12):
- central fixation,
- parafoveolar fixation,
- paramacular fixation,
- eccentric fixation.

Eccentric fixation is not stable, as the electrophysiological studies have shown. The eccentric fixation point changes during therapy, approaching the macula. Fixation reverts back to the true fovea, when one eye is covered. Aim of the treatment is to achieve the central fixation.

Anomalous Retinal Correspondence

Anomalous retinal correspondence (ARC) is present in both alternating and unilateral strabismus. Foveas of two eyes loose common visual direction and eccentric retinal point of the deviating eye (pseudo-fovea) corresponds with the fovea of the fellow eye. This is related also to the remaining corresponding points in the retina of two eyes.

Retinal correspondence may be divided into following groups:
1. Normal retinal correspondence.
2. Harmonious anomalous retinal correspondence.
3. Unharmonious anomalous retinal correspondence.
4. Lack of the retinal correspondence due to the complete image suppression in the deviating eye.

Harmonious ARC is the situation, where the position of the pseudo-fovea completely compensates for the angle of strabismus. An angle of the anomaly is the amount of the pseudo-foveal off-set. This angle is similar to the strabismic deviation (objective angle).

Unharmonious ARC is the term used to describe the situation, where the angle of strabismus does not match exactly the location of pseudo-fovea. The angle of deviation is larger than that of anomaly.

Most patients with unharmonious ARC suppress the target image and, therefore, do not experience diplopia.

Anomalous retinal correspondence is associated with good vision or small amblyopia.

In deviation greater than 30°, particularly alternating strabismus, anomalous correspondence usually is not produced as the image in the deviating eye is very weak and small suppression is sufficient. However, in the strabismus of the constant angle of 5° to 10° the image is relatively clear and its exclusion requires quite a suppression. In such cases anomalous correspondence is easier to develop, preventing diplopia, and suppression becomes weaker. Treatment of the anomalous retinal correspondence should be treated before the surgery to avoid postoperative diplopia.

STRABISMUS EXAMINATION

Properly performed strabismus examination and diagnosis are crucial as only early diagnosis and immediate treatment may lead to the complete recovery. There are several techniques of eye examination. They may be divided into the examination of ocular motor and ocular sensory functions.

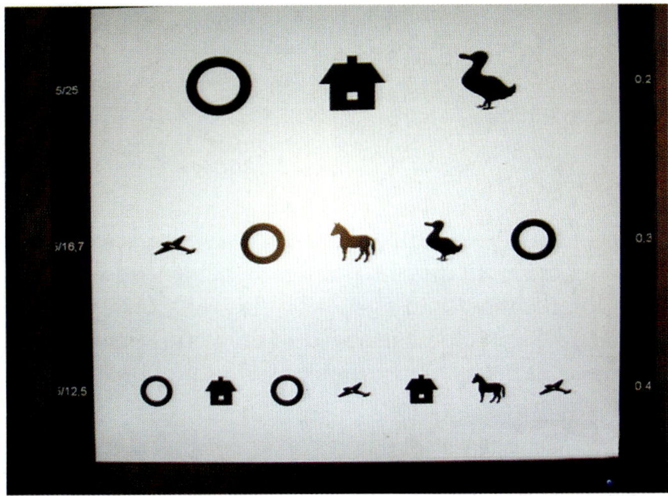

Fig. 16: The picture chart

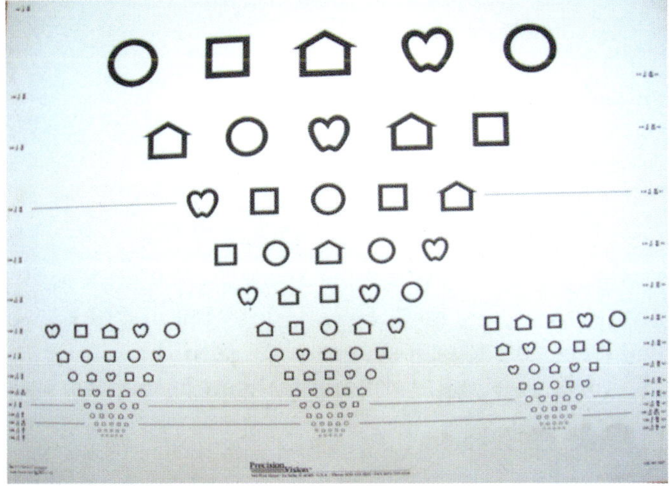

Fig. 17: Lea test

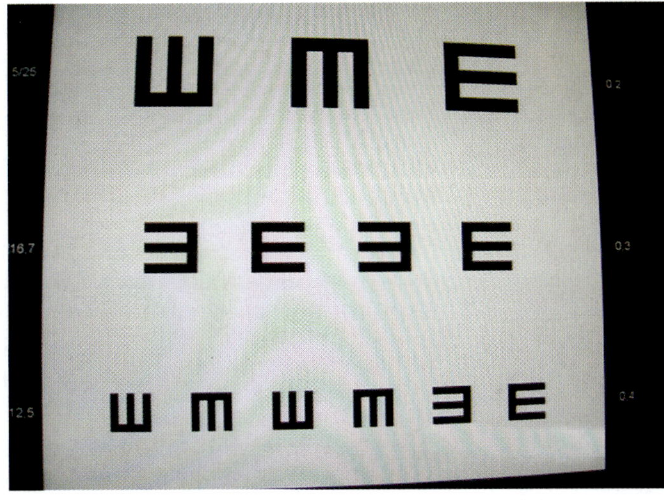

Fig. 18: Tumbling E-test

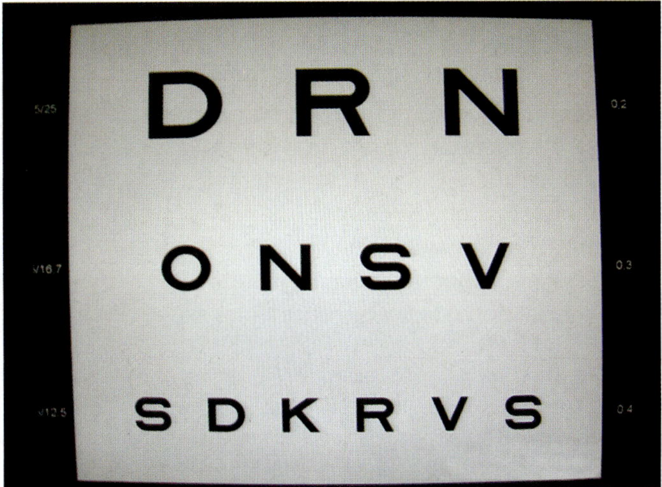

Fig. 19: Snellen test

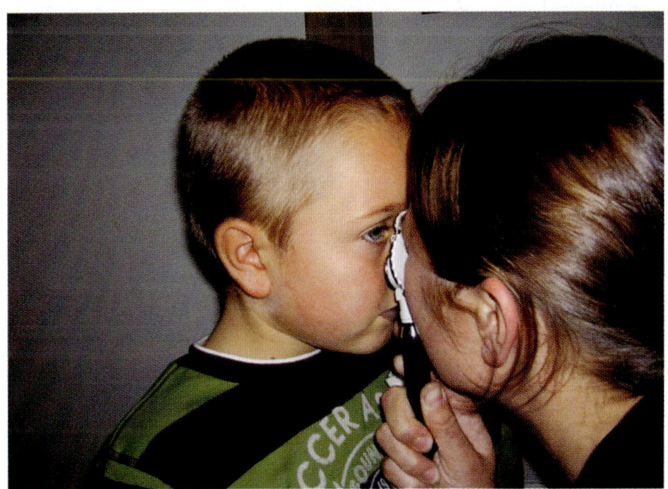

Fig. 20: Examination of fixation with use the visuscope

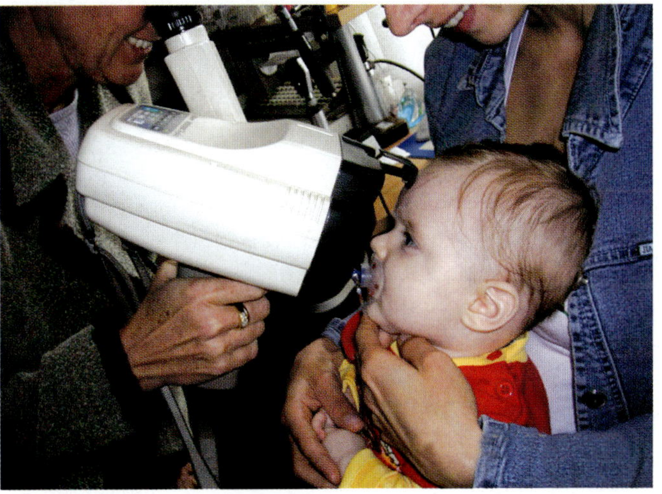

Fig. 21: Hand-held autokeratorefractometer being used in preverbal child

There are several techniques of examinations in the strabismus. In this chapter, only the most important and widely acknowledged techniques will be discussed. Each eye examination should be methodical and accurate. The goals of strabismus examination are to:

- Establishing a cause for strabismus.
- Diagnosing amblyopia.
- Measuring the deviation.
- Assessing binocular sensory status.

The examination is started with anamnesis and inspection.

HISTORY

Therefore, the following questions should be asked:

- Since when the child squints?
- What was the onset of strabismus: sudden or gradual?
- Is the strabismus constant or intermittent?
- Does the child complain for any problem?
- Was the child full-term baby and what was the course of delivery?
- What ophthalmologic and general diseases had the child?
- Are some ophthalmologic problems in the family?
- Was the child examined and treated ophthalmologically?

INSPECTION

Physical examination begins with the moment of child entering the room. Inspection may reveal direction of the squint eye deviation and approximate squint angle. The emphasis should be on the size of both eyeballs and their position in the orbits. Width of lid slits, lids motility and presence of the pathological synkineses are also looked for. Initially, ocular movements and presence or absence of nystagmus are assessed. Head posture, facial torsion, and chin position are also inspected:

- horizontal strabismus is compensated by the sinistro- or dextrotorsion in relation to the vertical axis.
- vertical strabismus is compensated by the chin lowering or elevation in relation to the horizontal axis.
- Oblique strabismus is compensated by head tilt to the right or left shoulder in relation to the sagittal axis.

The ocular torticollis, which does not lead to the facial asymmetry, should be differentiated with the myogenic torticollis resulting from the sternocleidomastoid muscle fibrosis and causing asymmetry of the face, reduction of head movements, and palpable induration of the muscle. Ocular torticollis is seen in the inferior oblique muscle overaction, in A or V syndromes (to achieve uniform visual field of the binocular vision), in nystagmus (compensative head posture with silence zone). Change of the head posture with the cover of one eye is the test confirming ocular torticollis.

VISUAL ACUITY

Visual acuity is evaluated for each eye separately and together, for both distant and near visions, and with and without glasses.

Visual acuity can be measured in the youngest children. In this case special measurement techniques are required such as:

- Observation.
- Optokinetic nystagmus.
- Visual evoked potentials.
- Forced choice preferential looking.
- Graded optotypes of special construction.
- Monocular fixation.

Observational Techniques

Age-dependent various visual reactions are observed. Child in the first month of life reacts to the faces being near and his pupillary light reactions are normal. By 6 to 8 weeks, an infant comes into the visional contact with his mother for the first time. It is difficult to evaluate visual acuity, basing on these reaction. It is known, however, that the vision develops normally. At 2 to 5 months of life blink response to the visual threat and fixation are well developed already. If the visual acuity of one eye is poorer than that of other eye, child will not allow to cover better-sighted eye. Normal visual development in children in the first year of life is presented in Table 2.

Table 2: Normal visual development

Age	*Visual development*
30 weeks gestation	Present pupillary light reaction
1 to 3 months	Stabilized ocular alignment Well developed saccases
2 to 4 months	Well developed fixation Blink response to visual threat OKN-temporal to nasal monocular response
3 to 7 months	OKN-nasal to temporal monocular response Accommodation appropriate to target Completed foveal maturation Well developed stereopsis
6 to 8 months	Well developed smooth pursuit
7 months to 2 years	Well developed contrast sensitivity Completed optic nerve myelination

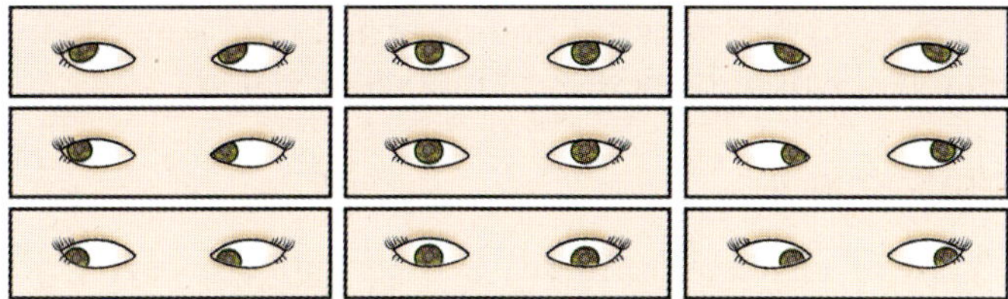

Fig. 22: Nine cardinal position of gaze

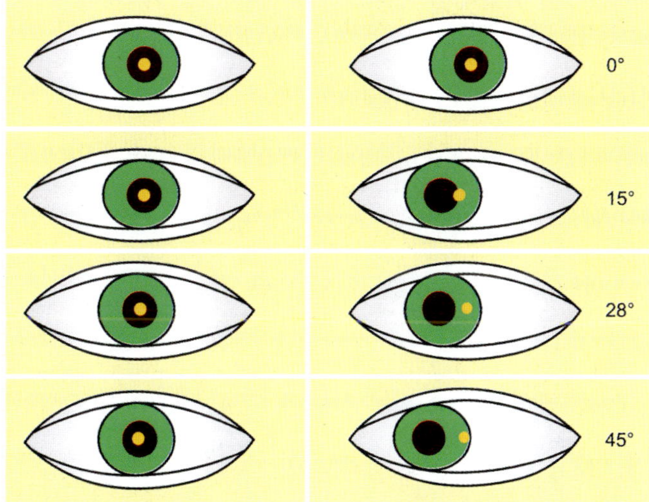

Fig. 23: Hirschberg test.

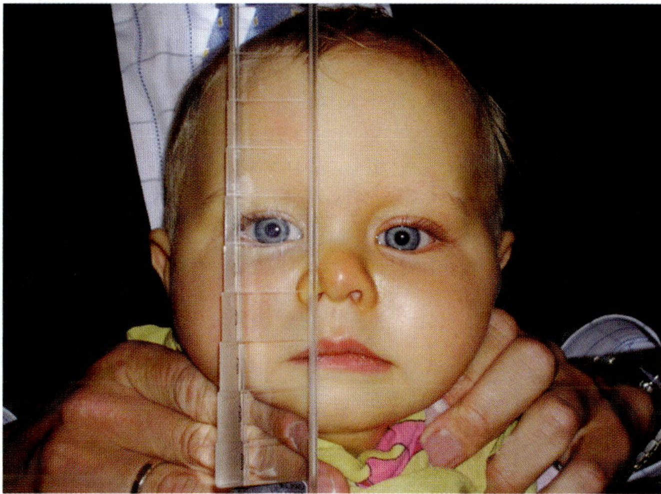

Fig. 24: Krimsky test

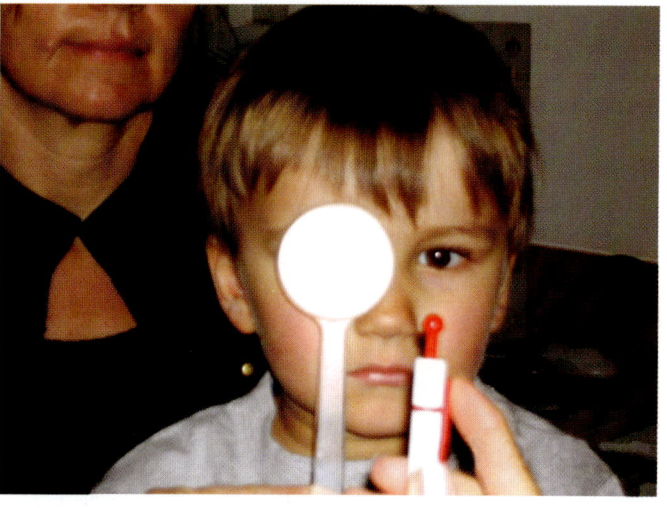

Fig. 25: Cover-uncover test

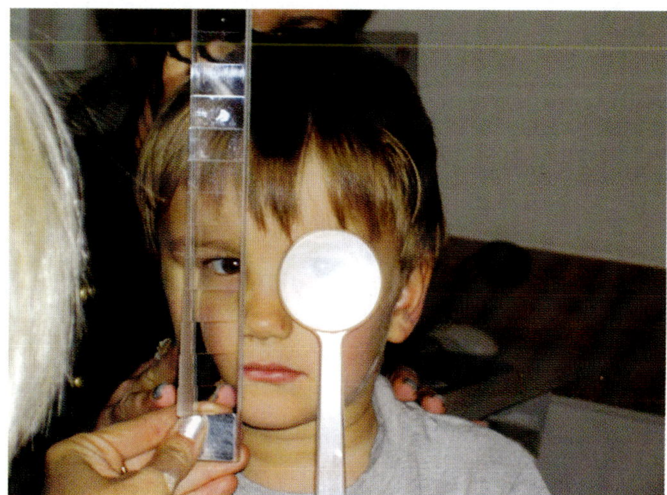

Fig. 26: Prism alternate cover test

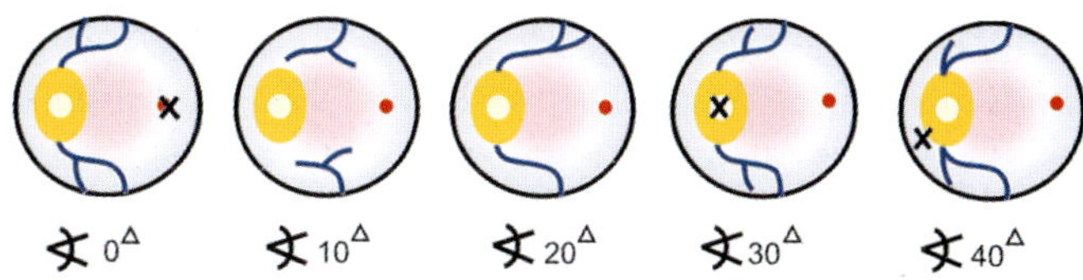

Fig. 27: The test evaluated angle of strabismus by examining fundus fixation

Optokinetic Nystagmus

This examination is performed in non-speaking children. This test comprises showing the child white-and-black strips moved on the special cylinder (Fig. 13). The higher density of strips is producing nystagmus in the child, the better visual acuity of the examined eye. Studying binocular vision, it was found that immediately after the birth visual acuity is poor and is about 6/120. It improves very rapidly, achieving 6/6 by about 24 to 30 months.

Visual Evoked Potentials

It is electrophysiological examination, which involves measurable EEG pattern from the electrodes localized on the scalp overlying occipital cortex and including use of the bright-flash stimuli, square-wave gratings, and phase-alternating checkboard. Several authors estimate that the visual acuity in newborns is 6/60, reaching 6/6 by 6 to 12 months of life. Visual evoked potentials testing are difficult due to the expensive and fragile equipment, and the lack of test standards.

Forced Choice Preferential Looking

This technique is based on the child's eye reaction. If the child prefers to look to the pattern stimulus rather than homogenous field, it means that he(she) sees. Using calibrated square-wave gratings for the test, visual acuity may be assessed. Visual acuity in the newborns is 6/120, reaching 6/6 by the 18 to 24 months (Fig. 14).

The diagram 1 (Fig. 15) presents visual acuity from the birth to 2.5 years of age, evaluated with the three above listed techniques.

Graded Optotypes

Visual acuity in older children is evaluated with the aid of standard Snellen acuity chart, picture chart (Fig.16)and single picture cards, Lea symbols (Fig. 17). Tumbling E test (Fig. 18), Snellen test (Fig. 19).

Monocular Fixation

Fixation of each eye separately is evaluated with visuscope in every child. Star of the device is clearly seen in the eye fundus by both the physician and examined child (Fig. 20). The child is asked to look straight into the star. Young children react spontaneously, fixing fovea on the mid-star, if they have central fixation. Visual acuity is good in such a case. If the patient does not fix with fovea, it indicates decreased visual acuity. Grading of fixation is given in the chapter "Pathophysiology of binocular vision".

REFRACTION

Grade of vision abnormality is determined in each child with the aid of automatic keratorefractometer. In newborns and young children hand-held autokeratorefractometer (Retinomax) is used (Fig. 21). The test is always performed following accommodation paralysis with 0.25-1% atropine administered twice a day for 3 days.

Ocular Motor Examination

Ocular motor function and the angle of eyes deviation, i.e. direction and value of the strabismus angle, are determined during the first visit.

Ocular Movements Examination

The range of eye movements is examined to find out, whether concomitant squint or paralytic squint is present in the patient. Examination is performed in nine cardinal gaze positions (Fig. 22)

Abnormal versions can be scored on the scale from +4 through 0 to -4, where 0 score indicates normal, +4 indicates maximum overaction, and -4 indicates severe underaction. To determine the oblique extraocular muscles action, the examined eye is being covered for a short time, enabling fixation of the normal eye. When the eye is uncovered, overaction of the muscle is clearly seen or is absent. Convergence should also be tested. Objective method is used in the young children, in case of deep amblyopia and lack of binocular vision. It is based on the measurement the distance between the point at which the eyes stop to converge. Measurements are made in the primary position and upright, and downright positions.

Subjective method is used exclusively in the patients with binocular vision, involving the determination of the convergence near point with the aid of diplopia.

Angle of convergence may be calculated with the formula:

$$\frac{\text{Half of interpupillary distance (DP/2)}}{\text{Distance of convergence (in meters)}}$$

Wilczek, basing on the above formula, made curves of the half convergence angle, enabling to find so-called convergence standard for various distances of pupils and various distances of convergence.

To evaluate precisely paralytic squint, testing of the forced duction test, diplopia examination, Hess screen,

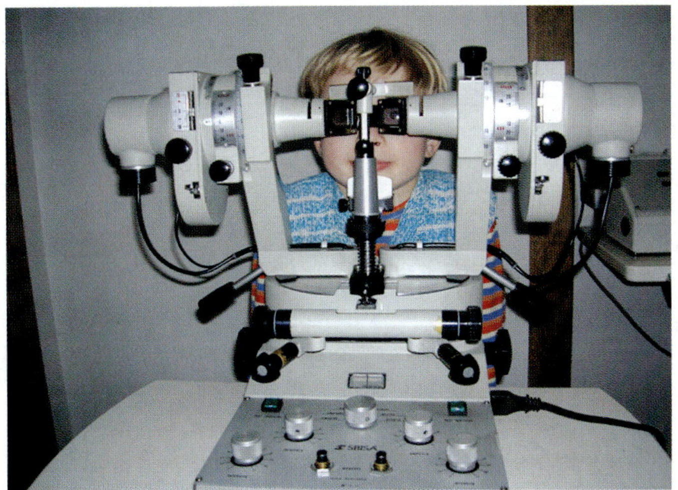

Fig. 28: Synoptophore

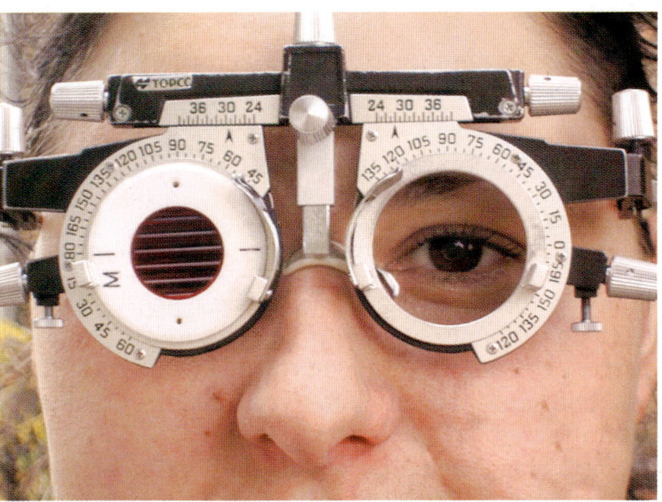

Fig. 30: Red Maddox rod test. Using in the special frame to evaluate ocular torsion

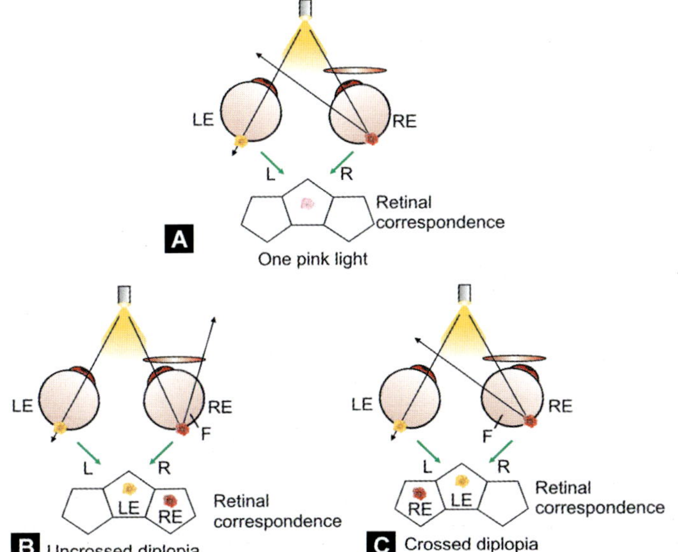

Figs 29A to C: Retinal correspondence-red filter test. A-Patient with straight eyes and normal retinal correspondence. B-Patient with esotropia and normal retinal correspondence. C-Patient with exotropia and normal retinal correspondence.

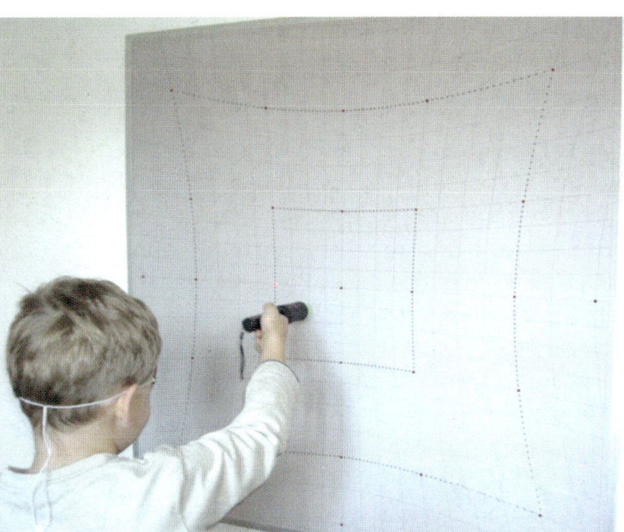

Fig. 31: Hess screen

Maddox rod test, oculomyodynamometry, and electromyography are used. However, paralytic squint is not a subject of this chapter.

Ocular Deviation Measurements

Hirschberg Method

Enables preliminary evaluation of the angle of strabismus. Reflection of the light projected straight ahead and near (0.5 m) on the both corneas is observed (Fig. 23). This test is performed mainly in newborns and young children, enabling rapid diagnosis of the type and range of the angle of strabismus.

Hirschberg method is relying on pupil size of 4 mm and assuming light displacement by 1 mm across the cornea, being equivalent to 8° of decentration. Kappa angle should always be taken into consideration. This angle may be assessed by projecting light source on the cornea of only one eye, covering fellow eye. The term angle kappa is related to the eye position in monocular vision and is associated with central fixation by the displaced fovea. The most frequently, this is caused by temporally displacement of the fovea in patient with retinopathy of prematurity. Displacement of the light reflex temporally to the papillary margin is an esotropia of 15 degrees, to the mid-iris indicates a deviation of 28 degrees, and at the limbus a deviation of 45 degrees.

Krimsky Test

It is modified Hirschberg method with the use of prisms. Angle of strabismus is evaluated, when the light is projected straight ahead, and subsequent prisms (prism bar) are placed before the fixing eye until symmetrical light reflexes are seen on the cornea of both eyes (Fig. 24).

The prism base is oriented appropriately to neutralize the deviation:

- Esotropia: prism base-out.
- Exotropia: prism base-in.
- Hypertropia: prism base-down.
- Hypotropia: prism base-up
- The results are expressed in prism diopter (PD). It is very convenient test for quick evaluation of the angle of strabismus, especially in the abnormal fixation of the squint eye and amblyopia.

Cover Tests

Cover-uncover or alternate cover tests serve to evaluate the type of strabismus.

Cover-uncover Test

Relies on the covering one eye and observation of the fellow eye. After uncovering the eye examiner observes whether fixation movement is present, indicating that this eye is the fixing one. Then, fellow eye is covered and its movements after uncover are observed. Ocular shift towards the temple indicates esotropia; the shift towards the nose—exotropia; ocular shift upward indicates hypotropia, while downward—hypertropia. The lack of fixation movements of the said eye despite the presence of strabismus suggests severe ambylopia or eccentric fixation. In such a case heterotrophy of one is diagnosed (Fig. 25)

Alternate Cover Test

Covering alternately one and then the other eye, fusion is broken. If the alternate cover test is positive and cover-uncover test negative, heterophoria is present. If, however, both these tests are positive, heterotropia is present. If the movement of uncovered eye is greater in the alternate cover test than in cover-uncover test, anomalous retinal correspondence (ARC) is present.

Prism Alternate Cover Test

This test is performed, when central fixation in both eyes is present. Objective angle of strabismus is evaluated. (Fig. 26).

To measure the angle of strabismus, eyes are covered alternatively and the prism bar is moved before one eye, watching fixation movement of the naked eye, until this movement has stopped. Strength of the prism at which fixation movement stops is the value of the angle of strabismus. Prism base is always directed opposite the eye deviation. The test is performed during distant vision of 6 m and near vision of 30 cm. If eccentric fixation is present in one eye, the value of angle of strabismus is assessed with Krimsky test or examining eye fundus through the prism. The patient views distant point with normal eye, and stronger prisms are placed before the deviating eye, examining eye fundus with the visuscope straight ahead (Baranowska-George).The prism corresponding with the angle of strabismus is the one through which the examiner sees fovea in line with the visuscope star (Fig. 27).

Synoptophore

It is an instrument serving to the examination and training of binocular vision. Objective and subjective angles of strabismus are measured with the aid of pictures for simultaneous perception (Fig. 28).

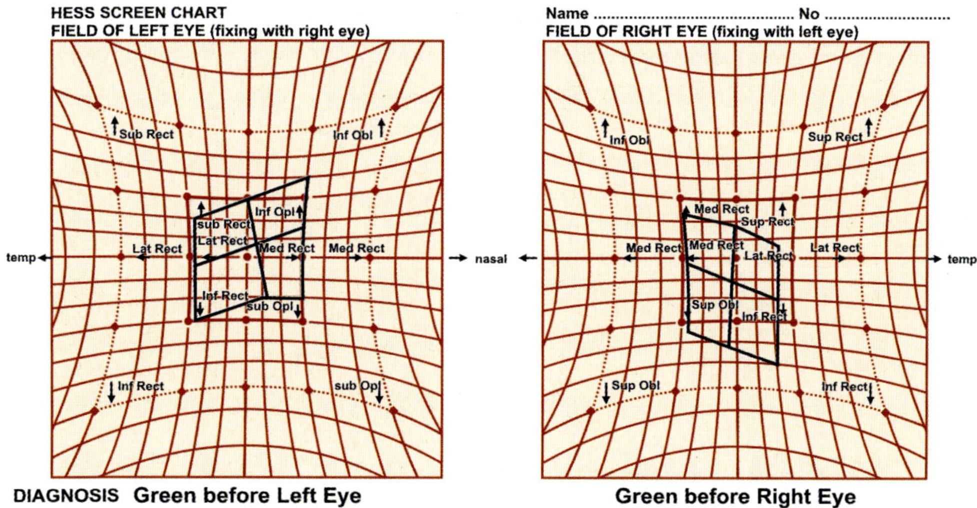

Fig. 32: The result of Hess screen examination in patient with left superior oblique underaction

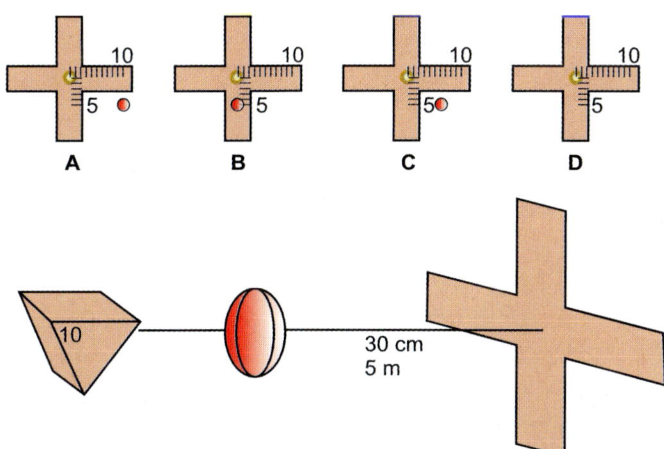

Fig. 33: The examination of the retinal correspondence with prism and red filter. Objective angle is 10 degree. A-NRC, B- harmonious ARC, C-nonharmonious ARC, D-suppression.

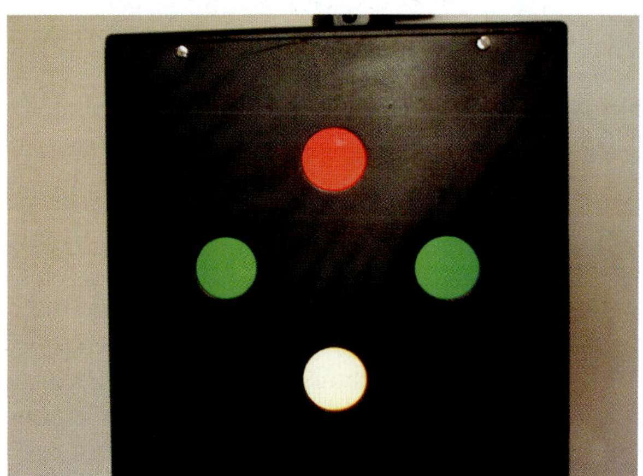

Fig. 34: Worth four-dot lamp

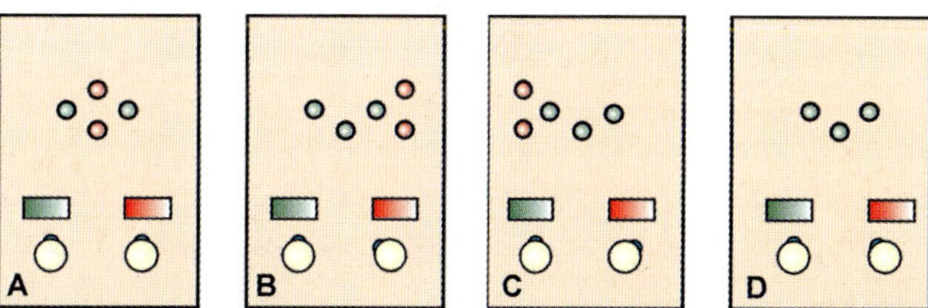

Fig. 35: Possible Worth four-dot test. A-normal binocular vision, B-esotropia with uncross images C-exotropia with cross images, D-suppression one eye

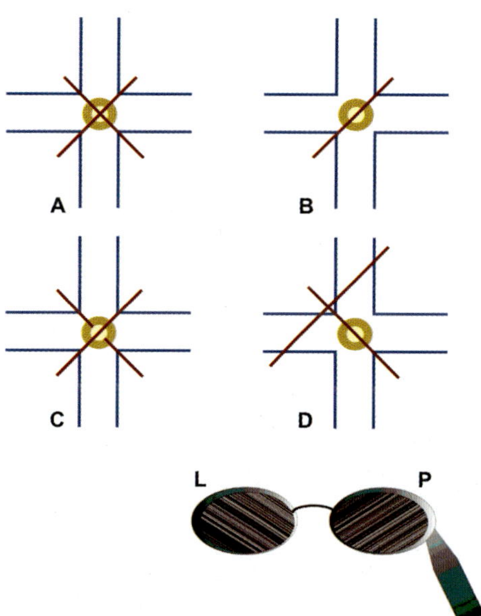

Fig. 36: Bagolini lenses

Objective angle of strabismus is measured by the disappearance of fixation movements of eyes fixing two supplementing pictures. The name of these pictures are the simultaneous perception pictures (e.g. lion in the cage). Subjective angle is the angle when the child places the lion into the cage. If both angles are identical, correspondence of both retinas is normal. If the value of the objective angle differs from that of subjective angle, anomalous retinal correspondence is present. The difference between subjective and objective angle of strabismus is called the angle of anomaly.

Red Filter Test

This test is suitable in case of the small angle of strabismus. If the simultaneous perception of the light source and normal retinal correspondence are found, the angle of strabismus may be measured with subjective technique. Dark red filter is placed over straight eye and the patient sees red light on the Maddox scale. With deviating eye the patient sees white light. So he sees two lights at the same time. Normal patient with straight eyes sees one pink light. The patient with esotropia sees double not crossed lights whereas the patients with exotropia sees two crossed lights (Fig. 29).

Consecutive prisms placed before the eye decreases the distance of the double images on the Maddox scale. Prism strength at which two images are fused into one is the value of the objective angle of strabismus, after considering the test distance.

Maddox Rod Test

Heterophoria may be detected with the aid of the test in which dark red rod is placed before one eye and the test is performed 5 m before Maddox cross. Fellow eye fixes the white light on the scale. Patient with ortophoria sees the red line running through the light point. If the red line is on another side of the light (crossed position), there is exophoria. If the red line is on the same side (uncrossed position), esophoria is present. The red line may rotate downward (hyperphoria), upward (hypophoria), outside (incyclophoria), inside (excyclophoria). Deviation of the eye is read on the Maddox scale in prism diopters (Fig. 30).

Forced Duction Test

A topical anesthetic eyedrops are given to the conjunctival sac of the patient's eye. Then, the conjunctiva in the limbus is grasped with forceps and an attempt to abduct the eyeball toward weakened muscle. Limitation or block of eyeball rotation means the mechanical restriction of movement.

Hess Screening

The most convenient is a gray screen covered with the net of tangent lines (Fig. 31). In the semi dark room the patient wearing red-green spectacles projects green vertical light streak with special Foster torch at 50 cm distance, covering it with red points lit on the screen by the examiner. The result is marked on the appropriate schemes (Fig. 32). Maximum deviation from the primary position to the direction of particular muscles overaction and underaction is evaluated.

SENSORY EXAMINATION

Normal binocular vision comprises of simultaneous perception, normal fusion amplitude, and stereoscopy. In the strabismus particular mechanisms are disturbed, changing retinal correspondence and frequently producing suppression of various degree.

Synoptophore Examination

Synoptophor consists of two tubes, which may be moved, in special holder. Examination of the simultaneous perception means the determination of the angle of strabismus and retinal correspondence assessment.

Fusion amplitude is evaluated with the use of nearly the same pictures, differing in only small details. Moving the arms of synoptophore until all details are seen clearly, fusion amplitude directed to the convergence and divergence is being determined. Normal values are given in the chapter "Binocular Vision".

Stereoscopy is examined with the use of slightly decentred special pictures. They are, therefore, projected on the dispart retinal point, but within Panum's area, giving the impression of depth and stereoscopy.

Anomalous Retinal Correspondence Examination with Prism

The test is performed with the use of Maddox scale at the distance of 5 m, and the near of 30 cm. The examined patient fixes the normal eye on the middle of the cross with the light, and vertical prism 10 to 20 PD and red filter are placed before the fellow eye. Objective angle is determined with prism cover test. In the strabismus with normal retinal correspondence subjective angle is equal to the objective angle. Red point is seen under the number corresponding to the objective angle. In the anomalous harmonious correspondence it is seen under the light in

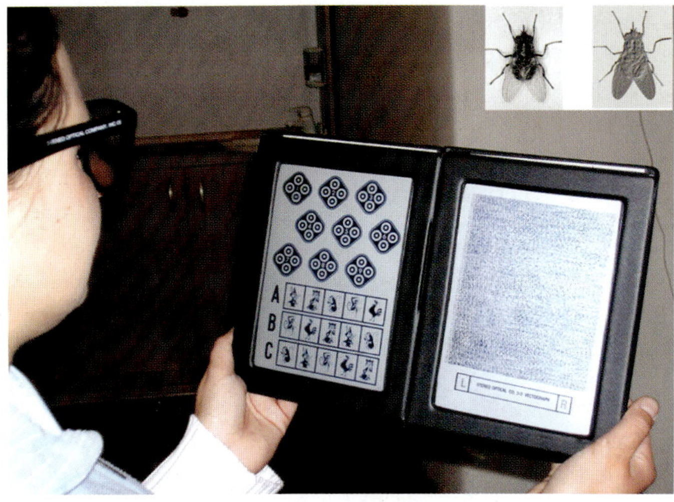

Fig. 37: Fly stereotest with Polaroid glasses

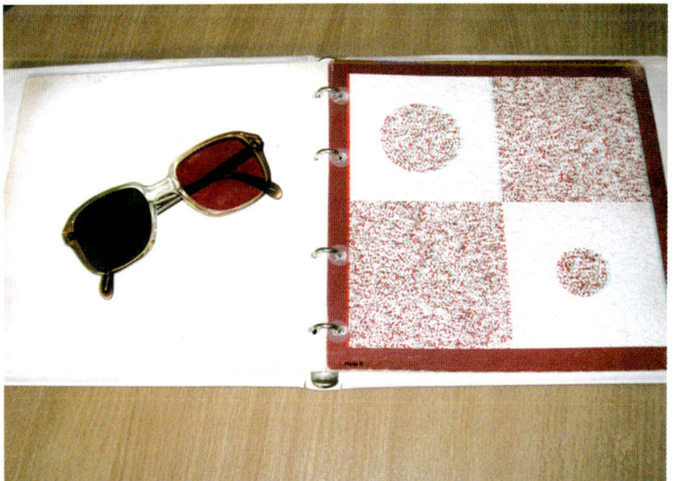

Fig. 38: TNO test with Polaroid glasses

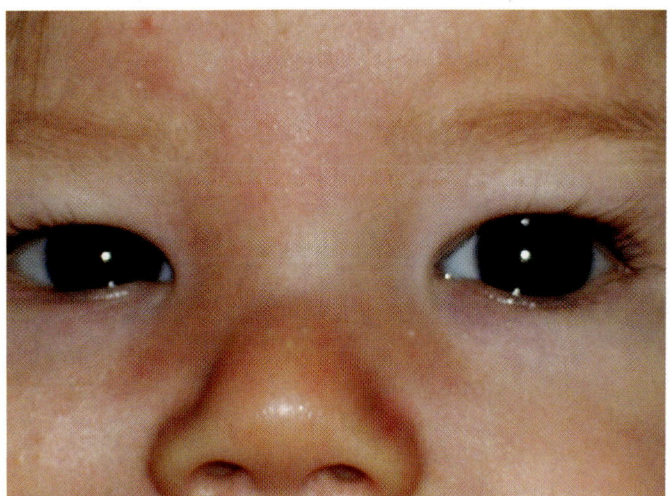

Fig. 39: Pseudostrabismus

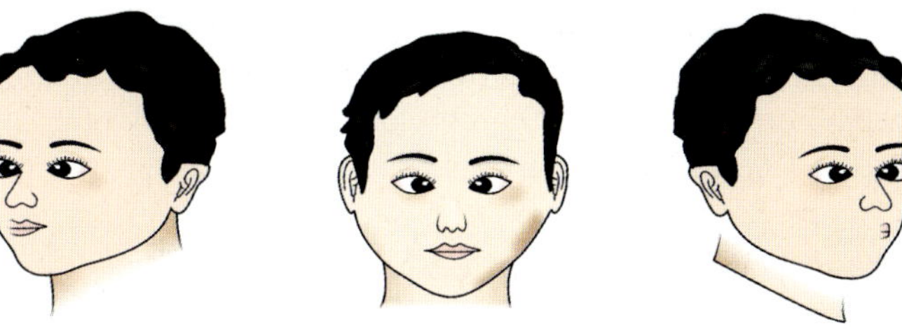

Fig. 40: Infantile esotropia showing alternating fixation

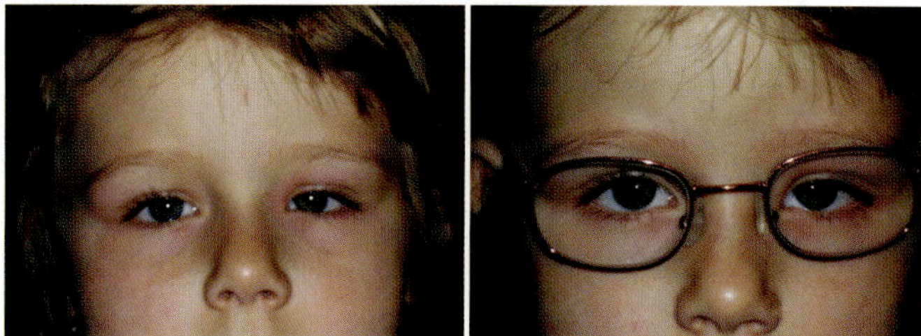

Fig. 41: Refractive accommodative esotropia with normal AC/A ratio

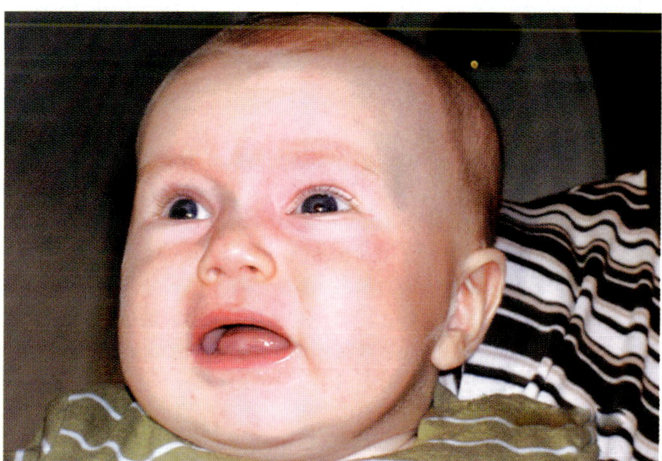

Fig. 42: Congenital exotropia – 6 month of age child

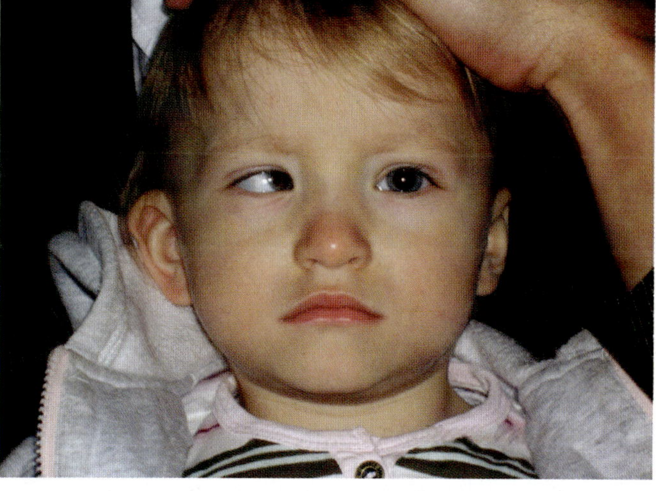

Fig. 43: 3-year old child with the right inferior oblique overaction

the middle of scale (subjective angle is 0°). In the anomalous unharmonious correspondence the red point indicates subjective angle lower than the objective angle. In case of suppression the red point is invisible (Fig. 33).

Possible Worth Four-dot Test

This test is strongly dissociating the vision. Red-green glasses are worn which permeable for only colors adequate for each eye and enables to see red-green lights arranged into the cross (Fig. 34).
Interpretation is dependent on the seen image:

- Visible four lights: normal binocular vision or microstrabismus of anomalous retinal correspondence.
- Visible only two red or green lights: suppression of one eye.
- Visible 5 lights: manifest squint with normal retinal correspondence or anomalous unharmonious correspondence (Fig. 35)

Bagolini Lenses

It is slightly dissociating test. This test is performed with the use of test striated glasses through which the patient sees light streak by each eye, viewing the light on the Maddox cross. Light streak is in the 45-degree meridian and another in the 135-degree meridian (Fig. 36).

Images of the light streaks images are interpreted as follows:

- Two streaks crossing at the center of the light: normal retinal correspondence without strabismus or microstrabismus with the anomalous harmonious retinal correspondence.
- Two streaks are crossed but one is broken in the center: scotoma of the fixation point.
- Two streaks: one running centrally, and another shifted: squint with either normal or anomalous unharmonious retinal correspondence.
- One streak is visible: suppression of the deviating eye.

Stereopsis Tests

Stereoscopic vision may be tested with various techniques. One of the oldest devices used for this purpose is Helmholtz apparatus with three needles or Howard-Dohlmann apparatus used for testing the pilots. Nowadays, stereoscopy is tested with the aid of stereotests. Two images of the same object are reproduced on the charts, which are polarized vertically. The patient, viewing through polarized glasses receives an impression of 3D image. The Titmus (fly test) stereotest is providing disparity between 3000 sec of arc and 40 sec of arc. at the 40 cm testing distance (Fig. 37).

More precise is TNO stereotest (Fig. 36), which uses random-dot stereograms viewed through the anaglyph red-green glasses and provides disparities between 480 and 15 sec of arc.

TYPES OF STRABISMUS

1. Pseudostrabismus.
2. Heterophoria (latent strabismus).
3. Heterotropia (concomitant strabismus).
4. Paralytic strabismus (incomitant strabismus).
5. Strabismus syndromes.

Concomitant strabismus should be distinguished from other types of strabismus. Only exact diagnosis of the pathology enables to undertake appropriate management leading the complete recovery.

PSEUDOSTRABISMUS

Pseudostrabismus is a condition, which only simulates squint. The eyes are straight, however, they appear to be crossed. Often we observed the abnormality of the eyeballs structure or its placement in the orbits or changes in the eye protective apparatus.

Pseudostrabismus is present, when the visual axis (connecting fixing object with the fovea) is different then the optic axis (the line running through the center of cornea and pupil). The angle at which these axes crossed is called gamma angle. Observed reflection of light from cornea is not in line with visual axis, simulating convergence, divergence, hypertropia or hypotropia. Gamma angle is measured with Maddox scale at 1 m distance. Covering one eye, examiner observes whether light reflection is in the center of pupil. If not, gamma angle is present. It is expressed by the necessary shift on the Maddox scale so as the reflex would be in the center. In very young children wide, flat bridge of the nose and small folds of the eyelid skin or narrow interpupillary distance are frequent. Such a state may simulate convergent strabismus. Pseudostrabismus is rarely seen also in high myopia.

In other cases (pseudoexotropia), wide interpupillary distance or presence of gamma angle resulting from the eyeball diseases (macular ectopia in the retinopathy of prematurity, or high hypermetropia) may be present (Fig. 39).

Detailed diagnosis with the aid of various tests should be made in every case to differentiate pseudostrabismus form the true strabismus. Pseudostrabismus does not require therapy and eye appearance frequently changes with the child's age.

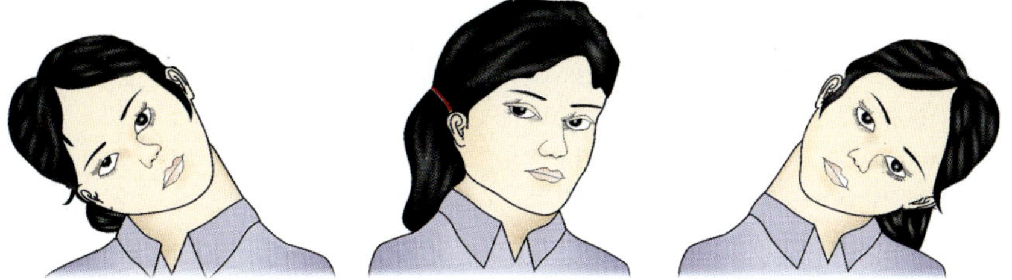

Fig. 44: Bielschowsky test is positive in patient with right superior oblique muscle paresis

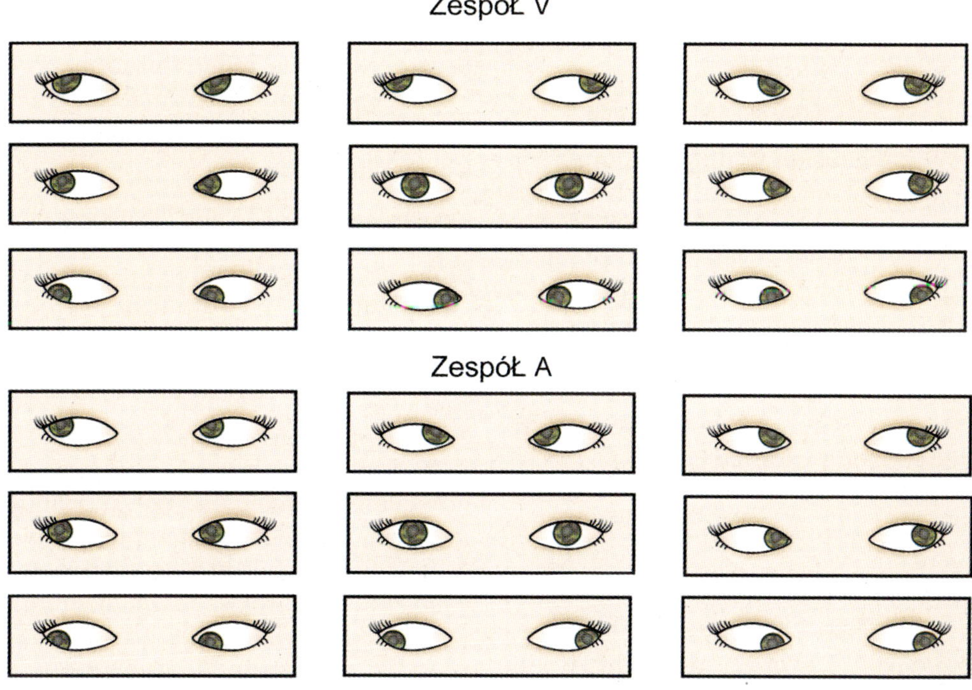

Fig. 45: V-pattern and A-pattern syndromes. Nine position of gaze is presented on each dysfunction

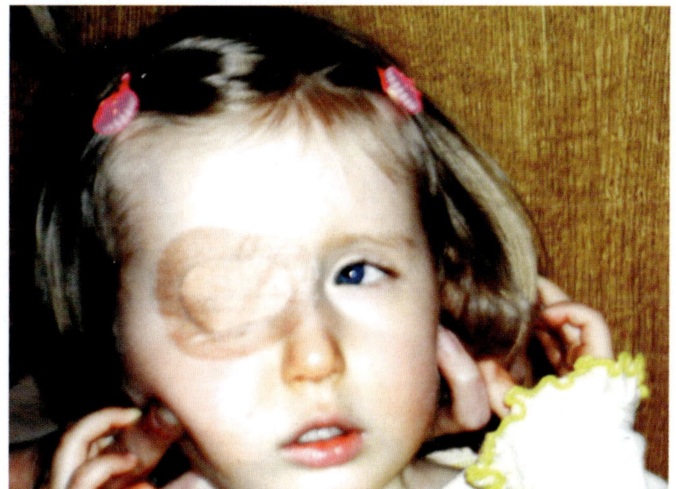

Fig. 46: Amblyopia management by sound eye patching

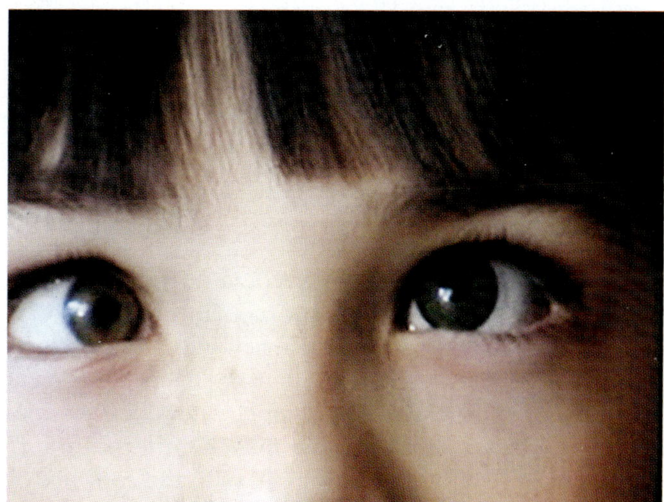

Fig. 47: Treatment of amblyopia with soft occlusion—color contact lens of left eye

HETEROPHORIA

In healthy children action of the extraocular muscles is balanced. It is so-called ortophoria. However, disturbances of such a balance are frequent and are generally called heterophoria. Deviation of the visual axis results from the fusion interruption, which is not able to maintain binocular vision any longer. Types of heterophoria, dependent on the direction of eye misalignment, are the following:

- Esophoria: deviation inward.
- Exophoria: deviation outward.
- Hyperphoria: deviation upward.
- Hypophoria: deviation downward.
- Incyclophoria:rotation inside.
- Excyclophoria: rotation outside

Factors weakening the fusion facilitate heterophoria progressing to the concomitant strabismus. Such a state is called decompensated heterophoria. It is the strabismus of a sudden onset with diplopia, lack of the symptoms of extraocular muscles paralysis and normal retinal correspondence. It requires immediate nonsurgical or surgical treatment to prevent stabilization of strabismus, diplopia, and constant fusion interruption with break of the binocular vision. Factors predisposing to decompensated heterophoria are listed below:

- Uncorrected refraction error
- Anisometropia.
- Transient cover of one eye.
- Emotional or physical shock.
- Fatigue or asthenia (severe infections).

In heterophoria with excessive and long-lasting overuse of the fusion mechanisms feeling of the eyes fatigue, sometimes headache, blurred near vision, especially with prolonged reading, and diplopia are seen. These are the signs of so-called asthenopia. Spectacles with prism facilitating actions of the weakened muscles are recommended. Eye exercises strengthening binocular vision are also effective. In rare cases, even surgical treatment is required.

CONCOMITANT STRABISMUS

Heterotropia may appear at any age of the child. It is characterized by the preserved eye mobility in all directions of gaze, the primary angle is equal to the secondary angle, diplopia is replaced by the compensation mechanisms in the form of suppression, amblyopia, anomalous retinal correspondence. Heterotropia may be alternating or unilateral, constant or intermittent, with the constant or variable angle of strabismus, and depending on the direction of deviation:

- Esotropia.
- Exotropia.
- Hypertropia.
- Hypotropia.
- Oblique muscle dysfunction
- A-pattern strabismus.
- V-pattern strabismus

ESOTROPIA

Esotropia is the most common type of strabismus, including congenital, accommodative, and cyclic forms.

Congenital Esotropia

Ocular Manifestation and Diagnosis

This form of strabismus is present since birth. It is characterized by the large and constant angle of strabismus. One eye and then the fellow eye fixes alternatively in the primary position. At side viewing cross fixation is present.The right eye is used in left gaze and the left eye is used in right gaze (Fig. 40)

Patients show limited abduction of both eyes; it may, however, be detected with alternate cover test and monocular abduction attempt. Positive result of the test differentiates between congenital esotropia and blockage nystagmus syndrome. Angle of strabismus is measured with the aid of Hirschberg method and Krimsky test. Usually, this angle is large, about 30-70 PD. Visual abnormality in the majority of children is mild. If in the primary position one eye is fixing all the time, amblyopia may develop in the fellow eye. In 75% of cases unilateral or alternate inferior oblique muscle overaction or dissociated vertical deviation (DVD) are seen.

Differential Diagnosis

Congenital esotropia should be differentiated between other syndromes:

- Nystagmus blockage syndrome
- Infantile accommodative esotropia
- Cyclic esotropia
- Mobius' syndrome
- Duane's syndrome
- Congenital fibrosis syndrome (fixed strabismus)
- Congenital myasthenia
- Congenital six nerve palsy

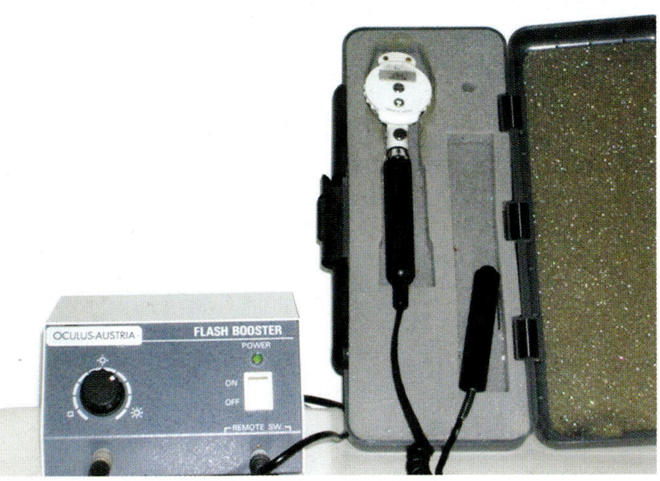

Fig. 48: Eutyscope

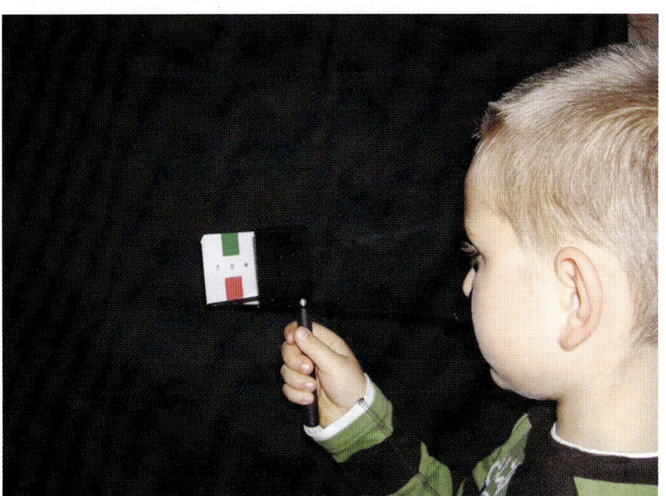

Fig. 51: 49.Diploscope

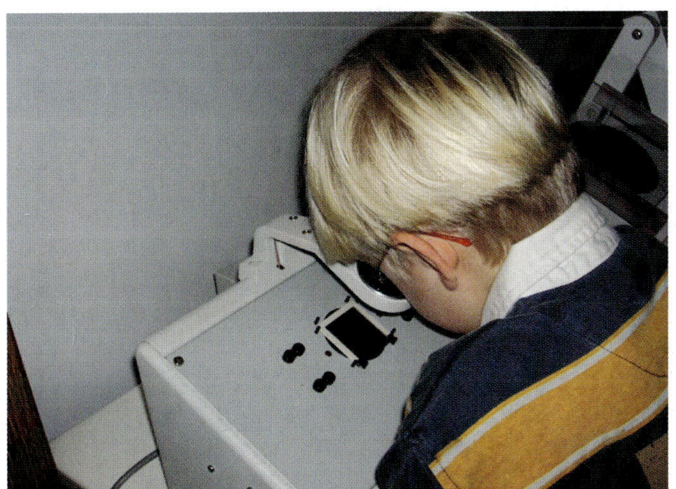

Fig. 49: Phenomenon of Haidinger using to pleoptic exercises improve visual acuity and fixation of the amblyopic eye

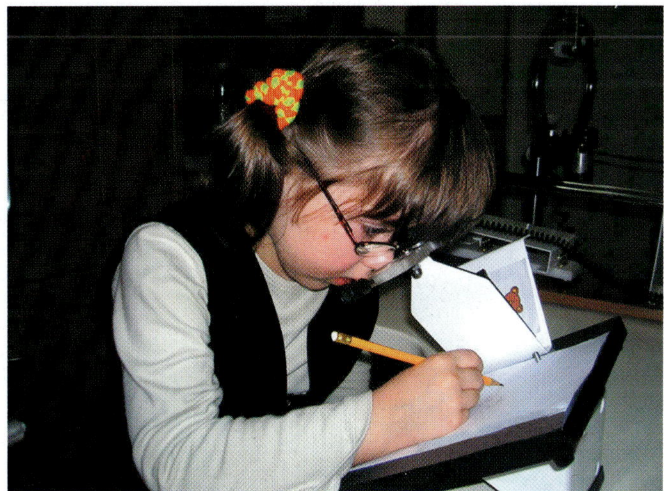

Fig. 52: Cheiroscope using to remove suppression and improve binocular vision

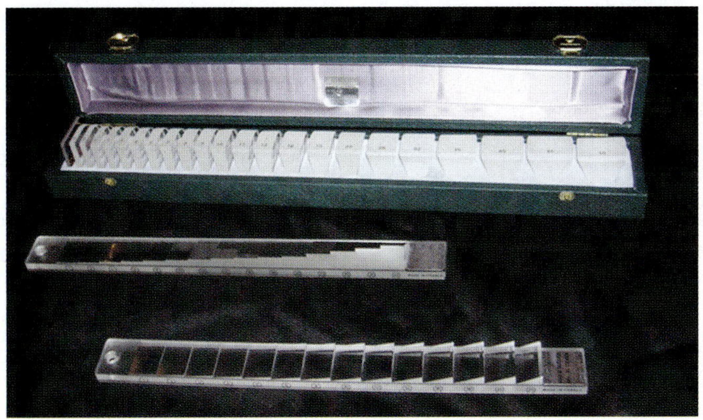

Fig. 50: The horizontal and vertical prism bar and separate prisms

Treatment

Only an early treatment of the congenital esotropia excellent visual acuity in each eye, single binocular vision in all directions of gaze and normal esthetic appearance may be achieved.

The first examination includes evaluation of refractive error and prescription of appropriate eye-glasses or contact lenses.

If amblyopia is present, it is initially treated with the full-time occlusion of the sound eye. Frequent follow-up visits are necessary, every few weeks, as the visual acuity may be quite easily evaluated and amblyopia more readily responds in younger child. The sound eye is covered the day long, and uncovered for two, six or eight hours daily parallel to the achieved improvement. Some researchers are inducing cycloplegia in the better-sighted eye, if it is hyperopic, using atropine for this purpose. When equal visual acuity is achieved in both eyes, the treatment of strabismus is started. Congenital esotropia usually is treated surgically. We may attempt to treat the child with the aid of prism-spectacles, completely correcting the angle of strabismus. However, therapy is longer and more inconvenient for both parents and child. Large angle of strabismus, which is seen in the congenital esotropia, between 30 PD to 70 PD, requires the use of Fresnel membrane prisms as smooth glasses would be too heavy. Fresnel membrane prisms are striated glasses and the child not always accepts such a correction. However, if these prisms are used early enough in the first week of life, the treatment may be effective and alignment of the eyes or correction of the angle of strabismus may be achieved in a short time. Small angle of strabismus may later be corrected with other therapies. Another effective therapy is the use of botulinum toxin, originally popularized by Scott. Botulinum toxin is injected intramuscularly into the medial rectus muscle of both eyes. Theoretical advantage of this technique is the achievement of incomitant deviation so that the patient could adapt face turn and obtain fusion. In some cases, multiple injections are required to sustain the effect. The injection is short-lasting, does not disturb the child as the short inhalation anesthesia (sevofluran).

In my experience, such a good result is achieved in about 55-60% of cases. If this procedure does not bring improvement, surgery is needed. Parks and von Noorden suggest that the goal of surgery is a delay of surgery until the child is over six months of age. Then, the development of fusion in the child who truly has the onset of esotropia at or shortly after birth.

Recommended surgery includes recession both medial rectus muscles in the range depending on the size of the angle of strabismus. If the angle after surgery larger than 10 PD remains, re-operation should be considered on the lateral muscles of one or both eyes or the use of prism-glasses, or botulinum toxin injections. This form of strabismus is sometimes accompanied by the overaction of the inferior oblique muscles. In such cases surgical recession of these muscles is needed to correct vertical deviation which in the low range over 2 to 3 PD breaks the binocular vision.

Sometimes, DVD may appear in some years after surgery. Main reason for DVD treatment is esthetic. If DVD is monocular or highly asymmetrical, surgical treatment is necessary as the binocular vision is impossible to obtain. This abnormality is treated surgically with superior rectus muscle recession with Cupper's sutures or inferior rectus muscle resection.

Accommodative Esotropia

Accommodative esotropia is a convergent deviation of the eyes dependent on the activation of accommodation reflex. The first cause is high hyperopia, greater than +4,oDsph. The second is an overconvergence associated with accommodation and high AC/A ratio. In many patients both these mechanisms are present and inter-related. Strabismus develops most frequently between 2 and 5 years of age and may be explained by the higher interest of child in near vision and reading, which provide stronger stimulus for accommodation, especially in case of non-compensated refractive error. Initially, strabismus is intermittent and angle of deviation is variable, usually larger at near. Retinal correspondence is normal as a rule but if the deviation appears at near, suppression or tendency to anomalous retinal correspondence is seen.

Ocular Manifestations and Diagnosis

The majority of authors distinguish three main types of accommodative esotropia:

- Refractive accommodative esotropia with normal AC/C ratio. Patients wearing the glasses do not squint at near and distance. Binocular vision is normal or slightly weakened. The squint is seen without glasses (Fig. 41).
- High AC/A ratio esotropia with anomalous accommodation to convergence. This type of strabismus develops in younger children, frequently in the first year of age. Children usually have small

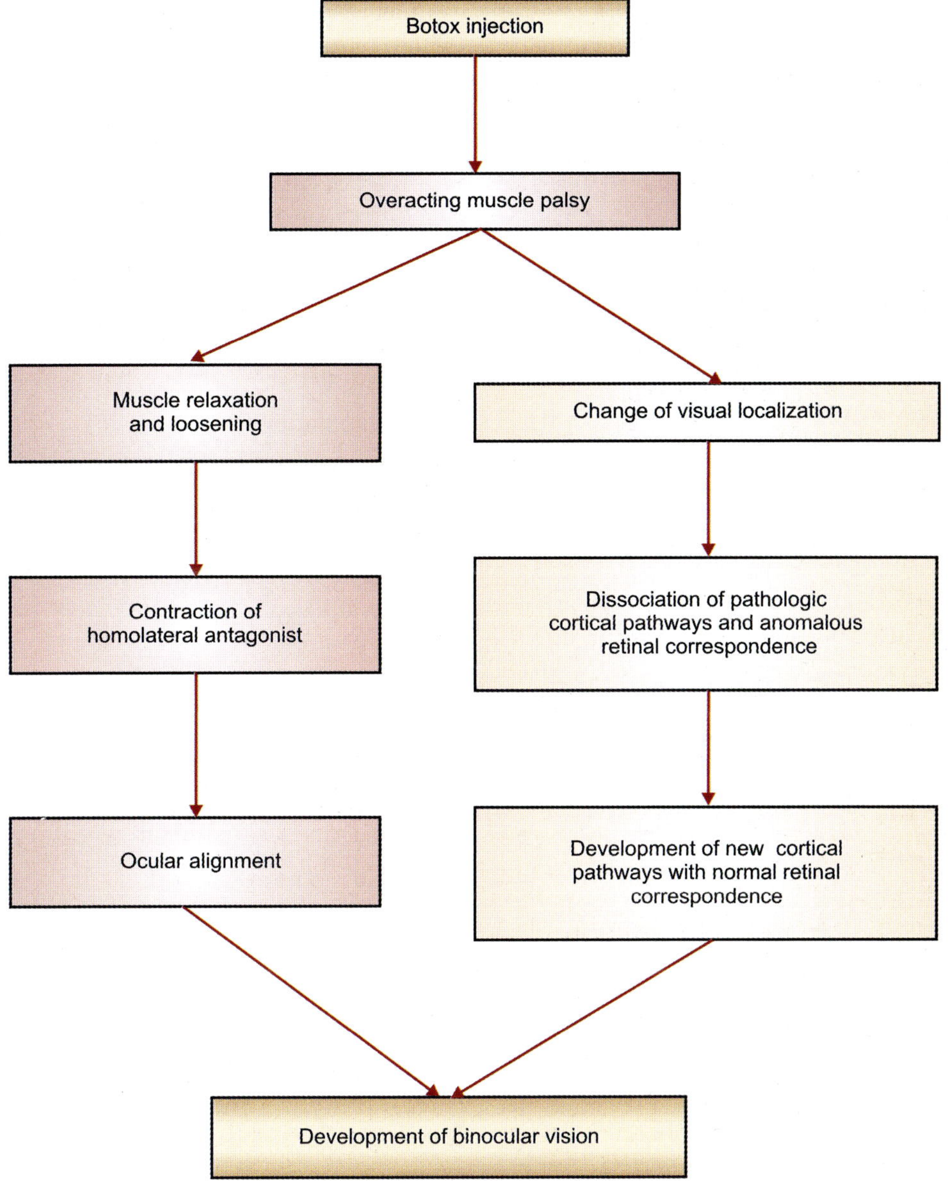

Fig. 53: Scheme of botulinum toxin action

hyperopia and its compensation leads to the straight eyes at distance, whereas esotropia remains at near. Amblyopia and binocular vision disturbances are seen more frequently in this type of esotropia.

– Partially accommodative esotropia. Spectacles significantly lower the angle of strabismus in this type of accommodative esotropia. However, marked residual deviation remains. If AC/A ratio is high, the angle of strabismus enlarges at near. If AC/A ratio is normal, the angle of strabismus is the same at near and at distant. Amblyopia and binocular vision disturbances are frequent in this type of esotropia. Partially accommodative esotropia is the most frequent type of the accommodative esotropia.

Treatment

Treatment of the accommodative esotropia is started with lowering excessive accommodation by the use of adequate spectacles with full correction of hyperopia. Normal or bifocal contact lenses may also be used. In cases of esotropia with high AC/A ratio bifocal spectacles with stronger correction at near by 2 - 3 Dsph are prescribed. High AC/A ratio may be corrected the use of topical miotic eyedrops (pilocarpine, phenylephrine). These medicine, producing peripheral stimulation of accommodation, lead to the elimination of the central stimulation of the ciliary muscle and consequently to the decrease in convergence. However, these medicines are rarely used because of their marked toxicity and local complications (iris cyst). If amblyopia is present, it is treated with obturation of the normal eye.

Partially accommodative esotropia requires the use of prisms or surgical treatment. Prisms compensating the angle of strabismus are prescribed and should be worn permanently. Moreover, therapy with a high hyper-correcting prismatic glasses for eye exercises (Baranowska-George, Berard) is used. It is called localization method based on the use hypercorrecting prismatic glasses to break pathological and fixed reflexes associated with anomalous retinal correspondence.

With therapy the angle of strabismus is lowered and retinal correspondence normalized. However, the treatment is long and requires high compliance of parents and treated child. Use of botulinum toxin injections to correct residue angle of strabismus is highly recommended and frequently lead to complete recovery. Surgery is reserved to cases in which the above described therapies are not enough. The range of surgery is often difficult to evaluate, especially in variable angle of strabismus. Only non-accommodative component of deviation is operated. Depending on the angle of strabismus, single medial rectus muscle recession is performed and, only sporadically bimedial rectus recession to enable the patient to stop wearing bifocal spectacles. Further visual rehabilitation in the form of orthoptic exercises is required, aimed at augmenting fusion with the wide amplitude, and decelerating and separating accommodation from convergence so that binocular vision is fixed and eyes are aligned.

Cyclic Esotropia

Cyclic estropia is very rare pathology. Its incidence has been estimated as 1 : 500 cases of strabismus. It may develop in any age but is the most frequent between 2 and 7 years of age. Cyclic esotropia is characterized by the alternate esotropia and eyes alignment in cycles every 24 to 48 hours. In orthoposition binocular vision and stereoscopy are normal, but they are disturbed during the cycle of deviation. Cyclic esotropia is usually progressive and esodeviation becomes permanent in the majority of cases after several months. Surgical therapy is effective in 75 to 90% of cases, and alignment is attained with a single operation. Very rare cases associated with central nervous system disease have been reported.

EXOTROPIA

Divergent strabismus (exotropia) is the disease in which outward deviation of the visual axes is seen. An onset of exotropia usually is late. Therefore, normal retinal correspondence and normal binocular vision with stereoscopy are present. There are three basic types of exotropia:

– Congenital exotropia.
– Intermittent exotropia.
– Constant exotropia.

Congenital Exotropia

This type is a rare condition. Most frequently it develops in children with congenital neurological abnormalities (cerebral palsy, craniofacial abnormalities, ocular albinism). Congenital exotropia is characterized by the large and constant angle of strabismus. In rare cases it is associated with larger refraction error. It frequently co-exists with V syndrome and DVD (Fig. 42).

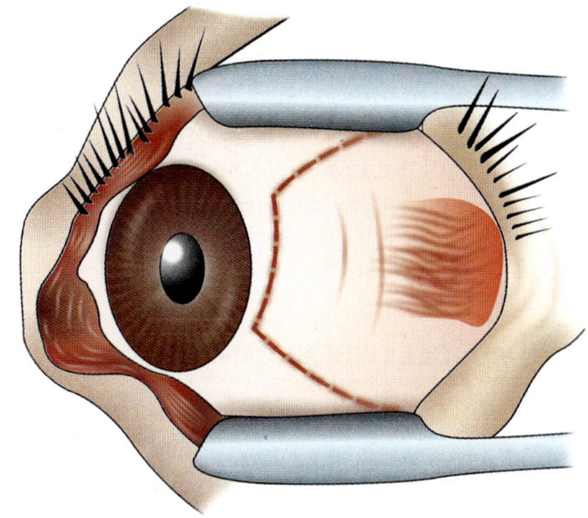

Fig. 54

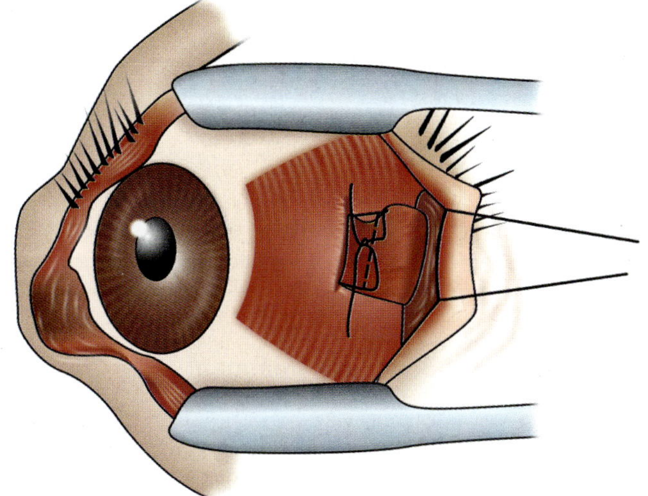

Fig. 57

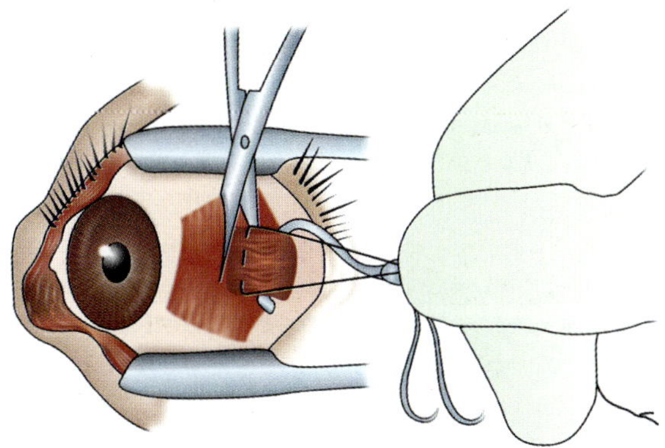

Fig. 55

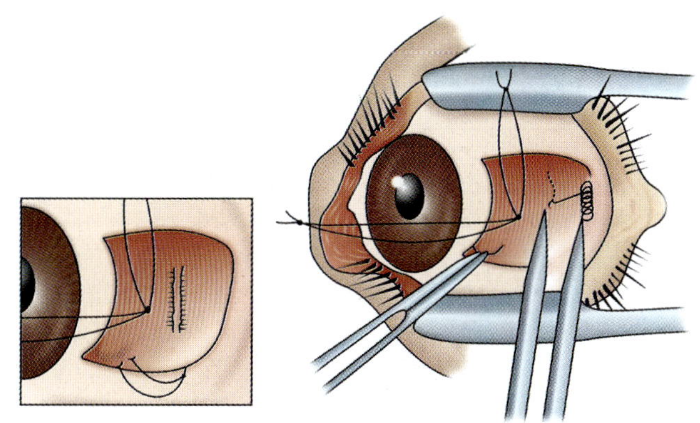

Fig. 58

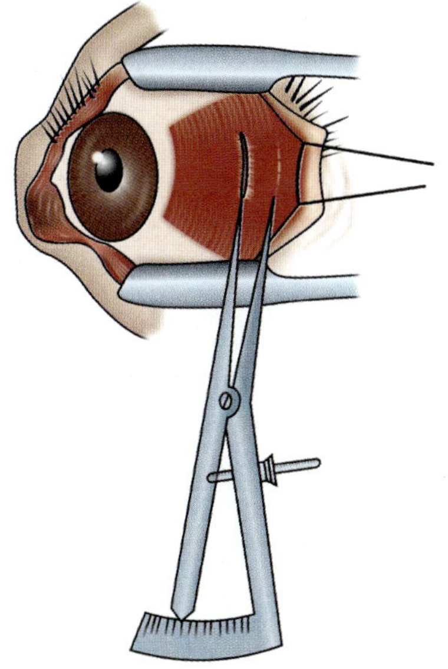

Fig. 56

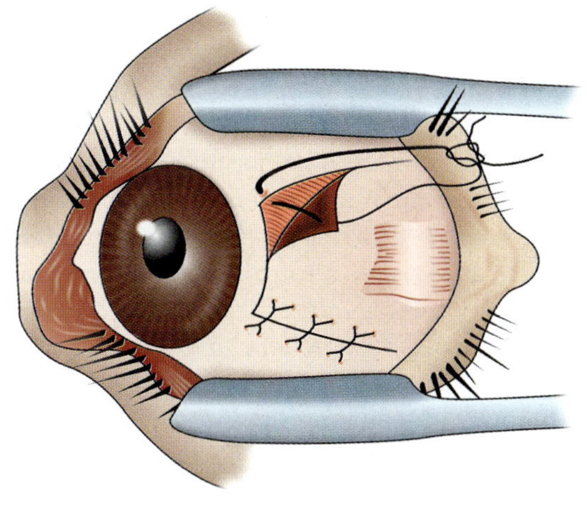

Fig. 59

Intermittent Exotropia

This type of exotropia is the most common type of exodeviation and it is often a progressive disease. Initially, marked exophoria is present and controlled by the fusion reflex. Fusion is often weak enough and disease or strong emotional or physical shocks may decompensated it, leading to divergent deviation. The long period of intermittent exotropia frequently leads to the constant exotropia.

Ocular Manifestations and Treatment

Intermittent exotropia may be classified into three types:

1. Basic intermittent exotropia, when distant and near deviations are nearly equal.
2. True divergence excess, which is characterized with distance deviation whereas at near fixation there is orthophoria with normal binocular vision. In the moment of eye deviation, with large angle of strabismus the most frequent is suppression or more rarely diplopia at small angle of strabismus.
3. Convergence insufficiency, concomitant divergent strabismus, when at distance fixation the eyes are aligned while at near fixation deviation with diplopia and fusion break. It often develops in teenagers, producing **astheopic symptoms**. In healthy men, near fusion point is about 5-8 cm whereas in exotropia it is even 10-30 cm. Range of fusion convergence is below 20 PD, and the norm is 30-35 PD. In many patients, there is no decreased convergence at the beginning of examination but on repeated testing they are easily fatigued.

Treatment

Effective treatment of the intermittent exotropia is confined to refractive correction and amblyopia therapy with obturation of the normal eye and pleoptic training. When equal visual acuity is achieved, deviation is treated with convergence exercises and orthoptic training, which aim to fix the fusion and to train convergence without excessive accommodation. Effective is also therapy with the use of prisms base-in, which neutralize the deviation, and exercises in hypercorrective prisms. Injections of the botulinum toxin are also beneficial, especially in case of variable angle of deviation. However, the prognosis is much poorer than in esotropia and dependent mainly on the child's age and duration of exotropia. Nonsurgical treatment is particularly beneficial in the convergence insufficiency. If the exercises alone do not restore the squint, surgical treatment is needed. In both intermittent and constant exotropia bilateral medial rectus muscles resection is performed, sometimes combined with unilateral or bilateral muscle recession of the lateral rectus, when the angle of strabismus is large, over 70 PD. In the true divergence excess the most frequently bilateral lateral rectus muscle recession or resection-recession of the muscles of one not fixing eye is performed.

OBLIQUE MUSCLE DYSFUNCTION

Unilateral or bilateral oblique muscle dysfunction comprises abnormal movements from the primary straight position to the tertiary position. Most frequently inferior oblique overactions primary or secondary to the superior oblique underaction are encountered. Inferior oblique underaction may also be combined with the superior oblique overaction. These abnormalities often co-exist with dissociated vertical divergence (DVD) or A-pattern or V-pattern syndromes.

About 50% of the horizontal strabismus cases are accompanied by the oblique dysfunction. Diagnosis of the oblique deviations are based on the detailed analysis of the eye movements, especially in the tertiary positions, Maddox rod test, examination with the Hess screening test, Bielschowsky test and forced duction test.

Inferior oblique overaction is the most frequent type of oblique deviations (Fig. 43).

It develops in case of even mild paresis superior oblique muscle or its underaction in the same eye. It is characterized by hyperdeviation in upgaze combined with excyclorotation and limitation of the downgaze in adduction. In unilateral disorders ocular torticollis is usually present to avoid diplopia. For example, if it is related to the right eye, head is tilted toward left shoulder, face is turned to the left, and chin is up. Bielschowsky head tilt test differentiates between the primary superior oblique muscle paresis and superior rectus muscle of the fellow eye paresis. Differentiation is of importance for the choice of surgical procedure.(Fig. 44)

Range and type of surgery depends on the size of deviation. The most frequent is weakening of the inferior oblique muscle, like a recession combined with anteriorization or myectomy.

Inferior oblique underaction is characterized by the limitation of elevation in adduction and incyclorotation. It develops spontaneously or more often with ipsilateral superior oblique overaction or contralateral inferior rectus palsy. To differentiate between oblique deviation and Brown's syndrome, forced duction test is performed.

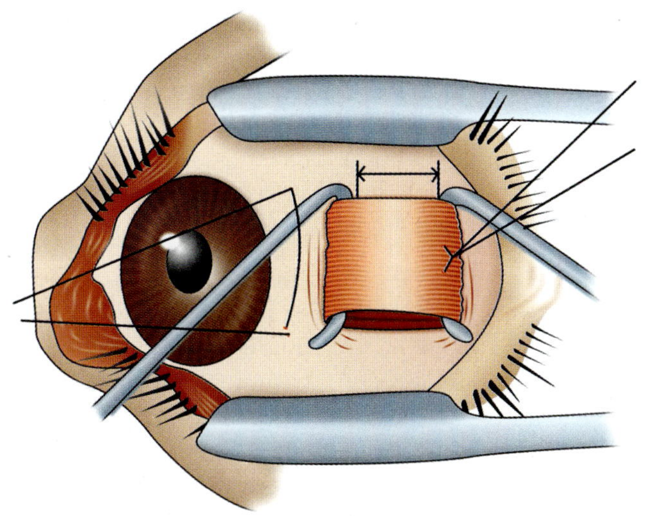

Fig. 60

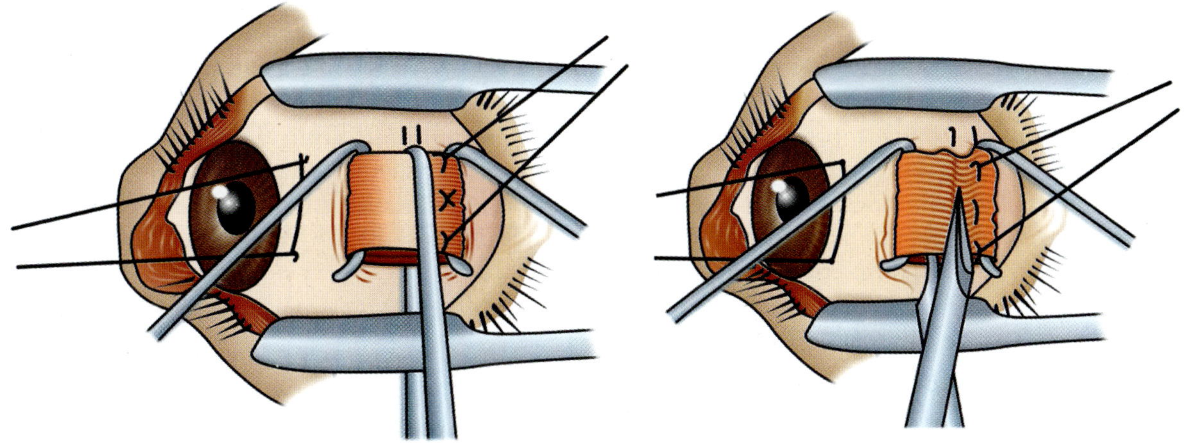

Fig. 61

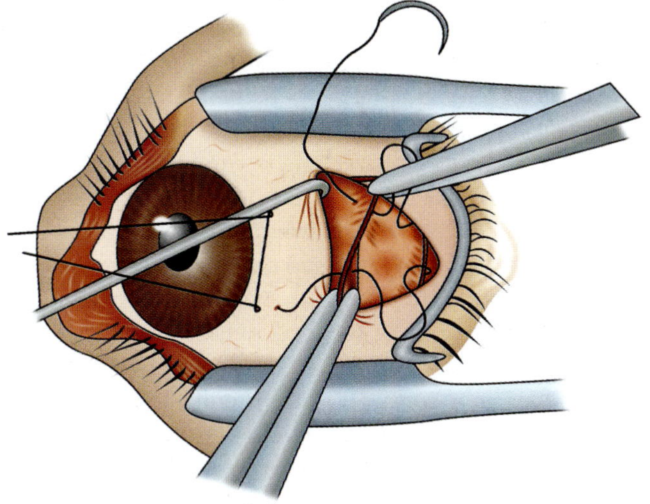

Fig. 62

Brown's syndrome is diagnosed if restriction of eye elevation in adduction or blockade of the superior oblique muscle in adduction is found.

The most effective is a surgery with the use of silicone tendon expander, recommended by Wright, allowing a controlled weakening of this muscle. Other clinicians recommend superior oblique tenotomy or superior oblique recession.

ALPHABET PATTERN STRABISMUS

Alphabet pattern strabismus is a horizontal deviation of the eyes: differing in upgaze from that in downgaze. There are two deviation patterns: A-pattern and V-pattern. Both may co-exist with orthotropia, esotropia or exotropia. Oblique muscles dysfunction is also frequent. They may be accompanied by deviations DVD. In the horizontal strabismus these deviations may be seen in 25% of cases.

V-pattern esotropia is characterized by more esodeviation in downgaze and often presents with a chin-down posture. Also high AC/A ratio and inferior oblique overaction is present.

V-pattern exotropia is much more exodeviation in upgaze and often presents with chin-up head posture. This form of alphabet pattern is more frequent and may be accompanied by the inferior oblique overactions. V-pattern syndrome is diagnosed, when difference from upgaze to downgaze is over 15 PD (Fig. 45). Binocular vision disorders are counteracted by the compensating head tilt.

Treatment

In V-pattern esotropia and V-pattern exotropia the lateral recti may be translated upward and the medial recti downward to a variable degree, if the function of oblique muscles is normal. Otherwise, inferior oblique overaction is reduced with the aid of weakening procedures.

A-pattern esotropia is esodeviation in which difference from the upgaze to downgaze is greater than 10 PD. It is characterized by the enlargement of the angle in upgaze with chin-up posture. In some patients overaction of the superior oblique muscle is present.

A-pattern exotropia is characterized by Lees exodeviation in upgaze and chin-down posture to maintain binocular vision. Difference from upgaze to downgaze is greater than 10 PD.

If the surgical treatment is indicated in A-pattern esotropia or A-pattern exotropia, superior oblique recession procedures and silicon tendon expander techniques have been available. If there is no superior oblique overaction, horizontal surgery along with lateral rectus translated downward, and translation of the medial rectus upward to a variable degree.

VERTICAL STRABISMUS FORMS

Hypertropia or hypotropia very rarely is a concomitant strabismus. Most frequently vertical deviations are secondary to dysfunction of other extraocular muscles, following muscular paresis or secondary to the surgical treatment of strabismus. Vertical deviations may present alone or concomitantly with the horizontal deviations. Dissociated vertical divergence (DVD) is a condition of dissociated strabismus complex involving movements in vertical, horizontal, and torsional planes. However, when the angle of strabismus develops in young children, is small and have prolonged duration, it may progress to the concomitant strabismus. In such cases it is characterized by all features of the concomitant strabismus and is subject to its laws (Hering, Scherington).

Incomitant vertical deviations are much more common than concomitant vertical deviations. Therefore, very important is the accurate differential diagnosis of both entities, first of all with the tests such as nine diagnostic gaze positions, duction and version testing.

CONCOMITANT STRABISMUS MANAGEMENT

Concomitant strabismus should be treated immediately after its detection, independent of the child's age. It is usually long-lasting process which requires a lot of patience and close cooperation of physician with the treated child and parents.

The treatment aims at achieving binocular vision at the full visual acuity with normal eyes alignment and motility. Full binocular vision comprises simultaneous perception, fusion with good amplitude, and stereoscopy with normal retinal correspondence. Naturally, the achievement of the ultimate goals of strabismus treatment is not always possible due to many reasons. Effective treatment requires the use of many procedures performed in the appropriate sequel: both nonsurgical and surgical.

Main principles of the strabismus treatment are the following:

1. Strabismus treatment should be started immediately after its detection.
2. The treatment aims at improving the vision in the deviating eye, producing central fixation and normal

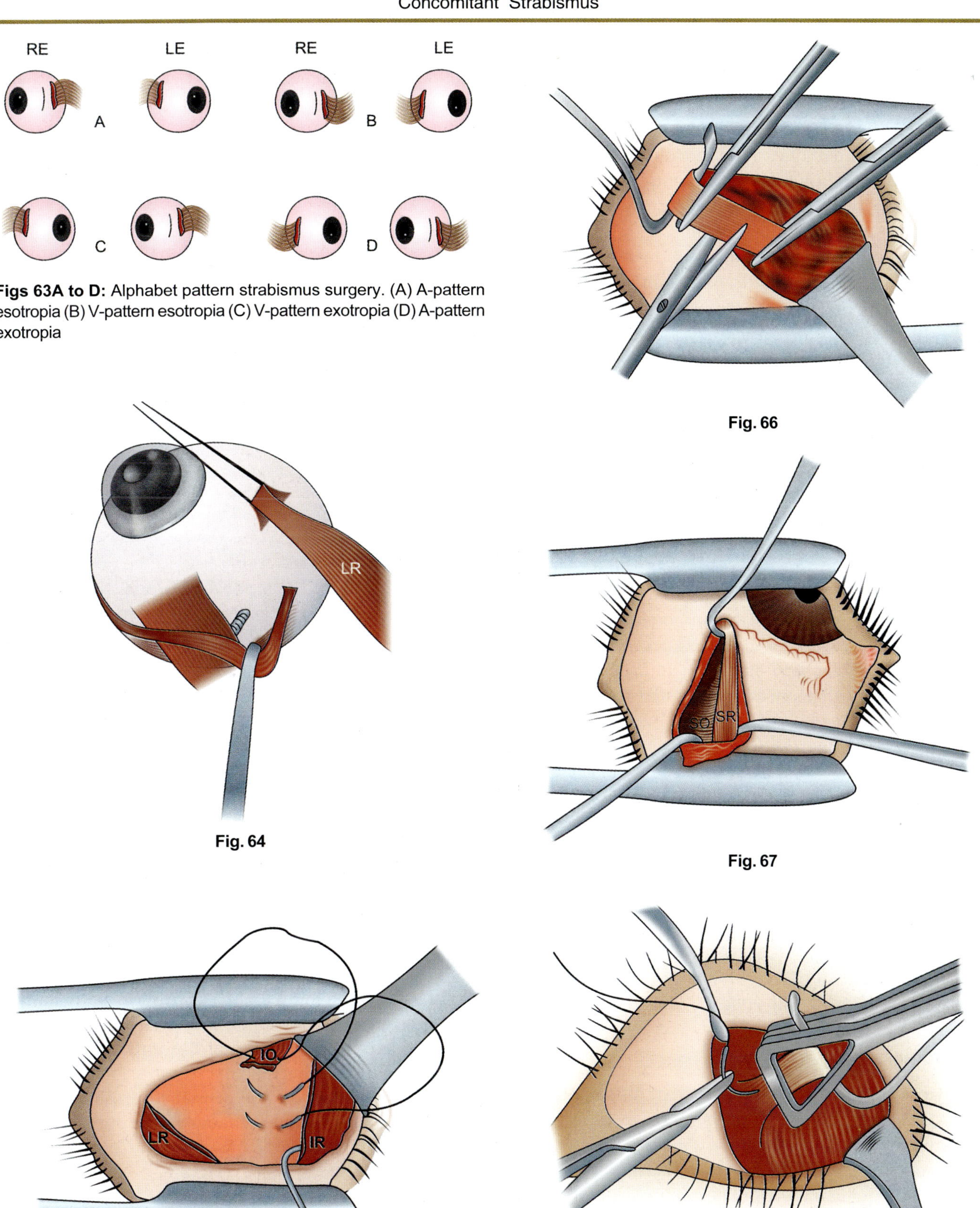

Figs 63A to D: Alphabet pattern strabismus surgery. (A) A-pattern esotropia (B) V-pattern esotropia (C) V-pattern exotropia (D) A-pattern exotropia

Fig. 64

Fig. 65

Fig. 66

Fig. 67

Fig. 68

visual localization with the aid of various therapeutical techniques.

3. Obtaining eye alignment with the use of prisms, botulinum toxin injections or surgery.
4. Ocular-motor exercises and binocular vision training in the adequate phase of treatment. These exercises aim to restore the normal retinal correspondence and binocular visual localization in the free space. An ultimate goal is achievement of the simultaneous perception and fusion with wide range and possibly stereoscopy.

NONSURGICAL STRABISMUS MANAGEMENT

Correction of Refraction Errors

Treatment of strabismus begins with the evaluation of refraction error and prescription of the appropriate spectacles or contact lenses. Refraction errors are the most common causes of the concomitant strabismus. Refraction is assessed with the automatic kerato-refractometer (in the younger children with Retinomax; (Fig. 21) following an application of 0.25 to 1% atropine eye drops for 3 days. This is necessary to paralyze accommodation.

Following refraction examination, fixation should be evaluated for each eye separately with the use of visuscope. Then, the anterior segment of each eye and eye fundus are evaluated.

Hypermetropia, myopia, and astigmatism are completely or nearly completely corrected to achieve good visual acuity and break pathological accommodative-convergence ratio. If anisometropia is present, especially more than 3 Dsph and 1.0 Dcyl, contact lenses are needed to allow the development of the binocular vision. As the rule, both contact lenses or spectacles should be worn permanently.

In some forms of the concomitant strabismus only wearing glasses is sufficient treatment. The best example is the accommodative esotropia.

Amblyopia

Amblyopia develops in children with anisometropia, unilateral concomitant strabismus or in case of the anatomical changes: congenital or acquired in the early childhood (congenital early-onset cataract, persistent hyperplastic primary vitreous, corneal opacity from glaucoma or dystrophy, lid masses, retinal dystrophy or inflammation). After treating anatomical changes, amblyopia ex anopsia is being treated.

Basic amblyopia therapy is the obturation of the sound eye that aims to force the fixation with deviating eye and improvement in the visual acuity in this eye. Obturation means not only total cover but also artificially weakened retinal image in one eye with the use of the visual acuity reductors (Bangerter's lenses) or penalizing method.

The best is total cover of the sound eye with special obturator, glued to the skin or, especially in the older children, use of appropriately color with black pupil soft contact lens (Figs 46 and 47).

The time of sound eye obturation is gradually shortened until the visual acuity has been the same in both eyes. In this stage of the treatment, visual acuity reductors from totally opaque to more and more transparent, changed with the improvement in the visual acuity in the amblyopic eye may be used or atropine solution may be applied.

Penalization Method

Penalization is a therapeutical method in which the sound eye has to be "punished" by the decrease in the visual acuity, which treats the amblyopia in the deviating eye, improves retinal correspondence and the angle of deviation. Classic penalizing method means that the fixing eye adapts to the distant vision only with the use of atropine and prescription of the corrective spectacles adjusted to the distant vision, dependent on the refraction error. Amblyopic eye is adapted to the near vision with the use of the stronger lens, adding +1 to +3.0 Dsph over complete refraction correction. With this therapy the child acquires proper binocular spatial orientation. Penalization decreases also accommodative factor that may lead to a decrease in or reduction of the angle of strabismus.

Some clinicians use different variations of the penalization method: penalization at near, at distance, complete, alternative, selective, reduced or maintaining.

Pleoptics

Additional treatments of amblyopia besides occlusion are pleoptic exercises. Their aim is to restore normal function of the deviating eye macula and domination over the peripheral retina so that macular suppression is removed, visual acuity improved and retinal correspondens,with good spatial localization is changed. Pleoptic techniques have been elaborated by Bangerter and Cuppers. In the treatment euthyscope is used.(Fig. 48).

It is a device with which orthoptist, observing eye fundus, dazzles peripheral retina with the place of anomalous fixation with simultaneous cover of the macula. Afterimage is produced with preserved macular

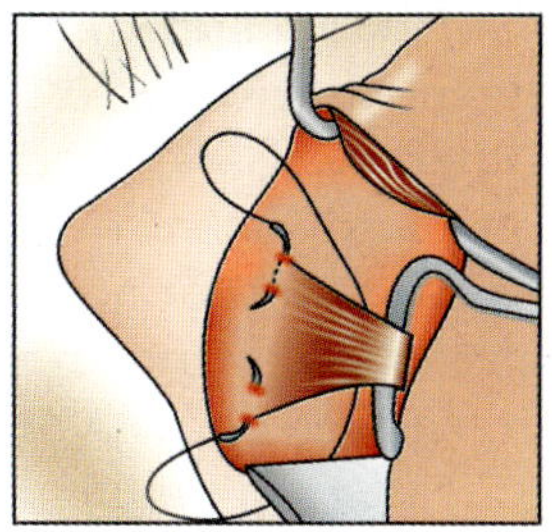

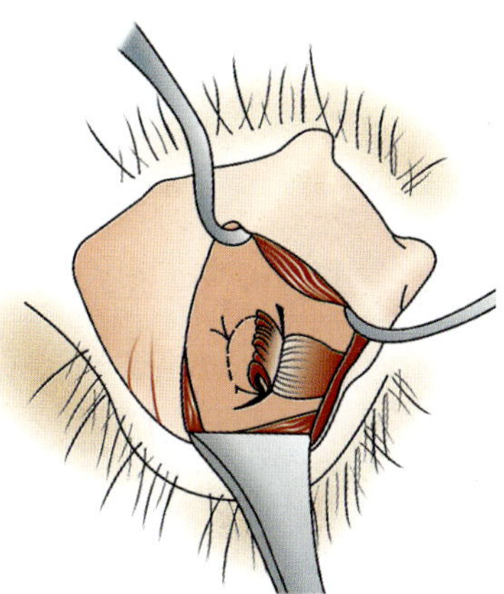

Fig. 69

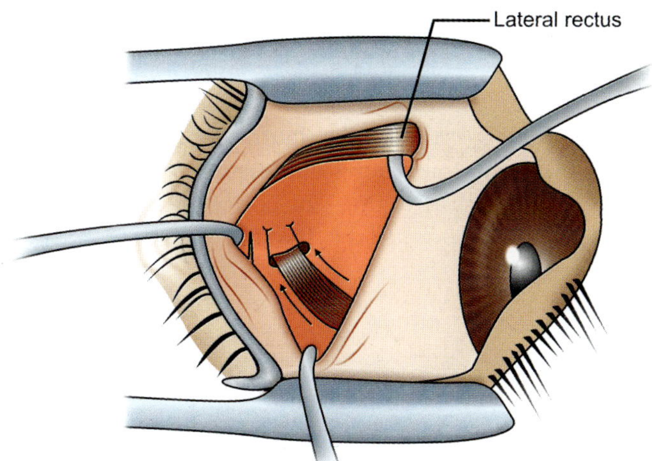

Fig. 70

vision, forcing the deviating eye to nearly central fixation. Localizing exercises of the deviating eye supplement the treatment. Haidinger phenomenon and Campbell apparatus are also used in the amblyopia treatment (Fig. 49).

Prisms

Immediately after the equalization of the visual acuity in both eyes and achievement of the central fixation, strabismus and anomalous retinal correspondence are treated. If the angle of strabismus is not large and does not exceed 20 PD, nonsurgical treatment may be started. To equalize the angle of strabismus, prisms of the strength equal to the angle of strabismus are used, with bases always directed inversely to the angle of deviation. In esotropia base-out prisms, in exotropia base-in prisms are used. Reduction of the angle of strabismus allows symmetrical stimulation of both retinas and formation of the normal binocular vision with normal straight binocular localization. As in the strabismus anomalous retinal correspondence is fixed, to dissociate fixed cortical pathways, prism hypercorrection is used. Hypercorrection prisms of the strength 2-6 times higher than the angle of strabismus are prescribed to the treated children. Alternatively covering the eyes, the child trains the vision at home. In such a way, pathological reflex leading to the persistent recurrence of strabismus is dissociated (Baranowska-George). However, the treatment is long-lasting and requires patience that is difficult to obtain in children.

Orthoptics

Binocular vision may be improved with the aid of orthoptic training. The treatment aims at restoring normal retinal correspondence and simultaneous foveal perception, fusion range, and sometimes stereoscopy. This training concerns first of all CNS. At the same time, exercises of the extraocular muscles are performed. Before the start of exercises, the eyes should be straighten with prisms, botulinum toxin injections or surgery. Straight eyes allow constant, symmetrical stimulation of the retinas of both eyeballs and fixation of the exercises effect in a free space under normal living conditions.

Simultaneous perception may be trained on synoptophore, using special images. Fusion amplitude is also trained with special, so-called fusional, images on synoptophore. Prism-bar may also be used for this purpose. Increasing the strength of prisms, diplopia is produced and so that fusion range in both convergence and divergence is widened (Fig. 50)

Other exercises, producing diplopia, also serve to fusion improvement, decrease in accommodation spasm and dissociation of accommodation and convergence, which is of importance in the treatment of accommodative esotropia. Stereograms, diploscope or reading with a rod (Fig. 51) are used for this purpose.

Exercises on cheiroscope are performed by the patients with suppression and normal retinal correspondence (Fig. 52) to remove suppression and stimulate binocular vision.

Stereoscopic exercises may be carried out on the synoptophore and various stereoscopes. Orthoptic exercises are indicated in case of all three stages of binocular vision insufficiency as well as the treatment of intermittent exotropia, deviations of the variable angle, in heterophorias. They are excellent visual rehabilitation following surgery.

Botulinum Toxin

Action of the botulinum toxin A, produced by anaerobic *Clostridium botulinum*, means relay on the blockade of acetylocholine release in presynaptic nerve endings in the neuro-muscular junction, paralyzing the muscle. In the eighties of the last century, Alan Scott introduced a method of concomitant and paralytic strabismus treatment. Injection of botulinum toxin into overactive muscle produces its temporary paresis or paralysis. Due to relaxation and elongation of the muscle overaction of its homolateral antagonist develops, leading to the positioning the eye in the contraposition to that in strabismus and temporary dissociation of the pathological reflex pathways with anomalous retinal correspondence. Scheme of the botulinum toxin action is shown in Figure 53. This method is effective, especially in the young children, as the achievement of eyes alignment in the binocular vision development process in infants facilitates fusion. These method of treatment is quick and safe for patient. There is always possibility to repeat injections or to perform surgery in cases of poor or without effect.

SURGICAL MANAGEMENT

The purpose of the concomitant strabismus surgical treatment is orthoposition with normal eyeballs motility. It allows single binocular vision with good fusion amplitude, reducing asthenoptic symptoms. Surgery frequently reduces abnormal head posture and improves patient's esthetic appearance. In the majority of cases, the objective of surgery is reduction of the constant static angle of strabismus with the aid of classic surgical techniques. Special surgical approach is needed in case of less frequent variable dynamic angle. To the surgical treatment of strabismus are qualified the patients in whom abnormal eyes position makes single binocular vision in the valuable segment of the visional field impossible and these in whom all nonsurgical methods of reducing eye deviations have failed.

Preoperative Evaluation and Diagnostic Approach

The most important examination is assessment of the angle of strabismus in the primary position when the patient looks at distance and near in both correction with spectacles and without it. Difference of the angle of strabismus at distance and near indicates anomalous AC/A ratio in the accommodative strabismus and the nystagmus blockage syndrome by convergence. After correction of the refractive error, indications to the surgery extend is frequently being decreased (accommodative esotropia, intermittent divergent deviation). Significant information is gained with measurements of the angle of strabismus at different positions of gaze. Increase or decrease in the upgaze or downgaze allows A-pattern or V-pattern syndromes diagnosis and taking it into consideration, when planning the surgery. Very important is also examination of eyeballs motility and deviation degree at nine diagnostic positions of gaze. Another examination is the forced duction test. Possible muscular contracture may thus be evaluated, allowing the choice of appropriate surgical technique. In case of the medial rectus muscle contracture, surgical strengthening lateral rectus muscle is required, followed by large recession of medial rectus muscle.

Evaluation of the lid slit is of esthetic importance. In case of narrow lid slit of the deviating eye, oculomotor muscle is slightly more weakened, leading to the protrusion of the eyeball, whereas at the wide lid slit an appropriate muscle is strengthend, and the eyeball is retracted.

Assessing indications to the surgery, binocular vision status is also taken into consideration. If after an operation there is possibility of the single binocular vision, a goals of it are straight eyes. Correction of small deviation or strabismus in adult patients may lead to the postoperative diplopia. Therefore, prism or biological test should be performed prior to surgery to exclude diplopia.

All diagnostic examinations are the base of patient qualification for the surgical treatment. Technique and extent of surgery should be established individually, depending upon the clinical findings.

How to establish the Extent of Surgery

There are various ways of establishing the extent of surgery. All provide only indicatory information. There are empirical rules and ways of calculation by how many millimeters muscles must be recessed or resected, depending on the angle of strabismus. Simple Stallard principle is frequently used: each millimeter recession or resection of the medial rectus muscle reduces the angle of strabismus by 4°, whereas each millimeter of the lateral rectus muscle recession or resection reduces the angle of strabismus by 2°. Combined surgery on two antagonist muscles is to increase the result by 20%. Cuppers thinks that muscle resection-recession ratio should be 2:1. Size of the eyeball should also be considered. If the eyeball is smaller, the same recession or resection gives considerably larger shortening of the arch of muscular contact with the eyeball in comparison with the eye of longer diameter.

In concomitant strabismus the best result of surgery with preservation of movements symmetry is, when the sum of retraction and pull to the opposite direction should be zero, and the same muscular tone as that before surgery is maintained.

Strabismus Surgery Techniques

Position of the eyes, dependent on the oculomotor muscles action, may be changed in two ways: muscle strengthening or weakening.

1. Weakening of the muscles:
   - Recession of muscle.
   - Elongation.
   - Myotomy.
   - Myectomy.
   - Posterior fixation suture.
2. Strengthening of muscle:
   - Resection of muscle.
   - Anteriorization.
   - Plication.

Rectus Muscles

To expose medial, lateral, superior, and inferior recti incision of the conjunctiva in the limbus with wing section in the quadrants encircling the muscle (Fig. 54). Then, sclera is exposed and Tenon's capsule is ruptured to introduce Graefe's muscular hook. The second Jameson's or square hook is introduced in order to precisely expose the muscle.

Table 3: Indications to the Surgery

Esotropia					
Symetrical surgery			*One eye surgery*		
ET angle	*Recess MR OU*	*or*	*Resect LR OU*	*Recess MR*	*and*	*Resect LR*
15 PD	3.o mm		4.0 mm	3.0 mm		4.0 mm
20 PD	3.5 mm		5.o mm	3.5 mm		5.0 mm
25 PD	4.0 mm		6.0 mm	4.0 mm		6.0 mm
30 PD	4.5 mm		7.0 mm	4.5 mm		7.0 mm
35 PD	5.0 mm		8.0 mm	5.0 mm		8.0 mm
40 PD	5.5 mm		8.0 mm	5.5 mm		8.0 mm
50 PD	6.0 mm		9.0 mm	6.0 mm		9.0 mm
Exotropia						
Symetrical surgery				*One eye surgery*		
XT angle	*Recess LR OU*	*or*	*Resect MR OU*	*Recess LR*	*and*	*Resect MR*
15 PD	4.0 mm		3.0 mm	4.0 mm		3.0 mm
20 PD	5.0 mm		4.0 mm	5.0 mm		4.0 mm
25 PD	6.0 mm		5.0 mm	6.0 mm		5.0 mm
30 PD	7.0 mm		6.0 mm	7.0 mm		6.0 mm
35 PD	7.5 mm			7.5 mm		6.0 mm
40 PD	8.0 mm			8.0 mm		6.5 mm
XT with profund amblyopia						
50 PD				9.0 mm		7.0 mm
60 PD				10.0 mm		8.0 mm
70 PD				10.0 mm		9.0 mm
80 PD				10.0 mm		10.0 mm

Insertion of the muscle onto the eyeball is being found after delicate removal of the muscle so that the Tenon's capsule is not damaged posteriorally. Recession or resection of the muscle is performed, depending on the form of strabismus.

Rectus Muscle Recession

Suture Vicryl 6.0 is placed on the muscle about 1 mm from its insertion into the sclera. Sutures are to be double knotted. Then, the muscle is cut off from the eyeball (Fig. 55).

Depending on the angle of strabismus, number of millimeters, by which the muscle needs to be recessed, are measured and new insertion is marked (Fig. 56).

Spatula needles from the double-armed sutures are passed to the sclera insertion line through half-thickness sclera. The needle should always be visible through the sclera to avoid accidental puncture (Fig. 57).

If adjustable sutures are used, a technique of the posterior fixation should be applied. In this procedure the needles are pulled backwards through the primary insertion and double knotted. Point corresponding to the recession of the muscle is measured on the sclera (Fig. 58).

Sutures are adjusted following several hours after surgery. Tightening or loosening of suture, orthoposition may be attained and diplopia prevented. The surgery is completed with suturing conjunctiva with single absorbable sutures 8.0 (Fig. 59).

Rectus Muscles Resection

After exposing the muscle, two hooks are applied to spread it flatly and widely (Fig. 60).

The number of millimeters of muscle shortening is measured with circle, and Vicryl 6.0 suture is placed on the muscle in the way described for muscle recession. Muscular fibers are crushed in their intersection with hemostat, and the muscle is cut off (Fig. 61).

Wescott's scissors are used to detach the muscle from the eyeball. Shortened muscle is very carefully resutured in the primary insertion site as the sclera is the thinnest under muscle insertion (Fig. 62). Sutures are knotted with 3-2-1 knots. Conjunctiva lying above is sutured with absorbable sutures 8.0.

Horizontal Muscle Transpositions for Alphabet Pattern Strabismus

Esotropia or exotropia may be accompanied by A-pattern or V-pattern deviations. If there is no underaction or overaction of the oblique muscles, beneficial for the decrease in the angle of strabismus is transposition of the horizontal muscles. The muscles are transposed vertically to strengthen or weaken their action at upgaze or downgaze. In the alphabet pattern strabismus one should remember that horizontal muscles are transposed to the direction requiring to be weakened.

In A-pattern esotropia both medial muscles should be recessed with transposition of their insertion upwards by 5-10 mm, whereas in V-pattern esotropia both medial muscles should be recessed with their insertions downwards (Fig. 63).

In V-pattern exotropia both lateral muscles are recessed and their insertions are transposed upwards, whereas in A-pattern exotropia both lateral muscles are recessed and transposed downward (Figs 63A to D)

Posterior Fixation Suture

This procedure is used to weaken horizontal recti. This technique, introduced by Cuppers, does not change the primary straight position of the eyes but weaken only motor activity of the muscle. Vicryl 6.0 sutures are placed 12-16 mm backwards the primary insertion of the muscle. Two U-shaped sutures are placed on the sclera and passed through the muscle, leaving its mid-portion to avoid blood vessels damage and perfusion decrease. This way, a new functional insertion is formed. This procedure is used in case of nystagmus, nystagmus blockage syndrome, DVD, strabismus of variable angle, and paralytic strabismus.

Inferior Oblique Muscle

Most frequently surgeries on the inferior oblique muscle are the procedures, which weaken the muscle: recession and myectomy.

Recession

To expose the inferior oblique muscle, conjunctiva is incised in the lower-temporal quadrant, about 8 mm from the limbus. Muscular fibers are isolated on the hook, and lateral and inferior recti are exposed (Fig. 64).

After suturing, the muscle is cut off with scissors from its insertion. Using Fink's localizer, which has a fork-shape of arms 6 mm long, being on the square, desired distance from the lower end of the lateral rectus muscle insertion is measured. Cut off muscle is resutured in this place (Fig. 65). Particular care is needed during this procedure due to adjacent macula.

Myectomy

The muscle is spread on two hooks, muscular fibers are crushed with hemostatic forceps, and the segment of muscle of about 8 mm long is being trimmed off. Cut ends of the muscle should carefully be coagulated. Myectomy is a simple and effective procedure in case of inferior oblique muscle overaction and also in DVD syndrome (Fig. 66).

Superior Oblique Muscle

Surgery on the superior oblique muscle is the most difficult. Proximity of the superior rectus muscle requires special caution during preparation of the muscle. Anatomy of the superior oblique tendon is different in the individual cases. Most safely, the superior oblique muscle is approached from the temple. Such an approach should be used for both muscle strengthening and weakening (Fig. 67).

Superior Oblique Tendon Plication

Superior oblique muscle underaction or paresis with accompanying excyclophoria is an indication to its strengthening. After exposing the muscle, its fibers are isolated on the hook and plicator is placed around the muscle (Fig. 68).

Size of plication is 8-15 mm, and plica is fixed with Vicryl 6.0 mattress suture. Thus, formed tendinous loop may be attached to the sclera (Fig. 69).

Modification of this procedure is transposition of the anterior segment of superior oblique muscle towards (Harada-Ito procedure) in cases with predominant excyclophoria with preserved movement downwards (Fig. 70).

Superior Oblique Tenotomy

In case of superior oblique muscle overaction with vertical disparation and incyclophoria the superior oblique muscle should be weakened. Most frequently tenotomy or posterior tenotomy with Wright silicone expander. The latter is particularly indicated in the treatment of Brown's syndrome.

Complications

Operative complications may relate anesthesia or surgical procedure. Most frequent are: hemorrhage, slip of the muscle from sutures and myostat or perforation of the sclera. Very rarely endophthalmitis or orbital cellulitis may develop. Conjunctival cyst, filled with clear liquid, may develop, when a fragment of the conjunctival epithelium will penetrate into the wound during its suturing. Sometimes, corneal throphic defects, so-called delle, appear, quickly covering with the epithelium within few days.

Postoperative complications include first of all overcorrection or undercorrection of deviation being treated nonsurgically. The patient should always be worn about such a complication before surgery. Anterior segment ischemic syndrome may result from the operation on multiple muscles of one eye. It is treated with topical and oral corticosteroids.

Diplopia after surgical treatment of strabismus is seen relatively often. Children rapidly overcome diplopia, forming the new area of suppression. Contrary to the adult patients, diplopia is children is not so annoying. In adults, prism test should always be performed before surgery to evaluate diplopia subjectively. It is also worth prescribing prisms glasses correcting the angle of strabismus to enable the patient making decision on surgery following shorter or longer wear of prismatic spectacles. Some clinicians administer botulinum toxin injections for the same purpose.

Outcomes

Children after strabismus surgical treatment are given antibiotic eye ointment and dressing is applied for 12-24 hours. Eye drops with antibiotic, sometimes combined with corticosteroids, are inserted into the operated eye for the consecutive 1-2 weeks. Patients should be carefully followed up for the first postoperative weeks to be assured that the infection or recurrent strabismus did not develop.

In order to increase higher efficacy and stability of surgery, adequate rehabilitation exercises should be performed immediately. These exercises ensure full motility of the operated muscles and facilitate attainment of the normal binocular vision.

FURTHER READING

1. Anderson JR. Latent nystagmus and alternating hyperphoria. Br J Ophthalmol 1954;38:217-31.
2. Atkinson J. Development of optokinetic nystagmus in the human infant and monkey infant: an analogue to development in kittens. In Freeman RD (Eds.): Developmental Neurobiology of Vision. New York, Plenum Press 1979.
3. Archer SM, Sondhi N, Helveston EM. Strabismus in infancy. Ophthalmology 1989;96:133-7.
4. Arthur BW, Smith JT, Scott WE. Long-term stability of alignment in the monofixation syndrome. J Pediatr Ophthalmol Strabismus 1989;26:224-31.
5. Baker JD, Parks MM. Early onset accommodative 1 esotropia. Am J Ophthalmol 1980;90:111 .
6. Baranowska-George T:Hypercorrection prismatique dans le traitement du symtome de surconvergence paraissant dans les strabismes convergents. Arch.Opht.(Paris) 1968;28:745-50.
7. Barlow HB, Blakemore C, Pettigrew JP. The neural mechanism of binocular depth discrimination. J Physiol (London) 1967;193:327-42.
8. Bechtoldt HP, Hutz CS. Stereopsis in young infants and stereopsis in an infant with congenital esotropia. J Pediatr Ophthalmol Strabismus 1979;16:49-54.
9. Benson PF. Transient unilateral external rectus muscle palsy in newborn infants. Br Med J 1962;1:1054-5.
10. Birch EE, Stager DR, Berry P, Everett ME. Prospective assessment of acuity and stereopsis in amblyopic infantile esotropes following early surgery. Invest Ophthalmol Vis Sci 1990;31:758-65.
11. Birch EE, Gwiazda J, Held R. Stereoacuity development of crossed and uncrossed disparities in human infants. Vision Res 1982;22:507.
12. Blakemore C, Cummings RM. Eye opening in kittens. VisionRes 1975;15:1417-8.
13. Blakemore C, Van Sluyters RC. Experimental analysis of amblyopia and strabismus. Br J Ophthalmol 1974; 58:176- 82.
14. Bower TGR. The object in the world of the infant. ScientificAm 1971;225:30-8.
15. Braddick O, et al. Cortical binocularity in infants. Nature 1980; 288:363-5.
16. Breinin GM. The nature of vergence revealed by electromyography. Arch Ophthalmol 1957;58:623-31.
17. Brown B. The convergence insufficiency masquerade. Am Orthoptic J 1990;40:94-7.
18. Buckley E, Seaber JH. Dyskinetic strabismus as a sign of cerebral palsy. Am J Ophthalmol 1981;91:652-7.
19. Burian HM, Smith DR. Comparative measurement of exodeviations at 30 and 100 feet. Trans Am Ophthalmol Soc 1971;69:188-99.
20. Burian HM, Spivey BE. The surgical management of exodeviations. Am J Ophthalmol 1965;59:603.
21. Campos EC. Binocularity in comitant strabismus:Binocular visual field studies. Doc Ophthalmol 1982;53:249.
22. Caputo AR, Guo S, Wagner R, Picciano MV. Preferred postoperative alignment after congenital esotropia surgery. Ann Ophthalmol 1990;22:269-72.
23. Cianda A. La esotropia en el lactante, diagnostico Y tratarniento. Arch Chil Oftalmol 1962;9:117.
24. Cheng KP, Hiles DA, Biglan AW, Pettapiece MC. Visual results after early surgical treatment of unilateral congenital cataract. Ophthalmology 1991;98:903-10.
25. Chimonidou E, Palimeris G, Koliopoulos J, Velissaropoulos Z. Family distribution of concomitant squint in Greece. Br J Ophthalmol 1977;61:27-9.
26. Chin NV, Gold AA, Breinin GM. Iris cysts and miotics. Arch Ophthalmol 1964;71:611.

27. Chrousos GA, O'Neill JF, et al. Accommodative deficiency in healthy young adults. J Pediatr Ophthalmol Strabismus 1988;25:176-9.
28. Cole MD, Hay A, Eagling EM. Cyclic esotropia in a patient with unilateral traumatic aphakia: case report. Br J Ophthalmol 1988;72:305-9.
29. Costenbader FD. Infantile esotropia. Trans Am Ophthalmol Soc 1961;59:397.
30. Crandall MA, Gerhard WC, Ellerhorst B. CAM (stripe) therapy for amblyopia, Perspec Ophthalmol 1981;5:51-55.
31. Crawford MLJ, Smith EL, Harwerth RS, von Noorden GK. Stereoblind monkeys have few binocular neurons. Invest Ophthalmol Vis Sci 1984;25:779-81.
32. Crawford MLJ, von Noorden GK. The effects of short-term experimental strabismus on the visual system in macaca mulatta. Invest Ophthalmol Vis Sci 1979;18:496-505.
33. Crawford MLJ, von Noorden GK. Optically induced concomitant strabismus in monkeys. Invest Ophthalmol Vis Sci 1980;19:1105.
34. Crone RA, Velzeboer CM J. Statistics on strabismus in the Amsterdam youth. Arch Ophthalmol 1956;55:455-70.
35. Cross HE, The heritablity of strabismus. Am Orthopt J 1975; 25:11-7.
36. Cynader M, Berman N, Hein A. Recovery of function in cat visual cortex following prolonged deprivation. Exp Brain Res 1976;25:139-56.
37. Cynader M. Prolonged sensitivity to monocular deprivation in dark-reared cats: effects of age and visual exposure. Dev Brain Res 1983;8:155-64.
38. Dayton GO, Jones MH, Steele B, Rose M. Developmental study of co-ordinated eye movements in the human infant. Arch Ophthalmol 1964;71:871-5.
39. Dell'Osso LF, Schmidt D, Daroff RB. Latent, manifest latent, and congenital nystagmus. Arch Ophthalmol 1979;97:1877-85.
40. Diamond GR, Katowitz JA, Whitaker LA, Quinn GE, Schaffer DB. Variations in extraocular muscle number and structure in craniofacial dysostosis. Am J Ophthalmol 1980;90:416-8.
41. Diamond GR:Strabismus,In:Ophtalmology, Mosby St.Louis, 2004;549-634.
42. Dickey CF, Metz HS, Stewart SA. The diagnosis of amblyopia in cross-fixation. J Pediatr Ophthalmol Strabismus 1991; 28:171-5.
43. Duane A. Studies in monocular and binociflar accommodation with their clinical applications. Am J Ophthalmol 1922;5:865-77.
44. Ellis FD, Schlaegel TF. Unexpected visual recovery: organic amblyopia? Am Orthoptic J 1991;31:7.
45. Fawer CL, Calarne A, Furrer M-T. Neurodevelopmental outcome at 12 months of age related to cerebral ultrasound appearances of high risk preterm infants. Early Hum Dev 1985; 11:123-32.
46. Fells P, Waddell E, Alvares M. Progressive, exaggerated A-pattern strabismus with presumed fibrosis of extraocular muscles. In: Reinecke RD (Ed): Strabismus II:Proceedings of the Fourth Meeting of The International Strabismological Association. Grune & Stratton, Orlando 1984;335-43.
47. Fink WE. The role of developmental anomalies in vertical muscle defects.' Am J Ophthalmol 1955;40:529-33.
48. Fitzgerald BA, Billson FA. Dissociated vertical deviation: evidence for abnormal visual pathway projection. Br J Ophthalmol 1984;68:801-6.
49. Fletcher MC, Silverman SJ, Boyd J, Callaway M. Biostatistical studies: comparison of the management of amblyopia by conventional patching, intensive hospital pleoptics, and intermittent office pleoptics. Am Orthopt J 1969;19-40.
50. Fox F, Albin RN, Shea SL, Dumais ST. Stereopsis in human infants. Science 1980;207:323-4.
51. France TD. The association of A pattern strabismus with hydrocephalus. Trans 3rd Int Orthoptic Congress 1975;287-92.
52. Francois J. Heredity in Ophthalmology. CV Mosby Co., St Louis 1961;255-69.
53. Friedman L, Biedner B, David R, Sachs V. Screening for refractive errors, strabismus and other ocular anomalies from ages 6 months to 3 years. J Pediatr Ophthalmol Strabismus 1980; 17:315-7.
54. Garey LJ, De Courten C:Structural development of the lateral geniculate nucleus and visual cortex in monkey and man. Behav Brain Res 1983;10:3-13.
55. Gobin MH. Sagittalization of the oblique muscles as a possible cause for the 'A', 'V, and 'X' phenomena. Br J Ophthalmol I968;52:13-8.
56. Gunter K, Von Noorden GK, Wong SY. Surgical results in nystagmus blockage syndrome. Ophthalmology 1986; 93:1028-32.
57. Harcourt B. Strabismus affecting children with multiple handicaps. Br J Ophthalmol 1974;58:272-9.
58. Harcourt B, Mein J, Johnson F. Natural history and associations of dissociated vertical divergence. Trans Ophthalmol Soc UK 1980;100:495-7.
59. Hardesty H. Management of intermittent exotropia. BinocVis Quart 1990;5:145.
60. Helveston EM. A-exotropia, alternating sursumduction and superior oblique overaction. Am J Ophthalmol 1969;67:377-80.
61. Helveston EM, Von Noorden GK. Microtropia: a newly dennedentity. Arch Ophthalmol 1967;78:272-81.
62. Helveston EM, Ellis FD, Plager DA, Miller KK. Early surgery for essential infantile esotropia. J Pediatr Ophthalmol Strabismus 1990;27:115-9.
63. Henderson JW, Iacobucci I. Occlusion in the preoperative treatment of exodeviations. Am Orthopt J 1965;15:42.
64. Hendrickson AE, Movshon JA, Eggers HM, et al. Effects of early unilateral blur on the macaque's visual system, II: anatomical observations. J Neurosci 1987;7:1327-39.
65. Hermann JS. Surgical therapy for convergence insufficiency. J Pediatr Ophthalmol Strabismus 1981;18:28.
66. Hiles DA, Davies GT, Costenbader FD. Long-term observations on unoperated intermittent exotropia. Arch Ophthalmol 1968; 80:436-42.
67. Hiles DA, Watson BA, Biglan AW. Characteristics of infantile esotropia following early bimedial rectus recession. Arch Ophthalmol 1980;98:697-703.
68. Hotchkiss MD, Miller NR, Clark AW, Green WR. Bilateral Duanes Retraction Syndrome. Arch Ophthalmol 1980; 98:870-4.
69. Hoyt CS. Nystagmus compensation (blockage) syndrome. Am J Ophthalmol 1977;83:423-4.

70. Hoyt CS. Abnormalities of the vestibulo-ocular response incongenital esotropia. Am J Ophthalmol 1982; 93:704-8.
71. Hoyt CS, Caltrider N. Hemispheric visually-evoked responses in congenital esotropia. J Pediatr Ophthalmol Strabismus 1984; 21:19-21.
72. Hoyt CS, Jastrebski GB, Marg E. Amblyopia and congenital esotropia visually evoked potential measurements. Arch Ophthalmol 1984;102:58-61.
73. Hubel DN, Wiesel TN. The period of susceptibility to the physiological effects of unilateral eye closure in kittens. J Physiol (London) 1970;206:419-36.
74. Ikeda H, Tremain K. Amblyopia and cortical binocularity. Trans Ophthalmol Soc UK 1980;100:452.
75. Ing MR. Early surgical alignment for congenital esotropia. Ophthalmology 1983;90:132-5.
76. Ing MR. Early surgical alignment for congenital esotropia. Trans Am Ophthalmol Soc 1981;79:625-63.
77. James R. Combined superior oblique muscle tendon resection and inferior oblique muscle recession for dissociated vertical deviation: A report of 25 cases. Binocular Vision 1987;2:137-51.
78. Jampolsky A. Ocular Deviations. Int Ophthalmol Clin 1964; 4:567-701.
79. Keith CG, Kitchen WH. Ocular morbidity in very low birth-weight infants. In: Reinecke RD (Ed): Strabismus II: Proceedings of the Fourth Meeting of the International Strabismological Association. Grune & Stratton, Orlando 1984;45-53.
80. Knapp P. A, V patterns. In: Dabezier OH (Ed): Symposium on Strabismus. CV Mosby 1971;St Louis pp. 242-54.
81. Kriss A, Timms C, Elston J, Taylor D. Pattern - and flash - evoked potentials in patients with dissociated vertical deviation. Doc Ophthalmol 1988;69:283-91.
82. Krzystkowa K, et al. Strabismus disorders, PZWL,. Warsaw 1997.
83. Krzystkowa K. The surgery of oculomotor muscles. In: Or?owski W (ed.): Modern ophthalmalmology, PZWL, Warsaw 1992;3:550-80.
84. Kushner BJ. The Role of Ocular torsion on the etiology of A+ V patterns. J Pediatr Ophthalmol Strabismus 1985;22:171-9.
85. Kushner BJ. Exotropic deviations: A functional classification and approach to treatment. Am Orthoptic J 1988;38:81-93.
86. Leguire LE, Rogers GL, Bremer DL. Visual-evoked response binocular summation in normal and strabismic infants. Invest Ophthalmol Vis Sci 1991;32:126-33.
87. Lewis TL, Maurer D, Brent HP. Effects of perceptual development of visual deprivation during infancy. Br J Ophthalmol 1986;70:214-20.
88. Ludwig IH, Parks MM, Getson PR, Kammerman LA. Rate of deterioration in accommodative esotropia correlated to the AC/A relationship. /Pediatr Ophthalmol Strabismus 1988; 25:8-13.
89. Ludwig IH, Parks MM, Getson PR. Long-term results of bifocal therapy for accommodative esotropia. J Pediatr Ophthalmol Strabismus 1989;26:264-70.
90. Magoon E. Chemodenervation of strabismic children. Ophthalmology 96:931-934 1989.ular optokinetic nystagmus in infants. Vis Res 1982;22:341.
91. Margolis S, Pachter BR, Breinin GM. Structural alterations of extraocular muscle associated with Apert's Syndrome. Br J Ophthalmol 1977;61:683-9.
92. Mazow ML, Musgrove K, Finkelman S. Acute accommodative and convergence insufficiency. Am Orthoptic J 1991;41:102-9.
93. McKusick VA. Mendelian Inheritance in Man. Johns Hopkins University Press, Baltimore & London 1978;359-60.
94. Moore S. The prognostic value of lateral gaze measurements in intermittent exotropia. Am Orthop J 1969;19:69.
95. Nashold BS, Seaber JH. Defects of Ocular motility after stereotactic midbrain lesions in Man. Arch Ophthalmol 1972; 88:245-8.
96. Nawratzi I, Jampolsky A. A regional hemiretinal difference in amblyopia. Am J Ophthalmol 1958;46:339.
97. Nixon RB, Helveston EM, Miller K, Archer SM Ellis FD. Incidence of strabismus in neonates. Am J Ophthalmol 1985; 100:798-801.
98. Olitsky SE,NelsonLB :Strabismus disorders:In Pediatric ophthalmology (ed.NelsonLB), Harley,'s,Philadelphia 1998;146-190.
99. Oliver M, et al. Compliance and results of treatment for amblyopia in children more than 8 years old. Am J Ophthalmol 1986;102:340-5.
100. Parks MM. Abnormal accommodative convergence in squint. Arch Ophthalmol 1958;59:364-80.
101. Parks MM. The overacting inferior oblique muscle. The XXXVI de Schweinitz Lecture. Am J Ophthalmol 1974;77:787-97.
102. Parks MM. Concomitant exodeviations. In Ocular motility and strabismus. New York 1975, Harper and Row, p. 113.
103. Parks MM. The monofixational syndrome. Trans Am Ophthalmol Soc 1969;67:609-57.
104. Parks MM. Congenital esotropia with a bifixation result, report of a case. Documenta Ophthalmologica 1984;58:109-14.
105. Pratt-Johnson JA. Central disruption of fusional amplitude. Br J Ophthalmol 1973;57:347-50.
106. Pratt-Johnson JA, Barlow JM, Tillson G. Early surgery in intermittent exotropia. Am J Ophthalmol 1977;84:689-94.
107. Pratt-Johnson JA, Tillson G. Acquired central disruption of fusional amplitude. Ophthalmology 1979, 86:2140.
108. Pratt-Johnson JA, Tillson G. Sensory outcome with non-surgical management of esotropia with convergence excess (A high accommodative convergence/accommodation ratio). Can J Ophthalmol 1984;19:220-3.
109. Prieto-Diaz J. Large bilateral medial rectus recession in early esotropia with bilateral limitation of abduction. J Pediatr Ophthalmol Strabismus 1980;17:101-5.
110. Prism Adaptation Research Group. Efficacy of prism adaptation in the surgical management of acquired esotropia. Arch Ophthalmol 1990;108:1248-56.
111. Raab E. Refractive amblyopia. Intl Ophthalmol Clin 1971; 11:155.
112. Rakic P. Prenatal genesis of connections subserving ocular dominance in rhesus monkey. Nature 1976;261:467.
113. Rabinowitz IM. Visual function in children with hydrocephalus. Trans Ophthalmol Soc UK 1974;104:353-65.
114. Reinecke RD, (ed.) Strabismus II: Proceedings of the 4th Meeting of the International Strabismological Association. Grune & Stratton, Orlando 1984;363-9.
115. Repka MX, Ray JM. The efficacy of optical and pharmacological penalization. Ophthalmology 1993;100:769-75.
116. Reisner SH, Perlman M, Bentovim N, Dubrawski C. Transient lateral rectus muscle paresis in the newborn infant. J Pediatr 1971;78:461-65.

117. Richard JM, Parks MM. Intermittent exotropia: Surgical results in different age groups. Ophthalmology 1983;90:172.
118. Ruttum M, Von Noorden GK. Orbital and facial arthropmetry in A and V pattern strabismus.
119. Schor CM, Levi DL. Disturbances of small field horizontal and vertical optokinetic nystagmus on amblyopia. Invest Ophthalmol Vis Sci 1980;19:668.
120. Scott WE. Temporary surgical overcorrection of infantile esotropia. Trans New Orleans Academy of Ophthalmology. New York 1986, Raven Press.
121. Scott WE, Keech R, Mash J. The postoperative results and stability of exodeviations. Arch Ophthalmol 1981, 99:1814.
122. Simons K, Reinecke RD. Amblyopia screening and stereopsis. In: Transactions of the New Orleans Academy of Ophthalmology. St Louis, CV Mosby 1978;15-50.
123. Sondhi N, Archer SM, Helveston EM. Development of normal ocular alignment. J Pediatr Ophthalmol Strabismus 1988, 25:210-211.
124. Stanworth A. Defects of ocular movement and fusion after head injury. Br J Ophthalmol 1974;58:266-71.
125. Starkiewicz W. Le methode localisatrice du traitment du strabisme. Bull Soc Franc Ophthalmol 1956, 69:343-347.
126. Steinberg M, Rendle-Short J. Vestibular dysfunction in young children with minor neurological impairment. Dev Med Child Neurol 1977;19:639-51.
127. Tamler E, Jampolsky A. Is divergence active? An electromyographic study. Am J Ophthalmol 1967;63:452-9.
128. Taylor DSI, Vaegan, Morris JA, Rogers RG, Warland J. Amblyopia in bilateral infantile and juvenile cataract. Trans Ophthalmol Soc UK 1979;99:170-5.
129. Timney B, Mitchell DE, Giffin F. The development of vision in cats after extended periods of dark-rearing. Exp Brain Res 1978;31:547-60.
130. Tsutsui J, Fukai S. Human Strabismic Cases Suggestive of asymmetric Projection of the visual pathway. In. Reinecke RD (Ed): Strabismus Proceedings of the Third Meeting of the International Strabismological Association. Grune & Stratton, New York 1978;79-88.
131. Tychen L and Lisberger SG. Maldevelopment of visual motion processing in humans who had strabismus with onset in infancy. J Neurosci 1986;6:2495-2508.
132. Tychsen L. Binocular vision. In Hart WM (Ed): Adlers Physiology of the Eye: Clinical Applications, 9th ed. St. Louis 1992, CV Mosby.
133. Urist MJ. The aetiology of the so-called A and V syndrome. Am J Ophthalmol 1958;46:835-44.
134. van Essen DC, Maunsell JHR. Hierarchical organization and functional streams in the visual cortex. Trends Neurosci 1983; 6:370-95.
135. Vereecken EP, Brabant P. Prognosis for vision in amblyopia after the loss of the good eye. Arch Ophthalmol 1984;102:220.
136. Werner DB., Scott WE. Amblyopia case reports-bilateral hypermetropic ametropic amblyopia. J Pediatric Ophthalmol Strabismus 1985;22:203-5.
137. Westall CA, Schor CM. Asymmetries of optokinetic nystagmus in amblyopia: the effect of selected retinal stimulation. Vision Res 1985;25:1431-8.
138. Westall Carol A, Woodhouse JM, Brown VA. OKN asymmetries and binocular function in amblyopia. Ophthalmol Physiol Opt 19899;269-76.
139. Wiggins RE, von Noorden GK. Monocular eye closure in sunlight. J Pediatr Ophthalmol Strabismus 1990;27:16.
140. Wiesel TN, Hubel DN. Effects of visual deprivation on morphology and physiology of cells in the cat's lateral geniculate body. J Neurophysiol 1963;26:978-93.
141. Wiesel TN, Hubel DN. Extent of recovery from the effects of visual deprivation in kittens. J Neurophysiol 1965(3);28:1060-72.
142. Wiesel TN, Hubel DN. Ordered arrangement of ocular dominance columns in monkeys lacking visual experience. J Comp Neurol 1974;158:307-18.
143. Wilczek M, Srzednicka K. Das Gesichtsfeld beim Schielen.Klin.Mbl.Augenhk 1964 145:713-6.
144. Wilczek M, Krzystkowa K. Strabismus management, PZWL, Warsaw 1971.
145. Wilson ME, Parks MM. Primary inferior oblique overaction in congenital esotropia, accommodative esotropia and intermittent exotropia. Ophthalmology 1989, 96:950-5.
146. von Noorden GK, Isaza A, Parks MM. Surgical treatment of congenital esotropia, Trans Am Acad Ophthalmol Otolaryngol 1979;76:1465.
147. von Noorden GK. Some aspects of exotropia. Paper presented before Meeting of Wilmer Resident's Association, Johns Hopkins Hospital. April 26 1966.
148. von Noorden GK. Divergence excess and simulated divergence excess. Diagnosis and surgical management. Ophthalmologica 1969;26:719.
149. von Noorden GK. Resection of both medial rectus muscles in organic convergence insufficiency. Am J Ophthalmol 1976;81:223-5.
150. von Noorden GK. Binocular vision and ocular motility. Theory and management of strabismus. St. Louis 1985, CV Mosby, p. 310.
151. von Noorden GK, Brown DJ, Parks M. Associated convergence and accommodative insufficiency. Doc Ophthalmol 1973; 34:393-403.
152. Von Noorden GK. Factors involved in the production of amblyopia. Br J Ophthalmol 1974;58:158-64.
153. Von Noorden GK. The nystagmus compensation (blockage) syndrome. Am J Ophthalmol 1976;82:283-90.
154. Von Noorden GK. Current concepts of infantile esotropia. Eye 1988;2:343-58.
155. Von Noorden GK, Avilla CW. Nystagmus Blockage Syndrome Revisited. In: Reinecke RD (ed.) Strabismus II: Proceedings of the fourth meeting of the International Strabismological Association. Grune & Stratton, Orlando 1984;75-82.
156. Von Noorden GK, Wong GM. Surgical results in nystagmus blockage syndrome. Ophthalmology 1986; 93:1028-31.
157. von Noorden GK, Crawford MLJ, Levacy RA. The lateral geniculate nucleus in human anisometropic amblyopia. Invest Ophthalmol Vis Sci 1983;24:788-90.
158. von Noorden GK, Crawford MLJ. The effects of total unilateral occlusion vs. lid suture on the visual system of infant monkeys. Invest Ophthalmol Vis Sci 1981;21:142-6.
159. Wright KW, Min BM, Park C. Comparison of superior oblique tendon expander to superior oblique tenotomy for the management of superior oblique overaction and Brown syndrome. J Pediatr Ophthalmol Strabismus 1992;29(2):92-7.
160. Wright KW:Strabismus and amblyopia In Pediatric ophthalmology and strabismus (ed.Wright KW) Mosby,St,louis 1995;89-209.

161. Wright KW, Bruce-Lyle L. Augmented surgery for esotropia associated with high hypermetropia. J Pediatr Ophthalmol Strabismus 1993;30:167-70.
162. Wright KW, Edelman PM, Terry A, et al. High grade stereo-acuity after early surgery for congenital esotropia. Arch Ophthalmol 1994;112:913-9.
163. Wright KW, Fox BES, Erikson KJ. PVEP evidence of true suppression in adult onset strabismus. J Pediatr Ophthalmol Strabismus 1990;27:196-201.
164. Wright KW, Christensen LE, Noguchi BA. Results of late surgery for presumed congenital cataracts. Am J Ophthalmol 1992;114:409-15.
165. Zak TA, Morin JD. Early surgery for infantile esotropia: results and influence of age upon results. Can J Ophthalmol 1982; 17:213-8.
166. Zubcov AA, et al. Latent nystagmus and strabismic amblyopia. Am J Ophthalmol 1981;103:87-89.

Chapter 11

Management of Paralytic Squint

Rohit Saxena, Swati Phuljhele, Ankur Sinha (India)

Paralytic strabismus is the only subset of strabismus with possible ominous implications particularly in acquired case and therefore should be differentiated from comitant squint.

CLASSIFICATION OF PARALYTIC SQUINT

1. Neurogenic-Supranuclear
   Nuclear
   Infranuclear
   e.g oculomotor, trochlear and abducent nerve palsies
2. Myogenic, e.g myotonic dystrophy, CPEO, myositis, Graves' disease
3. Neuromuscular junction disease, e.g Myasthenia gravis

   This chapter deals mainly with features and management of neurogenic causes namely oculomotor, trochlear and abducens cranial nerve palsies.

CLINICAL FEATURES OF PARALYTIC SQUINT

The following features are common to all paralytic squint irrespective of their cause or site of involvement:

- Diplopia
- Head posture
- Limitation of movement
- Incomitance in amount of deviation
- Associated Neurological Features

Table 1 summarizes the clinical features of the cranial nerve palsies.

INVESTIGATIONS

Congenital cranial nerve palsy does not require any specific investigation apart from routine work up for paralytic cases including diplopia charting, measurement of deviations in nine gazes, less charting. It is important to carry out investigations and neuroimaging in acquired

Table 1: Clinical features of the cranial nerve palsies

Third Nerve Palsy Complete (Fig. 1)	*Fourth Nerve Palsy (Fig. 2)*	*Sixth Nerve Palsy (Fig. 3)*
• Ptosis • Eye is down and out • Anisocoria may or may not be present *Partial* • Lesion is usually distal to cavernous sinus • Superior division palsy presents with ptosis and hypotropia • Inferior division involvement causes parlysis of IR, IO, MR along with internal ophthalmoplegia *Isolated Muscle palsy* • Direct trauma to orbit may cause isolated paralysis of the muscles • IR and SR are the common muscle to be paralyzed in isolation • Paralysis of isolated MR and IO is rarely seen	• Head tilt to the contralateral side • Asthenopia • Vertical diplopia more in downgaze • Tilting images • Hypertropia of the involved eye • Underaction of superior oblique muscle • Hypertropia increases on ipsilateral head tilt	• Esotropia • Horizontal diplopia more in the lateral gaze of the involved • Limitation of movement in abduction

Table 2: Indications for neuro-imaging in cranial nerve palsies

Third Nerve Palsy	*Fourth Nerve Palsy*	*Sixth Nerve Palsy*
• Pt < 40 years of age • More than 40 years of age with pupils involved • Aberrant regeneration with no history of trauma • Minor trauma presenting as III nerve palsy	• Isolated IV nerve palsy – No imaging required • Associated with neurological signs—MRI is done	• VI nerve palsy along with involvement of other cranial nerves • Isolated VI nerve palsy in patient with < 60 yrs of age • No improvement/ Worsening/ Development of other neurological signs in patients with systemic risk factors.

cases to identify the cause of paralysis. Systemic conditions like diabetes, hypertension, hyperlipidemia are important causes of mononeuropathy and should be investigated. Clinical localization of the lesion is important so as not to miss the lesion on neuroimaging. The indications of neuroimaging are given in Table 2.

NONSURGICAL MANAGEMENT

In cases of acquired paralytic strabismus, the management can be divided into two parts. During the acute phase of the disease the aim is to overcome the problem of diplopia till the deviation stabilizes and surgery can be performed.

Occlusion: In cases where the images are very much far apart the patient may be able to ignore one of the images and may not complain of diplopia, however, as the deviation decreases and the images come closer it is not easy to ignore and the problem of diplopia starts.

Patching, use of frosted gasses in spectacles, occluder patches for spectacles, pirate patches, occluder contact lenses, etc. are the various methods employed for patching depending upon the patient's demands and comfort.

Prisms: The use of prisms may provide benefit as it shifts the image to the desired direction depending upon the orientation and the power of the prism used. However, the role of prism is limited in cases where both the vertical and horizontal components of diplopia are present and in cases of complete third nerve palsies. The prisms may also find a role in postoperative cases where there is small amount of deviation left and patient complains of diplopia.

Botulinum Toxin

Botulinum Neurotoxin Type A is a neurotoxic agent that causes weakening of the muscle. It is used in paralytic to decrease the deviation and prevent the contracture of the antagonist muscle. The therapeutic effect of the toxin is dose related and peak effect is visible after 5 to 7 days of the injection. The effect is temporary lasting for 4 to 6 months after injection thus can provide a diplopia free period to the patient till spontaneous recovery occurs or definitive surgery can be performed. A dose of 2.5 to 5 IU is injected directly over the muscle with under guidance of electromyography (Figs 4A and B).

SURGICAL MANAGEMENT

The primary aim of all surgeries for paralytic strabismus is to increase the area of binocular single vision and reduce diplopia, particularly so in primary and downgazes, although the complete motility of the eye may not be restored in most cases of long-standing paralytic squints.

Third Nerve Palsy

Complete III Nerve Palsy

The aim of surgery in cases of complete external third nerve palsy is to align affected eye in primary position, though ocular movements cannot be restored. However in cases of complete external third nerve palsy where four of the six extraocular muscles are affected the conventional principle may not work and it is often not possible to align the affected eye even in primary position. Ptosis is another significant problem in these cases and a satisfactory Bell's reflex is a prerequisite for ptosis surgery.

LR recession and MR resection: Supramaximal recession of LR along with supramaximal resection of MR in the ipsilateral eye may work only in cases having some residual function of the medial rectus. The insertion of horizontal muscles during recession-resection surgery can

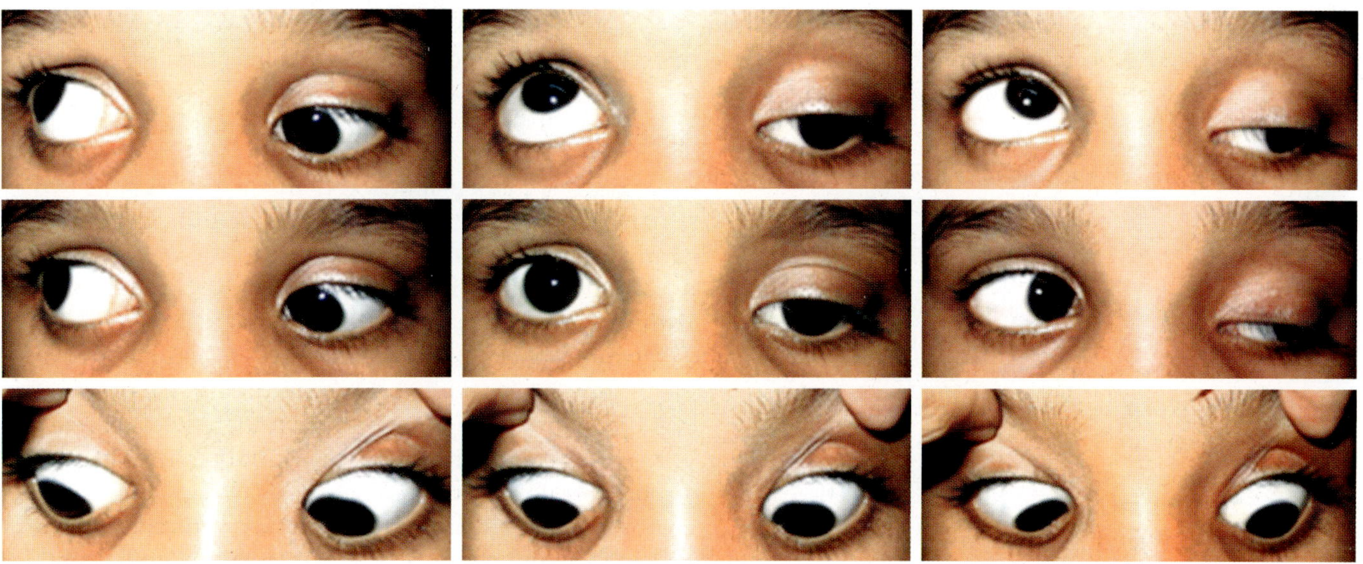

Fig. 1: A case of left III nerve palsy with aberrant regeneration (Note elevation of lid on adduction)

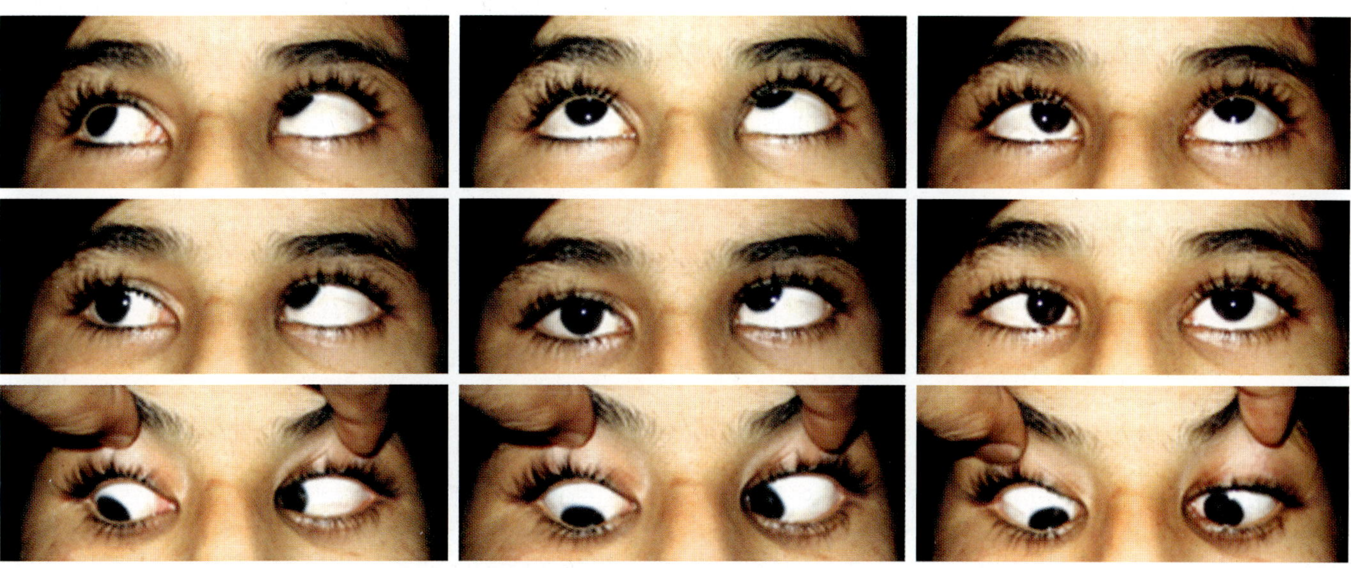

Fig. 2: A case of left IV nerve palsy

be shifted up or down to correct for vertical deviation. However in cases with inadequate or no medial rectus action, the deviation may recur due to unopposed lateral rectus action.

Transposition of SO oblique tendon to MR: The only muscle which can be utilized to counteract the force of lateral rectus is superior oblique; therefore it becomes important test for presence of superior oblique action in these cases. On attempted adduction or depression the eye intorts indicating the normal function of the fourth nerve. Transposition of tendon of superior oblique muscle by fracturing the trochlea and disinserting the muscle was described by Jackson. It is technically difficult as it requires skin incision at upper eyelid to fracture trochlea and disinsert tendon and carries a risk of severe orbital hemorrhage Scott modified this procedure by transposing superior oblique tendon without fracturing the trochlea.

A conjunctival incision circumferential to the limbus is made in the supranasal quadrant of the eye is given. The dissection is carried out to expose the insertion of SR and MR.

The SO muslce can be identified nasal to the SR muscle and is hooked under direct visualization to avoid injury to the vortex vein. The muscle is freed of its attachment and is prolapsed out of Tenon capsule. Tendon is pulled forward and a double arm nonabsorbable suture is woven into the tendon before the transaction and is cut as close to the insertion as possible.

The tendon is then transposed to superior side of MR muscle insertion and is secured to the sclera with non-absorbable suture. The limbal conjunctival incision is closed with 8-0 polyglactin suture.

Anchoring of the Globe on Medial Wall Periosteum

Anchoring the globe to nasal wall periosteum is now a well established surgery to treat complete third nerve palsy. Various materials have been used to anchor the globe like periosteal flaps, Superior oblique tendon, silicon bands, fascia lata, metal screw and 5-0 polyester sutures. Use of 5-0 polyester suture for anchoring the globe directly to periosteum appears to be less extensive and easier than procuring an apical periosteal flap and devoid of complications those seen with silicone band or screw system .

Most of the above mentioned procedures utilize skin approach for the exposure of medial canthal ligament of the medial wall periosteum. Authors have devised a new technique of approaching medial wall periosteum by using precarancular approach. This technique obviates the need for a skin incision and proves effective and cosmetically better as compared to other available techniques.

Technique (Figs 5A to I)

Using conventional limbal conjunctival incision 12-16 mm of lateral rectus recession is performed to ensure complete and free adduction.

Caruncular area is exposed using cotton sutures through skin near the medial canthus. Identify and dilate the two puncta and place Bowman's lacrimal probes to identify the canaculi and prevent injury. 0.2 to 0.5 ml of 1:1000 adrenaline with 2% Xylocaine is then injected in the caruncular area, to decrease intraoperative bleed and postoperative pain.

A curved superficial incision (approximately 7-8 mm) is made at junction of conjunctiva and canthal skin (Fig. 5A). After anatomical localization of the lacrimal system with the help of lacrimal probes, blunt dissection is performed posteriorly and nasally to expose the periosteum posterior to the posterior lacrimal crest (Fig. 5B). Through the exposed periosteum two double-armed 5-0 nonabsorbable coated braided polyester sutures are passed with enough tissue bite (Figs 5C and D).

Using a fornix-based limbal incision of Von Noorden; medial rectus muscle is hooked and dissected. Through this incision straight tenotomy scissors are passed towards the medial canthus. Once the tip of the scissors is seen through the medial canthal incision the intervening fibrous tissue is cut using spring scissors to produce a tunnel. Using the blunt tipped serrated forceps are passed from the side of the medial rectus the needles of the ethibond sutures are pulled out laterally adjacent to the medial rectus (Fig. 5E).

These sutures are then passed on the sclera on either end of medial rectus (Fig.5F), thus leaving the anterior ciliary vessels of the medial rectus undisturbed. Sutures are tightened (Fig. 5G) to leave esotropia of about 10-15 degrees intraoperatively (Fig.5H), as an exotropic drift is noted after fixation procedures. The conjunctival incisions are sutured separately using 8-0 vicryl (Fig. 5I).

The anchoring of the globe to the medial periosteal wall has lesser chances of anterior segment ischemia as only one anterior ciliary artery (through LR muscle) is disrupted leaving the blood supply through other muscles intact. Moreover it also provides a prospect of operating upon of vertical muscle to correct vertical deviation later on. Figure 6 shows a case of complete III nerve palsy before and after anchoring of the globe.

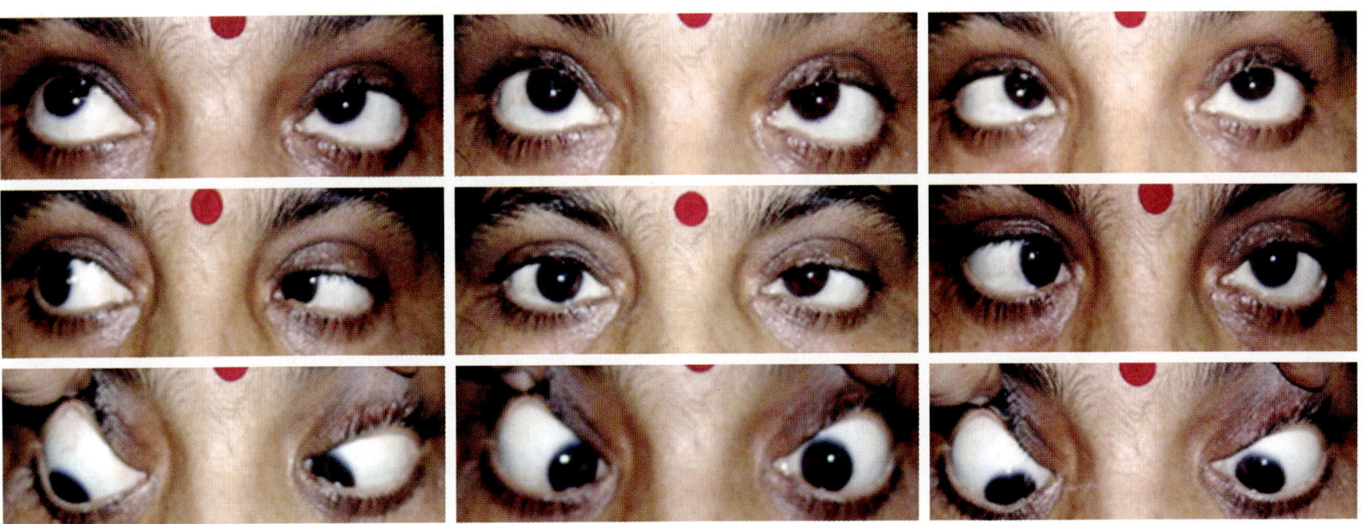

Fig. 3: A case of left VI nerve palsy

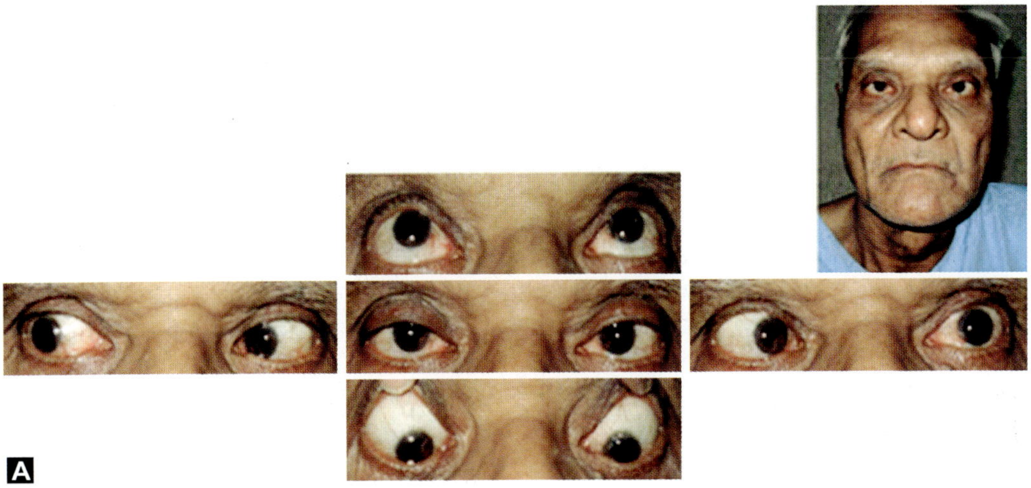

A

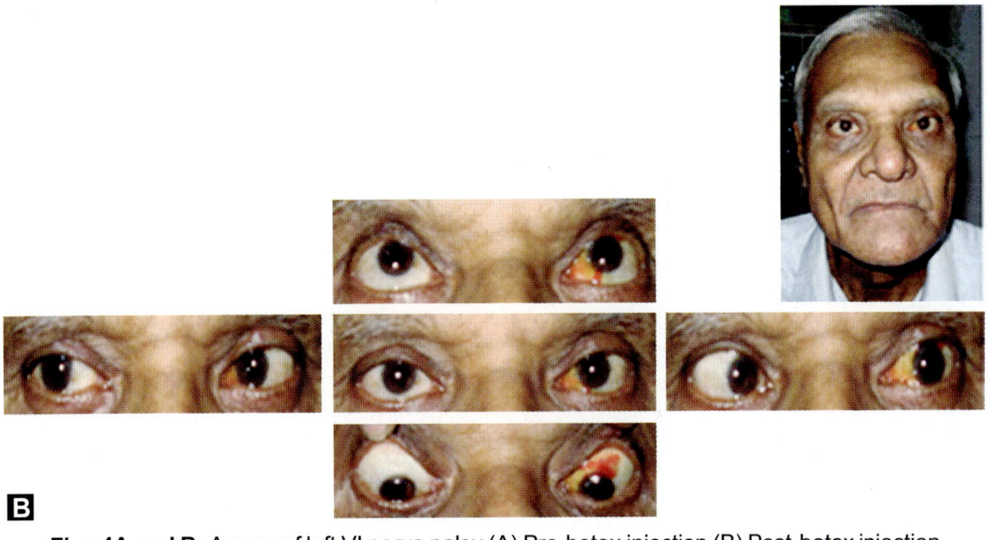

B

Figs 4A and B: A case of left VI nerve palsy (A) Pre-botox injection (B) Post-botox injection

Periosteal Fixation of Lateral Rectus Muscle

Large lateral rectus recession is usually a part of any surgical plan for a case of complete third nerve palsy but chances of recurrence in deviation is high since there is unopposed action of LR. A complete inactivation of lateral rectus force by orbital wall fixation could eliminate all residual lateral rectus function.

Technique (Fig. 7)

Using a limbal or fornix conjunctival incision LR muscle is exposed and isolated on a muscle hook. Blunt dissection is performed to outside the muscle to expose the adjacent periosteum approximately posterior to the orbital rim. The rectus muscle is then disinserted from the globe. A non absorbable suture is woven and locked through the insertional edge of the muscle before disinsertion to avoid slippage. The muscle is then attached to the adjacent orbital periosteum with two periosteal bites using pre-placed nonabsorbable suture. The above procedure can be combined with resection of MR muscle in the same sitting or as a second stage surgery to achieve better alignment.

Partial/Isolated Muscle Paralysis

The management of each patient varies according to differences in the extent of paresis and recovery.

Medial Rectus Muscle Palsy

The management in cases of isolated medial rectus palsy depends upon the amount of adduction and the muscle power regained by the medial rectus.

Horizontal muscle surgery: If the adduction is good (eyeball crosses the midline) and there is no contracture of the lateral rectus, then conventional recession-resection procedure on the horizontal recti can be performed. However, the amount of recession and resection would be larger than what is required for a comitant exotropia and supra-maximal recession-resection may be a good option. And as mentioned above it can be shifted downwards in case of associated hypertropia or vice versa. In cases with residual exotropia, contralateral eye surgery in the form of lateral rectus recession may be required.

Transposition surgery: In cases with very poor medial rectus function where the eye does not cross the midline with useful function of SR and IR transposition of vertical muscle to the MR can be viable options. The details of transposition surgery are discussed under the management of VI nerve palsy.

Superior Rectus Muscle Palsy

Most cases of superior rectus palsy are congenital and may have associated ptosis. If the hypotropia is not significant and there is no diplopia in downgaze it is better to avoid any surgical intervention. A significant deviation in the primary gaze as well as downgaze would require surgery.

Inferior rectus recession: A forced duction test is a must to rule out associated inferior rectus contracture. In presence of tight (contracture) IR it is necessary to perform the recession of the contracted muscle and most of the times this is sufficient to correct deviation in downgaze and primary gaze. A second stage surgery in form weakening of contralateral elevators can be performed for the residual deviation.

Knapp's procedure: In cases where inferior rectus is free, one can opt for a Knapp's procedure where both the horizontal muscles are disinserted and a full tendon transposition to the superior rectus muscle is done. Detail technique for transposition surgery is discussed under VI nerve palsy.

Inferior Rectus Muscle Palsy

In cases where the inferior rectus muscle paralysis is because of muscle entrapment in blow out fracture, the management is very challenging. Surgical plan is to explore the inferior orbital area. Repair of orbital floor and releasing entrapped IR itself may decrease hypertropia to certain extent. To attain the alignment in the primary gaze ipsilateral superior rectus recession can be performed. For the management of diplopia in downgaze contralateral faden operation of inferior rectus may be an option.

Inferior Oblique Muscle Palsy

The management of inferior oblique palsy is indicated in cases with marked vertical deviation and in cases with significant head posture.

If there is associated superior oblique overaction, a superior oblique weakening is the first surgery of choice. The weakening procedures of superior oblique include tenotomy, tenectomy, tendon Z plasty and tendon recession.

When the deviation is more than 15-20 prisms in primary gaze superior oblique weakening alone may not be sufficient. In such cases weakening of the yoke SR is required.

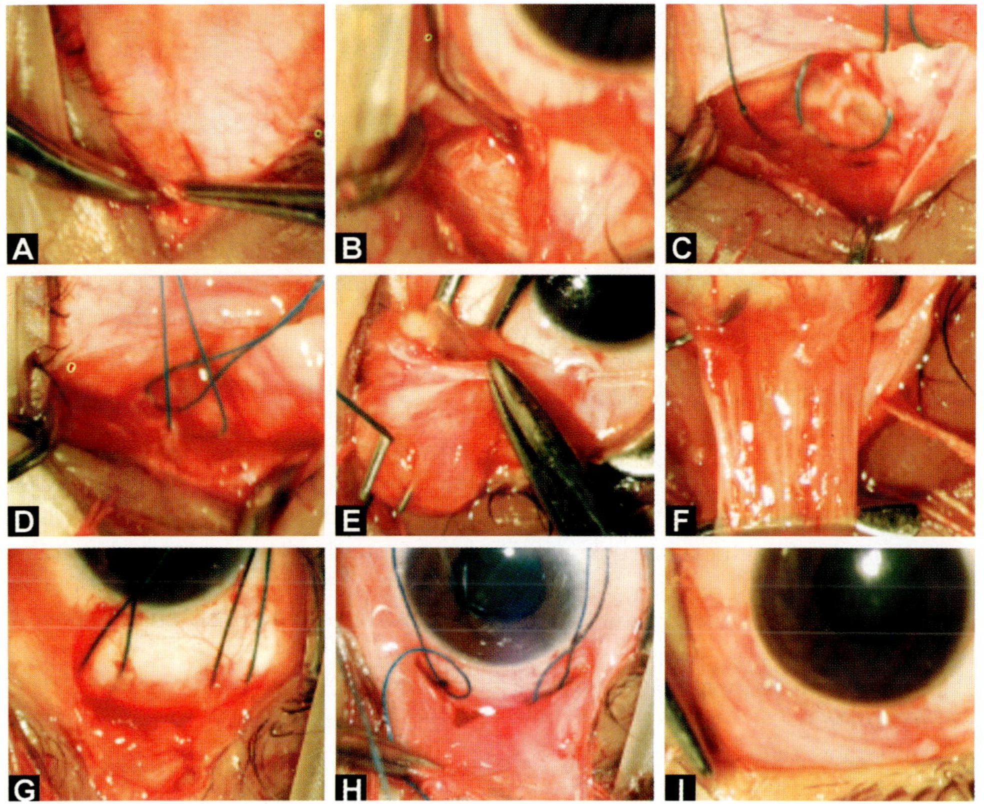

Figs 5A to I: Surgical steps showing precarancular approach for anchoring of globe to medial orbital wall *(published in Orbit, 25:205-208, 2006)*

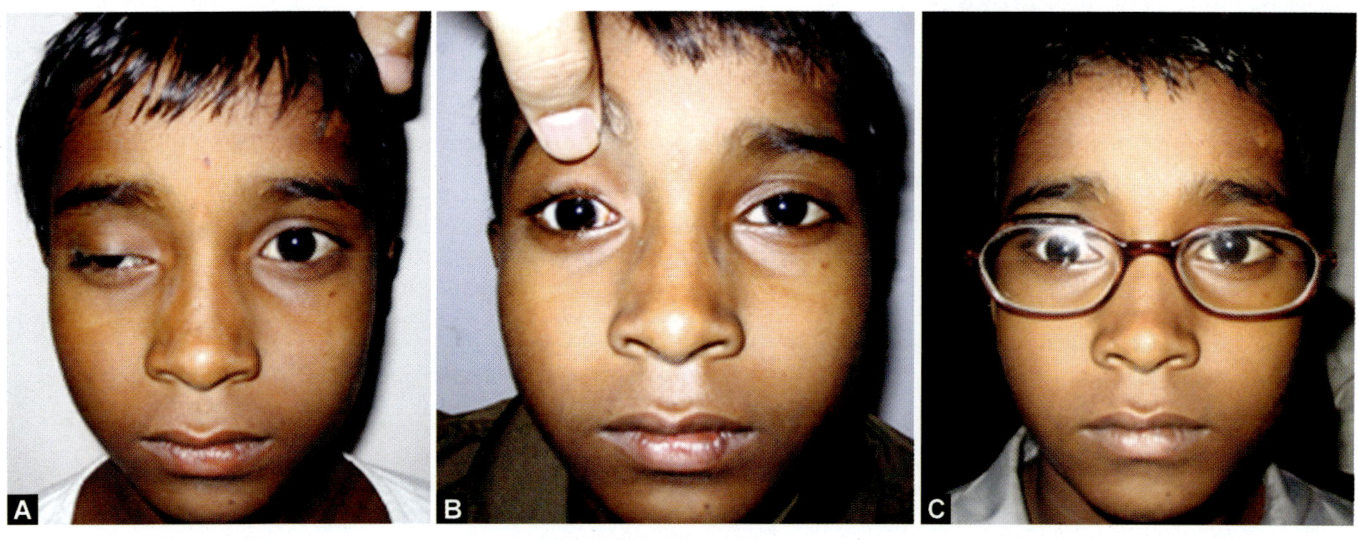

Preoperative | 2 months postoperatively | Six months postoperatively

Figs 6A to C: A case of complete III nerve palsy: Pre- and Post-anchor surgery

Inferior oblique strengthening procedure as a primary surgery is the least effective surgery and is indicated in cases where residual deviation is present even after the above procedures. Resection and tucking are two procedures used for IO strengthening.

Aberrant Regeneration

Patients with recovered III nerve palsy usually have aberrant regeneration if form of elevation of lid on adduction. This characteristic can be used to patients benefit by doing a large recession-resection surgery that will correct the exotropia as well as elevate the lid as result of increased innervation to MR muscle.

Fourth Nerve Palsy

The choice of surgical options is influenced by various factors:

1. Laxity of SO tendon
2. Presence of IO overaction
3. Amount of deviation in primary position
4. Gaze of maximum deviation

Knapp's classification and management protocol is one of the important landmarks in management of cases of fourth nerve palsy. The Knapp's management strategy depends upon the maximum deviation in different gazes. This has been summarized in Table 3.

Inferior Oblique Weakening Procedure

The weakening procedures for inferior oblique include myotomy, recession and anterior positioning.

Inferior Oblique Myotomy and Myectomy

For the exposure of inferior oblique muscle one can choose between the modification of Parks cul-de-sac incision (7-9 mm from limbus) in the inferotemporal quadrant or Von Noorden's limbal incision.

After the conjunctival incision is made in inferotemporal quadrant (Fig. 8A). Tenon's is cut and LR muscle is hooked with Green's squint hook. The conjunctiva in inferotemporal quadrant is retracted using two lens hooks or Desmarre's retractor. Inferior oblique muscle is hooked under direct visualization ensuring that all the fibers are included in the muscle hook (Figs 8B and C). Care must be taken of the vortex vein and the inferior division of the third nerve which is very close to the muscle.

The muscle is freed of its attachment of lateral rectus muscle and sclera (Fig. 8D). For myotomy the muscle is incised at its insertion and free part is allowed to retract. For myectomy at least 6-8 mm of muscle is exposed and two muscle clamps are placed at this distance. The segment of the muscle between the two clamps is removed and ends are cauterized. The posterior portion of the muscle is allowed to retract in the Tenon's space and conjunctiva is closed.

Inferior Oblique Recession and Anterior Positioning

A pure recession means that the muscle is retroplaced along the original course of the muscle, however in case of IO recession there is some amount of anterior positioning of the muscle.

After exposing the muscle as described above two single-arm or one double-arm suture is woven in muslce similar to that done in recession of a rectus muscle (Fig. 8E). The muscle is then reattached to any of the point described below depending upon the amount of recession and anterior positioning required.

Fink's method: Fink's point is a point 6 mm inferior and 6 mm posterior to the inferior end of insertion of lateral rectus muscle. The anterior end of recessed muscle is placed

Table 3: Management of IV nerve palsy (Von Noorden modification of Knapp's classification): For a case of left superior oblique palsy

Class	*Maximum deviation in gaze*	*Management*
1	Dextro-elevation (L/R maximum in this gaze)	Left inferior oblique recession
2	Dextro-depression	Left superior oblique tuck or Harada Ito's procedure + Right inferior rectus recession
3	All right gazes	If Hypertropia < 25 PD then left inferior oblique recession If hypertropia > 25 then add left superior oblique tuck
4	All down and right gazes	Treatment plan as in 3 with right inferior rectus recession or left superior rectus recession
5	All down gazes	Left superior oblique tuck with Right inferior rectus recession
6	Bilateral with a "V" pattern	Bilateral surgery as in class 5
7	All downgazes, primary gaze and dextroversion	Explore trochlea

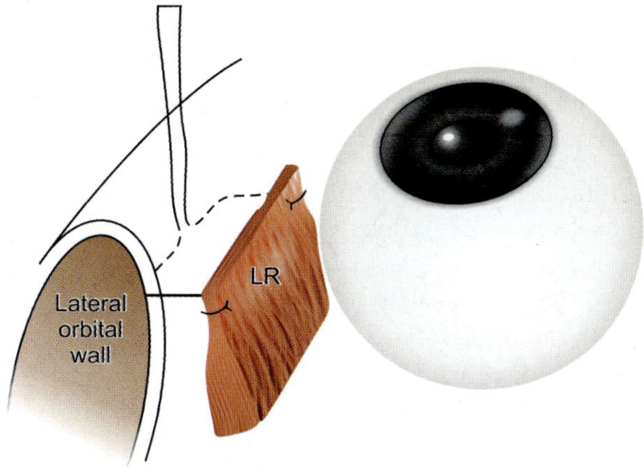

Fig. 7: Showing lateral rectus anchoring to periosteum of lateral orbital wall

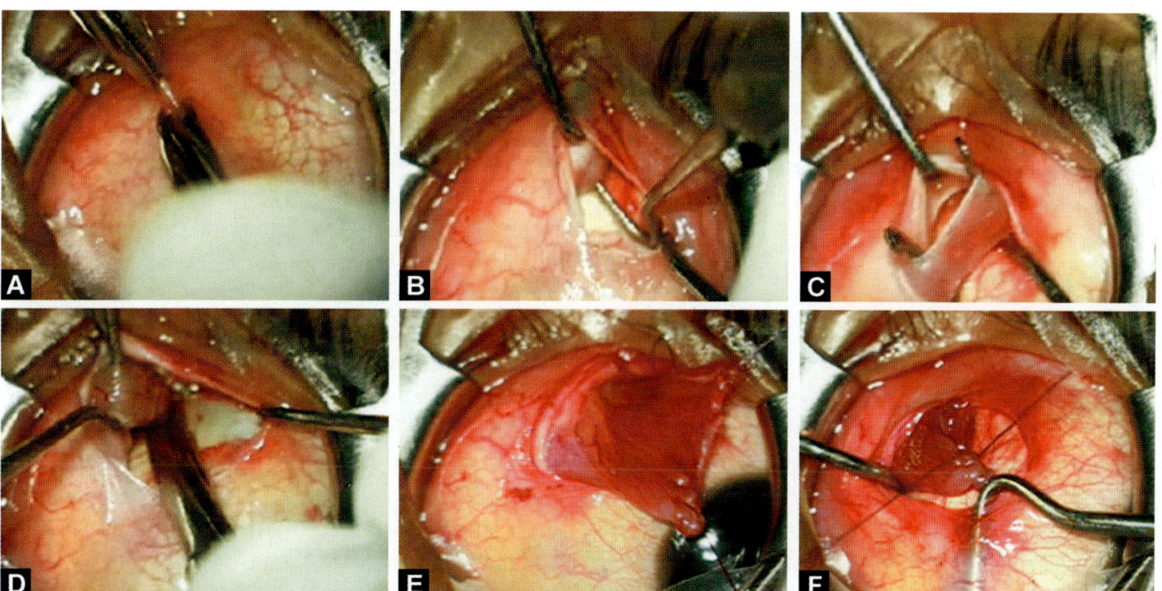

Figs 8A to F: Steps for inferior oblique recession (Modified Elliot & Nankin method)

at this point and the posterior point is approximately 5 mm posterior to it. This point corresponds to 8 mm recession and 1 mm anterior positioning of the muscle. For 10 mm recession one goes 2 mm inferior from the Fink's point and this acts as the anterior point of insertion of the muscle.

Park's method: A point 3 mm posterior and 2 mm lateral to the lateral end of insertion of the inferior rectus is labeled as "Scheie-Parks point". When the anterior end of recessed muscle is placed at this point it is considered equivalent to 10 mm recession. However even in this method there is anterior positioning of the muscle by 1.0-1.5 mm.

Elliot and Nankin's method and its modification: In the original description of Elliot and Nankin's method the anterior and the posterior end of the muscle are re-inserted at the lateral end of insertion of the inferior rectus muscle. This is a stronger weakening procedure than the Fink's or Park's method of recession. The recessed muscle starts acting as a stronger depressor, leading to an anti-elevation syndrome. To overcome this anomaly, the posterior end of the insertion is re-inserted 5-6 mm posterior to the lateral end of insertion of inferior rectus muscle. With this "modified Elliot and Nankin's method" the direction of the posterior fibers is maintained and the depressor action of the recessed muscle is eliminated (Fig. 8F)

Superior Oblique Strengthening

The two procedures commonly used for superior oblique strengthening are; SO tuck and Harada Ito. While tucking the SO tendon strengths the overall actions of the muscle the later procedure is done to bring only the torsional change without affecting the vertical action of the muscle. Thus, the procedure does not cause an iatrogenic Brown's syndrome.

Superior Oblique Tucking

A tucking surgery should be performed only in those cases where the tendons appear lax on performing traction test.

Superior oblique muscle is approached through the conjunctival incision along the temporal border of SR muscle. The tendon is hooked and isolated. Another muscle hook is then passed posterior to the insertion.

The tendon is then pulled temporally and the amount of laxity is assessed. While marking for the amount only half of the desired amount should be marked as the tendon folds upon itself. A nonabsorbable suture interwoven through the anterior and posterior end of the tendon and tendon is folded upon itself.

Forced duction test for elevation should be repeated before tying the final knot. In presence of restriction for elevation the amount of tucking should be decreased or it may lead to postoperative iatrogenic Brown's syndrome.

Harada Ito's Advancement of Superior Oblique

In procedure the anterior half of the SO tendon is disinserted and advanced anteriorly and laterally. This part of tendon is reinserted at 8 mm posteriorly to the upper end of the insertion of LR perpendicular to the upper border of LR muscle.

Sixth Nerve Palsy

The surgical decision is based upon the amount of abduction possible, amount of deviation in the primary gaze, muscle power of lateral rectus on active force generation test and contracture of medial rectus as on forced duction test.

Horizontal Muscle Surgery

In cases where there is moderate recovery of lateral rectus functions, horizontal muscle surgery in the form of medial rectus recession and lateral rectus resections may be an effective plan.

Vertical Rectus Transposition

In cases, where there is total sixth nerve palsy, recession-resection procedure may not work, and one may have to opt for, large recession of medial rectus along with a full or partial vertical rectus muscle transposition.

Tendon transposition can be either full tendon transposition or a partial tendon transposition. Figure 9 shows various types of transposition procedures. Since transposition of recti muscles is usually combined with recession of MR muscle the risk of anterior segment ischemia is high and vessel sparing surgery may be needed. While with partial tendon transposition there is low risk of anterior segment ischemia. To decrease the risk of anterior segment ischemia Jensen described the transposition of muscle by tying the superior and inferior half of LR muscle belly to temporal half of SR muscle and IR muscle respectively. Although this procedure claims to have less chance of anterior segment ischemia there is always a possibility of strangulation of vessels by the sutures. To decrease the risk of ischemia one can avoid the recession of the MR and chemodenervation with Botox

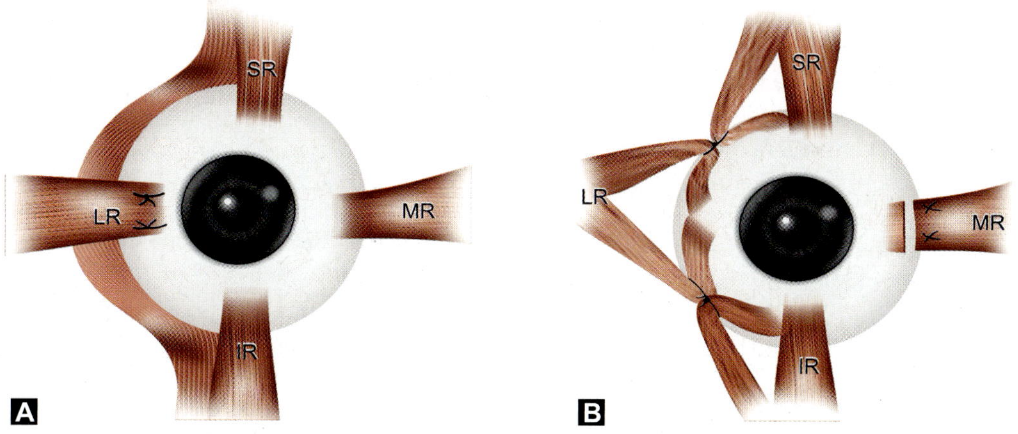

Figs 9A and B: Types of transposition (A) Hummelsheim (B) Jensen

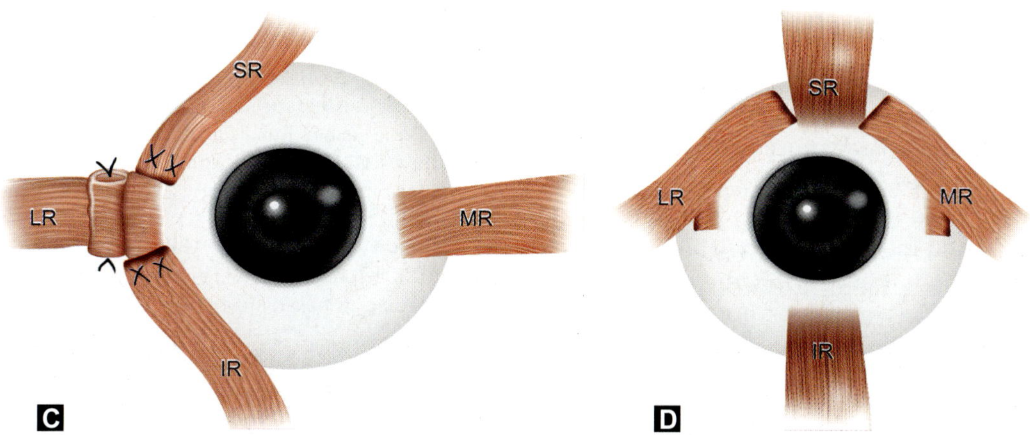

Figs 9C and D: Types of Transposition (C) O'Connor (D) Knapp

can be done, but in a long-standing case with fibrotic tight medial rectus the effect may not be significant.

The effect of transposition can be augmented with by bringing the transposed muscle closer to the palsied muscle and anchoring it to the adjacent sclera with the help of nonabsorbable suture as described by Foster and Buckley. This suture changes the direction of vector of the action of transposed muscle towards the new insertion site and thus augmenting the effect brought about by transposition.

Technique

The recession of MR is performed in a conventional method with limbal conjunctival incision so that conjunctival recession can be combined if indicated.

For transposition of SR a circumferential conjunctival incision is made 7 mm posterior to the limbus between LR and SR muscle. SR is hooked and is cleared of all its attachment to Tenon's, SO and adjacent tissue.

The muslce is now split into two halves till 15 mm posteriorly. A polyglactin 6-0 suture is woven through the lateral half of the muscle and this portion is disinserted. This half of the muscle is reinserted at the superior end of LR insertion.

The new insertion can be perpendicular to the LR muslce or can be concentric to the limbus. The effect of the transposition can be enhanced by placing a non-absorbable posterior suture 8 mm behind the new insertion of the transposed muscle. Same procedure is repeated for transposition of IR to the LR muscle.

Knapp's surgery is done by similar procedure where full tendons of MR and LR are disinserted and reinserted at the lateral and medial end of SR muscle insertion respectively. The muslce insertions are parallel to the insertion of SR and no foster suture is used (Fig. 9D).

Acknowledgement: The authors are grateful to Dr Pinto for the illustrative diagrams.

SUGGESTED READING

1. Bale JF Jr, Scott WE, Yuh W, Sato Y, Menezes A. Congenital fourth nerve palsy and occult cranium bifidum. Pediatr Neurol. 1988 Sep-Oct;4(5):320-1.
2. Bennett JL, Pelak VS. Palsies of the third, fourth, and sixth cranial nerves. Ophthalmol Clin North Am 2001 Mar;14(1):169-85, ix. Review.
3. Bicas HE. A surgically implanted elastic band to restore paralyzed ocular rotations. J Pediatr Ophthalmol Strabismus 1991;28:10-13.
4. Britt MT, Velez FG, Thacker N, Alcorn D, Foster RS, Rosenbaum AL. Partial rectus muscle-augmented transpositions in abduction deficiency. J AAPOS. 2003 Oct;7(5):325-32.
5. Cackett P, Fleck B, Mulhivill A. Bilateral fourth-nerve palsy occurring after shaking injury in infancy. J AAPOS. 2004 Jun;8(3):280-1.
6. Chang YH, Ma KT, Lee JB, Han SH. Anterior transposition of inferior oblique muscle for treatment of unilateral superior oblique muscle palsy with inferior oblique muscle overaction. Yonsei Med J. 2004 Aug 31;45(4):609-14.
7. Dalman NE, Schwarcz RM, Velez FG. Suture fixation system as globe tethers in severe paralytic strabismus. JAAPOS 2006;10:371-72.
8. EARL CJ. A case of bilateral congenital sixth nerve palsy.Guys Hosp Rep 1958;107(1):66-8.
9. Ehrt O, Boergen KP. A concept for the surgical treatment of trochlear palsy. Strabismus. 2004 Jun;12(2):75-83.
10. Federico G. Velez, Neepa Thacker, Michelle T. Britt, Deborah Alcorn, R. Scott Foster, and Arthur L. Rosenbaum. Rectus Muscle Orbital Wall Fixation: A Reversible Profound Weakening Procedure. J AAPOS 2004;8:473-80.
11. Genevois O, Beaumont R, Retout A, Quintyn JC. [Comparison of two surgical techniques for the treatment of superior oblique palsy] J Fr Ophthalmol. 2005 Apr;28(4):355-62. French.
12. Goldberg RA, Rosenbaum AL, Tong JT. Use of apically based periosteal flaps as globe tethers in severe paretic strabismus. Arch Ophthalmol. 2000 Mar; 118:431-7.
13. Harley RD. Paralytic strabismus in children. Etiologic incidence and management of third, fourth and sixth nerve palsies. Ophthalmology 1980; 87:24-43.
14. Harley RD. Paralytic strabismus in children. Etiologic incidence and management of the third, fourth, and sixth nerve palsies. Ophthalmology. 1980 Jan;87(1):24-43.
15. Hatz KB, Brodsky MC, Killer HE. When is isolated inferior oblique muscle surgery an appropriate treatment for superior oblique palsy? Eur J Ophthalmol 2006 Jan-Feb;16(1):10-6.
16. Helvesten EM (Ed). Surgical management of Strabismus. An Atlas of Strabismus Surgery. 4th edn. Mosby-Year Book Inc.; 1993.
17. Holmes JM, Mutyala S, Maus TL, Grill R, Hodge DO, Gray DT. Pediatric third, fourth, and sixth nerve palsies: A population-based study. Am J Ophthalmol. 1999 Apr;127(4):388-92.
18. Hong S, Chang YH, Han SH, Lee JB. Effect of full tendon transposition augmented with posterior intermuscular suture for paralytic strabismus. Am J Ophthalmol 2005 Sep;140(3):477-83.
19. Jackson E. In: Wiener M, Schie HG, (Eds). Surgery of the eye, 3rd edn. New York: Grune and Stratton, 1952;405.
20. Khan AO. Paradoxical head tilt during fixation with the affected eye in unilateral congenital fourth nerve palsy. J AAPOS. 2005 Apr;9(2):200-1.
21. Lee JP. Paralytic and incomitant strabismus. Curr Opin Ophthalmol 1996 Oct;7(5):19-23.
22. Mataftsi A, Strickler J, Klainguti G. Vertical and torsional correction in congenital superior oblique palsy by inferior oblique recession. Eur J Ophthalmol. 2006 Jan-Feb;16(1):3-9.
23. Mekari-Sabbagh ON, DaCunha RP. Crossed eyes in a six-year-old girl. Surv Ophthalmol. 2001 Jan-Feb;45(4):331-4.
24. Milea D, Laforet P, Eymard B. [Atypical ocular myasthenia gravis] Rev Neurol (Paris). 2005 May;161(5):543-8. French.

25. Moe KS. The precaruncular approach to the medial orbit. Arch Facial Plast Surg 2003 Nov-Dec;5(6):483-7.
26. Mohamed SR, Ainsworth JR. Vertical augmented transposition surgery. Eye 2004 Jan;18(1):81-4.
27. Mora J. An adjustable medial orbital wall suture for third nerve palsy. Clin Experiment Ophthalmol. 2004 Oct;32(5):460-1.
28. Morad Y, Kowal L, Scott AB. Lateral rectus muscle disinsertion and reattachment to the lateral orbital wall. Br J Ophthalmol 2005 Aug;89(8):983-5.
29. Morad Y, Nemet P. Medial transposition of the lateral rectus muscle in combined third and fourth nerve palsy. J AAPOS. 2000 Aug;4(4):246-7.
30. Nishida Y, Inatomi A, Aoki Y, Hayashi O, Iwami T, Oda S, Nakamura J, Kani K. A muscle transposition procedure for abducens palsy, in which the halves of the vertical rectus muscle bellies are sutured onto the sclera. Jpn J Ophthalmol 2003 May-Jun;47(3):281-6.
31. Nucci P. Superior oblique palsy: Promoting a simpler approach. Eur J Ophthalmol 2006 Jan-Feb;16(1):1-2. No abstract available.
32. Parvataneni M, Olitsky SE. Unilateral anterior transposition and resection of the inferior oblique muscle for the treatment of hypertropia. J Pediatr Ophthalmol Strabismus 2005 May-Jun;42(3):163-5.
33. Pinches E, Thompson D, Noordeen H, Liasis A, Nischal KK. Fourth and sixth cranial nerve injury after halo traction in children: A report of two cases.J AAPOS. 2004 Dec;8(6):580-5.
34. Prieto-Diaz J, Gallo EM. A case of cyclic superior oblique paresis. Binocul Vis Strabismus Q. 2005;20(1):27-32.
35. Rosenbuam AL, Santiago AP (Eds). Clinical Strabismus Management Principles and Surgical Techniques: WB Saunders Co; 1999.
36. Salazar-Leon JA, Ramirez-Ortiz MA, Salas-Vargas M. The surgical correction of paralytic strabismus using fascia lata. J Pediatr Ophthalmol Strabismus 1998 Jan-Feb;35(1):27-32.
37. Saunders RA, Rogers GL. Superior oblique transposition for third nerve palsy Ophthalmology 1982;89(4):310-6.
38. Saxena R, Sinha A, Sharma P, Pathak H, Menon V, Sethi H. Precaruncular periosteal anchor of medial rectus, a new technique in the management of complete external third nerve palsy. Orbit. 2006 Sep;25(3):205-8.
39. Schiavi C. Paralytic strabismus. Curr Opin Ophthalmol 2000 Oct;11(5):318-23.
40. Scott AB. Transposition of superior oblique. Am Orthoptic J 1977;27:11-4.
41. Sharma P, Gogoi M, Kedar S, Bhola R. Periosteal fixation in third-nerve palsy. J AAPOS. 2006 Aug;10(4):324-7. Dhaliwal A, West AL, Trobe JD, Musch DC.
42. Sharma P. Strabismus Simplified. 1st edn.1. Modern Publishers 1999.
43. Simon JW, Grajny A. Anterior segment ischemia following augmented 2-muscle transposition surgery. J AAPOS. 2004 Dec;8(6):586-7.
44. Srivastava KK, Sundaresh K, Vijayalakshmi P. A new surgical technique for ocular fixation in congenital third nerve palsy. J AAPOS. 2004 Aug;8(4):371-7.
45. Steffen H, Kolling GH. Single or combined oblique muscle surgery in acquired and congenital superior oblique palsy. Ann N Y Acad Sci. 2005 Apr;1039:583-7.
46. Straumann D, Steffen H, Landau K, Bergamin O, Mudgil AV, Walker MF, Guyton DL, Zee DS. Primary position and listing's law in acquired and congenital trochlear nerve palsy. Invest Ophthalmol Vis Sci. 2003 Oct;44(10):4282-92.
47. Third, fourth, and sixth cranial nerve palsies following closed head injury. J Neuroophthalmol 2006 Mar;26(1):4-10.
48. Tollefson MM, Mohney BG, Diehl NN, Burke JP. Incidence and types of childhood hypertropia: A population-based study. Ophthalmology. 2006 Jul;113(7):1142-5. Epub 2006 Apr 27.
49. Villasenor Solares J, Riemann BI, Romanelli Zuazo AC, Riemann CD. Ocular fixation to nasal periosteum with a superior oblique tendon in patients with third nerve palsy. J Pediatr Ophthalmol Strabismus 2000 Sep-Oct;37(5):260-5.
50. Von Noorden GK (Ed). Binocular Vision and Ocular Motility Theory and Management of Strabismus: Mosby-Year Book Inc.; 1996.
51. Von Noorder GK. Binocular vision and ocular motility. St Louis: Mosby 1996;422.
52. Yonghong J, Kanxing Z, Wei L, Xiao W, Jinghui W, Fanghua Z. Surgical management of large angle incomitant strabismus in patients with oculomotor nerve palsy. JAAPOS 2008;12: 49-53.

Chapter 12

Superior Oblique Surgery: Indications, Approach and Complications

Reena Sharma, Pradeep Sharma (India)

The superior oblique muscle is a fusiform muscle on the upper, medial side of the globe whose primary action is downward, lateral rotation of the eye. This muscle is innervated by the trochlear nerve (the fourth cranial nerve). It originates in the orbital apex and courses forward along the superior-medial wall of the orbit to the trochlea, where it becomes tendinous. After passing through the trochlea, the tendon reflects back temporally at an angle of 51 degrees with the medial wall of the orbit. It passes dorsally over the globe, underneath the SR muscle, and inserts in the posterotemporal sclera.

The primary (main) action of the superior oblique muscle is intorsion, the secondary action is depression (primarily in the adducted position) and the tertiary action is abduction (lateral rotation). The specific location of the insertion of the superior oblique tendon and the angle made by the course of the tendon and the antero-posterior axis of the globe determine how the muscle's force is distributed among these 3 functions.

INDICATIONS FOR SURGERY ON SUPERIOR OBLIQUE

A: For Weakening Superior Oblique

- A -Pattern strabismus with superior oblique overaction
- Strabismus deorsoadductorius
- Brown syndrome
- Skew deviation
- Inferior oblique palsy
- Superior oblique myokymia

Incision to Expose the Superior Oblique

There are two approaches to expose the superior oblique muscle, either nasal or temporal to the superior rectus muscle.

Superotemporal Approach

The muscle can be approached via a superotemporal incision. This exposes the superior oblique tendon at its insertion underneath the superior rectus. The incision is made in the conjunctiva at approximately the lateral aspect of the superior rectus muscle insertion 8 to 10 mm from and concentric with the limbus. The Tennon's is cut and sclera exposed. Blunt dissection is done to get a clear view. The superior rectus is then hooked using a muscle hook and pulled downwards. A lens hook is used to lift the lateral border of superior reactus and is pulled nasally to expose the superior oblique insertion. A Desmarre's retractor can also be used for the same purpose. This will reveal the fibers of the superior oblique tendon fusing with the sclera approximately at right angles to the superior rectus muscle insertion. These fibers are located about 6 to 12 mm posterior to the lateral end of the superior rectus insertion. Another lens hook is used to retract the tissues laterally. The superior oblique insertion is gently hooked in a sweeping fashion using a small muscle hook, gently moving it from anterior to posterior. A larger muscle hook is then used to hook the entire muscle taking care not to damage the vortex vein which lies very close. The muscle can then be manipulated as needed.

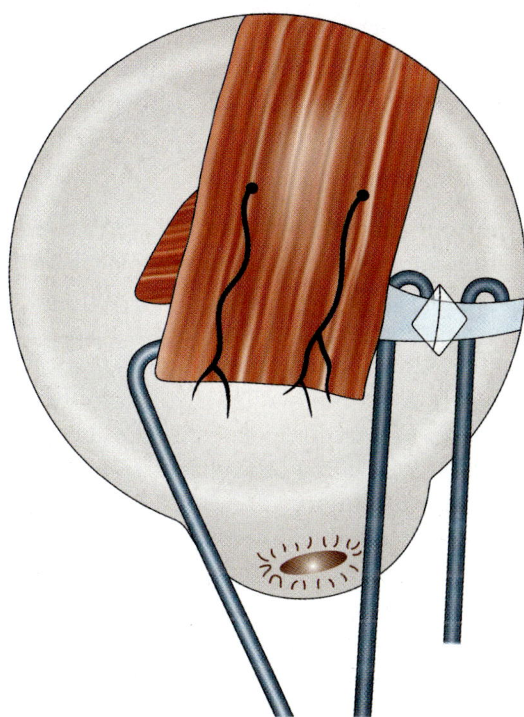

Fig. 1: Superior oblique tenectomy

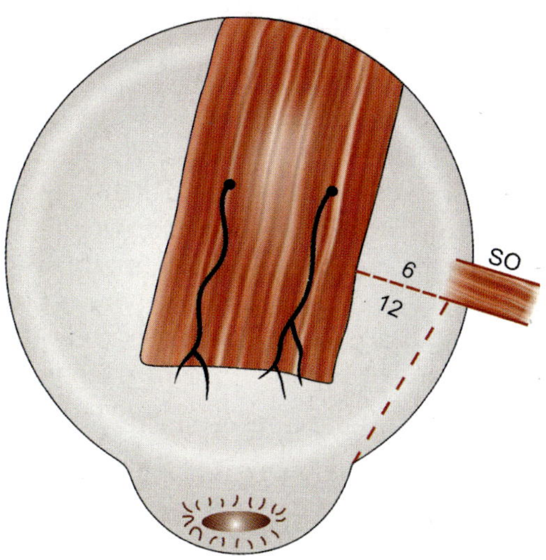

Fig. 3: Translational recession of superior oblique. The muscle disinserted from its insertion is sutured at a point 12 mm posterior to limbus and 6 mm nasal to nasal border of superior rectus muscle

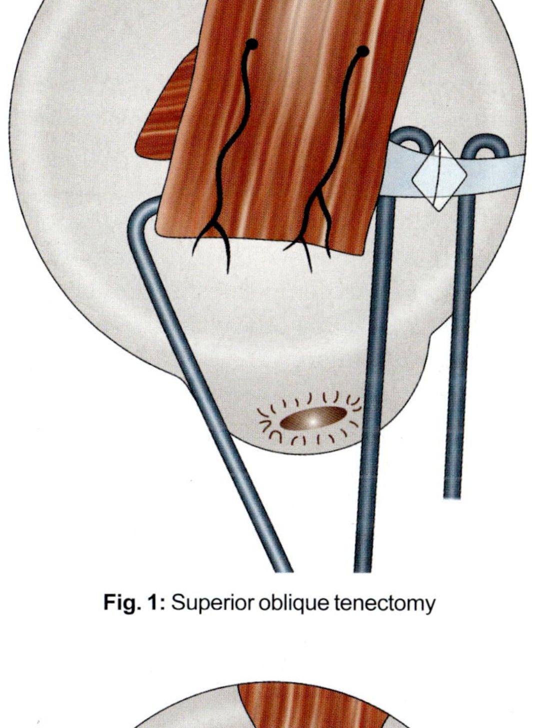

Fig. 2: Disinsertion of superior oblique. The muscle is cut at its insertion and allowed to retract

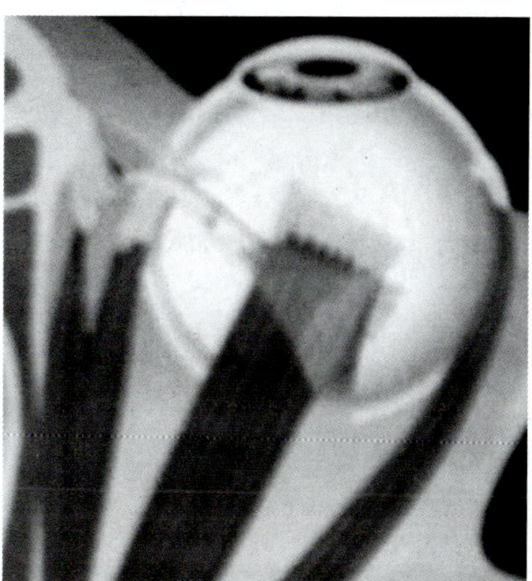

Fig. 4: A silicone expander used to lengthen the superior oblique tendon thereby weakening it

Superonasal Approach

The muscle can also be approached via a superonasal incision. The conjunctival incision is made in the superonasal fornix, midway between superior rectus and medial rectus. The Tenon's is cut and bare sclera exposed. Two muscle hooks are then used to hook the superior rectus and medial rectus. A lens hook or a Desmarre's retractor is then used to retract the conjunctiva and Tenon's posteriorly. A careful blunt dissection and close observation reveals a whitish band underneath the posterior Tenon. It is then exposed, hooked and dissected free from the surrounding structures.

Traction Testing of the Superior Oblique

Traction testing of the superior oblique tendon must be done in the operating room at the time of surgery to further identify tendon laxity. This test should especially be done in all patients with superior oblique palsy undergoing surgery.

It provides reliable information about the state of the superior oblique tendon; information that is essential for the design of the appropriate surgical procedure.

This test should again be repeated at conclusion of the surgery, to detect remaining laxity or an excessive tightness. If the test is positive, the muscle may need be reexposed and dealt with.

Weakening Procedures of the Superior Oblique

The complex anatomy of the superior oblique tendon and its proximity and attachment to the superior rectus and superior orbital fascia contributes to the differing results from the various weakening procedures used.

Procedures for Weakening Superior Oblique

- Tenotomy: temporal/nasal
- Tenectomy
- Z or L-tenotomy
- Posterior tenectomy/tenotomy (PTSO)
- Anterior tenectomy
- Loop tenotomy
- Silicon expander
- Recession/translational recession
- Differential recession of anterior fibers
- Retroplacement of trochlea

These procedures may be grouped as:

A. Generalized Weakening

These procedures weaken all the three actions of the muscle: intorsion, depression and abduction equally.

Tenotomy/tenectomy

The superior oblique is effectively weakened by a tenectomy, tenotomy, or recession. Minimal dissection and minimal disruption of the orbital fascial layers surrounding the superior oblique tendon help achieve the best results. The effect of tenotomy of superior oblique depends on how far the tendon is cut from the trochlea. Cutting the tendon closer to trochlea produces a greater weakening effect. On the other hand, size of tenectomy does not decide the amount of weakening effect.

Tenotomy/tenectomy can be done from either a superonasal or a superotemporal approach. The measurements are considered more reliable when done from its insertion using a superotemporal approach which is the preferred approach of the authors. The tendon gets retracted once the tenotomy is done. The conjunctival incision is then closed with vicryl 8-0 absorbable sutures.

Disinsertion

The superior oblique muscle can be disinserted by cutting it at its scleral insertion. This procedure is however unpredictable and carries a risk of iatrogenic superior oblique palsy.

Recession of the Superior Oblique

This procedure is believed to provide a more controlled weakening effect on superior oblique. Here, it is detached from its insertion and allowed to retract nasally underneath the superior rectus muscle for an intended amount of recession and the sutures are passed in the sclera 3-4 mm nasal to the superior rectus insertion. The sutures may be in a hang back fashion sutured to the previous insertion, that maybe a loop tenectomy.

Loop Tenectomy

A nonabsorbable suture like 5-0 Ethibond, is used to lengthen the tendon at the distal end of the superior oblique in a graded manner, and may be adjusted on the basis of intraoperative exaggerated forced duction testing.

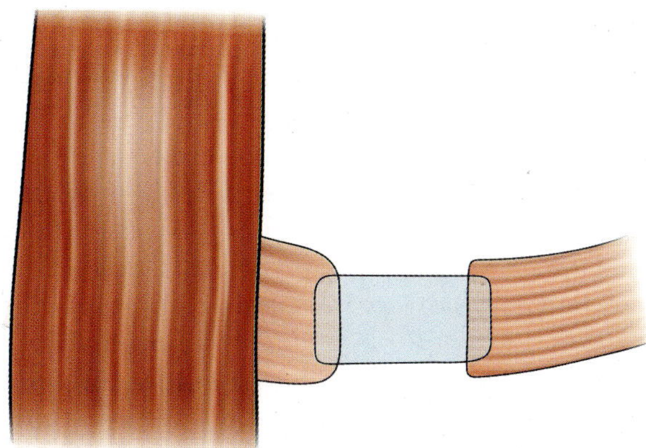

Fig. 5: The 'chicken suture' used to lengthen the superior oblique tendon by a required amount

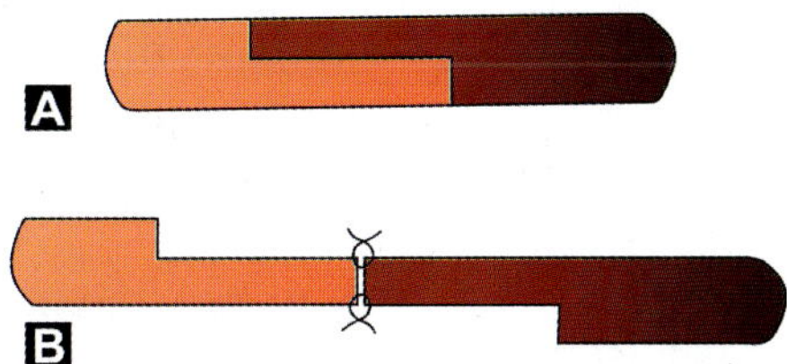

Fig. 6: Z tenotomy of superior oblique. The muscle is split in a z shape and sutured after appropriate lengthening

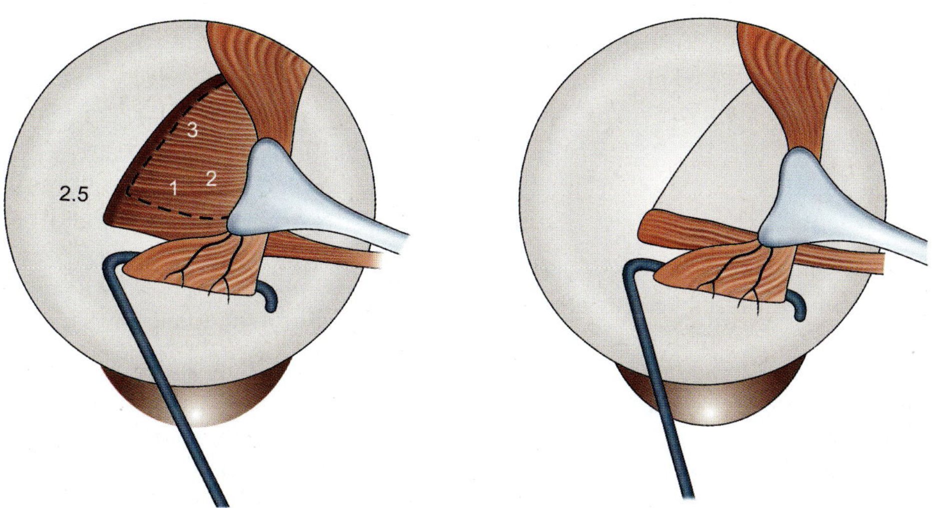

Fig. 7: Posterior tenectomy of superior oblique. The first figure shows the markings showing the anterior 2.5 mm marked. Second figure shows the remaining anterior tendon after posterior part of the muscle has been excised

Translational Recession

Since recession entails an anteropositioning which was noted to be causing an undesirable underaction of depression in abduction, Prieto Diaz proposed suturing the superior oblique tendon 6 mm nasal to the nasal border of SR and 12 mm from the limbus, a position allowing translatory movement. This prevents the underaction of depression in abduction and is called translational recession of the SO.

Superior Oblique Tendon Expander

A technique for treating Brown syndrome employs a band of silicone used as an expander to lengthen the superior oblique tendon nasal to the superior rectus. This technique has been used for all types of superior oblique overaction including Brown syndrome. It was described by Kenneth Wright.

The length of the expander used varies from 4 to 7 mm in 1 mm increments. The superior oblique tendon is isolated under direct vision nasal to the superior rectus. It is then dissected out. Two sutures are placed at mid tendon a few millimeters apart. The tendon is cut between these sutures. A No. 240 silicone band is secured with the needles of sutures. This increases the length of the tendon.

Autologous fascia lata has also been described for use as an expander to lengthen the superior oblique tendon.

The 'Chicken' Suture

This procedure creates controlled tendon expansion with a suture in place of the silicone spacer. This is for doing a guarded superior oblique lengthening employing a suture known as the 'chicken suture'.

Z or L-tenotomy

3-4 mm of the tendon is split and the ends are sutured with non-absorbable sutures—partial width tenotomy. Each 3 mm of split would cause 6 mm of elongation. The disadvantage or possible complication is: cross fibers of SO weak and diaphanous-may lead to complete tenotomy.

B. Selective Weakening

These procedures weaken selectively one of the actions of superior oblique with less to minimal effect on the remaining functions.

Posterior Tenectomy of Superior Oblique (PTSO)

This technique involves selective weakening of the depressor action of the muscle with minimal or no effect on the cyclotorsion. This therefore serves as a safeguard against the risk of postoperative complaint of torsional diplopia or head tilt.

In this procedure, the muscle is exposed in superotemporal quadrant. After exposing the insertion of the superior oblique tendon, the posterior part of the muscle is excised in the shape of a triangle with its base temporally, leaving anterior 2 mm fibers intact.

Advantages of posterior tenectomy include minimal-to-no postoperative superior oblique muscle underaction and no risk of foreign body extrusion, fibrosis, and scarring.

Anterior Tenectomy of Superior Oblique

Similarly the anterior fibers are tenotomized sparing the posterior fibers to selectively weaken the intorsion. This may be done for a torsional null in nystagmus surgery.

B: STRENGTHENING PROCEDURES FOR THE SUPERIOR OBLIQUE

Because the reflected tendon of the superior oblique has a limited potential amount of slack or redundancy, especially in acquired superior oblique palsy, tuck or resection of this tendon can cause an iatrogenic Brown's syndrome and should be done judiciously in selected cases.

Indications for Strengthening Superior Oblique

- Superior Oblique palsy
  - Vertical deviations:Tucking
  - Excycloductions: Mod. Harada-Ito
  - Nasal transpositioning in III N palsy

Sagittalization of the Superior Oblique (Harada-Ito Procedure)

The Harada-Ito procedure is a surgery designed to improve the excyclotorsion experienced by the patients with cranial nerve IV palsy. This involves anterior shift of the superior oblique tendon insertion. Harada and Ito described this technique whereby the anterior fibers are tented laterally. Fells modified it to separately disinsert the anterior fibers and advance them laterally. Metz used it as an adjustable procedure.

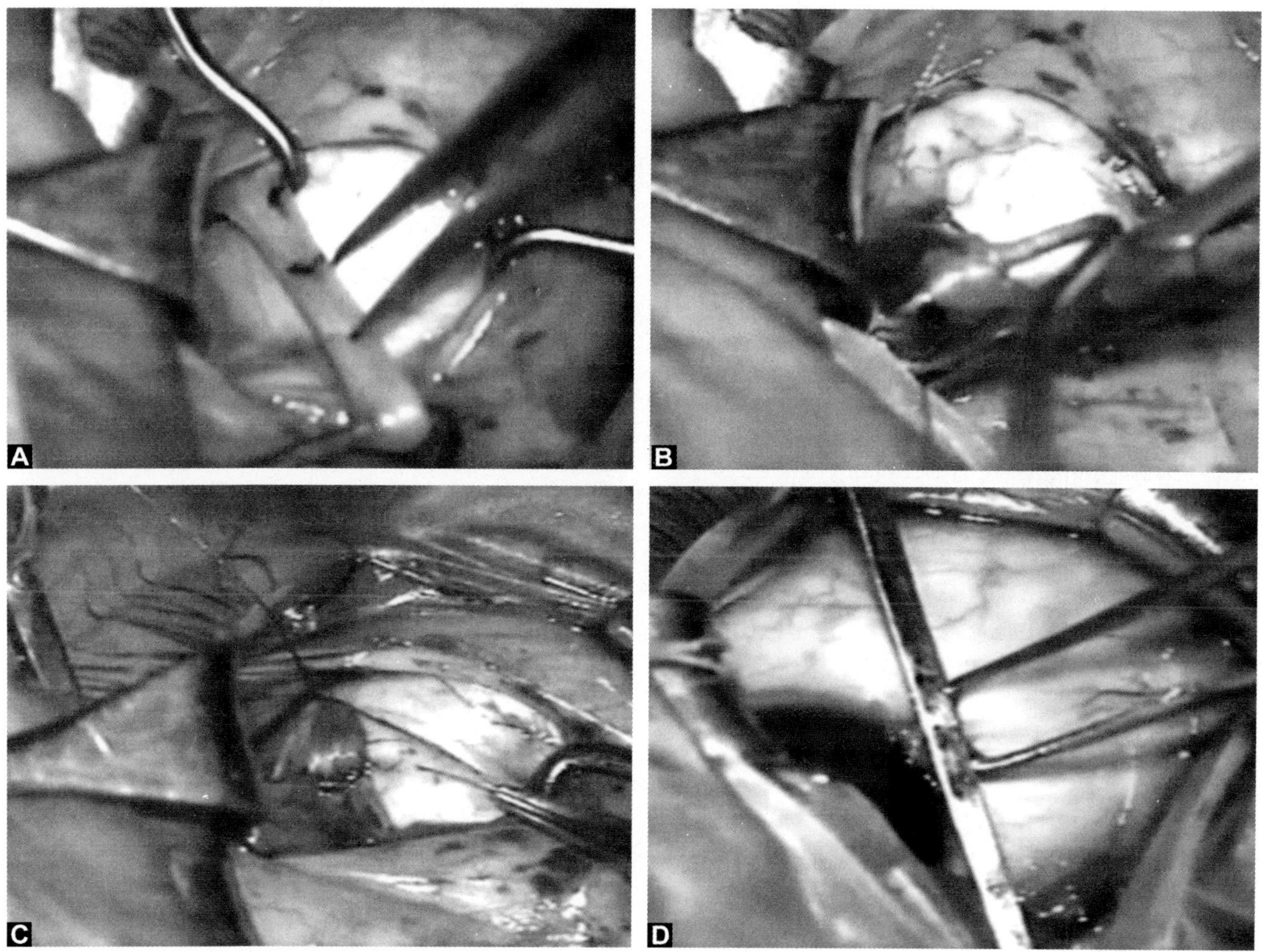

Figs 8A to D: Tucking of superior oblique muscle. (A) The tendon is exposed and the amount to be tucked is marked. (B) The tendon is then lifted using a muscle hook and clamped for the required length. (C) Sutures are passed at the site of clamp and the tucked muscle sutured to sclera. (D) At the end of procedure, the line passing between the two canthi should be below the lower limbus of elevated eye

The superior oblique tendon normally inserts in the posterotemporal quadrant of the top of the globe in a fan shaped manner. The anterior superior oblique fibers are probably more effective intorters and the posterior superior oblique fibers are more effective depressors.

In this procedure, the superior oblique tendon is split, and the anterior fibers — the fibers most responsible for incyclotorsion — are moved anteriorly and laterally. This selectively stretches and tightens these fibers, enhancing the incyclotorsion power of the superior oblique. The superior oblique tendon is exposed at its insertion and a small hook engages all or part of the insertion. The superior rectus is retracted medially, a 6-0 Vicryl or 6-0 non-absorbable suture is tied to the superior oblique tendon close to its insertion, the superior oblique tendon is split, and the anterior half of the superior oblique tendon is detached and is sutured to the sclera 5 to 10 mm anteriorly near the temporal aspect of the superior rectus or it may be placed more temporally for a greater effect.

The most common indication for the Harada-Ito procedure is bilateral acquired cranial nerve IV palsy following closed head trauma. In this clinical situation the vertical imbalance is often less symptomatically bothersome to the patient than the induced excyclotorsion. Patients with cranial nerve IV palsy whose complaints are not specifically limited to torsional diplopia, but instead also have significant vertical diplopia, are not good candidates for this procedure.

Superior Oblique Tuck at the Insertion

This procedure is done for a lax or redundant tendon. This can be confirmed by doing superior oblique traction test which reveals absence of the normal tug felt. This is seen in cases of congenital superior oblique palsy and usually not in acquired superior oblique palsy.

This is an effective and safe technique for strengthening the superior oblique. The muscle is exposed via a temporal incision for this procedure. The muscle is stretched and doublefolded on itself. The amount of tuck to be done is then marked on the tendon (half the amount is marked considering its doublefolded position). The sutures are then passed at the marked site. After the tuck has been secured, passive ductions (exaggerated forced duction test) should be performed. If the superior oblique traction test is too tight when compared with the fellow eye, the suture has to be released and the size of the tuck reduced. The endpoint is considered when the tendon is slightly tighter on the tucked side. The size of the tuck depends on the laxity of the tendon. The tucked part then may or may not be sutured to the sclera. Adjustable superior oblique tucking procedure has also been described. The eye should be able to be elevated such that the lower limbus just passes the line joining the two canthi (Figs 8A to D show the steps for tucking.)

This procedure maintains the normal action of the muscle and reduces the incidence, severity, and persistence of postoperative Brown syndrome if appropriate precautions are taken.

In general, the more vertical deviation to be treated and the more lax the superior oblique tendon, the greater is the amount of tuck required

Superior Oblique Resection and Advancement

Other techniques for strengthening or shortening the superior oblique tendon are resection, advancement, or resection and advancement.

The superior oblique tendon is exposed at the insertion. The tendon is engaged on a hook near its insertion and the superior rectus muscle is retracted medially. After the loose tendon is elevated, a double arm suture is placed at the intended amount of resection. The tendon is cut distal to the suture and the suture is passed through the tendon insertion. The distal tendon is excised. The tendon is tied securely to the insertion.

However, it is difficult to place sutures in the thin superior oblique tendon, therefore tucking is a preferred surgical option.

Transposition of the Superior Oblique Tendon

This is done in some cases of third nerve palsy, where the superior oblique tendon is transposed to the insertion of medial rectus muscle. This may be done with or without trochlear disruption.

Complications of Superior Oblique Surgery

1. Iatrogenic superior oblique palsy
2. Under correction/overcorrection
3. Injury to vortex vein
4. Upper lid edema and ptosis
5. Iatrogenic Brown syndrome—this occurs especially after superior oblique tuck or adhesions after use of a superior oblique expander.

Chapter 13

Management of A and V Patterns in Strabismus

Pradeep Sharma, Harinder Singh Sethi (India)

One of the most notable contributions in the understanding of strabismus was the emphasis on what has come to be known as the A and V patterns of strabismus. Recognition and proper evaluation of horizontal strabismus that becomes incomitant in vertical gaze is of paramount importance in the successful and effective management of the ocular deviation. Comitant horizontal deviations are those in which the angle of deviation is the same in all gaze positions. Incomitant horizontal deviations are those in which the angle of deviation varies in different gaze positions. Horizontal deviations may have *lateral* incomitances and *vertical* incomitances. In lateral incomitances, significant differences exist in the amount of horizontal deviation in primary gaze versus the side gazes, whereas, in vertical incomitances, significant differences exist in the amount of horizontal deviation in upgaze versus downgaze. These cases have been more descriptively called "Vertically Incomitant Horizontally Concomitant Strabismus" Graphically they have been called A,V,X, Y, lambda (λ) and diamond (◊) patterns depending on the pattern their deviations create.

When the eyes diverge more than 10 prism diopters (PD) from upgaze to downgaze, an A-pattern is present; when the eyes converge more than 15 PD from upgaze to downgaze, a V-pattern is present. Other types of vertical incomitances, which are less common, include X, Y, lambda(λ) and diamond (◊) patterns. The various alphabetic patterns are –

1. A-exotropia (exodeviation more in downgaze, less in upgaze) (Fig. 1)
2. A-esotropia (esodeviation less in downgaze, more in upgaze)
3. V-exotropia (exodeviation more in upgaze, less in downgaze) (Fig. 2)
4. V-esotropia (esodeviation less in upgaze, more in downgaze).
5. pure V-pattern with exodeviation in upgaze, esodeviation in downgaze and ortho-in primary position.
6. X-exotropia (exodeviation more in both up and down gazes)
7. Y-exotropia (exodeviation more in upgaze only).
8. λ-exotropia (exodeviation more in downgaze only), delta exotropia.
9. ◊ exotropia (Diamond exotropia): Exodeviation only in primary position not in up and down-gazes.

Prevalence

Since Urrets-Zavalia described them in 1948, A and V patterns have been commonly seen in at least one-third of esotropia and exotropia. V patterns are more common than the A patterns. While esodeviations are more common in the West the exodeviations are more common in the Indian and the African races. **V exotropia is by far the most common anomaly in our setup while V esotropia is so in the West.** The A esotropia is the least common type of pattern amongst the four main types, otherwise the diamond pattern is the least of all.

Etiology

A great deal has been written about the role of horizontal, vertical, and oblique muscle dysfunctions, facial characteristics, and abnormal muscle insertions. At this time, however, there is no unanimity concerning the pathophysiology of A and V patterns. From the differences in the various schools of thoughts, it appears none is singly/totally correct. It appears that multiple factors are responsible, different in different cases and more than one in some cases. The various factors that have been postulated are:

1. *Horizontal factors:* Urist championed the role of horizontal recti, assuming that lateral recti are more effective in upgaze and medial recti more effective in downgaze. An overaction of lateral recti causes V exotropia and underaction of medial recti causes A esotropia (Table 1). Cases with A-V pattern which do not have oblique muscle overactions could be responsible because of this factor. Based on this principle, Urist advocated surgery to correct the said anomaly, i.e. in case of overaction of the recti, recess them and in case of underaction resect them (Fig. 3).

Table 1: Alphabetic pattern in strabismus and overacting rectus muscles

Pattern	*Etiology*
V exotropia	overaction lateral recti
V esotropia	overaction of medial recti
A exotropia	underaction of lateral recti
A esotropia	underaction of medial recti

Vertical School

Brown stressed the role of vertical recti in the etiology of A-V patterns, the underlying mechanism known to be underaction or overaction of vertical recti, in which adduction is the tertiary action. Thus, weak superior recti would result in less adducting power in upgaze, causing V phenomenon. For example, if the superior rectus muscles are primarily underacting, their adductive effect in upward gaze will diminish; in fact, the eyes will diverge in upward gaze because of secondary overaction of the inferior oblique muscles. In downward gaze, secondary underaction of the superior obliques will cause decreased abduction and secondary overaction of the inferior rectus muscles, resulting in increased adduction of the eyes, which, according to Brown, would produce a V pattern. Brown's view is supported by the observation that secondary horizontal deviations with A and V patterns may develop following acquired paresis of vertical rectus muscles. While there is no doubt that the vertical rectus muscles contribute to adduction in elevation and depression of the globe, their action is, as a rule, normal in patients with A- and V-pattern strabismus.

Oblique School

Most strabismologists believe that dysfunction of the oblique muscles plays a major role in the etiology of A and V patterns since elevation in adduction is frequently associated with a V pattern and depression in adduction with an A pattern type of strabismus. This thinking is based on the fact that abduction is the tertiary action of the oblique muscles. Most of the A-V patterns have anomalies of oblique muscles and their respective surgery: weakening of overacting obliques and strengthening of underacting obliques does correct the respective patterns. More often it is the oblique overactions that are encountered, that is, inferior oblique overactions in V patterns and superior oblique overactions in A patterns are seen. Rarely underactions are also seen causing these patterns. Restrictive conditions like Brown's syndrome may show a Y pattern.

However, it seems logical to think that the actions of vertical recti and oblique muscles are linked inseparably. Thus, underacting superior recti would have underacting supenor obliques(ipsilateral antagonist of contralateral synergist). Thus, it would be more appropriate to have the vertical recti and obliques as a combined factor. This is the the cyclovertical school (Figs 4A and B and Table 2).

Table 2: Alphabetic pattern and overacting/underacting cyclovertical muscles

Pattern	*Overacting muscles*	*Underacting muscles*
'V' Pattern	Inferior oblique Inferior rectus	Superior oblique Superior rectus
'A' Pattern	Superior oblique Superior rectus	Inferior oblique Inferior rectus

Structural Factors (*Orbital*/Craniofacial Anomalies)

Variations in skull and orbital bones are known to have underaction or overaction of vertical oblique muscles. This may be due to variation in the site of origins and insertions of the inferior or superior obliques. It must be understood that the trochlea acts as the functional origin of the superior oblique. Thus in **sagittalization**: the oblique muscles become more parallel to the sagittal (antero-posterior) axis and in **desagittalization** (Fig. 5): the oblique muscle becomes more parallel to the coronal plane. This has been stressed by Gobin. If the superior oblique is desagittalised due to the retroplacement of trochlea (as in plagiocephaly), it becomes a poorer depressor and the inferior oblique becomes a stronger elevator relatively. Similarily a more frontally placed trochlea (as in hydrocephalus with frontal

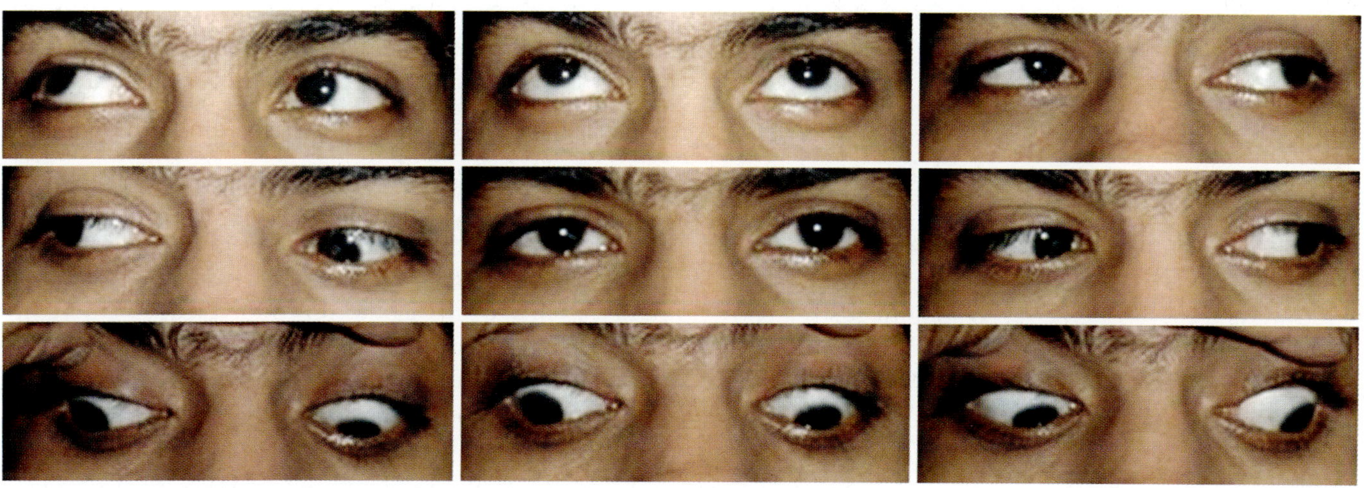

Fig. 1: A pattern exotropia with bilateral superior oblique overactions: Depression in adduction

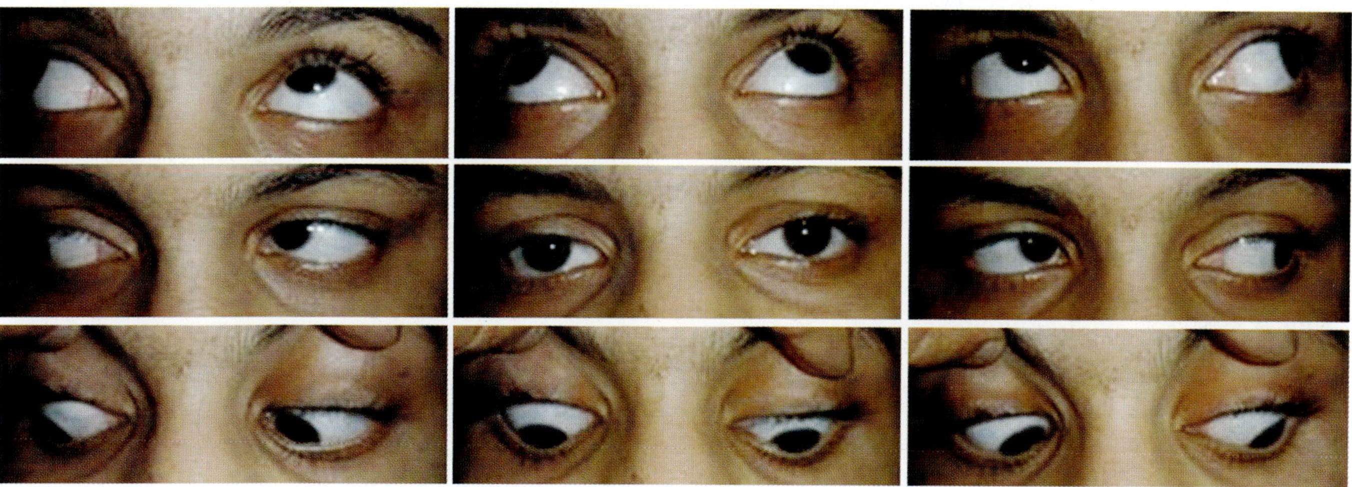

Fig. 2: V pattern exotropia with bilateral inferior oblique overactions: Elevations in adduction

bossing), becomes more sagittalized in relation to the inferior oblique making it a stronger elevator. This relative action of the obliques can cause A and V patterns.

Anomalies of Muscle Insertions

Anomalies of insertions of horizontal and vertical or oblique muscles are also known to cause A and V patterns. Because of obliquity, horizontal, vertical, and torsional vectors are created, which create more abduction in up or down gazes causing V or A phenomenon. In V patterns the insertions of medial recti have been reported to be higher than normal and those of lateral recti lower than normal. This will cause vertical vectors, making the horizontal vectors (for adduction or abduction), weaker or stronger in up and down positions creating these patterns. The vertical vectors add up to form torsional vector causing extorsion of the globes in V patterns and intorsion of globes in A patterns.

Effect of the Pulley Systems

The heterotopia of lateral rectus muscle pulleys has been postulated as one of the etiological reason behind A and V patterns. The heterotopia alters the vertical positions of the pulley, thus changing the course and the action of the lateral rectus muscle, which in turn produces elevation or depression in adduction of the fellow eye, depending on whether the pulley is displaced inferiorly or superiorly.

Hence, downward displacement of the lateral rectus pulley may cause a V-pattern strabismus and upward displacement may cause A pattern.

Clinical Findings and Diagnosis

Patient may present with the complaints of asthenopia and diplopia , since fusion may have to be maintained for a long time in certain positions of gaze. Anomalous head posture is common in patients with A and V patterns. Chin elevation or depression with a horizontal deviation should immediately alert the physician to search for vertical incomitance. The patient with A esotropia and V exotropia and fusion in downward gaze may have chin-up position. Conversely, V esotropia and A exotropia may cause chin depression. Many patients present with complaints of intermittent or permanent ocular deviation and are found to have vertical incomitance on examination.

The prevalence of amblyopia and other forms of sensorial adaptation with A and V patterns are reportedly not different from that with other forms of strabismus.

Measurements should be performed in the nine diagnostic positions of gaze. During examination, the full refractive correction be worn and accommodation controlled with appropriate targets during the measurements of the deviation. The horizontal deviations are measured in 25° upgaze and 35° downgaze in addition to the primary position. Sometimes it may be desirable to check in 45° downgaze position to exclude a significant A pattern. A 15 PD difference is taken as significant for a V pattern and a 10 PD difference is taken as significant for A pattern. For repeatable and reproducible measurements these positions are quantified with the help of a scale and a protractor on the lateral side of the head. A 35° chin-up and 25° chin-down position is used with a 6 m distance target for distance fixation measurement. For near fixation at 33 cm, either the head is similarly tilted or the target is suitably fixed. A **cephalodeviometer** has been devised using a mirror with markings drawn on it. The patient is made to wear a head band with a vertical marker, and head is suitably tilted for the required position.

It may be difficult to establish the presence of an A or V pattern in very young patients in whom a reliable prism cover test cannot be obtained in various gazes. In such cases, the head of the patient is moved passively up and down, while keeping child's attention directed at a distant fixation target. This makes it possible to evaluate any differences in the horizontal deviation between upward and downward gaze.

The fundus should always be evaluated for the torsional changes in A-V patterns especially with oblique overactions.

Treatment

While treating patient with A and V patterns, all factors should be considered. If the A/V pattern is significant and patient is symptomatic, it needs to be operated. All cases of esodeviation or exodeviations should be checked for A or V patterns.

In case of significant oblique overactions being present, the obliques should be weakened (recessed with or without anteropositioning). In case of underactions, the same should be strengthened (advancement of obliques or tucking in case of superior oblique). In the absence of oblique overactions, horizontal recti are operated (according to horizontal school). A *choice* as to either *weaken the lateral rectus* for V exotropia (as they are more effective in upgaze) or *strengthen the medial rectus* for A exotropia (as they are more effective in downgaze) can be made. Another option is *vertical transpositioning* of horizontal recti. Thirdly,

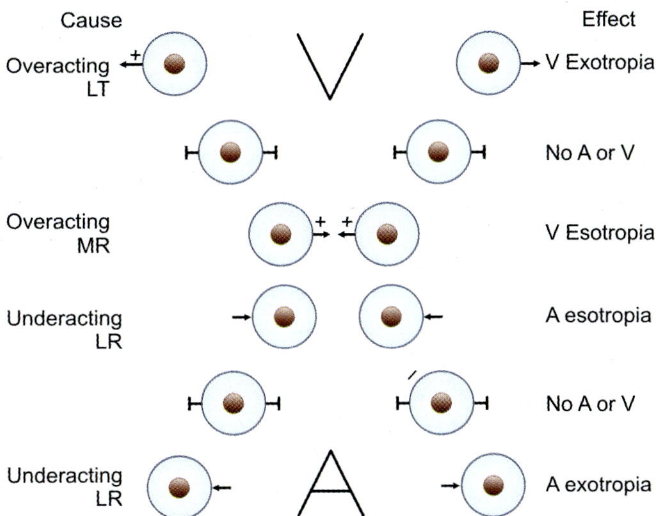

Fig. 3: Urist Horizontal School of Thought for A and V Phenomenon due to overacting lateral recti (V exo), overacting medial recti (V Eso), underacting Lateral recti (A Eso) and underacting medial recti (A eso)

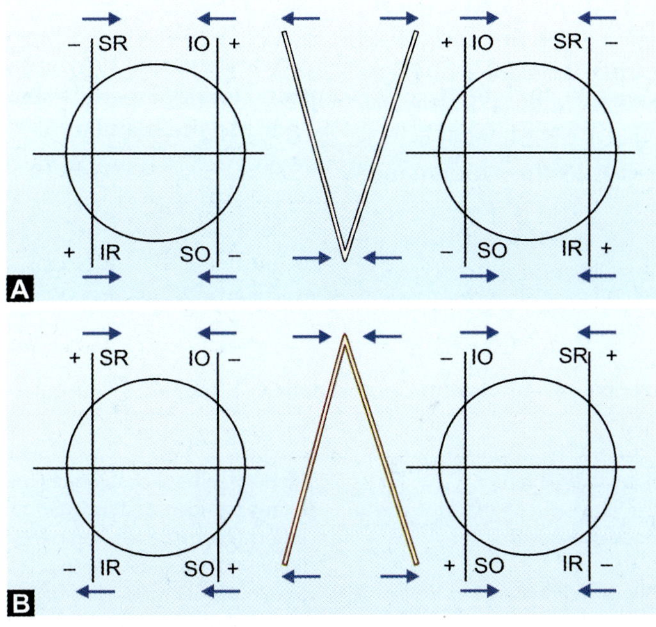

Figs 4A and B: (A) Cyclovertical Concept of V pattern caused by underacting (-) superiors (rectus and oblique, which are associated with overacting (+) inferiors (rectus and obliques). The combination is responsible for more abduction (less abduction) in upgaze and less abduction (more adduction) in downgaze (As indicated by arrows); (B) Cyclovertical Concept of A pattern caused by underacting (-) Inferiors (rectus and oblique), which are associated with overacting (+) superiors (rectus and obliques). The combination is responsible for less abduction (less adduction) in upgaze and more abduction (less adduction) in downgaze (As indicated by arrows)

differential (slanting) recession and resections can be done for added effect.

The deviation in the primary position determines the amount of surgery for the horizontal recti, whereas the amount of A or V and the associated oblique muscle status determines the oblique muscle surgery in case of oblique overaction or underaction. The various surgical procedures for correction of A and V phenomenon are summarized in Table 3.

It should be remembered that in V-esotropia esodeviation is more in downgaze so medial recti have to be weakened more in downgaze so shift them downwards (*The rule is: shift the muscle in the direction you want to weaken them*). The simple rule of the thumb is: For medial recti being recessed shift them towards the apex of the A or V phenomenon (up for A and down for V respectively) and reverse applies in case of lateral recti.

In addition the **slanting recession** or **differential recession** may be undertaken to correct A or V phenomenon. Similarly slanting resections can also be done. In slanting recessions the slant or differential recession determines the relative weakening effect. A slant of medial rectus with more recession of inferior and would correct a V esotropia. For A-esotropia, the slant is reversed (more recession of superior end). Similarly follow for lateral recti also in cases of exotropia. V exotropia demands more recession of upper end and A-exotropia demands more recession of lower end.

The **weakening procedures for inferior oblique** are graded (6, 8, 10 mm) recession for mild, moderate or severe inferior oblique over action, for 4+ (markedly severe) overactions the recession is combined with antero-positioning in the modified Elliot and Nankin's method. Myectomy is usually not recommended. For Superior oblique over actions, graded recession or graded lengthening of superior oblique by silicon expander is recommended. Bilateral posterior tenotomy/ tenectomy of superior oblique can also be done for mild to moderate superior oblique overactions. The horizontal shifting of vertical recti is rarely done. Nasal shifting of both superior rectus may be done in Y pattern. Nasal shifting of both inferior rectus may be done in collapsing an inverted Y or delta pattern.

CONCLUSION

From the above discussion, it appears reasonable to think that no single etiologic factor can explain all A and V patterns. An apparent overaction or underaction of oblique muscles is the most common clinical finding and surgery on these muscles has been quite successful in the elimination of these patterns. Whether this dysfunction is innervational and due to primary or secondary overaction, or anatomical as in the case of desagittalization of the muscle planes, or only apparent as in the case of ocular or orbital torsion, seems to be of secondary importance with regard to the management of these conditions. The best way to reach a therapeutic decision is to carefully measure the deviation and to search for apparently overacting or underacting oblique muscles. In the absence of such anomalies other surgical alternatives are available and are discussed as above.

Table 3: Horizontal deviation with A and V pattern : Suggested surgical procedures

	Pattern	*Surgical procedures*
1.	V - esotropia *with* inferior oblique overactions	Medial rectus recession or Recession-resection surgery+ Inferior oblique weakening
2.	V - exotropia *with* inferior oblique overaction	Lateral rectus recession or Recession-resection surgery + Iinferior oblique weakening
3.	A - esotropia *with* superior oblique overaction	Medial rectus recession or Recession-resection surgery + Superior oblique weakening
4.	A – exotropia *with* superior oblique overaction	Lateral rectus recession or Recession-resection surgery + Superior oblique weakening
5.	V - esotropia *without* oblique overaction	Bi-medial recession with MR down-shifted 5 mm
6.	V - exotropia *without* oblique overaction	Bi-lateral recession with LR up-shifted 5 mm
7.	A - esotropia *without* oblique overaction	Bi-medial recession with MR shifted up 5 mm
8.	A - exotropia *without* oblique overaction	Bi-lateral recession with LR shifted down 5 mm
9.	Pure V - Pattern (Exo up and eso down)	Bilateral inferior oblique weakening
10.	Pure A - pattern (Eso up and exo down)	Bilateral superior oblique weakening
11.	X - Pattern with superior and inferior oblique overaction	Weakening of both obliques of both sides.

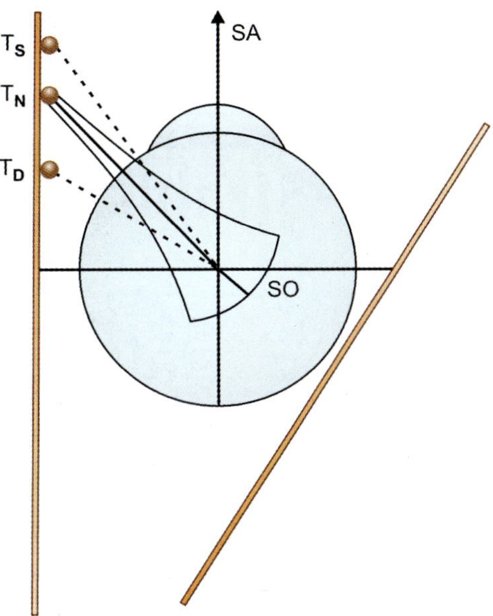

Fig. 5: Sagittalization and Desagittalization of superior obliques (SO)
SA: Sagittal axis
Trochlea: T_N = Normal position, Ts: Anteriorly placed trochlea = sagittalization, T_D : Posteriorly placed trochlea=desagittalization

SUGGESTED READING

1. Bagolini B, Campos E, Chiesi C. Plagiocephaly causing superior oblique deficiency and ocular torticollis. Arch Ophthalmol 1982;100:1093.
2. Boyd IAS, Leitch GT, Budd GE. A new treatment for A and V patterns in strabismus by slanting muscle insertions: A preliminary report. Can J Ophthalmol 1971;6:170.
3. Breinin GM. The. physiopathology of A and V patterns. In symposium, the A and V patterns in strabismus Trans. Am. Acad: Ophthalmol. Otolaryngol 1964;68:363.
4. Caldeira JA. Bilateral recession of the superior oblique in A pattern tropia. J Pediatr Ophthalmol Strabismus 1978;15:306.
5. Fink WH. The A and V Syndromes. Am Orthopt J 1959;9:105.
6. Gobin MH. Sagittalization of the oblique muscles as possible causes for the A, V and X phenomenan. Br J Ophthalmol 1968;52:13.
7. Knapp PA, V patterns. In Symposium on Strabismus. Transactions of the New Orleans Academy of Ophthalmology. St. Louis. 1971. Mosby-Year Book Inc.
8. Noorden GK von, Olson CL. Diagnosis and surgical man-agement of vertically incomitant horizontal strabismus. Am J Ophthalmol 1965;60:434.
9. Noorden GK von. Temporal transplantation of the inferior rectus muscle in V-esotropia. Am J Ophthalmol 1963;56:919.
10. Parks MM. The weakening surgical procedures for elimi-nating overaction of the inferior oblique muscles. Am J Ophthalmol 1972;73:107.
11. Payne JW, Noorden GK von. The ratio of accommodative convergence to accommodation in strabismus with A-and V-patterns. Arch Ophthalmol 1967;77:26.
12. Postie G. Etiopathogenic des Syndromes A et V. Bull. Mem. Soc Fr Ophthalmol 1965;78:240.
13. Ruttum M, Noorden GK. von. Orbital and facial anthropometry in A and V pattern strabismus. In Reinecke RD (Ed): Strabismus II New York. 1984 Grone and Stratton Inc.
14. Scott AB, Stella SL. Measurement of A and V patterns. J Pediatr Ophthalmol 1968;5:181.
15. Scott AB. A and V patterns in exotropia. An electromyo-graphic study of horizontal rectus muscles. Am J Ophthal-mol 1968;65:12.
16. Scott WE, Drummond GT, Keech RV. Vertical offsets of horizontal recti muscles in the management of A and V pattern strabismus. Aust NZ J Ophthalmol 1989;17:281.
17. Sharma P, Halder M, Prakash P. Effect of monocular vertical displacement of horizontal recti in AV. phenomena, Ind J Ophthalmol 1995;43: 9-11.
18. Sharma P, Halder M, Prakash P. Torsional changes in surgery for AV phenomena. Ind J Ophthalmol 45:31.
19. Sharma P. Strabismus Simplified. Modern Publishers, New Delhi 1999.
20. Urist MJ. Surgical treatment of esotropia with bilateral elevation in adduction. Arch Ophthalmol 1952;47:270.
21. Urist MJ. The etiology of the so called A and V syndromes. Am J. Ophthalmol 1958;46:835.

Chapter 14

Botulinum Toxin in Strabismus Management

Ewa Oleszczynska Prost (Poland)

Botulinum toxin (BTA) is very useful tool in the management of strabismus (Fig. 1)

BTA injection is rapid and relatively non-invasive. It may be repeated several times. It frequently produces complete cure or significant improvement. In case of the partial correction of the strabismus or nystagmus BTA use creates better conditions for the surgery which extension may significantly be reduced. It also facilitates further preservative treatment with prism glasses, correcting strabismus angle, and carrying exercises of binocular vision.

BOTULINUM TOXIN MODE OF ACTION

- Blocks acetylcholine release in presynaptic nerve endings in the neuromuscular junction, by antagonization of serotonin-mediated calcium ion release (Fig. 2).
- Paralyzes or cause temporal paresis of the human extraocular muscles by chemodenervation.
- Enables the antagonist muscles contraction.
- Produces an effect of permanent alignment change.
- Changes of visual localization by dissociation of pathologic cortical pathways and anomalous retinal correspondence.
- Enables development of new cortical pathways with normal retinal correspondence.

This method is effective, especially in young child, as the achievement of eyes alignment in the binocular vision development process in infants facilitates fusion.

INDICATIONS

Diagnostic Uses

- To assess whether diplopia will occur, if squint surgery is performed, especially in adults.
- To assess whether patient has useful binocular function, when orthoptic tests may fail to detect it.
- Following strabismus surgery in the past, whether reduced moment is due to an overweakened muscle or contracture of the ipsilateral antagonist.

Therapeutic Uses

- Unrecovered VI nerve palsies - Inject botulinum toxin to the medial rectus less than 6 months from the onset
- In long-standing paralysis of nerve VI - Inject botulinum toxin to the medial rectus with transposition the inferior and superior recti laterally.
- Decompensated heterophoria.
- Acute acquired esotropia.
- Congenital esotropia and exotropia - Only early intervention using simultaneous bimedial rectus muscle injection (esotropia) or bilateral rectus muscle injection (exotropia) of BTA can reestablish motor and sensory fusion with good long-term results.
- Accommodative esodeviation.
- Intermittent exotropia.
- Small esotropia and exotropia
- Consecutive esotropia and exotropia, especially with diplopia.
- Sensory strabismus.
- Nystagmus.
- Early cases of thyroid eye disease, with recent onset of strabismus.
- Cases of diplopia from orbital myositis.
- To make ptosis in sound eye in amblyopia treatment.

INJECTION TECHNIQUE

Botulinum toxin is administered on an outpatient basis:

- To adults under local anesthesia.

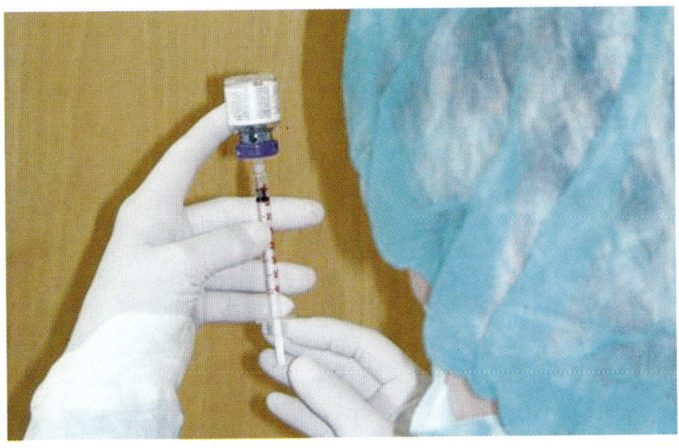

Fig. 1: Content of the vial is diluted with an appropriate volume of normal saline. One tenth of 1 ml of the diluted toxin is the recommended volume for injection and it is drawn up into a 1 ml tuberculin syringe

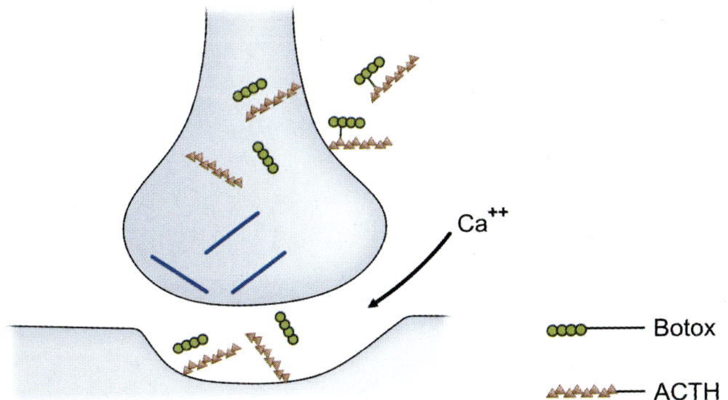

Fig. 2: The blockade of acetylcholine release in presynaptic nerve endings. Depolarization of the nerve membrane

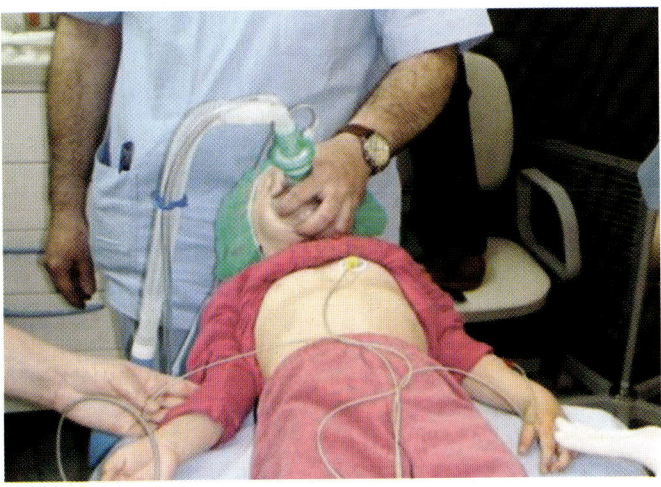

Fig. 3: Children may be sedated with short-acting inhalation anesthesia, e.g. using sevofluran, in the operating theater.

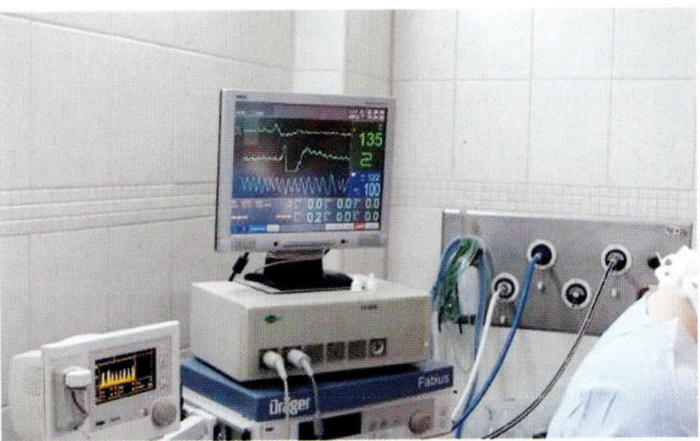

Fig. 4: Signal of bradycardia should be audible during traction of the muscle or needle insertion in ocular muscle

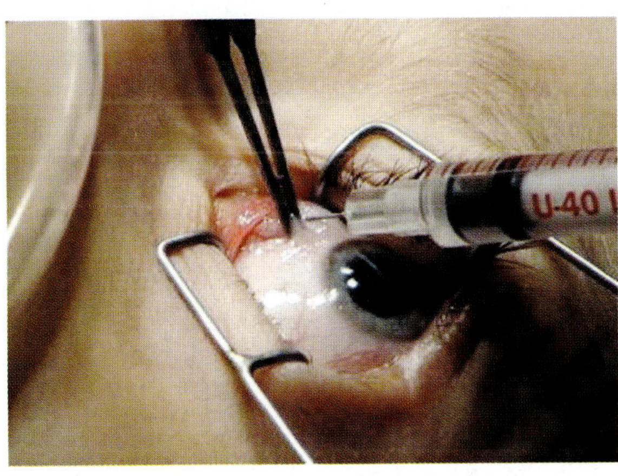

Fig. 5A: BTA injection technique in esotropia. Right medial rectus is injected with botulinum

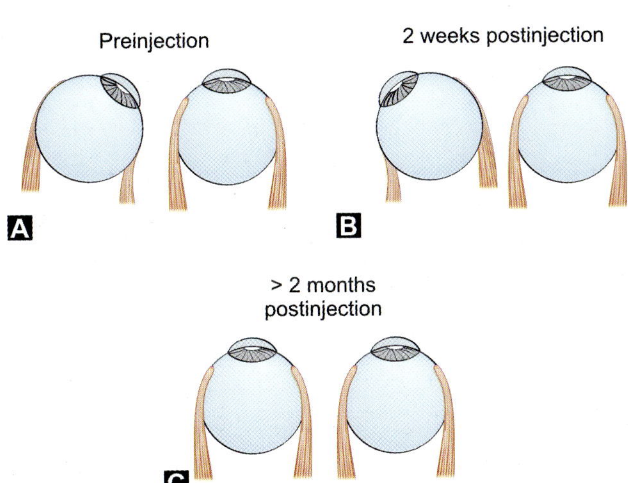

Fig. 5B: BTA mechanism of action in the covergent squint. (A) Esotropia +25PD; (B) Two weeks after injection, temporal paresis of the medial rectus muscle produced exodeviation; (C) An effect of BTA after three months, orthotropia.

- Children may be sedated with ketamine or better during short-lasting inhalation anesthesia (sevofluran) in the operating theater (Fig. 3).

Technique

- Body of extraocular muscle is pinched with the forceps through the conjunctiva.
- Needle is inserted subconjunctivally along the muscle anatomical line.
- Proper location of injection site is the junction between the posterior one-third and anterior two-thirds of the muscle.
- BTA is administered along the course of muscular fibers.
- Signal of bradycardia should be audible during traction of the muscle or needle insertion in ocular muscle (Fig. 4).
- Esodeviation - BTA is injected into both medial recti, the dose depends on the angle of strabismus and ranges from 2.5 U to 5U (Figs 5A and 5B).
- Exodeviation - BTA is injected into both lateral recti; the dose depends on the angle of strabismus and ranges from 2.5 U to 5U (Figs 6A and 6B).
- Hypertropia - BTA is injected into superior rectus; the dose depends on the angle of strabismus and ranges from 2.5 U to 5U (Fig. 7).
- Hypotropia - BTA is injected into superior rectus; the dose depends on the angle of strabismus and ranges from 2.5 U to 5U (Fig. 8).
- Horizontal nystagmus- BTA is injected to two inferior recti; the dose is 5 U.
- Vertical nystagmus - BTA is injected to two superior and two inferior recti; the dose is 5 U.
- Rotatory nystagmus - Retrobulbar needle is inserted through the skin at the inferolateral aspect of the orbit, it should be passed backward into the orbit, slightly medially and upwards; BTA dose is 10U.
- The needle should be kept *in situ* for about 50 seconds, so that the drug does not leak along the needle track and affect the other extraocular muscles.

COMPLICATIONS

- Transient ptosis.
- Subconjunctival hemorrhage
- Transient diplopia.
- Unwanted deviation due to spread of the toxin to another muscle
- Reduced accommodation—rarely.
- Dilated pupil—rarely.
- Scleral perforation—rarely (usually only in high risk cases, e.g. high myopes).

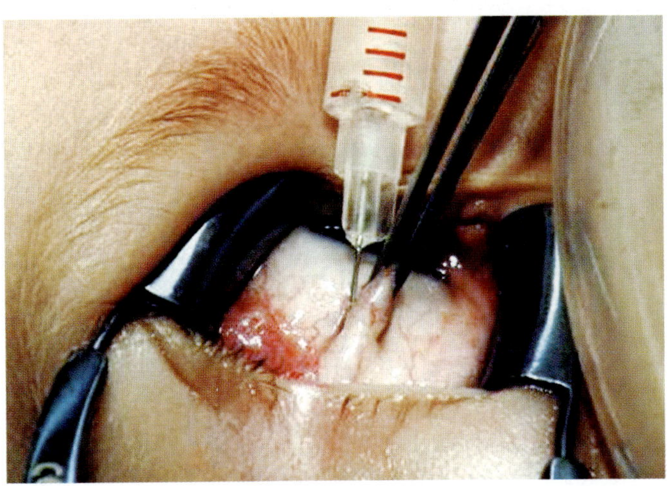

Fig. 6A: BTA injection technique in exotropia. Left lateral rectus is injected with botulinum

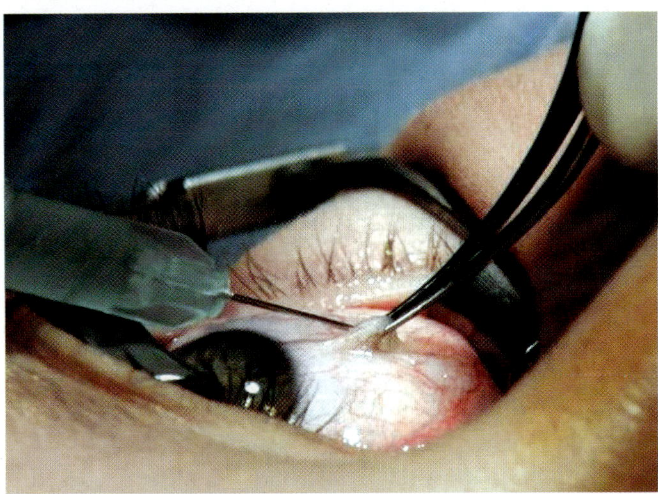

Fig. 7: BTA injection technique in hypotropia. Left inferior rectus is injected with botulinum

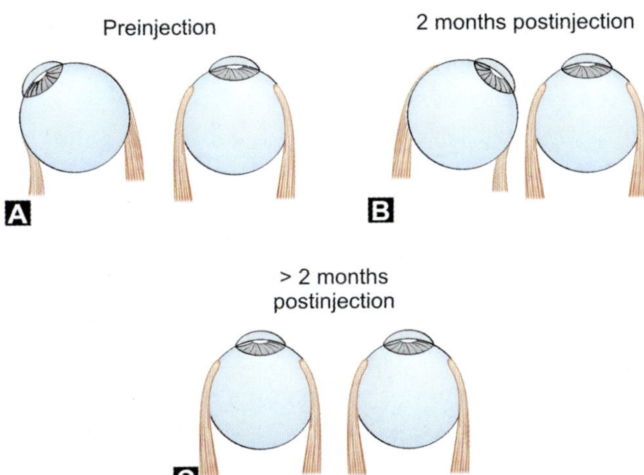

Fig. 6B: BTA mechanism of action in divergent squint. (A) exotropia - 48PD; (B) two weeks after injection,temporal paresis of the lateral rectus muscle produced esodeviation; (C) BTA effect after three month, orthotropia.

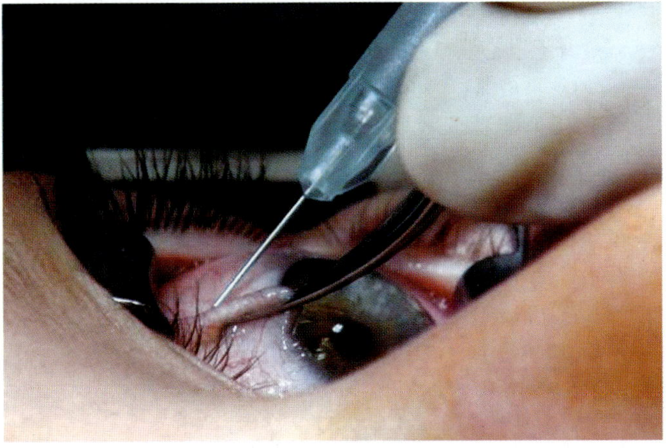

Fig. 8: BTA injection technique in hypertropia. Left superior rectus is injected with botulinum

Chapter 15

Management of Nystagmus

Rohit Saxena, Reena Sharma (India)

Nystagmus is defined as a rhythmic involuntary to-and-fro movement of the eyes. The term nystagmus is derived from the Greek word, "nystagmos", which was used to describe the wobbly head movements of a sleepy or inebriated individual. It has also been described as "dancing eyes" or "wriggly eyes".

These involuntary eye movements can occur from side to side, up and down, or in a circular pattern. As a result, the eyes are unable to hold steady on the objects being viewed. It may be accompanied by unusual head position and head nodding in an attempt to compensate for the condition. The prevalence of congenital nystagmus better termed as Infantile Nystagmus Syndrome (INS) is about 1 in every 1000 with unexplained preponderance in men. Eighty percent of nystagmus is congenital, and the remaining 20 percent is acquired.

CAUSES AND RISK FACTORS

It can be caused by multiple ocular or visual pathway problems but usually there is no identifiable cause. Some of the direct causes of nystagmus are:

1. Heredity
2. Poor vision during infancy
3. Oculocutaneous albinism
4. Eye disorders, such as optic nerve degeneration, congenital cataracts, congenital glaucoma, aniridia high myopia or severe astigmatism
5. Inner ear problems, such as infections or irritation
6. Diseases of the body, such as Meniere's disease (which involves balance problems), multiple sclerosis, or stroke
7. Injury to the head or involving the body's motor system
8. Use of certain medications, such as lithium or antiepileptic medications
9. Alcohol or drug use

Multiple neurological causes are increasingly being recognized as a cause of acquired nystagmus.

Symptoms

Nystagmus often occurs without any subjective symptoms. Symptoms that the patient might complain about include:

1. Head held in a turned position (head posture), to take advantage of the null position.
2. Oscillopsia (feeling that the world is shaking or moving) is primarily a complaint of patients with acquired nystagmus. The patient perceives the environment as moving in the direction of the fast phase of nystagmus.
3. Poor vision in patients with ocular abnormality.
4. Vertigo, nausea and vomiting are seen in patients with vestibular abnormality.
5. Neurological symptoms like weakness, sensory loss and cranial neuropathies are seen in patients with central nervous system lesions.

Features of Nystagmus

Nystagmus can be characterized by the following features:

1. *Types:* Pendular/Jerky: Pendular nystagmus is a smooth sinusoidal oscillation equal on two sides. Jerk nystagmus has a slow and a fast component.
2. *Direction:* Jerk nystagmus has a fast and a slow phase and the direction of nystagmus is according to the direction of the fast phase.
3. *Plane:* Horizontal, Vertical, Rotatory
4. *Amplitude:* Small ($<5°$), moderate ($5°$-$15°$), large ($>15°$)
5. *Frequency:* This is the no. of complete to & fro movements/sec.
   Slow (1-2Hz), medium (3-4Hz), fast ($\geq$ 5Hz)

Intensity of nystagmus: Amplitude × frequency

Nystagmus is graded according to the position of the eyes when it occurs:

Grade I – This is the type of nystagmus which is present only when the eyes are directed toward the fast component;

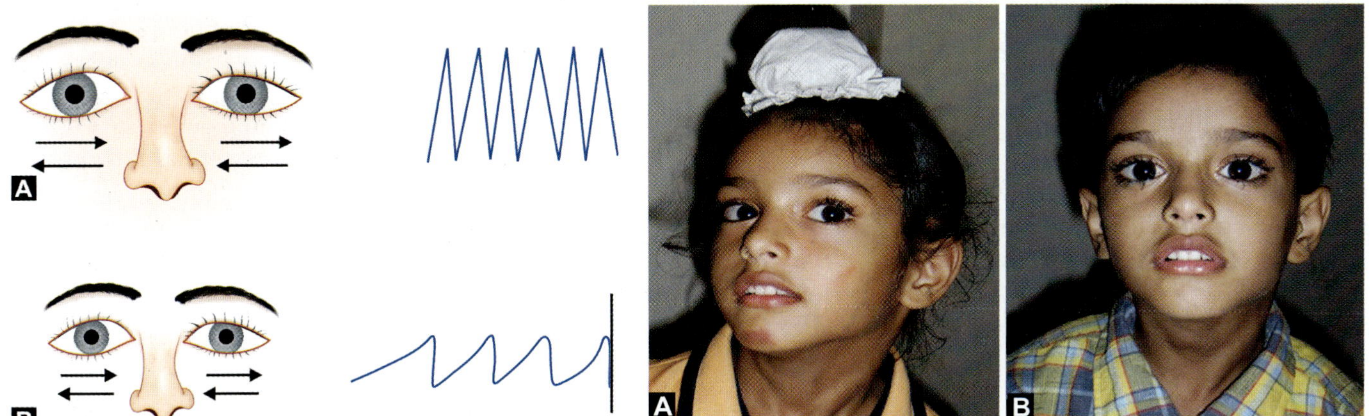

Figs 1A and B: (A) Pendular nystagmus (B) Jerk nystagmus

Figs 2A and B: (A) Preoperative head posture (B) Postoperative head posture

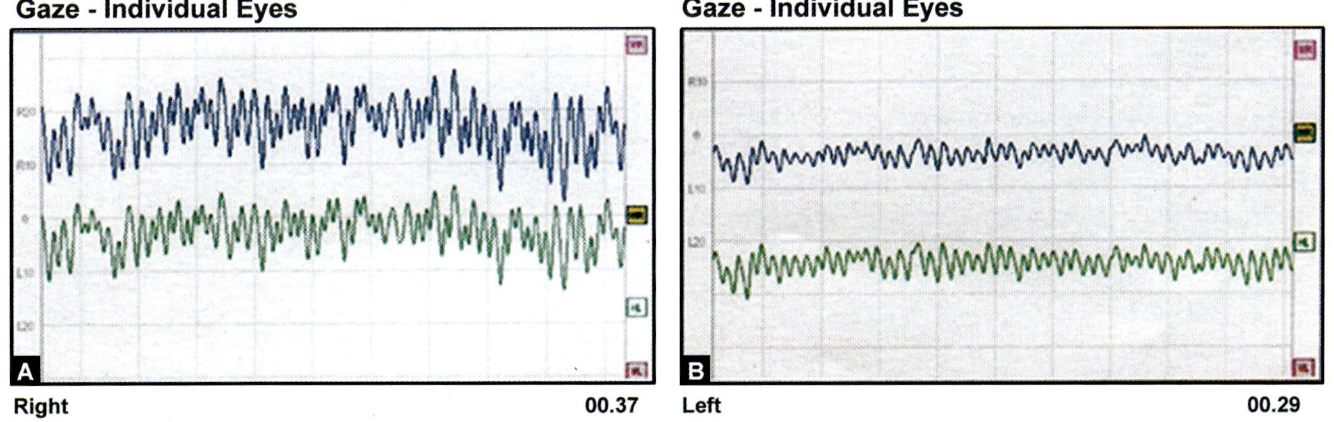

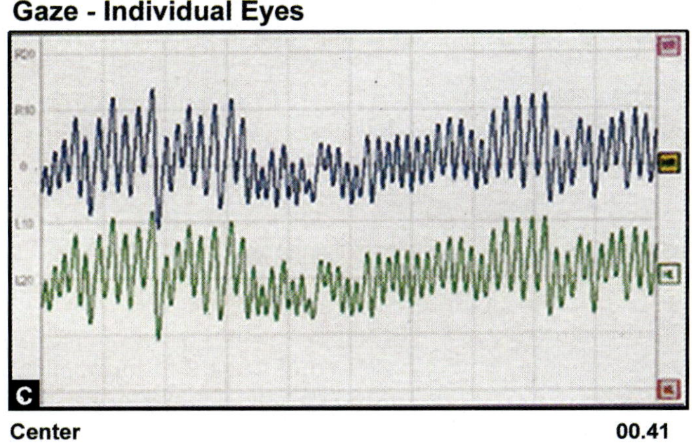

Figs 3A to C: (A) Dextroversion (B) Levoversion (C) Pre-operative ENG: Null in levovevsion

Grade II – This is the type of nystagmus which is present when the eyes are also in their primary position;

Grade III – This is the type of nystagmus which is present even when the eyes are directed toward the slow component.

Null zone: This is the field of gaze in which the intensity of the nystagmus is minimal. In most individuals with nystagmus, the severity of the eye movements can be reduced by positioning their eyes in a particular gaze. At this point, the nystagmus is the least with best visual acuity. It is important to identify the null zone if patient with nystagmus is to undergo surgery.

CEMAS Classification of Nystagmus Waveforms

The Classification of Eye Movement Abnormalities and Strabismus Working Group have recommended new names for nystagmus that begins during infancy. Three categories have been defined:

1. Infantile Nystagmus Syndrome (INS): It corresponds to what had previously been termed as motor or sensory forms of congenital nystagmus.

This type usually develops by 2 to 3 months of age. The trajectory is usually horizontal in direction though it may also have a vertical or torsional vector. It is often associated with other conditions such as albinism, congenital absence of the iris, underdeveloped optic nerves, and congenital cataract.

The important features of INS are:

- Binocular and associated (similar in both eyes)
- Uniplanar
- No oscillopsia
- Abolished in sleep
- Dampened by convergence
- Increase on fixation effort
- Distinct waveform: ascending slow-phase

2. Fusional Maldevelopment Nystagmus Syndrome (FMNS): It includes the forms of nystagmus earlier called manifest latent and latent nystagmus. This occurs in association with amblyopia and strabismus and is always congenital. This is a jerk nystagmus with either a linear or decreasing velocity slow phase identical to that of gaze-paretic nystagmus. Classically, "pure" or "true" latent nystagmus (LN) occurs only with uniocular fixation. There is no nystagmus with both eyes viewing, but when one eye is occluded, nystagmus develops in both eyes, with the fast phase toward the uncovered eye. True latent nystagmus is rare. Important features of FMNS include:

- Congenital, conjugate horizontal jerk nystagmus
- Increases under condition of monocular fixation
- When one eye is occluded, a jerk nystagmus develops in both eyes with a fast phase toward the uncovered eye
- Reverses direction with change in fixation
- Linear or decreasing velocity exponential slow phase
- Unknown cause
- Binocular vision better than uniocular vision
- Noted in early childhood in patients of congenital esotropia, DVD

3. Spasmus Nutans: It is a rare constellation of ocular oscillation, head nodding, and torticollis that begins in infancy (usually between 4 and 18 months of age) and disappears in childhood (usually before 3 years of age). The nystagmus is generally bilateral (but it can differ in each eye and may even be strictly monocular), and it oscillates in horizontal, torsional, or vertical directions. It may sometimes be mimicked by tumors of the optic nerve, chiasma, or third ventricle therefore neuro-imaging is necessary to rule them out. This type of nystagmus usually does not require any treatment.

Preoperative work-up

Patient history: A detailed history of the age of onset, symptoms, general health problems, medications and environmental factors needs to be taken. If the onset is acute, then usually the nystagmus is acquired.

A comprehensive eye examination is needed to identify the cause of poor vision which is often associated with the nystagmus.

Important points to remember during vision assessment in a patient with nystagmus include:

- Fogging of the other eye using either high plus lens or polarizing lens
- Give demanding visual tasks for distance and near
- See vision both for distance and near
- Assess monocular and binocular visual acuity
- Assess visual acuity with and without face turn.

Anterior and posterior segment examination: This is needed to find out the ocular associations and any cause for low vision.

Measurement of head posture: An orthopedic goniometer or a combination of a scale and a protractor can be used to measure the amount of face turn in nystagmus patients. A 'torticollometer' was proposed by Sradj for this measurement. This helps to decide the amount of surgical correction required.

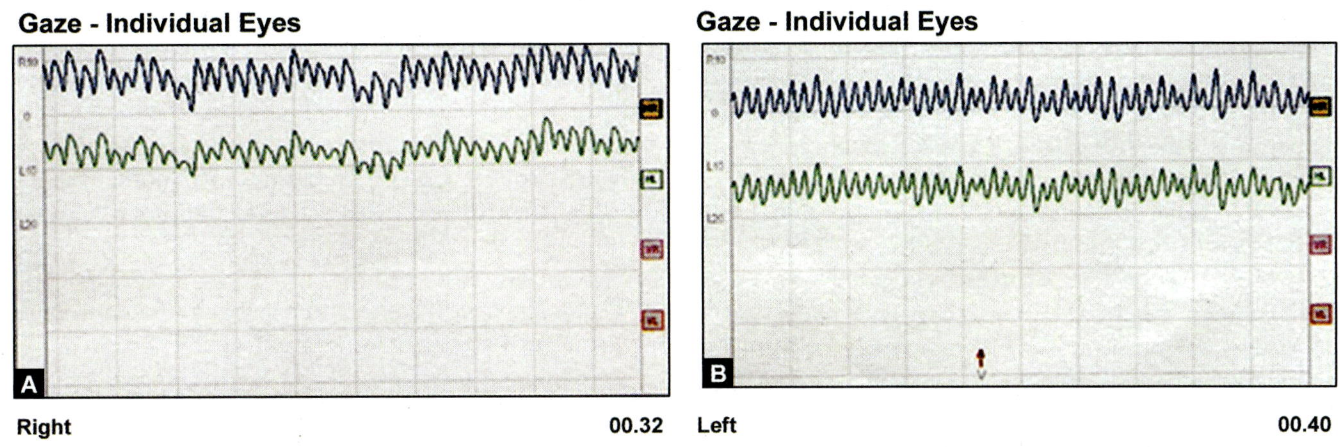

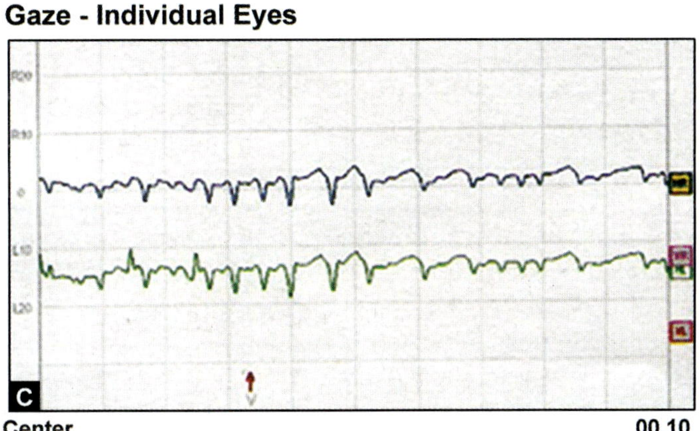

Figs 4A to C: (A) Dextroversion (B) Levoversion (C) Postoperative ENG: Null in primary gaze

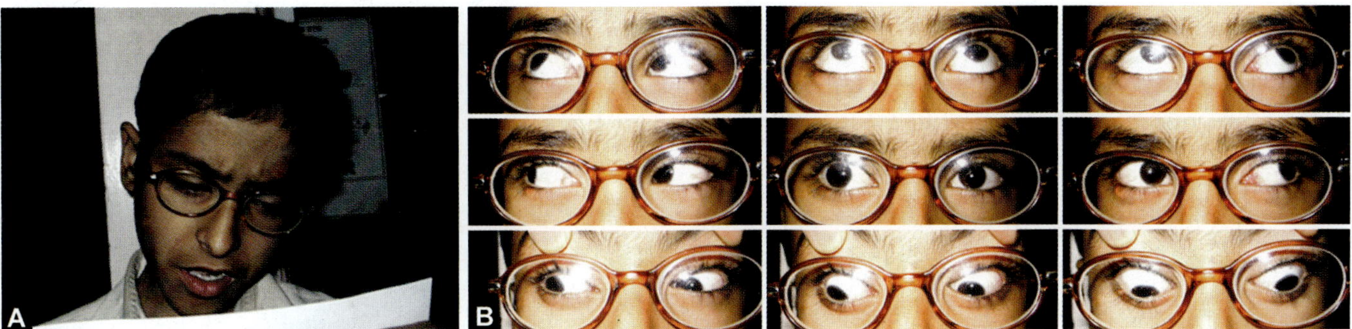

Figs 5A and B

Face-turns to one side or the other are the commonest type of posture, although minor degrees of head tilt or chin elevation or depression are seen. The typical head posture is in moderate but not extreme eccentric gaze, and nystagmus intensity will often increase again in gaze beyond this 'null zone'.

Care should be taken to identify the patients with *variable head-turns*, as these do not benefit from active treatment. They can have the rare condition of periodic alternating nystagmus. They can be identified by history or a careful examination. Head posture is used less frequently for near work so distance fixation targets should be used. It may not be present at all times and is usually seen when recognition of fine details is required.

Eye movement tracings: They can be used to verify the type of nystagmus and determine the details of the movements (electronystagmography and videonystagmography). They are especially useful in suspected PAN (periodic alternating nystagmus) cases. Using these modalities the nystagmus amplitude, frequency, intensity and velocity can be measured in various positions of gaze. This helps in localizing the null zone and documenting the changes during the postoperative period.

In a case of nystagmus neuroimaging is indicated in all cases of acquired nystagmus, Periodic alternating nystagmus, Seesaw nystagmus and Spasmus nutans syndrome.

Treatment

Nonsurgical Treatment

It is important to remember that congenital nystagmus can not be cured. However, certain interventions can help to dampen the nystagmus and help to improve visual acuity.

1. *Optical correction:* This is done to achieve the best corrected visual acuity. Low vision aids may be used when needed. Correction of significant refractive error in both children and adults with nystagmus is the single most powerful therapeutic intervention for improving vision.

   Over minus lenses stimulate accommodation and so can dampen the nystagmus to some extent. LASIK has also been recently done in myopic patients with nystagmus with good results.
2. *Amblyopia therapy:* Penalization/over plus spectacle lens can be given in better eye (manifest latent nystagmus) for the treatment of amblyopia.
3. *Contact lenses:* Contact Lenses help to improve vision in high refractive errors. They slow down eye movements, and because the optical center of the prescription is always centered on the eye with the contact lens, vision improves. They move with the eyes thus providing better image quality. Another theory is that the tactile feedback of feeling the contact lenses on the eyes may lead to better control of the movement and allow better vision.
4. *Botox injections:* These have been given either retrobulbar or directly in all 4 horizontal recti. They need to be repeated as the effect is short lasting, so is useful only for cases of acquired nystagmus.
5. *Medical management:* Baclofen has been used in the treatment of Periodic Alternating Nystagmus (PAN) with reported good results.

   Gabapentin, clonazepam, valproate and Memantine are few other drugs being used with promising results in selected nystagmus subtypes. No drug has been found to be effective in infantile nystagmus syndrome.
6. *Biofeedback training:* Attempts have been made to convert the movements of nystagmus into audible stimuli, so that on hearing these sounds, the patient may voluntarily increase the tone of his eye muscles thereby eliminating the nystagmus.
7. *Acupuncture:* It has also been successful for some patients. Afferent stimulation to the neck and face (acupuncture) may alter the behavior of the pathophysiological mechanism underlying congenital nystagmus by affecting the projections from these areas to the reticular formation and vestibular nucleus.

Nystagmus Surgery

Aims of surgical correction in a patient of nystagmus are:

1. To shift the null position from an eccentric position to primary gaze
2. To diminish the amplitude and frequency of nystagmus by improving the waveform, increase foveation time and broadening of the null position
3. To correct associated strabismus if present
4. To induce artificial divergence

Timing of surgery: There is no optimal time for surgery in patients with congenital nystagmus. It is best to wait till 4 or 5 years of age to allow maturation of binocular visual system. This will reduce the likelihood of permanent iatrogenic strabismus and loss of binocularity after surgery.

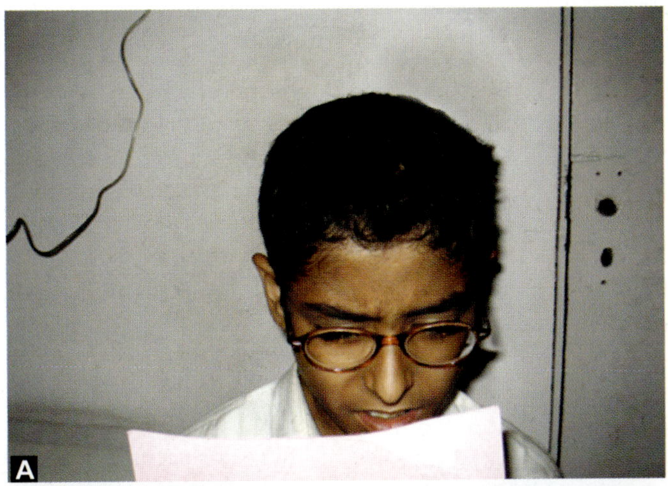

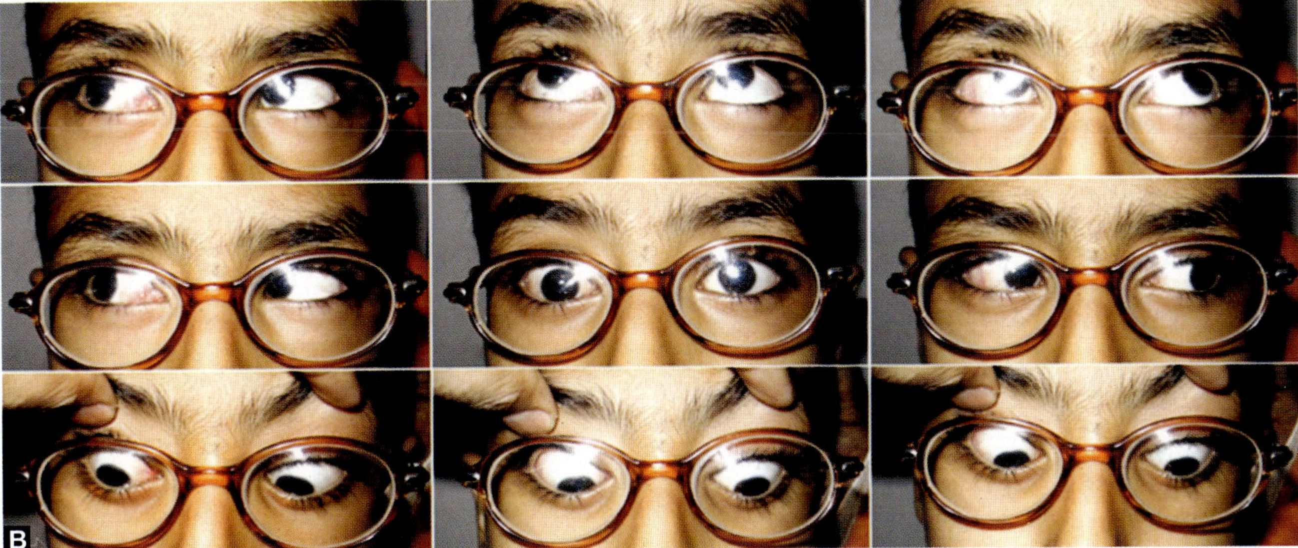

Figs 6A and B

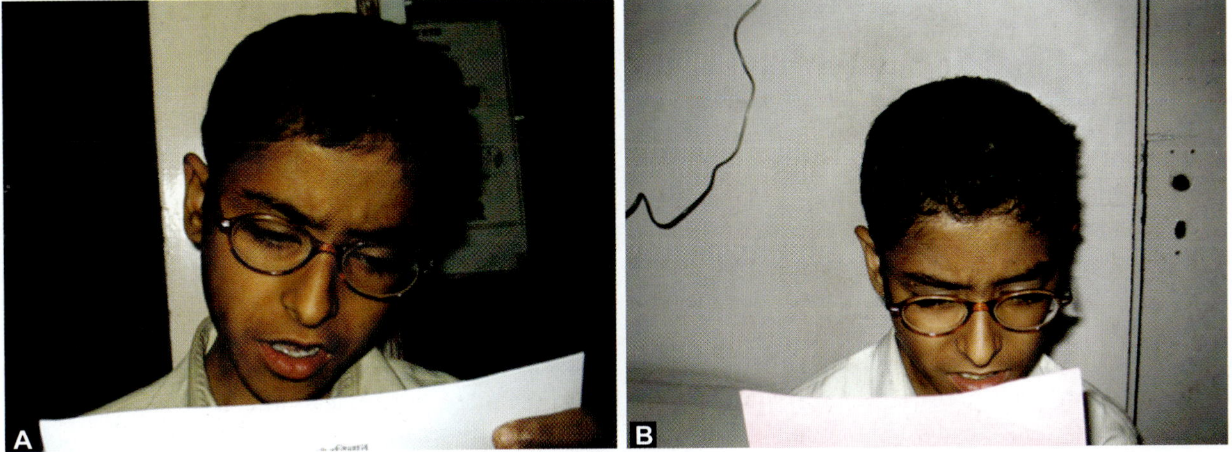

Figs 7A and B: Correction of head tilt (A) Anterior tenectomy of superior oblique (ant 2/3) (B) Advancement of anterior fibers of SO (IO weakening)

This also helps in the evaluation of the head posture as the child now goes to school and is involved in visually demanding tasks. In acquired nystagmus, one should wait for at least one year for evolution of nystagmus waveform and any resulting head posture.

Surgical Options

Treat Anomalous Head Positions

Surgery is usually done for a head posture of 20 degrees or more.

a. **Kestenbaum-Anderson surgery:** Kestenbaum described surgery on all four muscles, although he also suggested the two eyes should have sequential surgery. The procedure included recession resection of the four horizontal recti, recessing the muscles on the side of face turn and resecting the remaining ones. All muscles were operated for a measurement of 5 mm. Anderson proposed recession of the pair of rectus muscles whose action was in the direction of the face-turn. It is the Kestenbaum strategy, with modifications, that is normally performed today, and his name tends to be attached to this surgical approach used for nystagmus. 5 mm recessions and resections were not found to be adequate to improve the head posture in majority of the cases.
b. **Goto**: Goto concluded, after electro-oculographic studies in nystagmus patients that the horizontal rectus muscles that move the eyes away from the tonically deviated gaze are weak and, therefore, should be strengthened by resecting them.
c. **Modified (Parks') Kestenbaum Surgery (The classic maximum) –The 5, 6, 7, 8' procedure:** This is the most accepted modification of this surgery. It involves recession of medial rectus of 5 mm, and resection of lateral rectus of 8 mm in one eye along with recession of medial rectus of 6 mm, and resection of lateral rectus of 7 mm in the other eye. Therefore, each eye gets a total of 13 mm of surgery. This is adequate for head turns of upto 30°.
d. **Pratt-Johnson surgery:** Equal recessions and resections of all horizontal recti are done. Ten-millimetre recession/resection surgery produced the best correction of the face turn. This procedure has not received much attention.
e. **Augmented modified Kestenbaum surgery (augmented parks)**: Where the head-turn is up to 30°, the surgical amounts are increased by 40%—i.e. 7, 8.4, 9.8, 11.2 mm. Where the turn equals or exceeds 45°, they advocate 60% augmentation—i.e. 8, 9, 11.2, 12.8 mm. Head postures definitely improve but patients may develop some duction deficit.
f. **Augmented Anderson procedure** has been described by von Noorden where larger recession of the yoke muscles is preformed. For a face turn to the left, the lateral rectus muscle of the right eye is recessed by 12 mm and the medial rectus muscle of the left eye is recessed by 10 mm. The advantage of this procedure is that only one rectus muscle has been operated in either eye so operating another rectus muscle in either eye is still possible to correct for any residual deviation in the horizontal or the vertical direction. Also accidental surgery on a case of Periodic Alternating Nystagmus can easily be converted to all 4 recti recession by performing similar surgery on the remaining horizontal recti.

Improve Vision

In patients without a null position or null in primary position, the aim of surgery is largely directed at dampening the eye movements. Among the commonly used surgical methods are:

1. Surgically induced artificial exophoria: Bimedial recession is done to stimulate fusional convergence and thereby dampen the nystagmus.
2. Anterior tenotomy of horizontal rectus muscles (Hertle-Dell'Osso procedure): The surgery consists of a simple tenotomy, dissection, and suture of the involved extraocular muscles in place, with neither recession nor resection. The putative mechanism responsible for the damping effects of tenotomy is alteration of a proprioceptive tension-control loop.
3. Large recession of all horizontal rectus muscles: By retro placing the muscle insertion behind the equator and thus posterior to the tangential point, the leverage is decreased and given amount of muscle innervations will have less rotational effect on globe.

Other surgeries described in literature but no more popular include:

a. Fixation of extraocular muscles to the periosteum
b. Myopexy of all horizontal rectus muscles posterior to the equator.
c. Placement of retroequatorial encircling silicone band over all rectus muscles in both eyes.
d. Extirpation of horizontal rectus muscles.

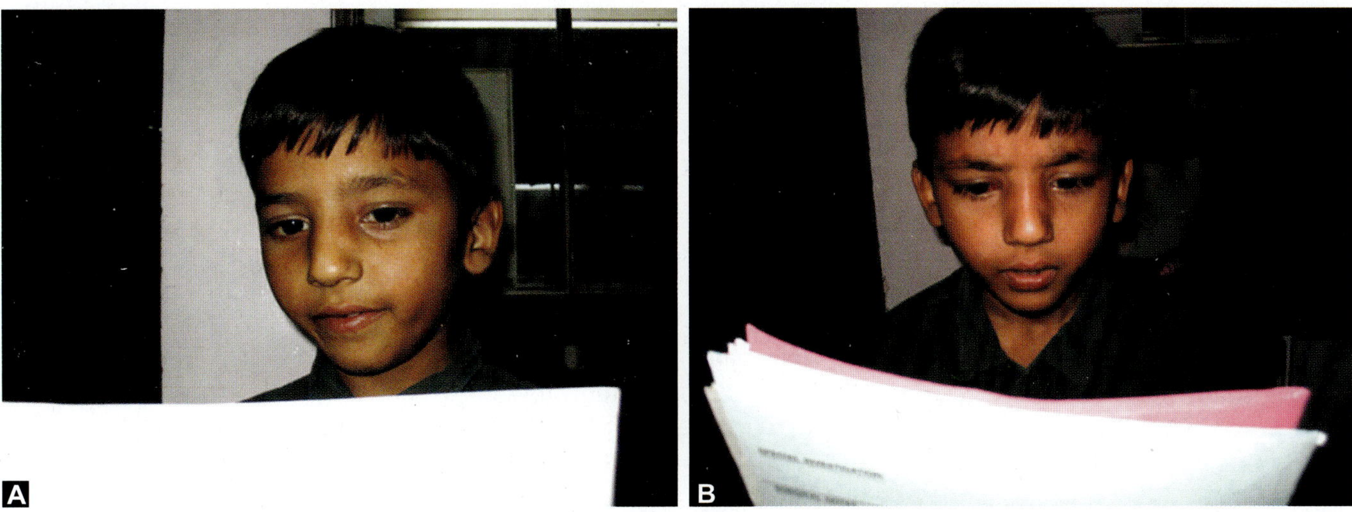

Figs 7A and B: (A) Null in levoversion (B) Corrected null: in 1° gaze

Artificial Divergence Surgery

A number of patients with nystagmus show an improvement in nystagmus amplitude on convergence. They have better near visual acuity. These patients can therefore benefit by a surgery which would stimulate convergence.

Before doing this surgery, base out prisms are given to the patient. Any decrease in the amplitude of nystagmus, suppression of nystagmus or an improvement in vision is recorded. The patients who show an improvement in this testing undergo the surgery which involves weakening of the two medial recti. A bimedial recession or bimedial faden (posterior fixation suture) is done. This induces a latent divergent ocular position (exophoria), which the patient will then overcome by exerting fusional convergence, thereby damping the nystagmus. Patients should have adequate fusional reserves to overcome the induced deviation, so preoperative testing with prisms is a must. The amount of recession is decided by the amount of base out prisms improve vision without inducing diplopia. Postoperative nonfusible diplopia is a major complication of surgery which may require reversible of the procedure.

Maximum Recession of Horizontal Rectus Muscles

It was first suggested by Bietti and Bagolini in 1960, but was then revived by von Noorden and Helveston. This procedure involves weakening of all four horizontal recti muscles. The weakening is achieved by recessing the two medial recti by 10 mm and the lateral recti by 12 mm. This reduces the amplitude of the nystagmus in these patients, all congenital nystagmus being either purely or largely horizontal in direction.

By retroplacing the muscle insertion behind the equator and thus posterior to the tangential point, the leverage is decreased and a given amount of muscle innervation will have less rotational effect on the globe. Large recessions cause reduction in horizontal rotations of the eye and therefore distinctly improve vision. No significant reduction in ductions is noted. The Snellen acuity is only slightly improved, but nearly all patients report a subjective improvement in visual acuity.

Anterior Tenotomy of Rectus Muscles

This type of surgery dampens the nystagmus in patients that do not have gaze-angle, convergence or static nulls (i.e. they have asymmetric (a) periodic alternating nystagmus—APAN) or do have a primary-position null. The surgery consists of a simple tenotomy, dissection, and suture of the involved extraocular muscles in place, with neither recession nor resection. The putative mechanism responsible for the damping effects of tenotomy is alteration of a proprioceptive tension-control loop. Dell'Osso et al described this procedure.

VERTICAL POSTURES AND HEAD TILTS

They are much less common, although many face-turns do have some amount of vertical head displacement. When chin elevation or depression is the main feature, the principle of surgery is to rotate the eyes in the direction of the head posture. Therefore, for chin depression, both inferior recti should be resected and both superior recti recessed by an amount of 4 mm.

For pure head tilt, the superior oblique on the side of the tilt should be weakened and the inferior oblique on the other side strengthened. Conrad and de Decker have described a surgery on all four oblique muscles. An alternative approach has been described by Spielmann described slanting of the insertions of all the rectus muscles of each eye.

Nystagmus Blockade Syndrome

Horizontal medial rectus muscle recession with or without posterior fixation sutures can be done in patients of nystagmus blockade syndrome. Prism adaptation can be done pre-operatively to determine the target angle for surgery that will not be associated with significant exotropia for distance.

ASSOCIATED STRABISMUS

In cases with strabismus along with nystagmus generalized doses are not possible and can be difficult to predict. One can either stage the procedure by operating for the nystagmus first in the dominant eye and for the strabismus later. Alternatively the doses for the nystagmus surgery can be "modified" to correct for the squint along with the nystagmus. If there is a distinct fixing eye, the head posture surgery can be done in that eye and the strabismus surgery in the non-dominant eye. Outcomes can be improved by using one or more adjustable sutures.

RESURGERY

Most authorities agree that the early response to surgery wears off in some cases, with recurrence of the head posture. Reoperation may be needed. Re-resection of the previously resected muscles and a posterior fixation procedure on the previously recessed muscles can be done.

Resurgery may also be needed in unsuspected cases of periodic alternating nystagmus who develop a face turn to the opposite side following the first surgery on two muscles.

The benefit of the various surgeries described is mainly cosmetic, either in terms of correction of anomalous head posture or decrease in the amplitude of nystagmus. Dell'Osso and Flynn have also additionally shown 'broadening of the null zone' postoperatively. Best corrected visual acuity usually remains same or improves by one to two lines after the surgery.

Of these various surgeries described above, the main surgical strategies that have received worldwide attention in management of congenital nystagmus are Kestenbaum-Anderson surgery and the Augmented Anderson procedure for compensatory head posture with null zone; artificial divergence surgery; maximum recession of horizontal rectus muscles and rectus muscle anterior tenotomy for improvement of vision.

BIBLIOGRAPHY

1. Anderson JR. Causes and treatment of congenital eccentric nystagmus. Br J Ophthalmol 1953;37:267-80.
2. Barbara A, Shehadeh-Masha'our R, Garzozi HJ. Laser ablation in eyes with congenital nystagmus. J Refract Surg. 2007 Jun;23(6):623-5.
3. Bietti GB, Bagolini B. Traitement médico-chirurgical du nystagmus. Année Ther Clin Ophthalmol 1960; 11: 268-93.
4. Biousse V, et al. The use of contact lenses to treat visually symptomatic congenital nystagmus. American Journal of Ophthalmology, Volume 137, Issue 5, May 2004, 972.
5. Blekher T, Yamada T, Yee RD, Abel LA. Effects of acupuncture on foveation characteristics in congenital nystagmus. Br J Ophthalmol 1998 Feb; 82(2):115-20.
6. Calhoun JH, Harley RD. Surgery for abnormal head position in congenital nystagmus. Trans Am Ophthalmol Soc. 1973; 71:70-83; discussion 84-7..
7. Colburn JE. Fixation of the external recuts muscle in nystagmus and paralysis. Am J Ophthalmol 1906; 23:85-8.
8. Dell'Osso LF, Flynn JT. Congenital nystagmus surgery: A quantitative evaluation of the effects. Arch Ophthalmol 1979;97:462-9.
9. Dell'Osso LF, Hertle RW, Williams RW, Jacobs JB. A new surgery for congenital nystagmus: Effects of tenotomy on an achiasmatic canine and the role of extraocular proprioception. J AAPOS 1999;3:166-82.
10. Dutton JJ, Fowler AM. Botulinum toxin in ophthalmology. Surv Ophthalmol. 2007 Jan-Feb; 52(1):13-31. Review.
11. Gräf M, Droutsas K, Kaufmann H. Surgery for nystagmus related head turn: Kestenbaum procedure and artificial divergence. Graefes Arch Clin Exp Ophthalmol 2001 Jun;239(5):334-41.
12. Gupta R, Sharma P, Menon V. A prospective clinical evaluation of augmented Anderson procedure for idiopathic infantile nystagmus. J AAPOS. 2006 Aug; 10(4):312-7.
13. Helveston EM, Ellis FD, Plager DA. Large recession of the horizontal recti for treatment of nystagmus. Ophthalmology 1991;98:1302-5.
14. Hertle RW. Examination and refractive management of patients with nystagmus. Surv Ophthalmol. 2000 Nov-Dec; 45(3): 215-22.

15. Mezawa M, Ishikawa S, Ukai K. Changes in waveform of congenital nystagmus associated with biofeedback treatment. Br J Ophthalmol. 1990 Aug;74(8):472-6.
16. Mitchell PR, Wheeler MB, Parks MM. Kestenbaum surgical procedure for torticollis secondary to congenital nystagmus. J Pediatr Ophthalmol Strabismus 1987;24: 87-92.
17. Nelson LB, Ervin-Mulvey LD, Calhoun JH, Harley RD, Keisler MS.Surgical management for abnormal head position in nystagmus: the augmented modified Kestenbaum procedure.Br J Ophthalmol. 1984 Nov;68(11):796-800.
18. Nystagmus surgery. In Strabismus surgery: Basic and advanced strategies by David A Plager, Edward G Buckley, Marshall M 2004;194..
19. Parks MM. Congenital nystagmus surgery. Am ortho J.1973;23:35-9.
20. Pratt-Johnson JA. Results of surgery to modify the null zone position in congenital nystagmus. Can J Ophthalmol 1991 Jun;26(4):219-23.
21. Sradj N. Torticollometry for direct measurement of head posture. Am Orthopt J 1984;34: 117-18.
22. von Noorden GK, Sprunger DT. Large rectus muscle recessions for the treatment of congenital nystagmus. Arch Ophthalmol 1991;109: 221-6.
23. von Noorden GK, Sprunger DT. Large rectus muscle recessions for the treatment of congenital nystagmus. Arch Ophthalmol 1991;109:221-6.

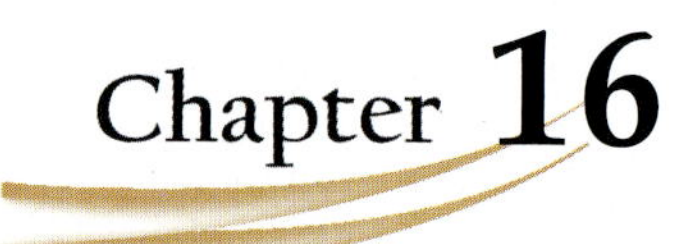

Infranuclear Disorders of Ocular Motility

JL Goyal, Sachin Mehta (India)

OCULOMOTOR NERVE PALSY

Presents with double vision, droopy eyelid with or without pain. However, pain does not distinguish between microvascular infarction and compression.

Features

External Ophthalmoplegia

- Complete palsy: Limitation of ocular movements in all fields of gaze except temporally
- Incomplete palsy: Partial limitation of ocular movement.
- Superior division palsy: Ptosis and inability to look up.
- Inferior division palsy: Inability to look nasally or inferiorly, pupil may be involved.

Internal Ophthalmoplegia

- Pupil involving: Fixed, dilated or minimally reactive pupil
- Pupil sparing: Pupil not dilated and reactive to light
- Relative pupil sparing: Pupil partially dilated and sluggishly reactive to light.

Others: An exotropia or hypotropia. Aberrant regeneration (elevation of the upper eyelid with gaze down or nasally, sometimes pupil constriction usually segmental when looking up, down or nasally).

Differential diagnosis: Myasthenia gravis, thyroid eye disease, chronic progressive external ophthalmoplegia, Orbital inflammatory pseudotumor, Internuclear ophthalmoplegia, Parinaud /dorsal midbrain syndrome.

Etiology

Pupil involving: Aneurysm (particularly a posterior communicating artery aneurysm), tumor, trauma, congenital, cavernous sinus mass, pituitary apoplexy, herpes zoster, leukemia.

- Pupil sparing: Ischemic microvascular disease, rarely cavernous sinus disease, GCA.
- Aberrant regeneration: Trauma, aneurysm, tumor, congenital. Not microvascular.

Workup

1. History: Onset and duration of diplopia? Recent trauma? Diabetes or hypertension.
2. Complete ocular examination: Check for pupillary involvement, motility restriction, ptosis, proptosis, orbicularis muscle weakness, and eyelid fatigue on sustained upgaze, signs of aberrant regeneration.
3. Neurologic examination: Assess other cranial nerves
4. Immediate imaging of the brain (gadolinium enhanced MRI) to rule out mass/aneurysm is indicated for
   a. Pupil involving III nerve palsy
   b. Pupil sparing III nerve palsy in the following group of patients
      - Patients younger than 50 years of age
      - Patients with incomplete third nerve palsies that may evolve into pupil involvement.
      - Patients with additional cranial nerve or neurologic abmormalities.
   c. All patients in whom aberrant regeneration develops, except after traumatic nerve palsy.
   d. Children younger than 10 years, regardless of the state of the pupil.
5. Cerebral angiography is indicated for all patients older than 10 years with pupil involving nerve palsies whose imaging study is negative.
6. Edrophonium chloride (Tensilon test) when myasthenia is suspected and pupil is not involved.
7. Blood pressure, FBS, glycosylated hemoglobin.
8. CBC with differential and ESR.

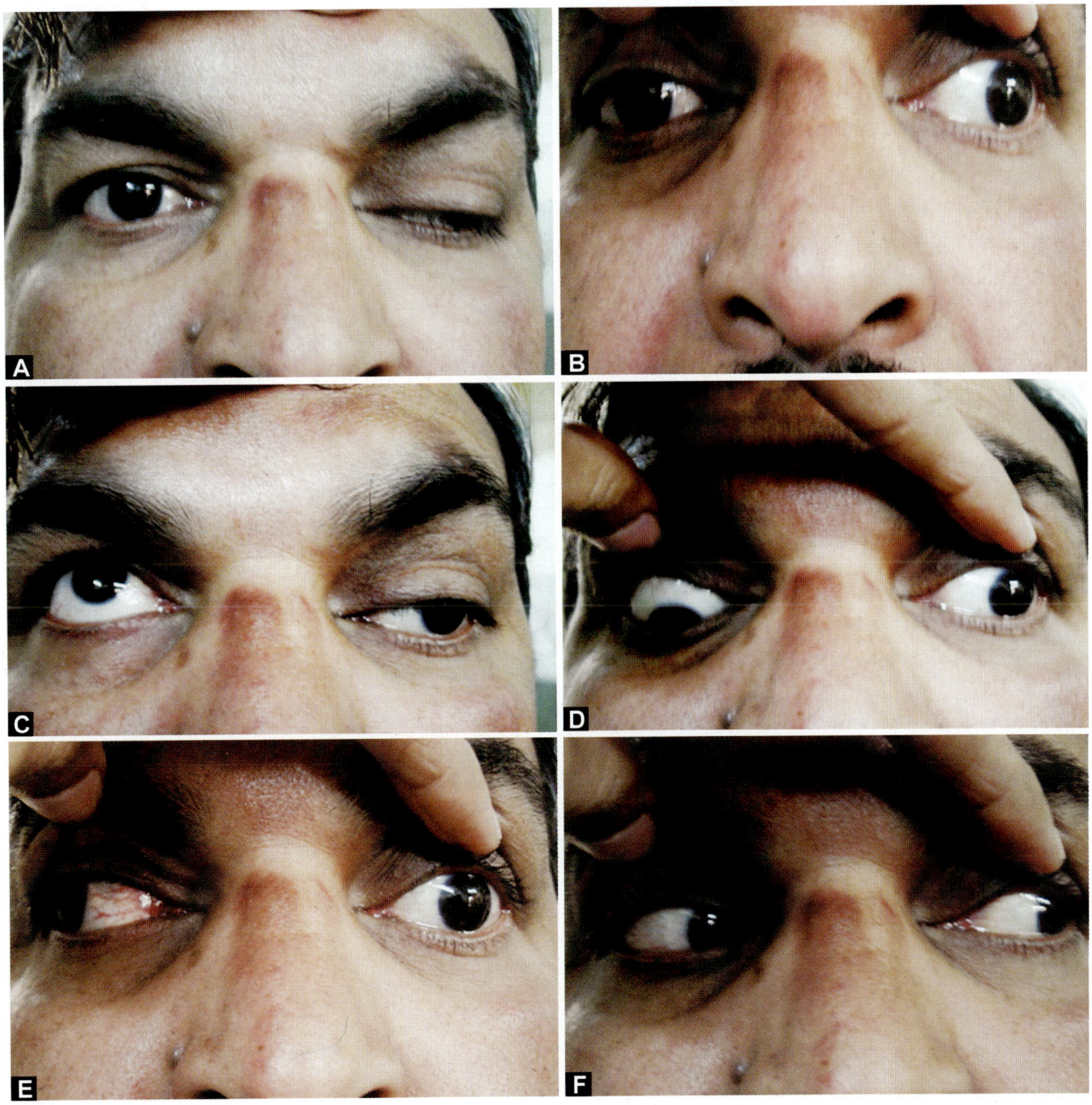

Figs 1A to F: Pupil sparing left third nerve palsy showing severe ptosis with complete ophthalmoplegia. There is total loss of motion on upgaze, downgaze, and on dextroversion with preserved levoversion

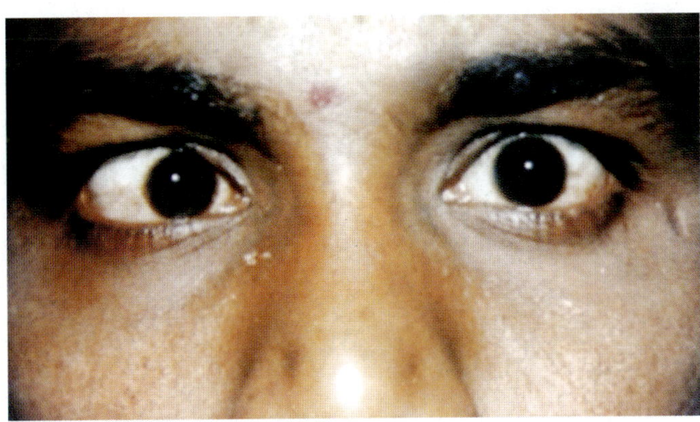

Fig. 2: Right abducens nerve palsy

Treatment

1. Treat the underlying abnormality.
2. If the nerve palsy is causing symptomatic diplopia, an occlusion patch may be placed over the involved eye.

Follow-up: Observe for delayed pupil involvement and then recheck every 4-6 weeks. If the palsy does not reverse by 3 months, the pupil dilates, additional neurologic abnormalities develop, aberrant regeneration develops or an incomplete III nerve palsy progresses, then an immediate MRI must be obtained. Refer to an internist for management of vasculopathic disease.

Abducens Nerve Palsy

Symptoms: Binocular horizontal diplopia most pronounced in the direction of the paretic lateral rectus muscle.

Signs: The affected eye has limited abduction with resultant esotropia.

Differential diagnosis: Thyroid eye disease, ocular myasthenia, orbital inflammatory disease, orbital trauma, Duane syndrome type I, Mobius syndrome, convergence spasm, divergence paralysis.

Etiology: Vasculopathic (diabetes, hypertension, atherosclerosis), trauma, idiopathic. Raised intracranial pressure, cavernous sinus mass. Benign postviral or postvaccination condition and petrositis causing a VI and VII nerve palsy (Gradenigo syndrome) in children.

Work-up

1. Hstory: History of systemic illness (diabetes, hypertension).
2. Complete neurologic and ophthalmic examination: examination of other cranial nerves. Optic disk examination to rule out papilledema.
3. BP, HbA1c and FBS.
4. MRI of the brain is indicated for following:
   - Younger than 40 years of age
   - VI nerve palsy associated with pain or other neurologic disease.
   - Bilateral VI nerve palsy
   - Papilledema

Treatment

1. Any underlying medical problem needs attention.
2. An occlusion patch may be placed over one eye to relieve symptomatic diplopia.
3. Prisms in glasses for chronic stable deviations.
4. Surgery can be considered for stable deviation that persists for more than 6 months.

SUGGESTED READING

1. Albert DM, Jackobeic FA. Principles and Practice of Ophthalmology: Clinical Practice; Philadelphia: Saunders, 1994.
2. Miller, Neil R. Newman, Nancy J. Walsh and Hoyt's Clinical Neuro-Ophthalmology, 6th Edition Lippincott Williams & Wilkins 2005.

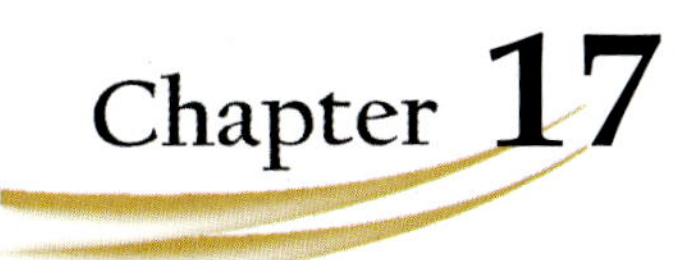

Dissociated Deviations

M Edward Wilson, Berdine M Burger (USA)

INTRODUCTION

Dissociated movements and misalignments of the eyes are grouped into what is known as the dissociated strabismus complex (DSC)[4,7,9,11]. Dissociated ocular deviations can be vertical (DVD), horizontal (DHD), or torsional (DTD). DSC obviates the semantic confusion that occurs when referring to a dissociated deviation as a DVD when, in some patients, the most prominent movement is horizontal or torsional. The DSC is commonly associated with congenital esotropia, but it may also be seen in association with other forms of strabismus.[3,8] In addition, it can be seen to develop whenever a child suffers from a permanent unilateral vision loss or in association with acquired tropias. All conditions have in common an absence of high-grade stereopsis (bifixation or macular binocular vision).

CLINICAL SIGNS AND SYMPTOMS

The classic DSC pattern is of a nonfixating eye slowly elevating, extorting, and abducting upon the spontaneous loss of binocular function or with cover testing. A reversal of these movements is seen with recovery and refixation. Latent nystagmus is also often seen on exam, but macular binocular vision with high-grade stereopsis is never present.

The DSC is nearly always bilateral but asymmetric.[5] Dissociated deviations may be controlled by binocular fusion mechanisms and remain latent, or the deviation may manifest spontaneously. When DSC becomes manifest, it does so intermittently, changing as the state of attention of the individual changes and variability is the rule. Although dissociated horizontal and torsional movements are being recognized with greater frequency, DVD remains the predominant manifestation in most cases of DSC.

INVESTIGATIONS

Placing base-down prisms before the higher eye or base-up prisms before the lower eye until all refixation movements are neutralized can quantitate a true hypertropia. The alternate cover test reveals these refixation movements to be upward in one eye and downward in the other eye. The absence of upward refixation movements in either eye on alternate cover testing usually distinguishes DVD from true vertical tropia. In addition, the upward deviation is very slow (2-40°/s) in DVD compared with true hypertropia (200-400°/s).[3]

When one is attempting to quantify DVD or DHD, each eye must be measured separately. Prisms are placed before the eye to be measured until it no longer drifts behind cover; this is the endpoint. A true neutralization is not reached. Manifestations of DSC vary and tend to decrease with prolonged occlusion. For these reasons a subjective 1+ to 4+ scale is sometimes used instead of an exact prism diopters measurement to describe each component of DSC and the largest deviation seen during the exam is usually the one graded. For a DVD < 10 prism diopters (PD), a 1+ designation is used. Deviations between 10 and 15 PD are labeled as 2+, 15-20 as 3+, and > 20 PD as 4+. If a true hypertropia and DVD coexist, prism and alternate cover test neutralization of the hypertropia should be made first. Use a rapid alternate cover test to measure the true hypertropia, not allowing the hypotropic eye time to dissociate behind the cover. The true hypertropia and the more marked DVD usually are present on the same side.

The Bielschowsky phenomenon[2,9] is unique to DSC. It can be demonstrated most easily when DVD and amblyopia are present. Downward movement of the elevated occluded nonfixating eye occurs when filters of increasing density are placed before the fixating eye.

DIFFERENTIAL DIAGNOSIS

DHD is distinguished from intermittent exotropia by the slow speed of the abducting movement, the association of DTD, and the absence of true neutralization with prisms. Close inspection also reveals that the DHD does not begin to drift until the formerly covered eye has returned to the primary position and picked up fixation. In contrast, exotropia produces simultaneous movement of one eye (as it is uncovered) toward fixation and the other eye (as it is covered) away from fixation. Many patients with DHD will reveal a micro-esotropia on rapid alternate cover testing, but slow alternate cover testing (allowing the eye with DHD to fully dissociate) reveals the exodeviated posture behind cover.

DSC can coexist with oblique muscle dysfunction.[8] In addition, it is well known that in adduction the nose may act as an occluder, allowing DVD to simulate inferior oblique muscle overaction (IOOA). A true hypertropia presents in side gaze but absent in primary gaze is evidence that oblique muscle dysfunction exists. The adducted eye would manifest a hypotropia when superior oblique muscle overaction (SOOA) is present and a hypertropia when IOOA exists. Oblique muscle dysfunction causes the DVD to appear incomitant. The IOOA reduces DVD in abduction, and SOOA reduces DVD in adduction. In other words, if DVD is evident in primary gaze but much less elevation is present behind cover when either eye is in abduction, bilateral IOOA should be suspected and a V pattern sought to confirm the diagnosis. If elevation behind cover is much less in adduction, SOOA should be suspected and an A pattern sought to verify the diagnosis.

Torticollis has been documented in up to 35% of patients with DVD when an ocular fixation preference is present.[1] When present, the head tilt usually is toward the side of the nonfixating eye with the more manifest DVD; thus, the DVD usually increases with forced tilt away from the eye with the more severe DVD and decreases on tilt toward the eye with more severe DVD. This tilting pattern is opposite from that seen in superior oblique muscle palsy, in which the hypertropia increases on ipsilateral tilt and decreases on contralateral tilt.

TREATMENT AND PROGNOSIS

Despite its ability to be disfiguring, most patients with DSC do not need treatment. If a DSC drift is seen only rarely, with fatigue, reassurance and observation is the best course of therapy. Available treatments are imperfect and none of them can eliminate DSC totally. Successful treatment merely reduces the frequency and magnitude of spontaneously manifest DSC so that it is rarely seen at home. Despite treatment, dissociated strabismus can almost always still be detected during alternate cover testing. No patient is cured of DSC and recurrence of manifest deviations is common even after aggressive treatment.

Nonsurgical treatment options to reduce the frequency of manifest DSC have met with limited success. Because DSC is usually asymmetric, switching the fixation preference to the eye that deviates most often may improve the patient's control of DSC and reduce how often the eyes are seen to drift. The Worth four-dot test can be used to verify this fixation switch.

DVD, when manifest frequently, can be treated surgically by several different approaches including superior rectus muscle recession, inferior oblique muscle anterior transposition, and inferior rectus muscle resection. DHD is not treated effectively by DVD surgery alone.[6] When prominent, DHD requires a special surgical strategy that usually involves recession of the lateral rectus muscle on the side of the manifest DHD.[10] The DTD is not treated surgically. Latent nystagmus can become manifest in patients with poorly controlled DSC. Treatment that restores DSC control and gross binocularity may also result in a manifest-latent nystagmus converting back to its latent status.

In conclusion, DSC should be used to refer to the entire complex of dissociated deviations, and subdivided into its vertical (DVD), horizontal (DHD), and torsional (DTD) axes when patient examination data are recorded. Latent nystagmus should be included as part of the complex. DSC does not occur in patients with macular binocular vision and high-grade stereopsis.

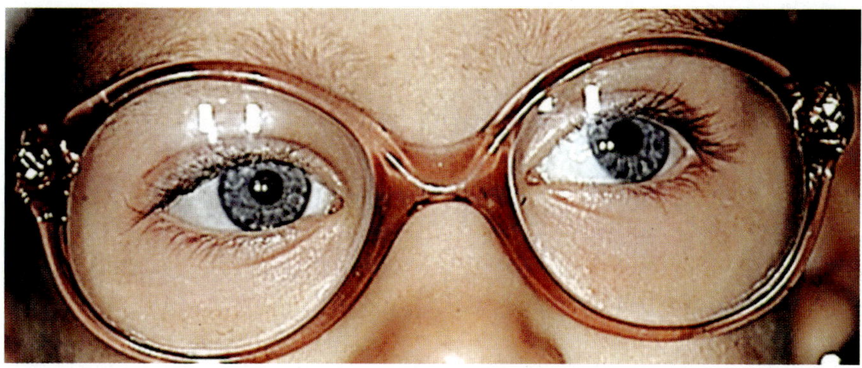

Fig. 1: DVE left eye with glasses

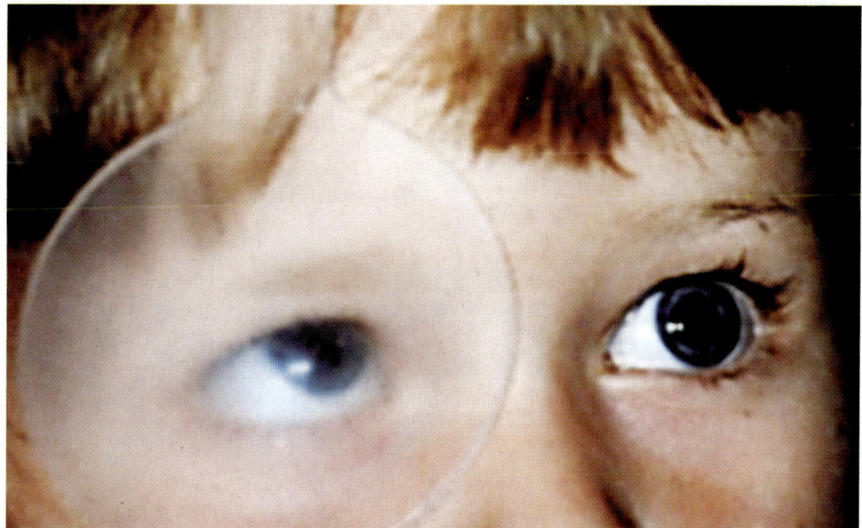

Fig. 2: DVD right eye with translucent occluder

REFERENCES

1. Bechtel RT. Kushner BJ, Morton GV. The relationship between dissociated vertical divergence (DVD) and head tilts. J Pediatr Ophthalmol Strabismus 1996;33:303-6.
2. Bielschowsky A. Lectures on motor abnormalities. Dartmouth College Publications, Hanover, 1940;p.17.
3. Helveston EM. Dissociated vertical deviation: A clinical and laboratory study. Trans Am Ophthalmol Soc 1980;78: 734-79.
4. Helveston EM. Surgical management of strabismus: A practical and updated approach, 5th edn. Wayenborgh Publishing, Oostende, Belgium, 2005;pp 88-9.
5. Noorden GK von (Ed).Binocular vision and ocular motility: theory and management of strabismus, 4th edn. Mosby, St Louis 1990;p. 341.
6. Wheeler DT, Enke ES, Scott WE. Surgical management of dissociated horizontal deviation associated with congenital esotropia. Binocul Vis Strabismus Q 1996;11: 256.
7. Wilson ME. The dissociated strabismus complex. Binocul Vis 1993; 8: 45.
8. Wilson ME, Parks MM. Primary inferior oblique overaction in congenital esotropia, accommodative esotropia, and intermittent exotropia. Ophthalmology 1989;96: 950-7.
9. Wilson ME, McClatchey SK. Dissociated horizontal deviation. J Pediatr Ophthalmol Strabismus 1991;28:90-5.
10. Wilson ME, Saunders RA, Berland JE.Dissociated horizontal deviation and accommodative esotropia: Treatment options when an eso- and an exodeviation co-exist. J Pediatr Ophthalmol Strabismus 1995;32:228-30.
11. Wilson ME, Hutchinson AK, Saunders RA (2000) Outcomes from surgical treatment for dissociated horizontal deviation. J AAPOS 4: 94-101.

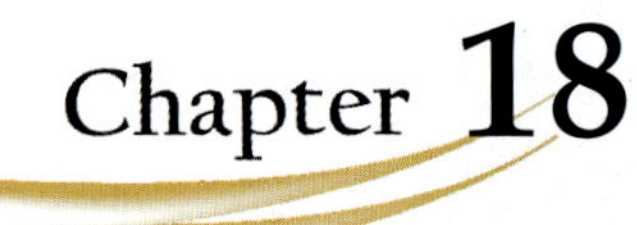

Chapter 18

Strabismus Surgery—An Update

Rohit Saxena, Ankur Sinha (India)

INTRODUCTION

The history of strabismus surgery dates back to 17th century, where John Taylor identified that the abnormal ocular alignment could be treated by dividing the extra-ocular muscle. Since then, strabismus surgery has traveled a long way and today most of the strabismologists are not satisfied with achieving only the ocular alignment.

The ideal and the dream goals of surgical management of strabismus are to achieve satisfactory cosmetic alignment (motor or cosmetic component) of the eyes along with maintenance and restoration normal single binocular vision in all the gazes (sensory or functional component). However, in most of the cases, where surgery is done, it is often possible to achieve only the motor alignment of the eyes.

SURGICAL ANATOMY OF THE MUSCLES

Recti Muscles

All the recti muscles originate from the tip of the orbital pyramid from a structure called annulus of Zinn. This is more or less a circular structure, surrounding the optic canal. The horizontal recti follow the course along the respective orbital walls. The superior rectus is separated from the roof by levator muscle and the inferior rectus is in contact with the orbital floor for only the inferior half. The insertion of all the recti is at different distance from the limbus and is in the form of a spiral called as "spiral of Tillaux". The medial rectus is closest to the limbus at 5.5 mm, followed by Inferior rectus at 6.5 mm, Lateral rectus at 6.9 mm and Superior rectus is at 7.7 mm which is farthest form the limbus. At the insertion the width of the muscle is about 10 mm and postoperatively this width must be maintained. Also during shifting of muscles, one should keep the muscles concentric to the limbus (both ends equidistant from limbus). Sclera is thinnest (0.3 mm) just behind the rectus insertion; care must be taken while passing the needles through the sclera to prevent perforation. Also for resection suturing retain an inside stump of 0.5 mm of the muscle. At all time during the surgery the integrity of the muscle sheath should be maintained. Also, during dissection prevent fat prolapse as postoperative adhesions can cause restrictive motility.

Superior Oblique Muscle

It arises from the body of sphenoid bone above and medial to optic foramen. Then it courses anteriorly in a line parallel to the upper part of the medial orbital wall and changes its direction (54° with the direct portion of muscle) at the trochlea, which is situated at the angle between the medial and the superior wall of the orbit. Trochlea is a 4-6 mm long tube, situated in the trochlear fossa of the frontal bone. It is considered as the functional origin of the superior oblique muscle. The post-trochlear portion of the muscle passes below the superior rectus muscle and fans out at the insertion. The anterior end of insertion 3-4.5 mm behind the lateral end of the superior rectus muscle and posterior end is approximately 13.6 mm from the medial end of superior rectus muscle. The posterior end of the oblique muscle is related to superior vortex vein.

Inferior Oblique Muscle

It is the smallest of all the extra-ocular muscles. It arises in the antero-inferior angle of the orbit from a shallow depression on the orbital plate of maxilla, just lateral to the entrance of the nasolacrimal duct. The muscle then courses between the inferior orbital wall and the inferior rectus muscle. The insertion of the inferior oblique lies on the postero-lateral aspect of the globe. The average width of insertion is approximately 9 mm. Its anterior end is approximately 10 mm behind the inferior end of insertion of the lateral rectus muscle; the posterior end is 1-2 mm in front of the macula.

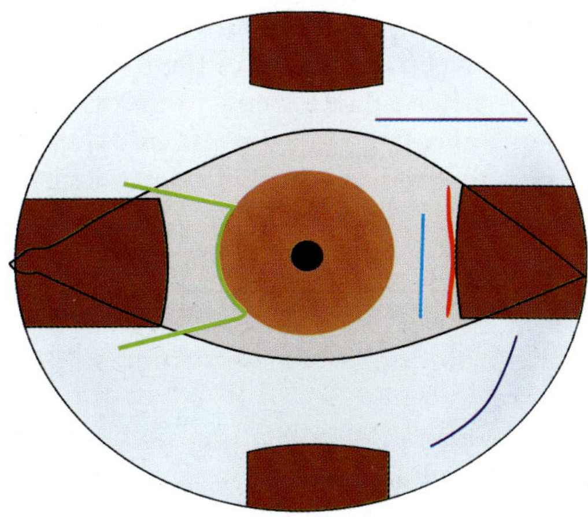

Fig. 1: Schematic diagram representing location of various techniques of muscle exposure for strabismus surgery. Red: Swan's technique. Purple: Park's and modified Park's incision. Green: Von Noorden's approach for muscle exposure. Light Blue: Prem Prakash's incision.

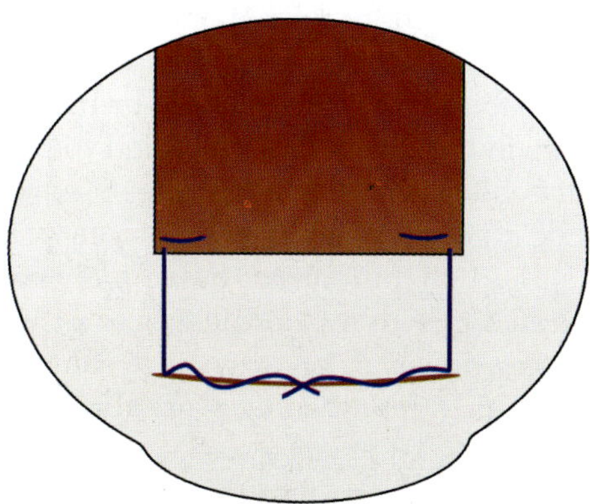

Fig. 3: Schematic diagram representing "Hang-back technique" for rectus muscle recession.

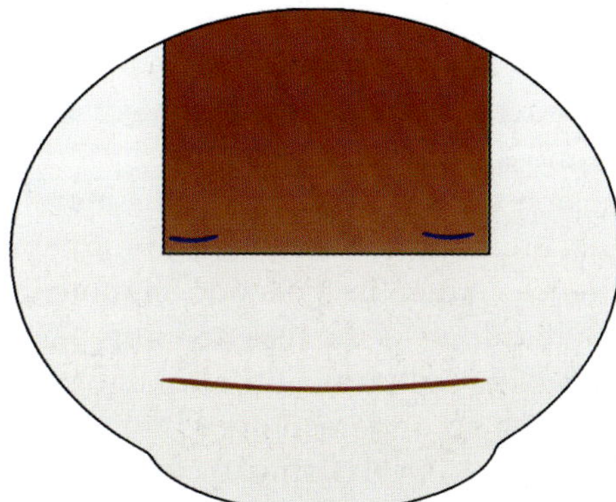

Fig. 2: Schematic diagram representing conventional recession technique.

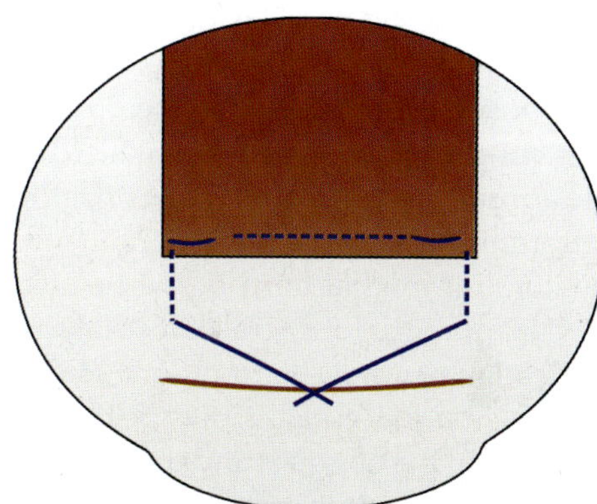

Fig. 4: Schematic diagram showing "Adjustable technique" for rectus muscle recession.

BASIC PRINCIPLES OF STRABISMUS SURGERY

There have been constant refinements and additions into the surgical technique, aiming at better predictable results and faster rehabilitation. There should be free movement of the tissues in the postoperative period to prevent any restrictive problems. This also increases predictability of surgery. For a good outcome of the surgery, the tissue handling should be minimized; tissue planes should be maintained along with a blood less field of vision. The basic principles, however, have remained same in the form of weakening and strengthening procedures.

TECHNIQUES OF MUSCLE EXPOSURE

The basic principle behind any technique of muscle exposure is to have minimum disturbance to the Tenon's capsule so as to prevent fibrosis. There are three basic techniques, which differ in their site of location of the incision with respect to the muscle and the palpebral aperture (Fig. 1).

1. **Swan's technique:** Here the incision is made directly over the muscle insertion. As the conjunctival incision and the site of the muscle surgery are close to each other the healing occurs with more of fibrosis, which may be cosmetically unacceptable.
2. **Park's cul-de-sac incision:** Originally described to be made approximately 4 mm above or below the cornea and 8 mm horizontally from the junction of middle and lateral or medial third of the cornea, depending upon the approach for lateral of medial surgery. A light modification of cul-de-sac incision, where the incision is placed circumferentially, may be used for approach for surgery of the obliques and the horizontal muscles. This incision is better cosmetically acceptable as the site of incision is hidden under the lids and may not be visible. However, the surgery through this type of incision needs more of experience as there is limited visibility of the anatomical landmarks.
3. **Von Noorden's limbal incision** in the palpebral aperture area: the use of this incision allows easy visibility and accessibility to the extra-ocular muscles and least disturbance with the orientation of the anatomical landmarks. Hence, this incision may be considered good for the beginners and in cases of re-surgeries. As the incision involves the limbal area, there may be increased bleeding from the limbal vessels and sometimes may need a gentle cautary to close the bleed.
4. **Prem Prakash's technique** of paralimbal incision: In this technique two paralimbal sutures are passed 2 mm and 4 mm from the limbus, the conjunctiva is incised between them. One of them is used to retract the globe while other to retract the conjunctiva. This technique allows good exposure also the bleeding is less as compared to Von Noorden's incision as the limbal vessels are not cut.

WEAKENING PROCEDURES OF THE RECTI

Weakening procedures of the Recti muscles

1. Recession
2. Fadenoperation (Retroequatorial myopexy)
3. Marginal myotomy
4. Myectomy
5. Free tenotomy

Recession

Recession or "measured retroplacement" (as termed by Helveston) is a procedure where the rectus muscle is first secured with the sutures and then disinserted from the original insertion and re-sutured on the sclera such that the new point of attachment is close to the point of origin (Fig. 2). The new point of attachment provides a new static alignment for the eye and hence acts as a corrective measure in cases of strabismus. As the distance between the origin and the insertion of the muscle is decreased the length-tension curve flattens and thus more changes in length are required to generate the same amount of resting tension, hence change in the static alignment. It is to be stressed that as long as the recessed muscle is with in its arc of contact, it would function, although weakened and there would be no underaction of the muscle. Once the muscle has been recessed beyond the arc of contact it would cease to function normally and one could expect an underaction of the muscle. Another point to be noted is that as long the muscle is not excessively recessed the saccadic velocity and the force generated by the muscle would not decrease and "weakening" as such may be labeled as a misnomer.

It is of importance to note that the insertions of the recti are in the form of a curved line rather than a straight line, hence it is important to measure the decided recession from the end of the muscle insertion as measuring the insertion from any other point would lead to under-recession and hence would effect the outcome of the surgery. While measuring the amount of recessions one should measure the distance in absolutely straight line so as to avoid vertical shift of horizontal muscles and horizontal shift of the vertical muscles.

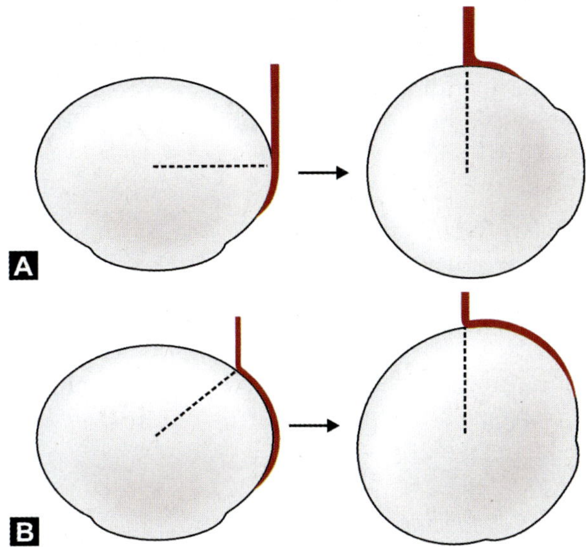

Figs 5A and B: Schematic diagram showing the mechanism how fadenoperation works. (A) showing the maximum excursion of the eye when the vector force of the muscle pulls the eye at right angles to the ocular surface. (B) demonstrates the decreased excursion of ocular rotation with the placement of faden suture.

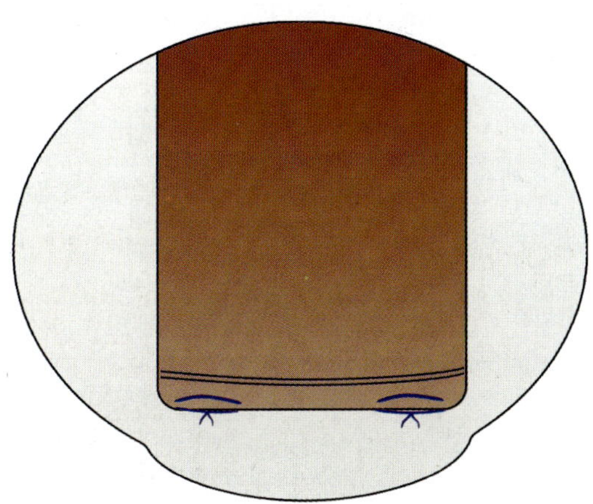

Fig. 6: Schematic diagram representing conventional resection technique

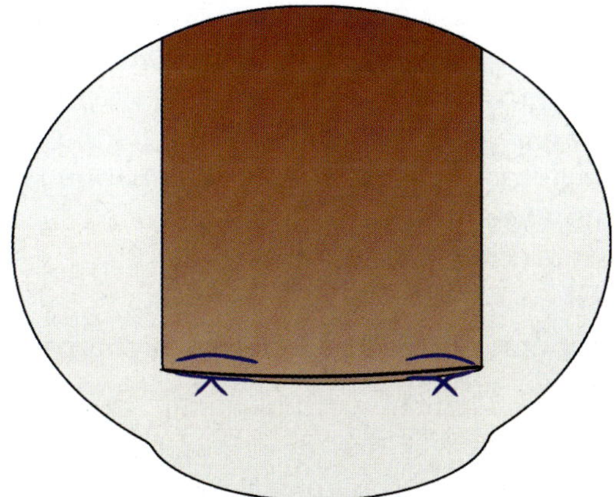

Fig. 7: Schematic diagram showing placation of the rectus muscle.

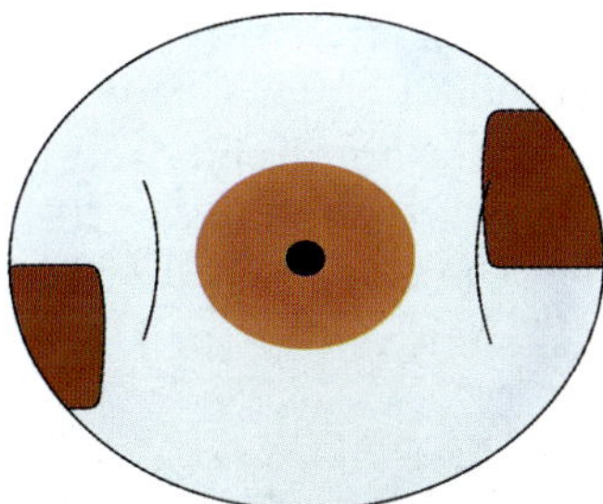

Fig. 8: Schematic diagram demonstrating recession with infraplacment and resection with supraplacement of the muscle by the half muscle width, for the management of pattern strabismus.

The amount of minimum and maximum recessions for various recti is different. As less than the minimum amount of recession may be nullified by the "resection" effect of the amount of muscle used for placement of sutures and fibrosis. If a recession is performed beyond the maximum limit and the new point of insertion is beyond the equator of the globe the muscle would act like a retractor and there would be gross underaction of the muscle action. However, in certain cases, supra-maximal surgery is performed. The maximum and minimum limit of recession for all the four recti is given in Table 1.

Table 1: Minimum and maximum recession of various recti muscle from their respective site of insertions

S No.	Muscle	Minimum limit of recession (mm)	Maximum limit of recession (mm)
1.	Medial Rectus	2.5-3.0	5.0-5.5
2.	Lateral Rectus	4	8.0-9.0
3.	Superior Rectus	2.5-3.0	5.0
4.	Inferior Rectus	2.5-3.0	5.0

It is known that the recessions of more than 5.0 mm of the vertical muscles may lead to changes in the palpebral aperture changes in the form of lid retraction in superior rectus surgery and lower lid ptosis in case of inferior rectus recession. However, larger superior rectus recessions have been performed as a surgical option for the management of "dissociated vertical deviation". While performing inferior rectus surgery it is of importance to have knowledge of its relationship with the ligament of Lockwood. Lower lid ptosis may be reduced if the intermuscular septa are divided on either side of the inferior rectus to as posterior as 10-14 mm from the insertion and carefully cutting the attachment with the Lockwood's ligament.

Hang-Back Recessions

As the name would suggest the muscle is allowed to hang posteriorly with the help of absorbable suture from the site of original insertion and hence the effect of recession is achieved (Fig. 3). This type of recession is simple and safe alternative to the conventional recession has been known to be equally effective. It is debated to be safe as it reduces the chances of scleral perforation as the needles are placed at the original site hence passed through thicker sclera and also the site is more anterior and is easily accessible. This may be of help when performing supra-maximal recessions and surgery in thin sclerae as in high myopes. Disadvantage of this type of recession may be that the muscle width at the new point of insertion may not be maintained and in large recessions there may be inadvertent vertical drift of the horizontal muscles and horizontal drift of the vertical muscles.

Hemi-Hang Back Recessions

This technique is a modification of the hang-back recession where the sutures are passed through a scleral tunnel before being inserted at the original site of insertion. This technique overcomes the disadvantage of hang-back recession by maintaining the width of the muscle recession and reducing the drift.

Adjustable Recessions

This technique allows postoperative adjustment of the recessed muscle and in an effort to provide accurate alignment this technique is rapidly gaining more popularity (Fig. 4). This is a modification of hemi-hang back procedure, where one and a half knot along with intervening suture (silk or ethibond) is tied at the site of original site of insertion. The intervening suture helps in re-opening the one and a half knot, thus allowing adjustment. The postoperative adjustment is done by tightening or loosening of the absorbable sutures. This can be done soon after the surgery (single stage) or 6-8 hours later (two-stage). This allows the surgeon to modify the result after the surgical outcome and thus give more accurate results. The patients with diplopia and the patients who are very demanding can actually guide the surgeon to titrate the outcome to perfection.

Fadenoperation (Retroequatorial Myopexy)

"Faden" is a German word meaning "string or suture". This operation was first described by Cüppers which involved fixing the rectus muscle on the sclera behind the equator (posterior to the arc of contact) and creating a new functional insertion of the muscle. A more descriptive terminology for this surgery would be *posterior fixation suture or retroequatorial myopexy*. This surgery aims at reducing the action of muscle in its field and does not have a bearing on the primary position or the movement on the opposite side. As the function insertion of the muscle is shifted posteriorly the angle of the "lever arm" which rotates the globe near zero and hence a new reference point is created, which decreases the ocular rotation. Since the muscle length and the tension are not altered the length

Table 2: Various indication of Fadenoperation

Condition where Fadenoperation may be performed	*Muscles operated upon*
Nystagmus blockade syndrome	Medial recti
Dissociated vertical deviation	Superior recti
Non-accommodative convergence excess type of esotropia	Medial recti
Manifest nystagmus (to decrease amplitude)	All four horizontal recti
Paralytic strabismus	Contralateral synergist
Duane's retraction syndrome	Contralateral medial rectus
Blow out fracture with inferior rectus injury	Contralateral inferior rectus
Thyroid ophthalmolopathy with inferior rectus contracture	Contralateral inferior rectus

tension curve remains same and hence does not affect the primary gaze. The restricted movement of the muscle in its field of action calls for an increased innervation and as per the Hering's law this increased innervations flows to the yolk muscle, which is indirectly strengthened, hence the primary alignment is maintained (Figs 5A and B). Indications of Fadenoperation have been given in Table 2. As the arc of contact of the different rectus muscles are different the distance between the site of insertion and the passage of posterior fixation suture is different (Table 3).

Table 3: The distance from the muscle insertion where the posterior fixation suture is passed in fadenoperation

S. No.	*Rectus muscle*	*Distance from point of insertion (mm)*
1.	Medial rectus	12-14
2.	Lateral rectus	16-20
3.	Superior rectus	14-16
4.	Inferior rectus	14-16

Adjustable Fadenoperation

As explained above that the fadenoperation limits the ocular rotation by changing the functional insertion and preventing the action of a part of muscle. Hence, fadenoperation should work even if this piece of the muscle is removed. Based on this principle the muscle equal to the location of posterior fixation suture is resected and this "resected muscle" is recessed using hang-back technique. Postoperatively the position of the muscle may be advanced or recessed depending upon the ocular alignment. In this manner fadenoperation can be combined with adjustable strabismus surgery.

Marginal Myotomy

In this process, the muscle is given multiple cuts alternatively to the alternate borders. This leads to increase in the effective length similar to "Z" plasty done by plastic surgeons.

Myectomy and Free Tenectomy or the Recti Muscles

These procedures do not find their role in management of Strabismus in the present era.

STRENGTHENING PROCEDURES OF THE RECTI MUSCLES

1. Resection
2. Tuck or Plication of muscle
3. Advancement
4. Cinching

Resection of Recti

In this procedure a part of muscle tendon the muscle is removed and the muscle is re-inserted at the original site of insertion (Fig. 6). While doing so, the length of the muscle is decreased and it shifts to a higher length-tension curve relationship. This shifting strengthens the muscle action. Although the surgical technique is simple, it often produces more reaction and "lumpiness" or "bogginess" at the surgical site, this often occurs with the resection of the medial rectus muscle, more so when large resections are done, which may lead to inclusion of some muscle fibers in the resected tendon. Inferior rectus resection may lead to narrowing of the palpebral aperture similarly superior rectus resection may lead to ptosis of the upper lid. Lateral rectus resections may carry a risk of inadvertently including inferior oblique during the surgery. As with the recession, the minimum and maximum limit of resection of each rectus muscle is defined (Table 4). Resection also has a disadvantage of compromising on the ciliary circulation as the vessels are cut during the surgery; hence some people advocated use of tuck of the recti muscles.

Tuck or Placation

This is another form of strengthening the muscle, here the ciliary vessels are spared as the muscle is not shortened, and instead the tendinous part of the muscle is double folded /breasted (Fig. 7).

Table 4: Minimum and maximum resection of various recti muscle

S No.	Muscle	Minimum limit of recession (mm)	Maximum limit of recession (mm)
1.	Medial rectus	3.0	6.0
2.	Lateral rectus	4.5	9.0
3.	Superior rectus	2.5-3.0	5.0
4.	Inferior rectus	2.5-3.0	5.0

Advancement

This is another alternative to resection as a strengthening procedure. In this procedure the muscle is not shortened but the new site of insertion is shifted closer to limbus. This may lead to "lumpy" and congested appearance in the paralimbal area, which is more pronounced when the surgery is performed on horizontal recti, as the site would be visible in the palpebral area. However, this is an important tool for the management of consecutive strabismus, where not only the previous surgery needs to be undone, also there is a need for strengthening the muscle. While opting for this procedure there is no loss of the muscle tissue.

Cinching

It may be labeled as a modification of placation surgery. Has similar advantage as of placation of disturbing the ciliary circulation to minimum and reducing the risk of anterior segment ischemia.

RESECTION-RECESSION PROCEDURES ON HORIZONTAL MUSCLES AND THEIR MODIFICATIONS (FIG. 8)

Recession and Resection (R and R)

For the surgical management of moderate to large angle horizontal strabismus, the surgeon often has two choices. First is a bilateral weakening procedure in the form of bilateral recession. Second, opt for a recession-resection procedure, where one muscle is weakened while the other is strengthened. In bilateral recessions none of the muscle tendon is excised and has a theoretical advantage of being fully reversible. However, there is no additive effect of both muscles being operated together. This type of surgical plan is more suitable for children under general anesthesia. Recession-Resection procedure is done on one eye. When the two recti are operated upon at the same sitting, they provide an additive effect of approximately 25%, over and above what each muscle must have given when operated separately. This type of surgical plan is suited for adult strabismus where local anesthesia in the form of peribulbar is used. Even in pediatric strabismus, where the angle of strabismus is large R and R surgery can provide larger correction hence may be the procedure of choice.

Vertical Displacement of Horizontal Muscles

These procedures are recommended in cases of vertical incomitance in the form of "A" or "V" patterns. The people following horizontal school of thought propagated vertical displacement of horizontal recti as a method of surgical option. In the present era, if the "V" pattern is associated with the overaction of the inferior oblique muscle, then one should plan an inferior oblique weakening procedure, similarly for overacting superior oblique muscles with "A" pattern superior oblique surgery is warranted. However, shifting procedures still find a place where "A" or "V" pattern is not caused by oblique overaction or the magnitude of "A" or "V" is large enough to be corrected by the weakening procedure of the respective oblique muscle.

If the medial rectus is downshifted, the distance between the new insertion and origin in the downgaze is less as compared to the distance in upgaze, thus the muscle is a weaker adductor in downgaze as compared to its adductor action in upgaze. Similarly, upshifting or lateral rectus muscle would lead to relative weakening of the abductor action in the upgaze as compared to its action in downgaze. Based upon the above theory vertical muscles are shifted up or down depending upon the muscle being operated and whether it is done for a "A" or "V" pattern.

Slanted Recession-resection Procedure

This procedure involves differential recession-resection of the two ends of the horizontal recti. For "A" pattern medial rectus is recessed more at the upper end and resected more at the lower end, similarly lateral rectus is recessed more at the lower ends and resected more at the upper end of the muscle. In the similar manner one can plan differential recession-resections for "V" pattern.

INFERIOR OBLIQUE SURGERY

Various workers have described different type (Transcutaneous tenectomy, disinsertion at the scleral insertion, recession, myotomy, myectomy, denervation etc) of surgery on inferior oblique. It was Parks, whose effort to compare four different types of surgeries revealed that recession is the most effective and long lasting procedure and extirpation and denervation may be effective in markedly overacting muscle.

Weakening Procedures of Inferior Oblique Muscle

1. Generalized weakening
   a. Recession
   b. Myectomy
   c. Disinsertion
   d. Denervation
   e. Extirpation
2. Selective weakening
   a. Anterior positioning with recession
   b. Pure anterior positioning
   c. Total anterior positioning
   d. Recession of anterior fibers

Technique of Muscle Exposure

For the exposure of inferior oblique muscle the historical approach of transcutaneous incision is not used and the preferred approach is through the conjunctiva. One can choose between the modification of Parks cul-de-sac incision (7-9 mm from limbus) in the infero-temporal quadrant and Von Noorden's limbal incision. After the conjunctival incision is made the lateral rectus is secured using the Green's squint hook and the conjunctiva is retracted using two lens hooks or Desmarre's retractor and under direct visualization the muscle is lifted using lens hook or Jameson's squint hook. Care must be taken of the vortex vein and the inferior division of the third nerve which is very close to the muscle. Once the muscle is secured and it is ensured that no posterior fibers are left then the desired surgery can be performed.

Myotomy

In the present era, this surgery has a very limited place in the management of the overacting inferior oblique. If myotomy is to be done it is now done at the insertion and through a conjunctiva approach. The proponents of this surgery believe that the surgery is "self-adjusting" to the amount of overaction. The points against this weakening procedure is that once the muscle is cut and left it contracts and re-inserts on its own at a point over which the surgeon does not have a control.

Myectomy

After the muscle is secured, two clamps are placed 4-8 mm apart and the muscle between the clamps is excised and cauterized to prevent hemorrhage and possible re-attachment. It is also thought to be a "self-adjusting" type of a surgery, again there is no control of the surgeon over the amount of recession. If re-surgery is required then it is difficult to locate the muscle.

Denervation

The nerve supplying the inferior oblique muscle runs along the posterior edge of the muscle, which can be identified and cauterized and cut. This induces paralysis of the muscle and hence the overaction is obliterated. Such procedures are not commonly used in the present era.

Extirpation of the Muscle

As the literal meaning suggests the muscle is identified, isolated and the entire mass of the muscle is excised and hence the muscle action is lost permanently. Alike denervation, this procedure has a very limited role in present day strabismus surgery. However, the need of such destructive procedures may arise in cases where the muscle action persists even after maximal recession or myectomy.

Pure Recession, Recession with Anterior Positioning and Pure Anterior Positioning of Inferior Oblique

Technically speaking a pure recession means that the muscle is retroplaced along the original course of the muscle, however in case of IO recession there is some amount of anterior positioning of the muscle.

Fink's method: Fink's point is a point 6 mm inferior and 6 mm posterior to the inferior end of insertion of lateral rectus muscle. The anterior end of recessed muscle is placed at this point and the posterior point is approximately 5 mm posterior to it. It is calculated using dissection on cadeveric eyes that this point corresponds to 8 mm recession and 1 mm anterior positioning of the muscle. For 10 mm recession one goes 2 mm inferior from the Fink's point and this act as the anterior point of insertion of the muscle.

Park's method: A point 3 mm posterior and 2 mm lateral to the lateral end of insertion of the inferior rectus is labeled as "Scheie-Parks point". When the anterior end of recessed muscle is placed at this point it is considered equivalent to 10 mm recession. However even in this method there is anterior positioning of the muscle by 1.0-1.5 mm.

Elliot and Nankin's method and its modification: In the original description of Elliot and Nankin's method the anterior and the posterior end of the muscle are re-inserted at the lateral end of insertion of the inferior rectus muscle. This is a stronger weakening procedure than the Fink's or Park's method of recession. When this procedure was performed, there was a acute change in the direction of the posterior fibers of the muscle and due to the fascial attachments the posterior end of the re-inserted inferior oblique muscle acted as depressor and hence the recessed muscle was acting as a stronger depressor, leading to restricted elevation in abduction. To overcome this anomaly, the posterior end of the insertion is re-inserted 5-6 mm posterior to the lateral end of insertion of inferior rectus muscle. With this "modified Elliot and Nankin's method" the direction of the posterior fibers is maintained and the depressor action of the recessed muscle is eliminated.

Pure anterior positioning: This method of inferior oblique weakening has an effect equivalent to 8 mm recession of Fink's method and the advantage of this method is that there are no torsional changes with this method. In this method the anterior end of the re-inserted inferior oblique muscle is placed at the inferior end of insertion of lateral rectus muscle and the posterior end is inserted 5-6 mm behind.

Total anterior positioning: In this procedure the whole of the width of the inferior oblique muscle is re-inserted anterior to the inferior rectus muscle. As with Elliot and Nankin's method the fascial attachment with the ligament of Lockwood may act as the new functional origin of the muscle and the anteriorly positioned muscle acts as a depressor of the globe. This disadvantage of the surgery may act as an advantage when the inferior oblique weakening surgery is performed for inferior oblique overaction is present with dissociated vertical deviation.

Recession of Anterior fibers of inferior oblique: Looking at the functions of the inferior oblique muscle, one would understand that the posterior fibers of the muscle are elevator and abductor and the anterior fibers are responsible for the extorsional action. Recession of the anterior fibers of the inferior oblique may be required as a part of torsional Kestenbaum surgery. In this technique, the anterior half of the fibers of the inferior oblique muscle are isolated and recessed for about 12-14 mm.

Strengthening Procedures of Inferior Oblique

The need for strengthening inferior oblique rarely arises. It is done in cases of inferior oblique palsy where the weakening of the yolk muscle, i.e. the superior rectus fails to provide adequate alignment.

Inferior Oblique Tuck

After the muscle is exposed and secured a double breasting or tuck of inferior oblique is performed using a non absorbable suture (e.g. 5-0 ethibond). At least 10 mm of muscle should be included in the tuck.

Resection with Advancement of Inferior Oblique

This is another option for strengthening of inferior oblique. In this technique the sutures are placed at the inferior border of lateral rectus (i.e. approx. 5.0 mm from the insertion of the inferior oblique). The muscle is then cut this leads to resection of 5.0 mm. The muscle is then re-inserted at the superior border of the lateral rectus muscle such that the anterior end of insertion is 12 mm posterior to the point of insertion of lateral rectus muscle. This produces 5.0 mm of advancement; hence resection with advancement produces 10.0 mm resection effect of inferior oblique.

SUPERIOR OBLIQUE SURGERIES

Weakening procedures for superior oblique.

1. Generalized weakening procedures
   a. Tenotomy and tenectomy
   b. Recession
   c. Translational recession
   d. L-lengthening
   e. Expander procedures "silicon" and "chicken suture
2. Selective weakening procedures
   a. Posterior tenotomy
   b. Posterior tenectomy
   c. Recession of anterior fibers
   d. Anterior positioning

Superior Oblique Tenectomy and Tenotomy

The initial description of tenectomy was that of a blind sweep using a supero-nasal approach, this approach led to high rate of complications. With the use of direct visualization techniques the success rate of complete tenectomy has increased and the complication rate has decreased.

Tenectomy or tenotomy procedures are indicated in cases of Brown's syndrome, "A" pattern strabismus, overacting superior oblique muscles (primary and secondary to inferior oblique palsy), and superior oblique myokymia.

The conjunctiva is incised in the superonasal quadrant making a circumferential incision, 8 mm form the limbus. The muscle tendon is then identified and secured on a muscle hook. Under direct visualization the tendon is either cut (tenotomy) or a part of tendon is excised (tenectomy). The cut end of tendon is then allowed to retract.

Recession of Superior Oblique

This is a more controlled and a lesser weakening procedure as compared to tenectomy and tenotomy of superior oblique. Through a temporal approach the superior oblique tendon is secured over a muscle hook, a 6-0 double armed vicryl suture is woven along the tendon approximately 4 mm from the insertion. The muscle is then disinserted and allowed to retract beneath the superior rectus muscle for a distance of 8-20 mm and the sutures are then tied at the muscle insertion. This is something like a hang-back recession of a rectus muscle.

Posterior Tenectomy of Superior Oblique Muscle

The posterior fibers of the tendon of the superior oblique muscle are responsible for the abductor and depressor functions while anterior fibers are responsible for incyclotorsion. The removal of posterior fibers could thus lead in decrease in the abductor and depressor actions without having an effect on torsion. Prieto-Diaz first described the selective weakening procedure of posterior tenectomy of superior oblique. This surgery may help to correct moderate of "A" pattern (up to 20 PD) in cases of overacting superior oblique muscle. In this procedure the incision is made in the supero-temporal quadrant 8 mm from the limbus in circumferential or radial fashion. Using Desmarre's retractor or the lens hook the superior rectus muscle is retracted medially, and one could find white shiny fibers of the tendon of superior oblique. The fibers are then dissected free of the intermuscular septum. Under direct visualization the posterior fibers of the tendon are identified and approximately 8 mm of tendon length is removed, leaving only 1-2 mm of anterior fibers. The remaining muscle is then allowed to retract and the conjunctiva is sutured using absorbable suture. It is important to note that the supero-temporal vortex vein lies close to the posterior edge of the insertion of the tendon, and care must be taken to avoid injury to it. Incomplete identification of the posterior fibers may lead to incomplete tenectomy and hence the overaction may persist.

Superior Oblique Expander

For significant superior oblique overactions leading to "A" pattern strabismus, tenectomy could result in over correction and extorsion leading to troublesome diplopia. Hence, a graded weakening procedure in the form of silicon expander was first described by Wright. We have been using this form of technique to correct "Browns Syndrome" and an "A" pattern of 20-55 PD.

The conjunctival incision is placed as in PTSO. After making sure all the muscle fibers are secured, a double armed 5-0 ethibond (non-absorbable) suture is woven through the whole length of the tendon. A similar suture is woven approximately 4 mm from the first suture, after securing both the ends the muscle tendon is cut in between them. Now 8 mm long piece of silicone band (size 240) is placed and the non-absorbable sutures are passed through the two ends and sutured snugly. An intraoperative exaggerated forced duction test is performed to assess the tightness of the superior oblique muscle.

The tissue handling in such cases should be very gentle as excessive dissection could lead to fibrosis and restriction.

STRENGTHENING PROCEDURES OF SUPERIOR OBLIQUE

Superior Oblique Tuck

It is something like double breasting of the muscle tendon. The indications of such procedure are very limited; it is usually done for superior oblique palsy without inferior oblique overaction or as a secondary procedure when weakening procedure of inferior oblique has not yielded a satisfactory outcome. The aim of this surgery is to correct vertical and torsional misalignment in primary and down gaze and provide enlarged binocular single field of vision, and correct anomalous head posture.

It can correct approximately 10-15 PD of vertical deviation, 10-12 PD of torsional misalignment and 15-20 PD of esotropia in downgaze.

The exposure of the muscle tendon requires same incision as that for PTSO. The muscle is secured, half the desired amount of tuck required to be done is marked using a calipers and the muscle tendon is then double folded over itself and sutured using a 5-0 non-absorbable suture, such that the folded portion is under the tendon.

As with SO expander an intraoperative exaggerated forced duction test is performed to assess the tightness of the superior oblique muscle, a tuck having produced a tight superior oblique could result in post-surgical Brown's syndrome.

Harada-Ito Procedure

This is a selective strengthening procedure of superior oblique, involving only the anterior fibers responsible for intorsion. In this procedure anterior lateralization of the anterior fibers of the superior oblique is done as a treatment of extorsion. Originally, the procedure involved splitting of the tendon 5 mm behind the muscle insertion and the anterior fibers are sutured 5 mm anterior to the insertion of superior oblique tendon.

The Fells modification of the technique involves, splitting of the anterior fibers of the superior oblique tendon and then these fibers are sutured close to the upper border of the lateral rectus muscle.

The conjunctival incision is made as in PTSO; a double armed 6-0 vicryl suture is passed along the insertion of the superior oblique tendon. The anterior fibers are then disinserted and advanced 6-8 mm towards the lateral rectus re-inserted there.

Complications of Strabismus Surgery

As with any other surgery, strabismus surgery is not immune to complications. It is said rightly "there are only two ways of avoiding complications, one is to avoid surgery and the second is to deny the presence of complications". It also imperative to note that, with repeated surgeries the rate of complication can be reduced but cannot be made zero. Although there is a long list of complications that can occur during the strabismus surgery, most of them are listed in Tables 5 and 6 and a few of them explained below.

Complications due to General Anesthesia and Local Anesthesia

It is rightly said that "surgery may be major or minor, anesthesia is always major". Anesthesia can lead to a large number of complications; few of them are mentioned in Table 5 and below.

Bradycardia: one of the most commonly encountered problem while operating a pediatric strabismus under general anesthesia. Stretching of the medial rectus muscle often leads to oculo-cardiac reflex, due to vegal stimulation the heart rate slows down and leads to a significant bradycardia. This is reduced if a sub-Tenon's block is used along with the anesthesia during the surgery.

Table 5: Complications of strabismus surgery due to anesthesia

S. No.	*Complications due to general anesthesia and local anesthesia*
1.	Bradycardia
2.	Aspiration pneumonitis
3.	Malignant hyperthermia
4.	Allergy or hypersensitivity to drugs
5.	Postoperative nausea and vomiting
6.	Toxicity of local anesthetic agents
7.	Cardiac arrest

Table 6: Intraoperative and postoperative complications of strabismus surgery.

S. No.	*Intraoperative and postoperative complications*
1.	Operating the wrong muscle/wrong surgery
2.	Operating the wrong eye
3.	Loss of vision
4.	Orbital hemorrhages
5.	Scleral perforation
6.	Lost or slipped muscle
7.	Hyphema
8.	Posterior chamber hemorrhage
9.	Muscle tendon rupture
10.	Central sag
11.	Tenon's prolapse
12.	Loose suture or partial thickness suture
13.	Postoperative infection
14.	Inflammation
15.	Undercorrection and overcorrection
16.	Postoperative diplopia
17.	Conjunctival granulomas and cysts

Toxicity of local anesthetic agents: The risk of toxicity is more when both the eye of the patient is being operated for squint.

Intraoperative and Postoperative Complications

Operating the wrong muscle/wrong surgery: There could be globe rotation under the anesthesia, while using the fornix incision, the surgeon may misidentify the muscle and a wrong muscle may be operated. There is a chance that a muscle to be recessed is resected and vise versa can occur if the surgical notes are not looked into just before starting the surgery. These situations may lead to surprises in the immediate post-surgical day, to avoid these one should develop a habit of going through the patient records before the surgery.

Operating the wrong eye: This complication can occur when performing a surgery under general anesthesia, as the patient is not aware of the eye which being operated. Under local anesthesia the patient is aware of the surgery and often can object of the wrong eye is blocked for surgery. In cases of horizontal comitant strabismus, operating wrong eye would not have a bearing on the outcome as both the eyes work as a single system with respect to ocular alignment and motility. Hence, it is imperative to always check the operative notes and surgical decision.

Loss of vision: The causes of loss of vision as a complication of strabismus surgery include retinal detachment, vitreous hemorrhage, endophthalmitis, cataract, lens subluxation, hyphema etc. These can occur as a consequence of a mechanical or microbiological event following inadvertent scleral perforation at time of dissection or suture placement. This dreadful complication can be prevented by following proper surgical technique.

Scleral perforation: This is not an uncommon complication and can lead to loss of vitreous and other posterior segment problems. This can be avoided by carefully passing the sutures during the strabismus surgery and ensuring that the tip of the needle is always visible and the direction of needle is tangential to the sclera.

Lost or slipped muscle and Muscle tendon rupture: This is seen in cases with a long standing squint and tight rectus muscle. Most frequently lost muscle is a medial rectus in cases of long standing convergent squint. Care must be taken while passing sutures through such tight muscles, so as not to apply much traction leading to pitting and loss of the muscle in the orbit.

Hyphema: A rare complication of strabismus surgery, has been reported after superior oblique tendon tuck, as a result of abnormal vessels at the anterior chamber angle. The hyphema clears in due course of time with conservative management.

Posterior chamber hemorrhage: Another rare complication has been reported due to a scleral perforation involving a retinal vessel. This can be avoided by taking shallow scleral bites.

Undercorrection and overcorrection: These are probably the most common "complications" noted following strabismus surgery. Many of these are transient and can be corrected by optical means (prisms, lenses). However, large undercorrection or overcorrection associated with limited motility may need an urgent intervention in view of a lost muscle.

Anterior segment ischemia: Much of the anterior segment circulation derives from ciliary arteries which are affected by surgery involving the extraocular muscles. This occasionally leads to a peculiar complication called anterior segment ischemia manifesting with a significant anterior chamber reaction, iris atrophy, and various degrees of cataract formation. Its occurrence following strabismus surgery is correlated with the number of operated muscles and the general circulation characteristics of the patient.

SUGGESTED READING

1. Apt L, Call NB. Inferior oblique muscle recession.Am J Ophthalmol 1978 Jan;85(1):95-100.
2. Caldeira JA. V-pattern esotropia: a review; and a study of the outcome after bilateral recession of the inferior oblique muscle: a retrospective study of 78 consecutive patients. Binocul Vis Strabismus Q. 2003;18(1):35-48; discussion 49-50.
3. Capo H, Repka MX, Guyton DL. Hang-back lateral rectus recessions for exotropia. J Pediatr Ophthalmol Strabismus. 1989 Jan-Feb;26(1):31-4.
4. Chia A, Seenyen L, Long QB. Surgical experiences with two-muscle surgery for the treatment of intermittent exotropia. J AAPOS. 2006;10(3):206-11.
5. Cibis GW. Comitant strabismus. Curr Opin Ophthalmol. 1998 Oct;9(5):15-9.
6. Greenberg MF, Pollard ZF. Treatment of inferior oblique paresis with superior oblique silicone tendon expander. J AAPOS 2005 Aug;9(4):341-5.
7. Guthrie ME, Wright KW. Congenital esotropia. Ophthalmol Clin North Am 2001 Sep;14(3):419-24.
8. Helvesten EM (Ed). Surgical Management of Strabismus. An Atlas of Strabismus Surgery. 4th edn. Mosby-year book Inc.; 1993.
9. Mohan K, Sharma A, Pandav SS. Unilateral lateral rectus muscle recession and medial rectus muscle resection with or without advancement for postoperative consecutive exotropia. J AAPOS. 2006;10(3):220-4.
10. Morris RJ, Luff AJ. Adjustable sutures in squint surgery.Br J Ophthalmol 1992 Sep;76(9):560-2.
11. Murray T. Eye muscle surgery. Curr Opin Ophthalmol. 2000 Oct;11(5):336-41.
12. Nelson LB, Wagner RS, Simon JW, Harley RD. Congenital esotropia. Surv Ophthalmol. 1987 May-Jun;31(6):363-83.
13. Potter WS 3rd, Nelson LB, Handa JT. Hemihang-back recession: description of the technique and review of the literature. Ophthalmic Surg 1990 Oct;21(10):711-5.
14. Prieto-Diaz J. Posterior tenectomy of the superior oblique. Pediatr Ophthalmol Strabismus 1979 Sep-Oct;16(5):321-3.
15. Repka MX, Guyton DL. Comparison of hang-back medial rectus recession with conventional recession. Ophthalmology. 1988 Jun;95(6):782-7.
16. Rosenbuam AL, Santiago AP (Eds). Clinical Strabismus Management Principles and Surgical Techniques: WB Saunders Co; 1999.
17. Sharma P, Khokhar S, Thanikachalam. Evaluation of superior oblique weakening procedures. J Pediatr Ophthalmol Strabismus 1999 Jul-Aug;36(4):189-95.
18. Sharma P. Strabismus Simplified. Ed.1. Modern Publishers 1999.
19. Strominger MB, Richards R. Adjustable sutures in pediatric ophthalmology and strabismus. J Ophthalmic Nurs Technol. 2000 May-Jun;19(3):142-7.
20. Suh DW, Guyton DL, Hunter DG. An adjustable superior oblique tendon spacer with the use of nonabsorbable suture. J AAPOS. 2001 Jun;5(3):164-71.
21. Von Noorden GK. ed. Binocular Vision and Ocular Motility Theory and Management of Strabismus: Mosby-Year Book Inc.; 1996.
22. Wright KW, Hwang JM. Surgical techniques of strabismus. Curr Opin Ophthalmol. 1993 Nov;4(5):19-24.

Chapter 19

Special Forms of Strabismus

Rohit Saxena, Swati Phuljhele, Ashish Kakkar (India)

A. BROWN SYNDROME

Brown syndrome is characterized by deficit in elevation during adduction, which is restrictive in nature. The consistent features of Brown's syndrome are absence of elevation in adduction, normal elevation in abduction, positive exaggerated FDT for SO and divergence (Y or V) pattern in upgaze. The variable features are mild limitation of elevation from primary position, downshoot in adduction, widening of lid fissure, hypotropia in primary position, compensatory head posture (chin up, contralateral face turn) and intortion in upgaze.

Congenital abnormality In congenital cases the abnormality primarily lies in the tendon and/or tendon-trochlear complex. The anomaly may be in form of short tendon, inelastic sheath around tendon, trochlear deformity as in thick trochlea or presence of bursa like structure between the tendon and trochlea.

Acquired Brown syndrome occurs as result of inflammation secondary to infection or surgery. There is formation of adhesions between trochlea and tendon which prevent the slippage of tendon through trochlea. There could be thickening of SO tendon is seen in inflammatory cases. Direct damage to trochlea may occur as a result of trauma to orbit.

The important causes of acquired Brown's syndrome include surgeries such as SO tucking, scleral buckle, glaucoma valve surgery, sinus surgery; infection or inflammation like Graves, ophthalmopathy, and sinusitis

Clinical Features

Brown's syndrome is usually unilateral, 10% of cases may be bilateral. There is no sex or laterality predisposition. Selected cases may resolve spontaneously while other may present in intermittent or constant form depending upon the etiology of the syndrome.

Brown's syndrome can be classified as follows:

Mild – There is no hypotropia of the involved eye in the primary or adducted position. The limitation is present only in elevation in adduction.

Moderate – Hypotropia in secondary position and there may be downshoot on adduction (Fig. 1).

Severe – When hypotropia is present even in the primary position.

Differential Diagnosis

1. True inferior oblique palsy – FDT for SO will be negative
2. Monocular elevation deficiency – The elevation in abduction is generally more marked than in adduction.
3. Blow out fracture leading to entrapment of IR muscle – the elevation deficient will be similar in abduction and adduction or worse in abduction. Other associated findings like infra-orbital paresthesia, enophthalmos etc. help in distinguishing the two conditions.

Management

I. Nonsurgical Management

Selected cases, most commonly acquired, may undergo spontaneous resolution, and this should be kept in mind while planning for intervention in a case of Brown syndrome. The nonsurgical options include: elevation in adduction exercises, oral or local corticosteroids at trochlear area for inflammation.

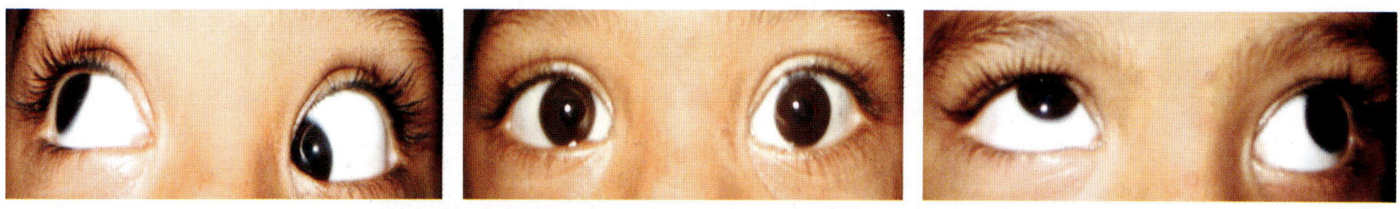

Fig. 1: A case of Brown's syndrome with downshoot on adduction

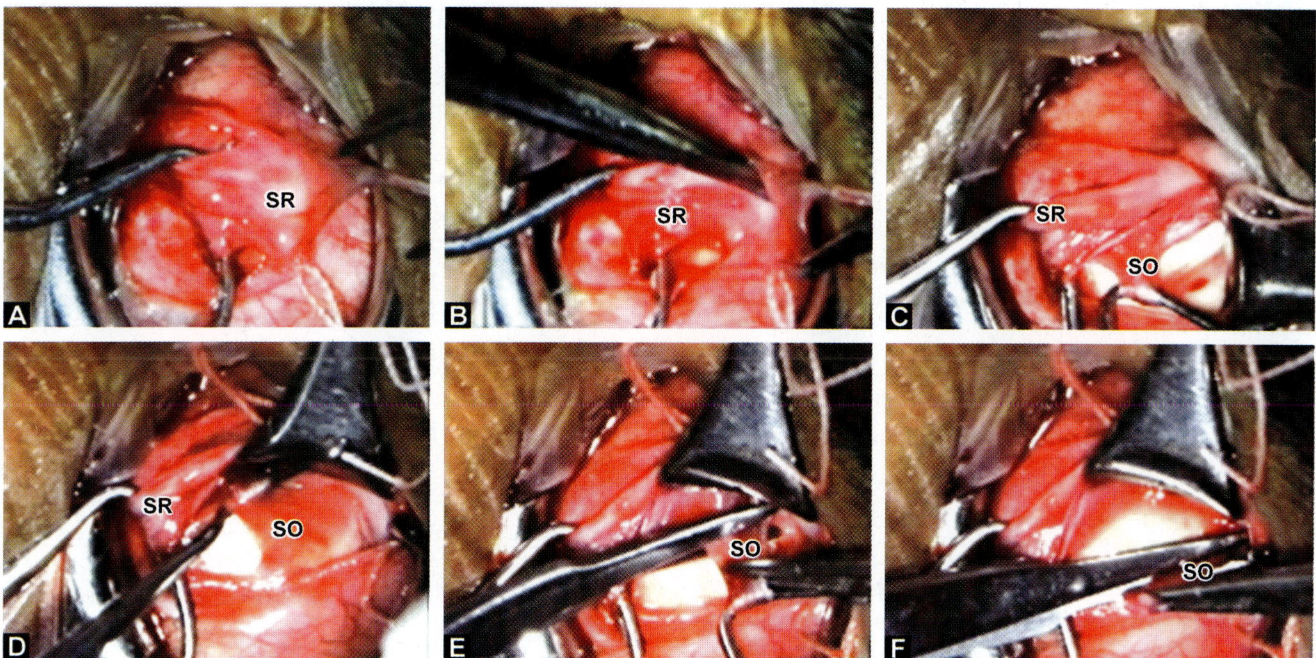

Figs 2A to F: Steps for free tenectomy of superior oblique muscle (temporal approach)

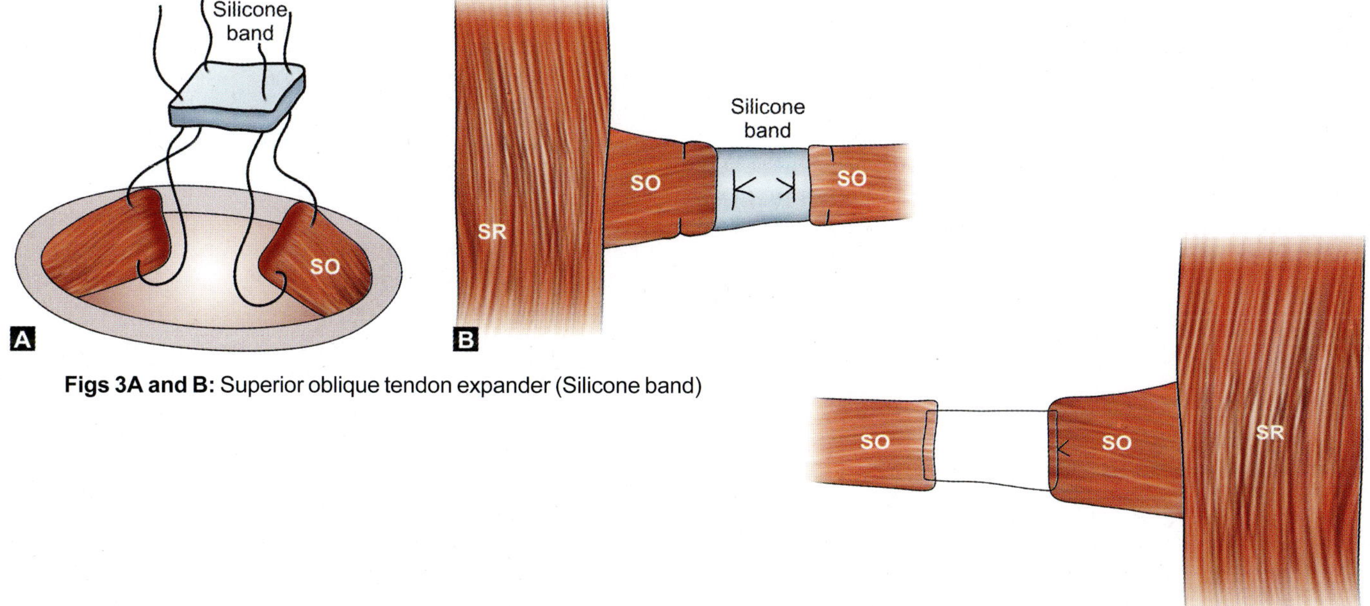

Figs 3A and B: Superior oblique tendon expander (Silicone band)

Fig. 3C: Superior oblique tendon expander (chicken suture)

II. Surgical Management

Surgical intervention in cases of acquired inflammatory condition should be deferred till underlying disease is controlled. The indications of surgery are:

1. Severe and constant case of congenital Brown syndrome
2. Brown syndrome plus that includes primary position hypotropia or downshoot
3. Presence of head posture

The main principle is to relieve the restriction by weakening the SO muscle that includes procedures like tenectomy, tenotomy, tendon recession, tendon expander.

Superior oblique insertion can be approached either from nasal side or temporal side of the SR muscle. Whichever approach a surgeon chooses one should try to disrupt orbital fascial layer as minimally as possible. Secondly, postoperative forced duction test should be done to ensure that the elevation of the eye is unrestricted after surgery.

Tenotomy or Tenectomy through Nasal Approach

A conjunctival incision is made in the supero-nasal quadrant, 8 mm posterior to the limbus extending 6 mm circumferentially.

The posterior lip of incision is retracted with lens hook and SO tendon is then identified as a whitish band of approximately 3 mm. SO tendon is hooked under direct visualization without disturbing the surrounding Tenon's tissue and vortex vein. Alternately one can engage SR and MR muscle on muscle for better visualization of SO tendon. Once hooked the tendon is then isolated from its attachments and fascia.

The surgeon has the choice to either cut the tendon (Tenotomy) or remove a section of tendon (Tenectomy) depending on the amount of weakening desired. However, it must be ensured that all the fibers of the tendon are isolated and removed or it may lead to postoperative undercorrection. It has been seen that the closer the distance of the site of tenotomy or tenectomy from the trochlea the greater the weakening effect.

The free part of tendon is allowed to retract in its sheath. The conjunctival incision is closed with 8-0 vicryl suture.

Temporal Approach

A 6 mm radial conjunctival incision is made in the supero-temporal quadrant or a limbal incision can be used to approach to SR muscle (Fig. 2A).

SR muscle is hooked and freed of its attachment on lateral border (Fig. 2B). The muscle is retracted nasally with another hook and a third hook is used to retract the conjunctiva.

Insertion of SO tendon can be identified as fibers fusing with sclera approximately at right angles to lateral border of SR. The SO tendon is now hooked under direct visualization ensuring that all the fibers of SO tendon are isolated on the hook (Fig. 2C). The SO tendon is brought temporally and freed from intermuscular membrane fibers (Fig. 2D) and inferior muscle capsule beneath SR. Tendon is cut as nasally as possible (Fig. 2E) and left to retract. A tenotomy closer to insertion leads to less weakening and closer to trochea produces more weakening. The base of the disinserted portion of the tendon is excised (Fig. 2F) and the conjunctiva is closed with 8-0 vicryl suture.

Superior Oblique Tendon Expander

The results of SO tenotomy or tenectomy are unpredictable. Under-correction is a common complication if all the fibers are not transected or tenotomy is performed closer to the insertion. However, after a complete tenotomy iatrogenic SO palsy has been reported in 30-85% of cases. Using an expander for SO tendon provides graded weakening proportional to the length of the expander and moreover the surgery is reversible.

Technique: Superior oblique tendon is isolated nasal to superior rectus as described above while maintaining the integrity of orbital fascia and sheath. This is important for the free movement of expander within the sheath.

Once the tendon is isolated on the hook a double-arm nonabsorbable suture is passed through the width of the tendon few mm apart from the nasal border of the SR muscle. Similarly another suture is woven 2 mm apart from the first one (Fig. 3A).

The SO tendon is cut between the sutures. A no.240 silicone band is secured with needles of both double arm nonabsorbable sutures (Fig. 3A). The size of band may vary between 4 to 7 mm depending upon the amount of weakening desired. The sutures are tied to secure silicone expander between cut ends of SO and lengthen it (Fig. 3B). Orbital fascia is closed over band with 8-0 Vicryl.

A similar effect can be obtained by replacing silicone band with a nonabsorbable suture. Instead of using two double arm sutures, single suture is woven within few mm of tendon. The tendon is cut between the sutures leaving a large loop intervening loop (Fig. 3C).

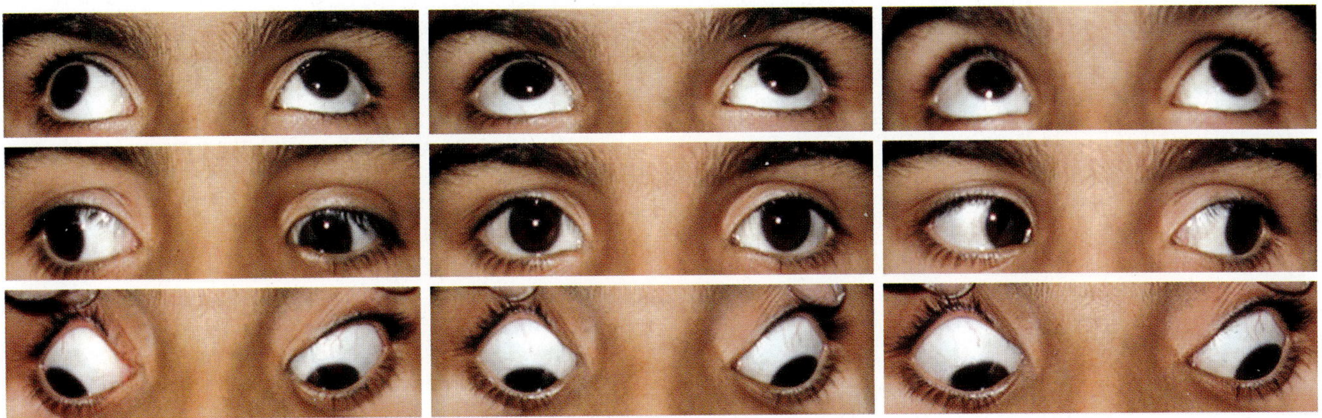

Fig. 4: A case of L DRS (type II) Note: Normal abduction, limitation of adduction and downshoot

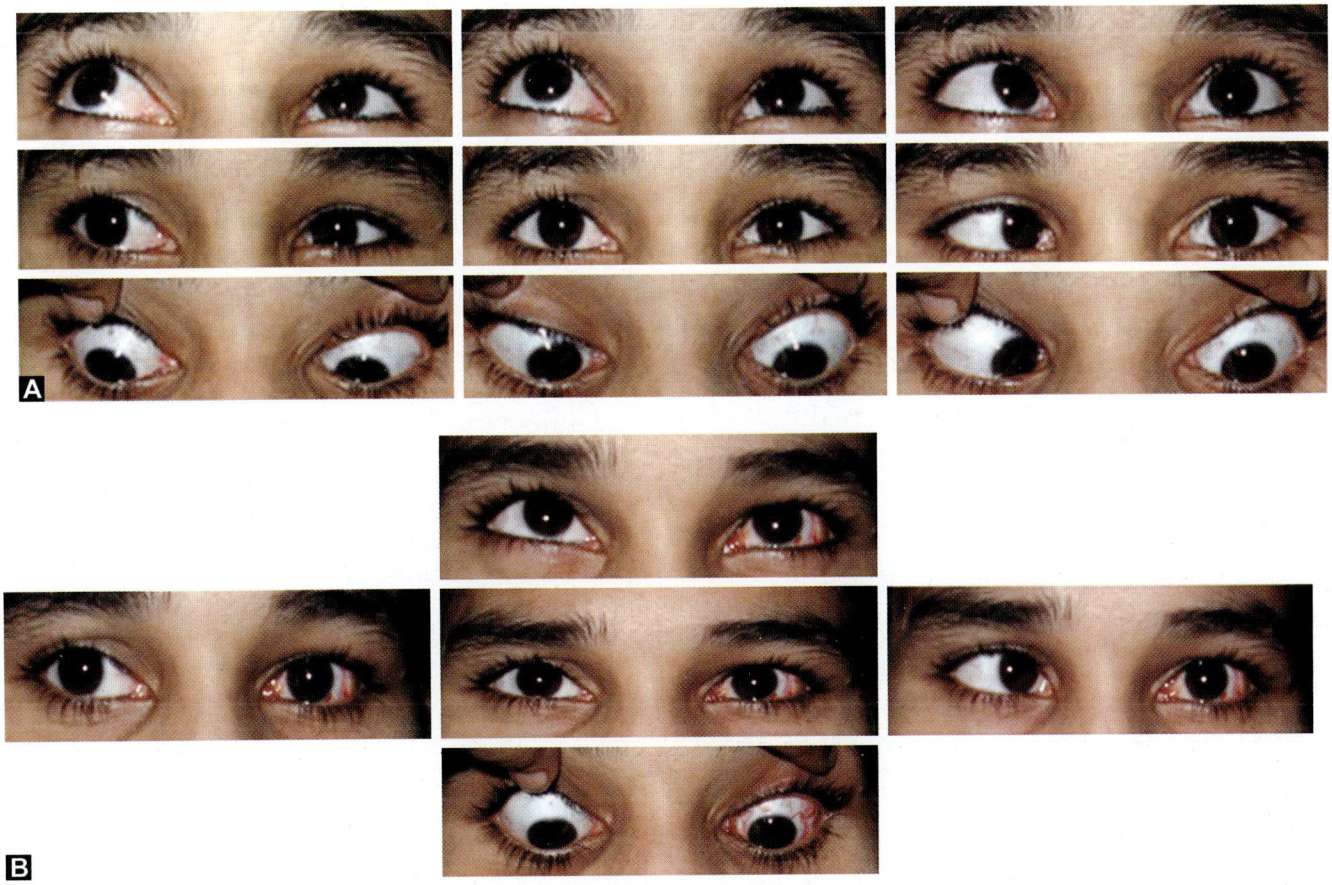

A

B

Figs 5A and B: A case of L DRS with retraction (A) Preoperative (B) Postoperative; note decrease in amount of retraction in primary position and adduction

Recession

SO tendon is engaged at its insertion temporal to lateral border of SR. A double arm 5-0 Mersilene or 6-0 Vicryl suture is placed through SO tendon 4 mm from its insertion and knot is tied. Muscle is transected between suture and tendon's insertion. Tendon is allowed to retract beneath the SR for distance of 8 to 20 mm and sutured at tendon insertion.

Complications of Surgery

Superior oblique palsy is the most common complication of the surgery for Brown syndrome especially with free tenotomy or tenectomy surgeries. Therefore, some surgeons advocate simultaneous inferior oblique recessions. Under-correction is more commonly seen with SO tendon expansion techniques and also when some residual fibers of the tendon is left attached at the insertion during tenotomy. Adhesions in superonasal quadrant can affect the final outcome of the surgery. In cases where silicon expanders/spacers are used, there is always the possibility of extrusion of the spacer. Moreover, these can form adhesions with the surrounding Tenon's fascia leading to restriction of downgaze. The chance of extrusion can be minimized by avoiding long spacers, maintaining appropriate surgical planes, and closing Tenon's and conjunctiva in separate layers. Postoperative complications also include ptosis and intraoperative damage to SR muscle.

Acknowledgement: The authors are grateful to Dr Pinto for the illustrative diagrams.

SUGGESTED READING

1. Brown HW. True and simulated superior oblique tendon sheath syndromes. Doc Ophthalmol. Feb 21 1973;34(1):123-36.
2. Cho YA, Kim S, Graef MH. Surgical outcomes in correction of Brown syndrome. Korean J Ophthalmol. 2006 Mar;20(1):33-40.
3. Helvesten EM (Ed). Surgical Management of Strabismus. An Atlas of Strabismus Surgery. (4the edn) Mosby-Year Book Inc 1993.
4. Parks MM, Brown M. Superior oblique tendon sheath syndrome of Brown. Am J Ophthalmol. Jan 1975;79(1):82-6.
5. Rosenbuam AL, Santiago AP (Eds). Clinical Strabismus Management Principles and Surgical Techniques: WB Saunders Co; 1999.
6. Von Noorden GK. (Ed). Binocular Vision and Ocular Motility Theory and Management of Strabismus: Mosby-year book Inc.; 1996.
7. Wright KW, Min BM, Park C. Comparison of superior oblique tendon expander to superior oblique tenotomy for the management of superior oblique overaction and Brown syndrome. J Pediatr Ophtalmol Strabismus. 1992;29:92.
8. Wright KW. Superior oblique silicone expander for Brown syndrome and superior oblique overaction. J Pediatr Ophtalmol Strabismus. 1991;28:101.

B . MANAGEMENT OF DUANE'S RETRACTION SYNDROME

Duane's Retraction syndrome is a form of congenital restrictive strabismus which is caused by musculofacial innervational anomalies. Various etiologic factors may play role in this syndrome, and can be classified as structural anomalies and abnormal innervation.

Structural Anomalies

1. Posterior insertion of MR may lead to retraction.
2. A slip originated from the orbital apex and is inserted 6 mm behind the medial rectus muscle.
3. Degenerative changes in lateral rectus that leads to fibrosis and contracture.

Abnormal Innervation

The injury at the time of embryogenesis leads to aplasia or hypoplasia of sixth nerve nucleus and nerve aberrant supply to LR by third nerve. In cases of Duane's the LR may exhibit a spectrum of abnormal innervational pattern ranging from paradoxical to the subnormal innervation. Abnormal simultaneous innervation can also be seen with superior rectus and inferior oblique.

Clinical Features

Duane's is predominantly found in females. It is unilateral in 75% cases with left eye preponderance, 25% cases may be bilateral.

Characteristics

1. Severe limitation of abduction.
2. Limitation of adduction.
3. Globe retraction and narrowing of palpebral aperture on adduction.
4. Upshoot or downshoot in adduction.

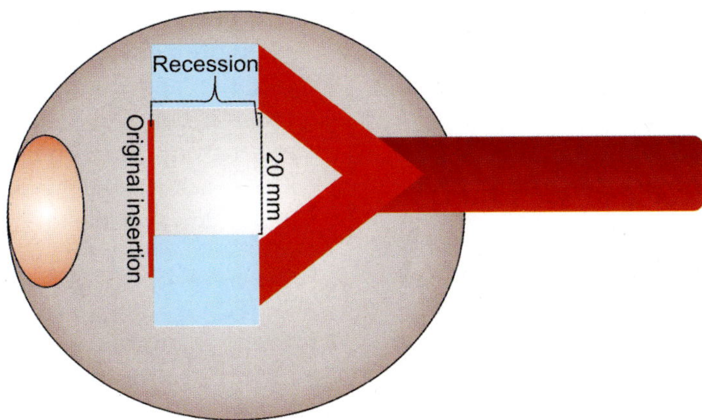

Fig. 6: Y split of LR muscle

Classification

Type I – Classic esodeviation with anomalous LR on adduction with no normal LR function on abduction.

- Most common type of Esotropia
- Limitation of abduction

Type II – Both anomalous LR and normal LR activity is present (Fig. 4)

- Exotropia
- Normal or subnormal abduction
- Limitation of adduction

Type III

- Severe restriction of both abduction and adduction
- Minimal esotropia /exotropia/ near orthophoria
- Retraction on both abduction and adduction

A clear distinction between different types may not be possible and mixed pattern is not unusual. Certain cases may present with fusion when the patient is orthotropic in primary position or may have head posture to maintain binocularity when the deviation is present in primary position. **Acquired DRS** may follow trauma, myositis or metastasis or any other infiltration.

Differential Diagnosis

1. LR palsy
2. Crossed fixation of infantile esotropia
3. Entrapment of MR in cases of orbital wall fracture.

Management

The management of Duane's syndrome depends upon its clinical pattern and presentation. The **indications** for surgery are:

1. Presence of compensatory head posture
2. For cosmetic improvement in cases of marked deviation and when disfiguring globe retraction and palpebral changes are seen.

Type I DRS with Minimal or no Retraction

In these cases absence of retraction indicates that LR muscle has either no or minimal anomalous innervation, hence correction of esotropia in primary position is the main concern and recession of MR muscle would be adequate. Some surgeons advocate recession MR of the other eye to produce a fixation duress. This would help in reducing incomitance of esotropia in contralateral gaze. One can consider a Faden suture on the MR muscle of the better eye instead of the recession.

In no circumstances LR resection is an option for a case of DRS however one may consider transposition of vertical recti to the LR muscle in absence of any severe LR anomaly, to increase the range of abduction. In presence of severe LR anomaly this may actually worsen the retraction. If at all required in presence of severe LR anomaly sixth nerve palsy is created followed which partial width transposition is done.

Type I DRS with Retraction (Figs 5A and B)

Presence of retraction suggests that both the muscles are receiving innervation on adduction and the anomalous LR muscle needs to be dealt with. While weakening of LR muscle would take care of retraction it would definitely increase the amount of esotropia in primary gaze. Hence, differential recession of both the ipsilateral horizontal recti is done to correct the esotropia in primary position. Recession of MR muscle of other eye can be done, if required, depending upon the amount of deviation at primary position.

Exo-DRS (DRS Type II) with/without Retraction

In these cases the LR may receive anomalous as well as some normal innervation. Hence, recession of LR of the involved eye would correct the exotropia in primary position and simultaneously would also decrease the activity of abnormal innervation. The amount of recession depends upon the amount of retraction and amount of exodeviation. Since the LR receives subnormal innervation a modest recession would be enough to correct exotropia in primary position; however, large recession is required in cases where retraction or enophthalmos is severe.

DRS with Upshoot or Downshoot

The LR in these cases of DRS is shortened and contracted. Consequently on adduction thus when MR contracts the shortened LR does not allow globe to adduct freely resulting in slippage of globe. The various options for managing this condition are:

a. Recession of MR & LR of the affected eye
b. Posterior fixation suture on the LR of the affected eye
c. Y – splitting of LR with or without recession on the ipsilateral side
d. Lowering the insertion of LR for upshoots, and
e. Recession of Vertical Recti

a. *Recession of horizontal muscles:*
   Since the inflexible LR is responsible for the slippage of the globe it becomes necessary to recess the LR, however, the resultant esotropia needs to be counter balanced by recession of the MR. If upshoot and downshoot are complicated by the presence of esotropia then the above surgery should be supplemented with recession of good eye MR.
b. *Bifurcation of LR (Y split) with or without recession (Fig. 6):*
   The splitting and spreading the muscle into two halves stabilizes the globe and prevents it from slipping up or down in the contralateral gaze and at the same time reduces the retraction in primary position.

   The muscle is split into two parts from its insertion as far posterior as possible and each half is reinserted superior and inferior to the original insertion with around 20 mm of distance between them. The Y split may or may not be combined with recession, although if co-existing exotropia is present or retraction is severe it may be advisable to recesses each half by 5 to 10 mm.

Technique

It is better to approach LR muscle in these cases through a limbal approach as good exposure and complete dissection is vital for the successful outcome of the surgery. After isolating the LR muscle in the usual way, it is then split longitudinally for approximately 15 mm. Two single arm sutures are passed in each half and both of them are disinserted. Two halves are then reinserted at least 20 mm away from each other and 10 mm above and below the original insertion. When this is combined with the recession the two halves are reinserted at the desired position posterior to the original insertion.

Type III DRS with relatively Immobile Globe

Both LR and MR is contracted in these cases and patients usually present with restriction of movement on adduction as well as abduction with severe retraction. Patients usually are orthotropic in primary position with or without minimal head posture therefore surgery is not indicated in these cases. However in presence of severe retraction both LR and MR need to recessed in large amount. The amount of recession depends upon the severity of the retraction and presence of any primary deviation.

Bilateral DRS

In patients with bilateral DRS with fusion (binocularity) the eyes may be aligned in primary position with straight head or there may be presence of deviation along with head posture. In these cases all four horizontal recti need to be recessed depending upon the deviation in primary position. In cases where there is no binocularity the patients either has marked eso or exo deviation is primary position. These cases are treated as unilateral DRS and balancing of MR and LR forces is done depending on the deviation governed by the dominant eye.

SUGGESTED READING

1. Alexandrakis G, Saunders RA. Duane retraction syndrome. Ophthalmol Clin North Am 2001;14(3):407-17.
2. Farvardin M, Rad AH, Ashrafzadeh A. Results of bilateral medial rectus muscle recession in unilateral esotropic Duane syndrome. J AAPOS 2009;13(4):339-42.
3. Heo H, Park SW. Rectus muscle posterior tenon fixation as an inactivation procedure. Am J Ophthalmol 2008;146(2):310-7.
4. Mims JL 3rd.Describing Duane's (Retraction Syndrome). Binocul Vis Strabismus Q. 2002;17(2):86-8.
5. Mohan K, Sharma A, Pandav SS. Differences in epidemiological and clinical characteristics between various types of Duane retraction syndrome in 331 patients. J AAPOS 2008; 12(6): 576-80.
6. Rosenbuam AL, Santiago AP (Eds). Clinical Strabismus Management Principles and Surgical Techniques: WB Saunders Co; 1999.

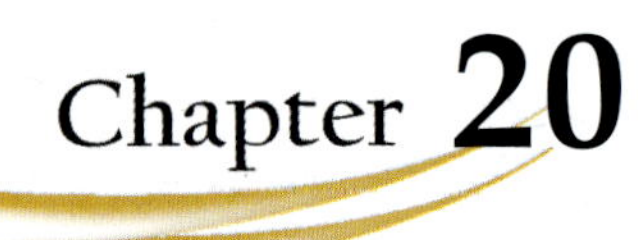

Post-traumatic Strabismus

B Shukla, P Bhasin (India)

After ocular trauma strabismus is not a common finding. Shukla[1] in a study of 1600 cases found cranial nerve involvement in 57 cases. Of these there were 12 cases of VII nerve palsy. If these are excluded the involvement of III, IV, VI nerve palsy would be in 45 cases (2.8%) (Fig. 1 to 3). Many studies have shown the ocular cranial nerve involvement in head injuries. Thus, Rucker[2] found it in 13.9% cases and Rush[3] in 19.7% cases. It is quite possible that there might be involvement of both as orbits and eyeballs cannot be strictly excluded from head injury.

Prakash[4] and Menon[5] have also reported the involvement of head trauma as a cause of cranial nerve palsies (III, IV, VI N). They have not mentioned as to how many cases of cranial nerve palsies were due to ocular trauma or whether ocular trauma was also a part of head injury. After head trauma they found the VI N to be commonly affected.

Table 1: Distribution of ocular cranial nerve involvement after ocular trauma

Cranial nerve	*Number*	*Percent*
IIIrd N	29	64.45
IVth N	05	11.11
VIth N	11	24.44
Total	45	100.00

Thus, the III cranial nerve was found to be most commonly involved. For obvious reasons all cases of post-traumatic strabismus are of paralytic nature. In most cases the squint appeared shortly after injury. However in Flew cases it appeared late after development of contracture in the muscles. Hence, the management in most cases in conservative up to 6-8 months. Surgery may be planned for residual squint after this period.

Traumatic squint can result from:

1. Disintegration of extraocular muscles.
2. Intramuscular edema or hemorrhage.
3. Entrapment of muscles in bony fractures.
4. Direct injury to the extraocular muscles or their nerve supply.

The management will also differ according to the pathology involved.

1. TRAUMATIC DISINSERTION

This may be due to intraorbital penetration of sharp objects like a knife or after some surgical procedures like excision of pterygium or limbal dermoid removal. The muscles may be partially or totally disinserted from its attachment on the globe. This can be diagnosed by forced duction test (FDT), ultrasound, EMG or CT scan. The disinserted muscle should be re-attached to its original insertion.

2. INTRAMUSCULAR HEMORRHAGE

This is usually caused by a blunt object to the orbit or to the muscle. The muscle gets swollen due to blood and is unable to contract or relax properly. The treatment in conservative by anti-inflammatory and anti-hemorrhagic drugs. Cold compression may be of some help and rest to the movement of eyeball should be given.

3. ENTRAPMENT OF MUSCLE

This is the result of fracture of the orbital walls. It is commonly seen in blow out fractures where the floor of the orbit gives way and inferior rectus muscle gets entrapped at the fracture site. If there is diploma in the primary and downward position surgical intervention is indicated with release of muscle and repair of floor of orbit by silastic plates.

4. DIRECT TRAUMA

This is usually due to blunt objects causing traumatic inflammation to the muscles and their nerve supply. Anti-inflammatory and steroids would be useful in such cases. These injuries usually recover soon.

During the recovery period it may be useful to occlude one eye to prevent intractable diploma or prescribe prismatic glasses to minimize it. Alternate occlusion should be done to prevent amblyopia. On the whole prognosis is good in these cases and surgery is rarely required.

REFERENCES

1. Shukla B. Epidemiology of Ocular Trauma, Ist edn., Jaypee Brothers Medical Publishers, New Delhi 2002;p. 82.
2. Recker CW, Amer J Ophthal 1996;61:1293-8.
3. Rush JA, Young BR, Arch Ophthal 1981;99:76.
4. Prakash P, Reddy SK. Ind J of Orthopt and Pleoptics 1979;15:1.
5. Menon V, Singh J, Prakash P. Ind. J Ophthal 1983;32:447-53.

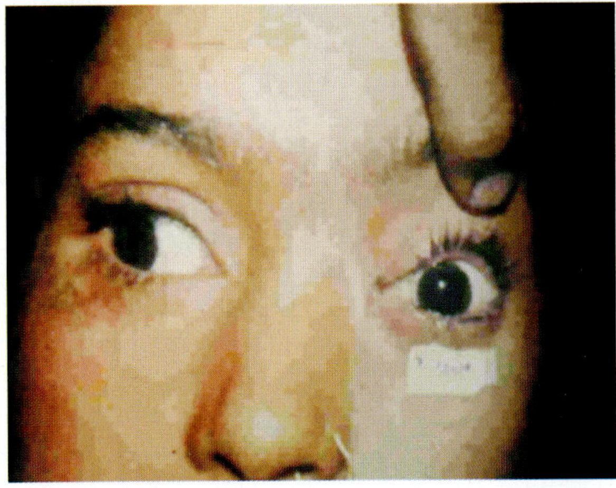

Fig. 2: LE immobile on dextroversi with dilated and fixed pupil

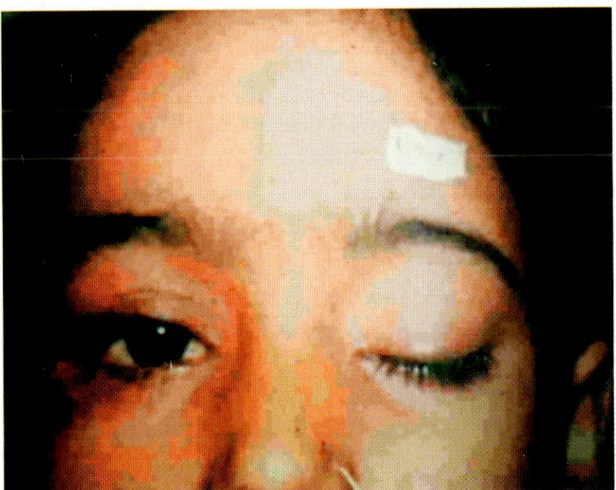

Fig. 1: IIIrd N palsy with ptosis LE

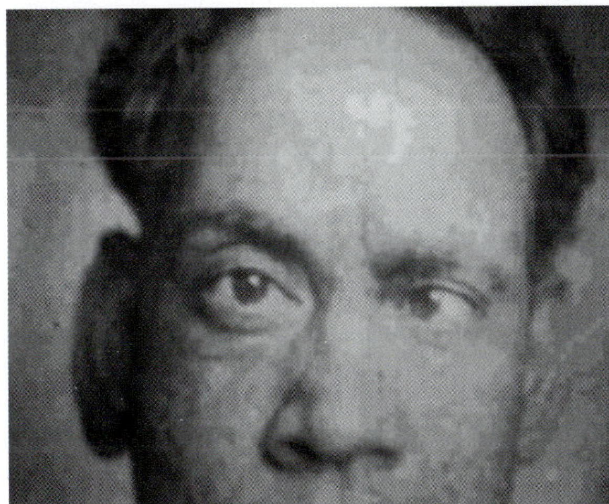

Fig. 3: VIth N palsy after jeep accident

Section II: Recent Advances and Innovative Techniques in Strabismus Surgery

Chapter 21

Newer Surgical Procedures in Strabismus

Paromita Datta, Pradeep Sharma (India)

Strabismus surgery seems to have been unchanged for the last several decades. But that is not true as we see the slow and steady evolution of surgical procedures for the more complex procedures earlier denied any treatment. It has been a constant crusade against the complicated and complex situations and has made the job of the strabismologist more interesting. Some of these are reviewed here. *We acknowledge the individual contributions of the authors who have published their innovative work and thank them for the illustrations that are reproduced here.*

Surgery of the inferior oblique muscle (IO) has undergone significant changes in the past 160 years. Many investigators have contributed to our understanding of the action of this muscle and to the surgical options that have developed. Recent anatomic findings have helped explain the effects of the anterior transposition procedure and allow further development of our surgical armamentarium for vertical strabismus problems. Further nasal transposition of that insertion should reduce or eliminate the incidence of the antielevation syndrome. If transposed far nasally, the IO could convert to an intorter, as well as to an antielevator and tonic depressor.

The surgical correction of strabismus in third-nerve paralysis is one of the most formidable challenges in the field of strabismus because even the modest goal of restoring the eyeball to the primary position, and maintaining it there over the course of time, has proved extremely difficult to achieve. Unfortunately, there is no agreement on the choice and efficacy of a given surgical modality, which has spawned several innovative suggestions, none of which has found widespread acceptance.

A rectus muscle may be functionally inactivated by reattachment of its insertion to the orbital periosteum. In third-nerve palsy, maximal weakening of the lateral rectus muscle is required to prevent persistent or recurrent exotropia because of the lateral rectus force being unopposed by any medial rectus muscle force. Lateral rectus inactivation may balance the absence of medial rectus force and reduce the exotropic drift postoperatively. In Duane syndrome subjects with marked co-contraction, limitation to adduction, severe globe retraction, enophthalmos, and pseudoptosis in primary position, in whom functional inactivation of the abnormal lateral rectus muscle eliminate the effects of co-contraction.

Extraocular rectus muscles transpositions may be indicated when limitations to ocular rotations are secondary to minimal or absent muscle force. Similar to patients with near complete or complete sixth cranial nerve palsies, Duane's syndrome patients with severe abduction deficit may present with a compensatory face turn and esotropia in primary position. Surgical goals for both patients with a chronic lateral rectus paralysis and Duane's syndrome include decreasing or eliminating head turn; centring and expanding single binocular visual fields; and increasing abduction while preserving adduction.

NEWER INFERIOR OBLIQUE WEAKENING PROCEDURES

The action of the IO muscle in the primary position is extorsion and elevation. Overaction of the IO muscle is characterized by increased adduction.

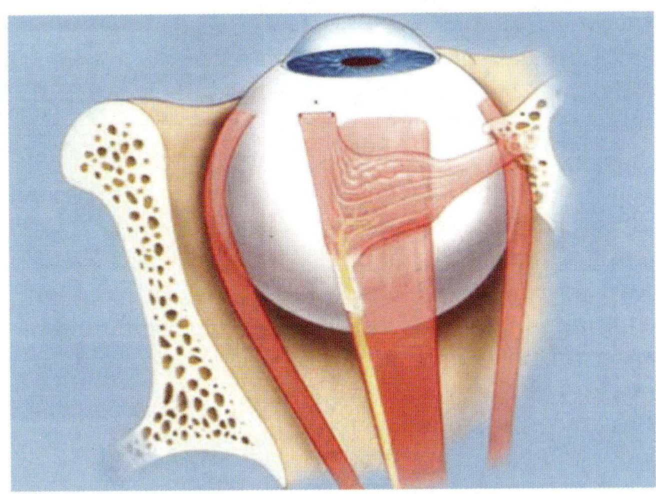

Fig. 1: Traditional AT procedure

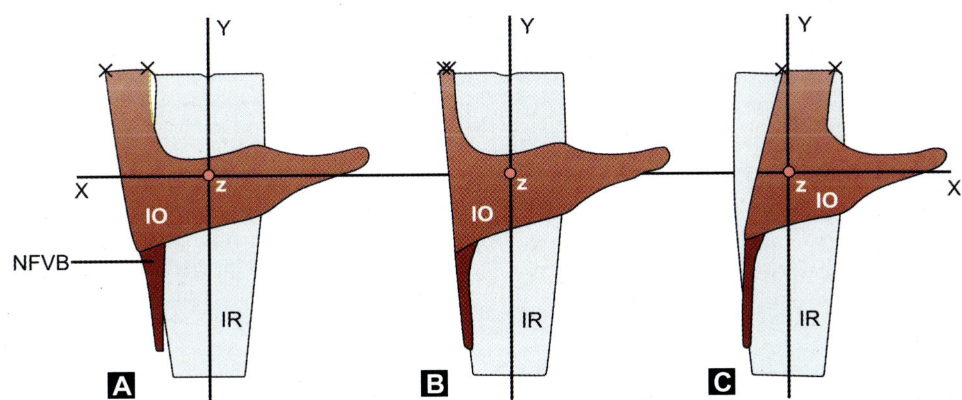

Fig. 2: Schematic representation (inferior view) of the traditional anterior transposition of the 10 muscle. (B) Placing the new IO muscle insertion close to the temporal border of the IR muscle decreases the risk of AES[9] (C) Placing the new insertion even further nasally should decrease the risk of AES even more.[13] The axes z, y, and z are the axes of Fick and correspond to the directions of rotation of the globe. 10-inferior oblique; IR-inferior rectus; AES-antielevation syndrome

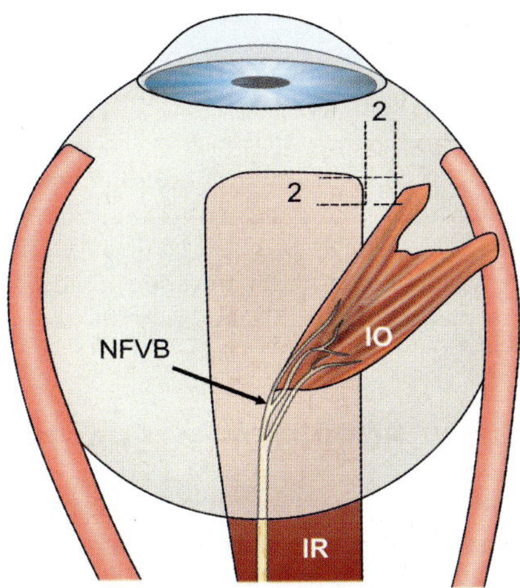

Fig. 3: Representation of the eye (viewed from below) with the IO muscle in its new position after ANT, 2 mm nasal and 2 mm posterior to the insertion of the IR muscle. The neurofibrovascular bundle (NFVB) acts as functional origin of the anteriorized IO muscle. IO–inferior oblique; ANT–anterior and nasal transposition

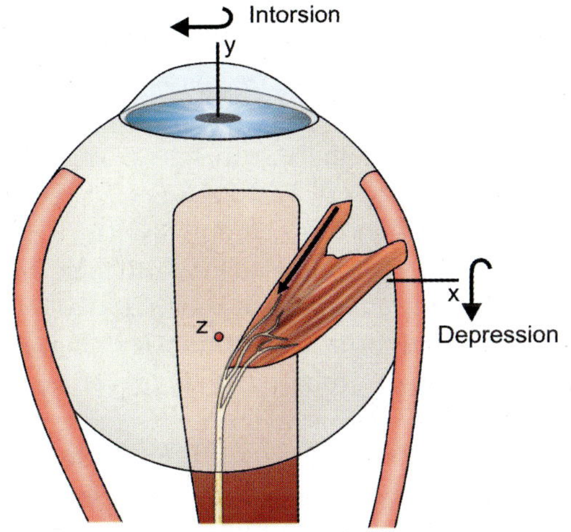

Fig. 4: The IO muscle after ANT, Contraction of the IO muscle creates a torque vactor (black arrow) that causes the globe to depress and intort (open arrows) around the x- and y-axes, respectively. IO–inferior muscle; ANT–anterior and nasal transposition

Anterior transposition of the inferior oblique (IO) muscle has been widely used for the treatment of increased adduction (traditionally termed "IO over-action") associated with dissociated vertical deviation (DVD). The AT procedure (Fig. 1) was developed in the 1980s and 1990s. Initially, Alan Scott,[2] Apt and Call,[1] and Elliott and Nankin[3] described an AT procedure that was designed to bring the insertion closer to the frontal plane containing the origin of the IO to enhance the weakening effect. Mims[6] found that this procedure eliminated the need for dissociated vertical deviation surgery in the vast majority of cases. Thus, a technique of correcting both IO overaction and dissociated vertical deviation could be accomplished with one muscle procedure in each eye.

A recognized risk of IO muscle anteriorization is that it may cause a limitation in increased abduction, resulting in an apparent IO muscle overaction in the contralateral eye, often accompanied by Y-pattern exodeviation. This was named and described by Kushner as "anti-elevation syndrome" (AES). [4]

Stager[7,8] postulated that the functional origin of the posterior fibers of the temporal portion of the IO muscle (the posterior temporal fibers) after the anterior transposition procedure is formed by the myoneural junction of the neurobrovascular bundle (NFVB).The insertion is temporal to the Y-axis of Fick (torsional movement), anterior to the X-axis (vertical movement), and temporal to the Z-axis (horizontal movement (Fig. 2A).This theory also explains why AES occurs less frequently if the new insertion of the IO muscle is placed close to the temporal border of the insertion of the inferior rectus (IR) muscle and thus close to the Y-and Z-axes (Fig. 2B). Stager[8] suggested that placing the new IO muscle insertion even further nasally, just anterior to the mid-portion or the nasal half of the IR muscle insertion, decreases the risk of AES even more because the functional origin and the posterior and temporal fibers of the IO muscle would then be superimposed with the Y- and Z-axes (Fig. 2C), thus eliminating extorsion and abduction.

A new technique was proposed in which the IO muscle is transposed not only anteriorly but also nasal to the nasal border of the insertion of the IR muscle[10] (Fig. 3).This anterior and nasal transposition (ANT) procedure places the insertion of the IO muscle to the Y-axis and anterior to the X-axis, thereby converting the IO muscle from an extorter and elevator in adduction to an intorter and tonic depressor in adduction (Fig. 4).

ANT of the IO muscles may be an effective procedure to weaken and reverse the action of the IO muscle when other IO muscle weakening procedures fail, and it also may be used for severe or recurrent IO muscle over action. It is an effective procedure for increased adduction, torsion, and head tilt. It may be indicated when other techniques have failed or are deemed destined to fail, e.g. the SO for patients in whom muscle is absent. This procedure has been found to be most effective in unilateral absence of the SO tendon.

It is likely to benefit patients with severe congenital fourth nerve palsy in which standard IO muscle weakening procedures have been ineffective.[11]

(Figures 2, 3 and 4 from *Stager DR Jr, Beauchamp GR, Wright W, Felius J, Anterior and nasal transposition of the inferior oblique muscles. J AAPOS 2003; 7:167–173)*.

REFERENCES

1. Apt L, Call NB. Inferior oblique muscle recession. Am J Ophthalmol 1978;85:95-100.
2. Scott AB. Planning inferior oblique muscle surgery. In: Third international strabismus symposium. New York: Grune & Stratton; 1978. p. 347-54.
3. Elliott RL, Nankin SJ. Anterior transposition of the inferior oblique. J Pediatr Ophthalmol 1981;18:35-8.
4. Kushner BJ. Restriction of elevation in abduction after inferior oblique anteriorization. J AAPOS 1997;1:55-62.
5. Stein LA, Ellis FJ. Apparent contralateral inferior oblique muscle overaction after unilateral inferior oblique weakening procedures. JAAPOS 1997;1:2-7.
6. Mims JL III, Wood RC. Antielevation syndrome after bilateral anterior transposition of the inferior oblique muscles: incidence and prevention. J AAPOS 1999;3:333-6.
7. Stager DR. The neurobrovascular bundle of the inferior oblique muscle as its ancillary origin. Trans Am Ophthalmol Soc 1996;94:1073-94.
8. Stager DR. Costenbader lecture. Anatomy and surgery of the inferior oblique muscle: recent findings. J AAPOS 2001;5: 203-8.
9. Kushner BJ. Torsion as a contributing cause of the anti-elevation syndrome. J AAPOS 2001;5:172-7.
10. Stager DR Jr, Beauchamp GR, Wright W, Felius J. Anterior and nasal transposition of the inferior oblique muscles. J AAPOS 2003;7:167–73.
11. Hussein MA, Stager DR Sr., Beauchamp GR, Stager DR Jr., Felius J. Anterior and nasal transposition of the inferior oblique muscles in patients with missing superior oblique tendons. J AAPOS 2007;11:29-33.

PERIOSTEAL ANCHORING OF LATERAL RECTUS

Surgical treatment of third nerve palsy, sensory exotropia and strabismus secondary to anomalous innervation of the rectus muscles, frequently requires large rectus muscle recessions in an attempt to maintain alignment in the primary position and reduce the effects of misinnervation. A rectus muscle may be functionally inactivated when its

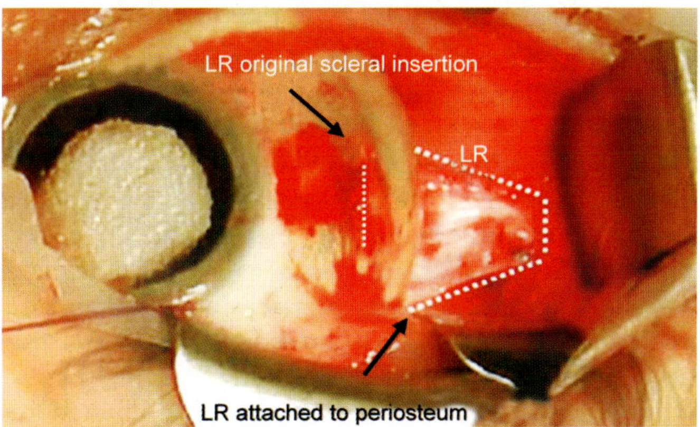

Fig. 5

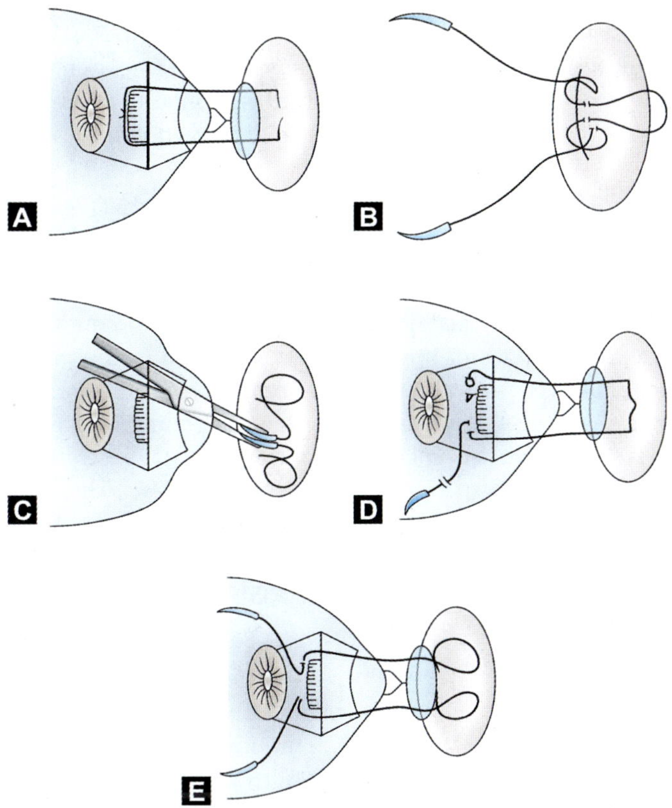

Figs 6A to E: Schematic drawing (showing right eye for the top end) (A) Incision on the lateral nasal wall as media for the deoryocystorhinostomy procedure. The fomix based conjunctival flap for exposure of the medial rectus muscle also is seen. (B) The dissection is carried out till the periosteum is exposed at the antarior acrimal crest. (C) The double-armed sutures are secured to the periosteum and brought out into the subTenon space using an artery forceps (the Bowman lacrimal probe is not shown in the drawing). (D) The sutures are secured to the sclera anterior to the medical rectus insertion. (E) The sutures are tightened so as to create a small esotropia (IO pd). (*Courtesy: Sharma P, Gogoi M, Kedar, S, Bhola R. Periosteal Fixation in Third-Nerve Palsy. (JAAPOS 2006;10:324-327)*)

insertion is attached to the orbital periosteum. Advantages of this procedure over extirpation and free tenotomy include permanent disinsertion of the muscle from globe and reversibility.

In third-nerve palsy, maximal weakening of the lateral rectus muscle is required to prevent persistent or recurrent exotropia because of the lateral rectus force being unopposed by any medial rectus muscle force. Lateral rectus inactivation may balance the absence of medial rectus force and reduce the exotropic drift postoperatively. Residual abduction may be caused by periocular connective tissue contracture due to a long-standing deviation and the abducting action of the oblique muscles combined with poor adducting power. Functional inactivation of the lateral rectus muscle should be combined with a medial fixation procedure such as an apically based periosteal flap fixation or superior oblique transposition to achieve permanent ocular alignment in the primary position. Lateral rectus inactivation of function is not required for most cases of Duane syndrome, but may be beneficial only for those subjects with severe lateral rectus contraction on attempted adduction.

SURGICAL PROCEDURE

A limbal or fornix conjunctival incision is made in the area of the rectus muscle undergoing surgery. The muscle is cleaned of surrounding connective tissue and isolated on a muscle hook. Blunt dissection is performed to expose the adjacent periosteum approximately 5 mm posterior to the orbital rim, outside the muscle cone. The rectus muscle is disinserted from the globe. A 6-O blue-dyed monofilament suture is woven and locked through the insertional edge of the muscle. The rectus muscle is attached to the adjacent orbital periosteum with two periosteal bites using pre-placed non-absorbable suture (Fig. 5).

REFERENCE

1. Velez FG, Thacker N, Britt MT, Alcorn D, Foster RS, Rosenbaum AL. Rectus Muscle Orbital Wall Fixation: A Reversible Profound Weakening Procedure. J AAPOS 2004;8:473-480 (Fig. from same article.)

VERTICAL RECTUS TRANSPOSITIONS

Vertical rectus transposition (VRT) surgery for the treatment of paralytic strabismus was first described by Hummelshein in 1907.[1] He transposed the lateral halves of the superior and inferior rectus muscles to the lateral rectus insertion as a method to improve abduction in a patient with Abducens Nerve palsy. In 1964, Jensen reported a different technique in which he split the superior and inferior rectus muscles into medial and lateral halves and then united them with the upper and lower halves of the lateral rectus muscle in the region of the equator.[2] However, cases of anterior segment ischemia have been reported utilizing this procedure.[3]

Carlson and Jampolsky described an adjustable partial tendon transposition that permitted self-adjustment of the vertical axis of the united temporal halves of the transposed halves of the vertical rectus muscle. This allowed for adjustment of the abducting effect of the transposition.[4] Full tendon VRT was not described until 1959 by Schillinger.[5] An adjustable suture technique to correct induced vertical deviations caused by full tendon transposition was reported by Laby and Rosenbaum in 1994.[6]

In 1997, Foster described the modication of posterior augmentation of vertical rectus full tendon transposition using nonabsorbable sutures to enhance lateralization of each transposed rectus muscle.[7]

Lateral augmentation seems to provide maximal transposition force. The efficacy of VRT is due to a vector shift of available mechanical forces generated from the primary position innervation of the transposed muscles.[8]

PHYSIOLOGY AND MECHANICS

Innervational plasticity does not occur. There is no innervational "relearning" of the transposed muscles and increased recruitment of the transposed muscles into the field of action of the paretic muscle does not occur. The increased rotational ability is due to relaxation of the antagonist combined with the "tonic" primary position innervation of the transposed muscles. The transposed muscles continue to fire at a low level and no change occurs in firing in the direction of gaze.[9]

SURGICAL TECHNIQUE

The rectus muscle is transposed along the spiral of Tillaux with the temporal edge of the vertical rectus adjacent to the corresponding edge of the lateral rectus insertion. A temporary knot is tied in the muscle. Forced duction testing is performed to detect any restriction to full rotation in the gaze field opposite the transposed muscle. If restriction is present, the transposed muscle can be easily recessed 1.0 or 2.0 mm until the restriction is relieved. The suture is then permanently tied.

The technique for partial rectus muscle transposition involves longitudinally splitting superior and inferior rectus muscles in half and extending the incision 9.0 mm

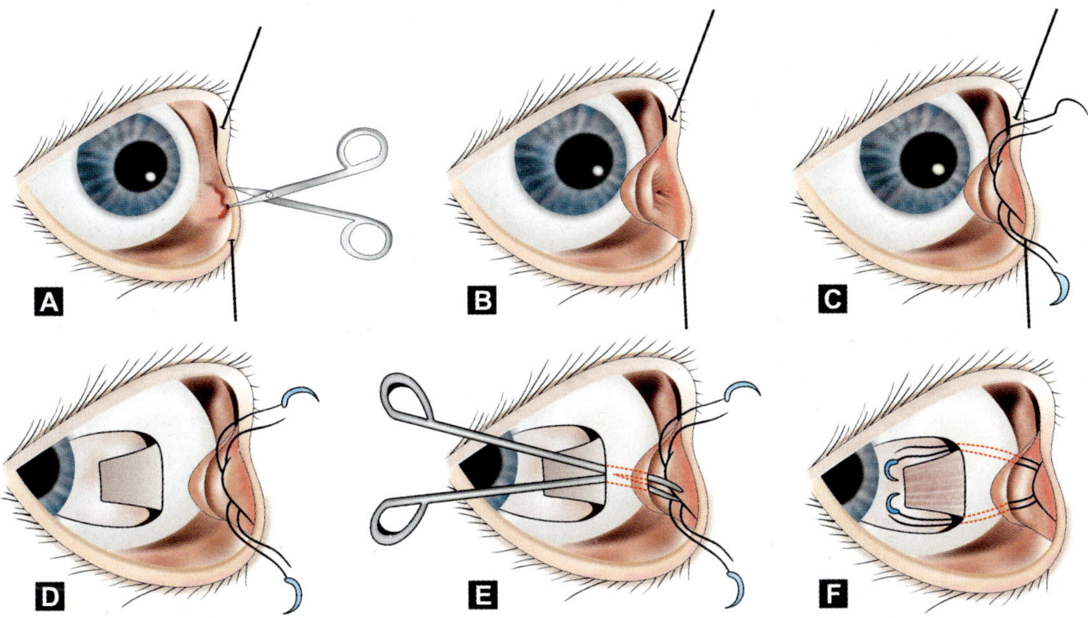

Figs 7A to F: Surgical steps for anchoring of the globe through a precaruncular approach. (A) Incision is made at the precaruncular conjunctiva; lacrimal probes are placed to protect the canaliculi from inadvertent transaction. B. Dissection is continued medially. Fibers of the posterior medial canthal lendon are separated to reach the periosteum posterior to the posterior lacrimal crest. (C). Nonabsorbable sutures are passed through the periosteum posterior to the posterior lacrimal crest (D). Medial rectus insertion is exposed using limbal conjunctival approach. (E) Sutures are held with the needle tips and brought out in the sub-Tenon's space using artery forceps. (F) sutures are passed on the sciera on either end of the medial rectus muscle. *(Courtesy:Saxena R, Sinha A, Sharma P, Pathak H, Menon V, Sethi H. Precaruncular periosteal anchor of medial rectus muscle, a new technique in the management of complete external third nerve palsy. (JAAPOS 2009;13:578-582))*

posteriorly. If each rectus muscle has a ciliary vessel that is near the nasal border of the muscle, more than 50% of the muscle may be transposed temporally.[11] However, care must be taken to transpose equal amounts of each vertical rectus (**Split VRT**) muscle in an attempt to avoid inducing a vertical imbalance. Posterior fixation of each transposed section can be accomplished 8.0 mm posterior to the insertion.

VRT should be reserved for cases in which there is complete loss of rectus muscle function resulting from rectus muscle palsy. This requires clinical differentiation of rectus muscle palsy from paresis where some residual muscle function remains. If function remains, rectus muscle resection rather than transposition is preferred. However, if residual rectus muscle function is not present, a resection procedure is contraindicated. It is better to preserve the ciliary vessel circulation provided by the paralyzed rectus muscle to reduce the risk of anterior segment ischemia if VRT procedures are subsequently performed.

The most important factor determining the efficacy of transposition procedures for VI nerve palsy or Duane syndrome is the state of contracture of the antagonist medial rectus muscle. If forced duction testing shows no restriction to abduction, it is reasonable to expect a good to excellent result from almost any type of transposition procedure. If forced duction testing indicates that the medial rectus muscle is contracted, one option is to inject Botox in combination with the VRT.[10]

VRT results in excellent alignment in the primary position and restores a useful binocular visual field of about 50% of normal. The efficacy of the surgery and the size of the binocular field obtained are directly related to the contracture of the antagonist. Improved rotation in the field of the paretic muscle is due to relaxation of the antagonist combined with tonic vertical rectus muscle forces. There is no true muscle recruitment. Thus, the rotation into the paretic field is of fairly slow velocity and may not be useful when rapid pursuit or saccadic movement is required. The procedure carries a small risk of anterior segment ischemia and induced vertical deviation.

REFERENCES

1. Hummelshein E. Uber Schnentransplantation am Ague. Ophthal Gesselschft 1907;34:248.
2. Jensen CDF. Rectus muscle union: a new operation for paralysis of the rectus muscles. Trans Pac Coast Ophthalmol Surg 1964;45:359.

3. Frey T. Anterior segment ischemia caused by Jensen's procedure. J Ocul Ther Surg 1985;3:242.
4. Carlson MR, Jampolsky A. An adjustable transposition procedure for abduction deficiencies. Am J Ophthalmol 1979;87:382.
5. Schillinger RJ. A new type of tendon transplant operation for abducens paralysis. J Int Coll Surg 1959;31:593.
6. Laby DM, Rosenbaum AL. Adjustable vertical rectus muscle transposition surgery. J Pediatr Ophthalmol Strabismus 1994;31:75.
7. Foster RS. Vertical muscle transposition augmented with lateral fixation. J Am Assoc Pediatr Ophthalmol Strabismus 1997;1:20.
8. Metz HS, Scott AB. Innervational plasticity of the oculomotor system. Arch Ophthalmol 1970;84:86.
9. Metz HS, Scott AB, O'Meara D, et al. Ocular saccades in lateral rectus palsy. Arch Ophthalmol 1970;8:453.
10. Rosenbaum AL, Kushner BJ, Kirschen D. Vertical rectus muscle transposition and botulinum toxin (Oculinum) to medial rectus for abducens palsy. Arch Ophthalmol 1989;107:820.
11. Britt M, Velez F, Alcorn D, Foster S, Rosenbaum AL. Partial rectus muscle augmented transpositions in abduction deficiencies. J AAPOS 2003;7:325-32.
12. Molarte AB, Rosenbaum AL. Vertical rectus muscle transposition surgery for Duane syndrome. J Pediatr Ophthalmol Strabismus 1990;27:171.
13. Velez F, Rosenbaum AL. Augmented transposition surgery in Duane syndrome. J AAPOS 2001;5:105-13
14. Thacker N, Britt M, Velez F, Rosenbaum AL. Surgical management of severe co-contraction, globe retraction and pseudoptosis in Duane syndrome. J AAPOS 2004;8:362-7.

PERIOSTEAL FIXATION OF THE GLOBE IN THIRD NERVE PALSY

Severe paretic strabismus in the form of complete external third (oculomotor) nerve palsy is one of the greatest challenges facing strabismus surgeons. This condition often leaves the eye in fixed hypotropic and exotropic positions (down and out) , and achieving even modest correction is difficult. Various treatment options have been tried in the past. Horizontal muscle surgery may work only in cases having residual function of the medial rectus muscle.

In cases with inadequate or no medial rectus muscle action, the deviation may recur due to unopposed lateral rectus muscle action, often requiring globe fixation procedures. Various approaches to anchoring surgery have been described.

The conventional procedure for the correction of the horizontal strabismus in total third-nerve palsy is supra-maximal horizontal muscle surgery[1,2] along with second eye surgery or pharmacologic weakening. Upshift (supra-placement) of their tendons by approximately 1 mm for each 2 PD of hypotropia in primary position also has been performed. [3] Multiple surgeries very often are required, including on the second eye, and not infrequently the result is under-correction and postoperative drift in the direction of the preoperative deviation. These modalities, utilized alone have been found to be generally inadequate. Several additional procedures have been advocated. These include mattress suture eye fixation temporally at the junction of the middle and lateral third of the upper eyelid,[4] various transposition procedures on the superior oblique muscle, with or without trochleotomy (such as the Scott procedure),[5-8] and through-the-lid traction sutures placed through the insertions of the superior and inferior rectus muscles, which are then brought out through the extreme medial fornices and skin of the upper and lower eyelids, and left in place for 6 weeks.[9]A modified Hummelsheim procedure also has been used, but it has very limited role in total third-nerve palsies because the vertical rectus muscles that could be transposed are already paralyzed.[10] Myectomy of the lateral rectus muscle without suturing it to globe has been described recently.[11] Periosteal fixation of the lateral rectus muscle has been described. Although results have been reported satisfactory, none of these procedures have found widespread acceptance.

The amount of recession of the lateral rectus muscle is determined by the preoperative deviation and the extent of paresis; up to 12 mm recession may be required for success in chronic cases in which lateral rectus muscle contracture is noted. The concept of anchoring the eyeball to the nasal periosteum is not new. It has been described previously for the treatment of third-nerve palsy, using fascia lata.[12] Its advantages are that it uses autogenous material and is less expensive, but it involves harvesting from a second site and takes longer to perform. Also, it cannot be performed in children younger than the age of 2 years because the fascia lata is not adequately developed, and residual exotropia to the extent of 30 PD has been described, especially in large-angle deviations. The technique of directly anchoring the eyeball to the periosteum with Ethibond [17] is technically easier to perform and is less traumatic, unlike the apical periosteal flap technique.[14] Like fascia lata, Ethibond has the advantages of tensile strength, durability, and tolerability by tissues.

The scope for lateral rectus muscle recessions significantly larger than 12 mm is limited. Another option could be to induce a larger initial eso-overcorrection of 12-15 PD base out to counteract the postoperative exodrift. Because late under-corrections are caused by residual lateral rectus muscle action, an alternative approach could be to disinsert the lateral rectus muscle and attach it to the periosteum of the lateral orbital wall.[15,16] An additional correction that can be affected at the same time is the vertical component in the hypotropic eye, which is achieved by exposing the superior portion of the lacrimal fossa periosteum so that the double-armed sutures may be placed at the upper part of the anterior lacrimal crest.

SURGICAL PROCEDURE

Using a limbal conjunctival approach, a conventional (not a hangback) 12-mm recession or more to ensure no restriction on Forced duction test of the lateral rectus muscle is performed. The nasal periosteum is then exposed as in a dacryocystorhinostomy procedure through a vertical skin incision approximately 15 mm long, 11 mm nasal to the medial canthus (Fig. 7A). Blunt dissection is performed until the periosteum at the anterior lacrimal crest is reached (Fig. 7B). A vertical incision is made into the periosteum at the anterior lacrimal crest such that it extends superiorly above the level of the medial rectus muscle insertion. The anterior edge of the periosteum is elevated from the underlying bone. The posterior edge of the periosteum is reflected laterally along with the lacrimal sac to avoid any accidental injury to the sac. The double-armed spatulated needles of the 5-O double-armed polyester are then passed through the anterior edge of the incised periosteum and secured firmly. The needle ends are brought out into the sub-Tenon space through the medial orbital tissue (Fig. 7C) by a special technique. After a medial limbal conjunctival incision to reach the medial rectus insertion, a small buttonhole in the medial orbital fascia upto the exposed periosteum is created by blunt scissors. Next, an artery clamp is passed through it and the 2 needles are "fed" into the artery clamp, such that the sharp ends are in-sheathed in the long axis of the artery clamp (Fig. 7D). The artery clamp is then pulled toward the medial rectus muscle, bringing out the 2 needles into the sub-Tenon's space. The needles are then passed through the insertion of the medial rectus muscle at its superior and inferior ends (Fig. 7E). Medial rectus muscle resection is not performed. Utmost care has to be taken to preserve the integrity of the lacrimal drainage system by passing lacrimal probes during these steps of the surgery and maintaining the separations between the sutures such that they correspond to the width of the medial rectus muscle insertion. It is ensured that the medial canthal tendon area, through which the common canaliculus passes, is avoided. The sutures are then tightened enough to align the eyeballs in primary position creating a slight esotropia of approximately 8-10 PD. The forced duction test is repeated. In presence of a positive forced duction test for adduction, a conjunctival recession may have to be added. The conjunctiva is closed at the limbus with interrupted 8-O absorbable polyglactic (Vicryl).

Most surgeons differ in their approach to the medial orbital wall. A skin incision gives good exposure of structures at the medial canthal area; however, the chemosis and fullness of the medial canthal region persists postoperatively for months.[17,18] An approach to the medial wall through an incision in the medial Tenon's capsule has also been described.[20] The precaruncular approach[19] was initially described by Moe.[21] The technique obviates the need for skin incision, reduces the risk of inadvertent injury to the globe, medial canthal tendon, or angular vessels, and avoids the extensive dissection required to fashion periosteal flaps. This approach follows an avascular path directly to the medial orbital wall.[19,22] It heals rapidly, with minimal postoperative morbidity.[23]

REFERENCES

1. Wiener M. Correction of defects due to third nerve paralysis. Arch Ophthalmol 1928;57:597.
2. von Noorden GK. Surgical therapy of paralytic strabismus. In: von Noorden GK, Campos EC. (editors): Binocular Vision and Ocular Motility. Theory and management of strabismus. 6th ed. St. Louis (MO): Mosby Inc; 2002. p. 445.
3. Biglan AW, Walden PG. Results following surgical management of oculomotor nerve palsy with a modified Knapp procedure. Ophthal Surg 1985;16:759-64.
4. Callahan A. The arrangement of the conjunctiva in surgery for ocular motor paralysis and strabismus. Arch Ophthalmol 1961;66:117-22.
5. Young TL, Conahan BM, Summers CG, Egbert JE. Anterior transposition of the superior oblique tendon in the treatment of oculomotor nerve palsy and its influence on postoperative hypertropia. J Pediatr Ophthalmol Strabismus 2000;37:149-55.
6. Metz HS, Yee D. Third nerve palsy: Superior oblique transposition surgery. Ann Ophthalmol 1973;5:215-8.
7. Maruo T, Iwashige H, Kubota N, et al. Results of surgery for paralytic exotropia due to oculomotor palsy. Ophthalmologica 1996; 210:163-7.
8. Saunders RA. Superior oblique transposition for third nerve palsy. Ophthalmology 1982;89:310-6.
9. Daniell MD, Gregson RM, Lee JP. Management of fixed divergent squint in third nerve palsy using traction sutures. Aust NZJ Ophthalmol 1996; 24:261-5.
10. Brooks SE, Olitsky SE, deB Ribeiro G. Augmented Hummelsheim procedure for paralytic strabismus. J Pediatr Ophthalmol Strabismus 2000;37:189-95; quiz 226-7.
11. Sato M, Maeda M, Ohmura T, Miyazaki Y. Myectomy of lateral rectus muscle for third nerve palsy. Jpn J Ophthalmol 2000;44:555-8.
12. Salazar-Leon Jo, Ramirez-Ortiz MA, Salas-Vargas M. The surgical correction of paralytic strabismus using fascia lata [Erratum appears in J Pediatr Ophthalmol Strabismus 35:269]. J Pediatr Ophthalmol Strabismus 1998;35:27-32.
13. Srivastava KK, Sundaresh K, Vijayalakshmi P. A new surgical technique for ocular fixation in congenital third nerve palsy. J AAPOS 2004;8:371-7.

14. Goldberg RA, Rosenbaum AL, Tong JT. Use of apically based periosteal flaps as globe tethers in severe paretic strabismus. Arch Ophthalmol 2000;118:2431-7.
15. Morad Y, Kowal L, Scott AB. Lateral rectus muscle disinsertion and reattachment to the lateral orbital wall. Br J Ophthalmol 2005;89:983-5.
16. Velez FG, Thacker N, Britt, MT, Alcorn D, Foster RS, Rosenbaum AL. Rectus muscle orbital wall fixation: A reversible profound weakening procedure. J AAPOS 2004;8:473-80.
17. Sharma P, Gogoi M, Kedar, S, Bhola R. Periosteal Fixation inThird-NervePalsy. JAAPOS 2006; 10:324-27.
18. Srivastava KK, Sundaresh K, Vijayalakshmi P. A new surgical technique for ocular fixation in congenital third nerve palsy. JAAPOS 2004;8:371-7.
19. Saxena R, Sinha A, Sharma P, Pathak H, Menon V, Sethi H. Precaruncular periosteal anchor of medial rectus muscle: a new technique in the management of complete external third nerve palsy. Orbit 2006;25:205-8.
20. Mora J. An adjustable medial orbital wall suture for third nerve palsy. Clin Exp Ophthalmol 2004;32:460-61.
21. Moe KS. The precaruncular approach to the medial orbit. Arch Facial Plast Surg 2003;5:483-7.
22. Kothari M, Kothari D. Periosteal fixation in third-nerve palsy [letter]. JAAPOS 2007;11:207.
23. Saxena R, Sinha A , Sharma P, Phuljhele S, Menon V. Precaruncular approach for medial orbital wall periosteal anchoring of the globe in oculomotor nerve palsy. JAAPOS 2009;13:578-82.

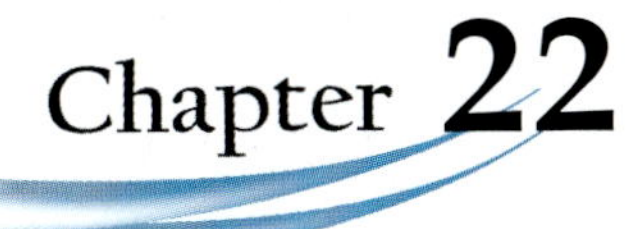

Update on Strabismus Surgery in Children

Brigitte Pajic-Eggspuehler (Switzerland)

INFANTILE ESOTROPIA

Esotropia presenting during the first 6 months of life is termed infantile esotropia and is divided into the following categories:

- Congenital esotropia
- Infantile accommodative esotropia

Congenital Esotropia

Congenital esotropia is characterized with large constant esotropia (usually >40PD), onset birth to 6 months of age, amblyopia common (50-60%) and associated motor phenomenon (usually present after 1 year of age):

- Inferior oblique overaction (IOOA)
- Dissociated vertical deviation (DVD)
- Latent nystagmus

Preoperative Evaluation

a. *Degree of amblyopia:* First treat amblyopia before surgery by patching the dominant eye until the patient holds fixation well with the non-dominant eye.
b. *Cycloplegic refraction:* Cyclogyl® (Cyclopentolati Hydrochloridum) 0.5% is used in infants less than 5 years old and 1% in older children. Full hypermetropic correction, especially in hyperopia or astigmatism is proposed to be prescribed.
c. *Limitation of abduction:* Abduction should be full or only slightly limited. Inferior oblique overaction and V-pattern have to be investigated.
d. *Angle of strabismus:* Angle at near and distance have to be measured with prism alternate cover test if possible. For verification or if prism cover testing is unobtainable we propose to use the Krimsky test.

Timing for Congenital Esotropia Surgery

The optimal age for surgery for infantile esotropia is controversial. In Europe, most references recommend congenital esotropia surgery not before 4 years of age.

Recent studies, especially in North America, suggest that early surgery may provide a better binocular outcome than after 6 months of age.

In 2003, the European multicentric "Early vs. late infantile strabismus surgery study" (ELISSS) compared the results of two different patient groups at 6 years of age, one having undergone early surgery, between the 6th and the 24th month of life, the other later, between the 32th and the 60th month of life. In the early surgery group a slightly better binocular function was seen whereas the vast majority of cases the level of binocular functions was subnormal or anomalous binocularity. At age of six years, 13.5% of the early vs. 3.9% of the late group recognized the Titmus Housefly. 3.0% of the early and 3.9% of the late group had stereopsis beyond Titmus Housefly.

Furthermore, an extremely early intervention increases the risk of including cases where the diagnosis is not fully established, in particular certain intermittent forms of strabismus which explains some of the excellent binocular results.

In 50-60% of cases different quality of stereopsis can be found in congenital esotropia, examined with Bagolini-Striateglasses-Test, independent of the age of being operated.[1-9]

Non-negligible is also the fact that very early surgery does increase the risk of a greater number of surgeries to achieve an equivalent postoperative angle. In the "early vs. late infantile strabismus surgery study" the number of surgeries per child was in the early group 1.18 (SD 0.67) and 0.99 (SD 0.64) in the late group. These are all good reasons for not performing surgery before 4 years. The indications for early surgery, defined between 6 months and 1 year of age, are setting for the following reasons:

- No hypermetropic correction or well-ported glasses
- Good cooperation between parents regarding amblyopia treatment
- Strong wish of parents for early surgery.

Surgical Approach for Congenital Esotropia

The choice of the technique and selected muscles is depended on behavior of angle of strabismus in different directions of gaze and distances.

The angle of strabismus for distance and near is the basis of dosage, measured with best correction using the alternate cover test.

Usually the first choice procedure is a bilateral medial rectus muscle myopexia called Cüppers-Faden procedure. The myopexia consists of suture placed through a rectus muscle, securing the muscle to posterior sclera, usually 13-14 mm posterior the muscle insertion (Figs 1 to 4). This procedure reduces the moment arm when the eye rotates toward the fadenned muscle. It has minimal effect in primary position, but progressively reduces the rotational force when the eye rotates toward the operated muscle (Figs 5A to C). If the deviation at distance is over 18PD the bilateral medial rectus muscle myopexia is combined with a bilateral medial rectus muscle recessions.

In congenital esotropia the myopexia procedure shows superior results than bilateral medial rectus muscle recessions or recession-resection procedure, it is said medial rectus muscle recession and lateral rectus muscle resection or plication.[7]

The advantage of a bilateral medial rectus muscle myopexia is a manifest convergence excess diminution and decreasing of the strabological angle fluctuation. Furthermore postoperative, frequency of divergence diminishes.

For the dosage of operation the bulb length is a very important fact. It is not enough to take the refraction alone. The situation of the vortex vein as reference point for a dosage of 13 mm is not precise enough. There exists no systematic measurement of localization of vortex vein. More precise is to perform a biometry.

Infantile Accommodative Esotropia

Infantile accommodative esotropia is characterized by an acquired esotropia, by onset at 2 months to 1 year of age, by a hypermetropia of more than +2.5D, by a moderate up to a large esotropia (20 to 50 PD) and by a variable often intermittent angle.

The treatment is a full hypermetropic correction determined by a cycloplegic refraction, usually more than +3.0D, given as soon as the esodeviation is identified.

There are three possible responses to prescribing hypermetropic spectacle correction for acquired accommodative esotropia.

a. *Esotropia fully corrected for distance and near:* Single vision spectacles are sufficient. No bifocals are needed.
b. *Distance corrected, but there is residual esotropia at near (high AC/A ratio):* If the full hypermetropic correction accurates the distance deviation resulting in fusion contemporary a residual esotropia persists at near that cannot be fused (usually >10PD), then we propose to prescribe a bifocal add (usually +2.5 to +3.5 add to start) to obtain fusion while leaving a small near esophoria (E<5PD). Leaving a small esophoria at near will help build up fusional divergence amplitudes. Surgery is not required. A flat-top bifocal that splits the pupil is preferable until the child learns to use the bifocal well.
c. *Residual esotropia for distance and near, partially accommodative esotropia:* If after prescribing the full hypermetropic correction, a distance esotropia persists that cannot be fused (usually >10PD), then surgery is indicated. The surgical goal for partially accommodative esotropia is not to operate the patient out of glasses, but to achieve alignment and fusion with full hypermetropic correction. The treatment of choice is a bilateral medial rectus recession. A prism adaptation test should be performed before surgery. The idea behind prism adaptation is that prism neutralization done over a long period of time will bring out the full latent deviation and reduce surgical undercorrection. It can also help to determine if the patient has fusion potential. We take press-on prisms. The patient wears them for 1 week, then returns for re-measurement. The prisms are increased if there is a residual distance esotropia left. News prisms are put on for another 1 week. This process is repeated until the angle is stable. Surgery is based on the full prism adapted angle. After surgery, repeat cycloplegic refraction and prescribtion of new glasses have been done if necessary. Patients with a preoperative high AC/A ratio will often have a residual esotropia at near after surgery and may require a bifocal add. If postoperative consecutive exotropia results, first reduce hypermetropic correction to stimulate accommodate convergence. If consecutive

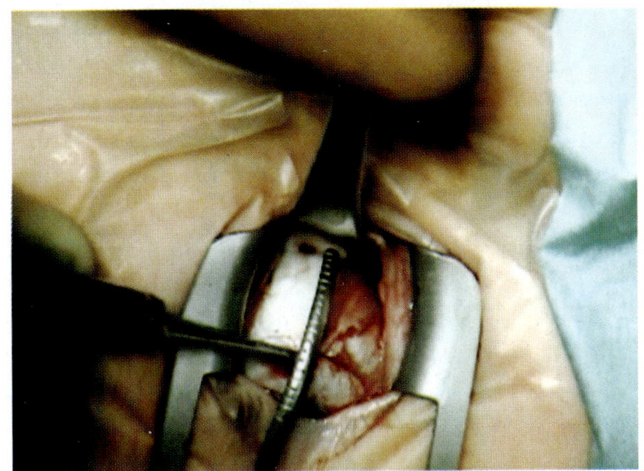

Fig. 1: The medial rectus muscle is isolated. With a scale the distance of 13-14 mm posterior to the muscle insertion is marked

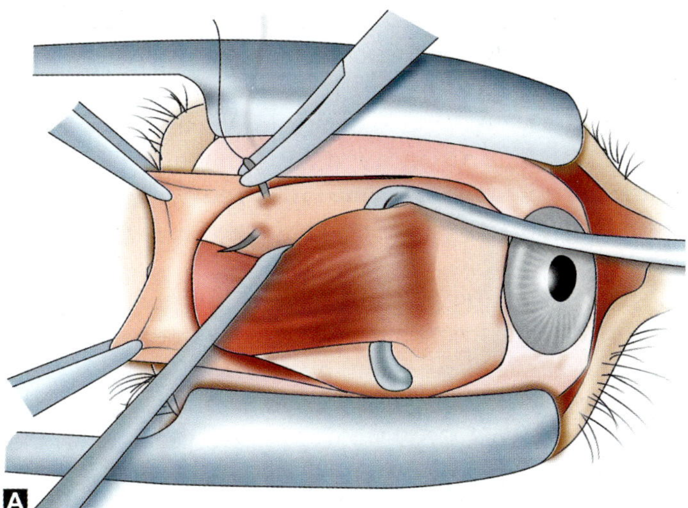

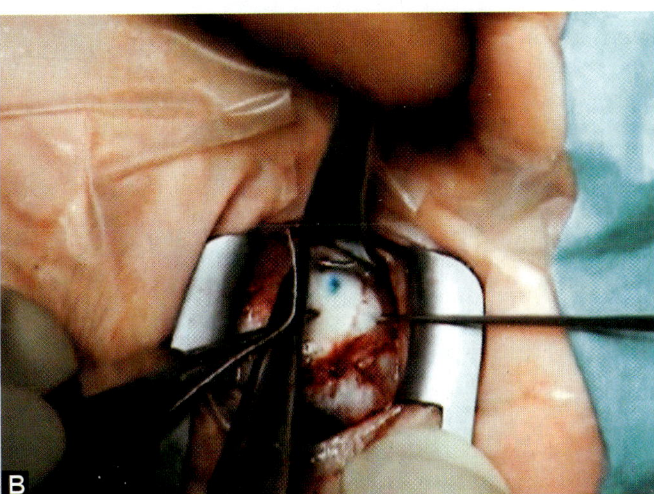

Figs 2A and B: A 5-0 Suturamid suture on a spatula needle is secured through the sclera

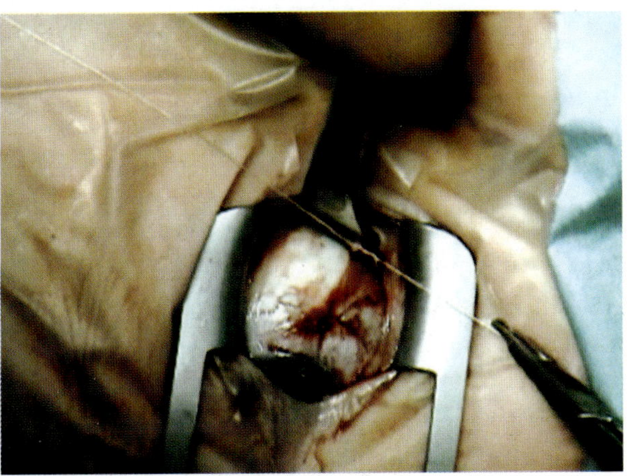

Fig. 3: The suture is knotted firmly to secure the muscle to sclera

Fig. 4: Both sutures are fixed in place incorporating the lateral 1/3 of each border of the medial rectus muscle 13 mm posterior to the muscle insertion

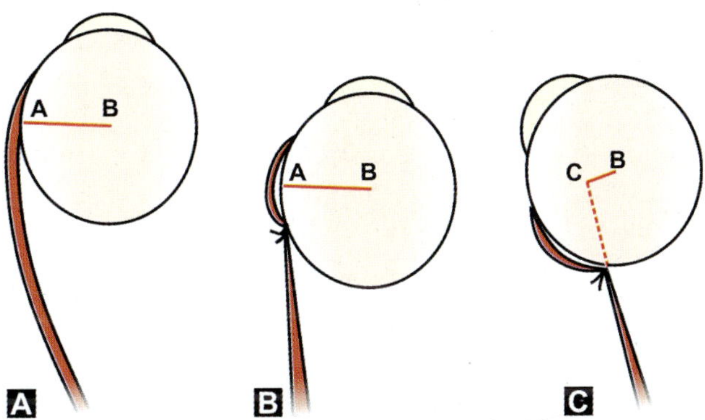

Figs 5A to C: (A) Shows the normal length of the moment arm when the eye is in primary position The moment arm equals the radius of the eye (line A-B). (B) Shows a faden fixing a rectus muscle 13-14 mm posterior to the muscle's insertion. The length of the moment arm remains unchanged with the eye in primary position (line A-B). (C) Shows the eye rotated toward the fadenned muscle. When the eye rotates towards the fadenned muscle, the moment arm is significantly shortened (line C-B)

exotropia persists after reduction of the plus lens, then consider re-surgery consisting of bilateral lateral rectus recessions. Examine the ductions before re-surgery to exclude a slipped medial rectus muscle.

LATE ONSET STRABISMUS

First of all a paralytic strabismus presenting signs of a neurological process as myasthenia gravis, chronic progressive external ophthalmoplegia (CPEO) or intracranial tumor have to be excluded.

Normosensory Strabismus

Full correction after cycloplegic refraction has to be prescribed. If an esotropia of more than 10PD for distance and near persists after wearing the full hypermetropic correction for 6 weeks, then surgery is indicated. Surgery should be performed within 2-3 months to avoid a sensory adaptation to the angle of strabismus. An early intervention can result in restoration of high-grade binocular fusion.

Non-accommodative Acquired Esotropia

Children are usually emmetropic, may be myopic. The onset is after 2 years, sometimes even in late adulthood. Ductions are full. Most often a case of comitant acquired esotropia is simply a preexisting esophoria that has broken down into a tropia. Therapy is a combined surgery: medial rectus muscle recession and lateral rectus muscle resection. Try using prism adaptation to determine the full target angle, especially if there is a difference between the distance and near deviation. Very often assimilate the angle for distance and near under prism adaptation test. If there persists a difference after prism adaptation test one can choose a different division of muscle recession and resection. If angle for near is higher than for distance, increase the amount of recession. If angle for distance is higher than increase the amount of resection. We propose to operate for the full prism adapted angle.

EXOTROPIA

Intermittent Exotropia

The intermittent exotropia is the most common form of exotropia. Usually it presents after 1 year of age. The precise etiology is unknown. Patients with intermittent exotropia have a large exophoria that intermittently breaks down to an exotropia. When fusing, they have high-grade stereopsis and when tropic, they usually suppress one image. Some patients, however, will experience diplopia. The exotropia is typically manifest when the children are fatigued, daydreaming or ill. Approximately 80% of intermittent exotropia patients will show progressive loss of fusion control and an increase in the exotropia over months to years. Often there is a distinctive glare, because intense light leads to a higher rate of their manifestation. Indications for surgery are:

- Increasing tropia phase with diminished fusion control
- Exotropia that is manifested more than 50% of waking hours
- Poor fusion recovery on cover/uncover testing
- Asthenopic difficulty

For measuring the deviation use prolonged prism alternate cover testing for far distance fixation and near fixation. For patients with a divergence excess pattern consider the "patch test". The "patch test" consists of patching one eye for at least 60 minutes, then measuring the deviation at distance and near without allowing the patient to re-establish fusion. Prolonged occlusion of one eye suspends tonic fusional convergence and discloses the full exophoria.

Because of the risk for developing postoperative amblyopia and losing binocular fusion, especially young children (under 4 years old) must be followed closely to check for development of postoperative amblyopia.

The preferred age of surgery is 5 to 6 years unless the patient demonstrates progressive loss of fusion control.

Surgical Treatment

There are not only conservative therapeutical strategies but also surgical options as follow:

- Bilateral lateral rectus recessions
- Bilateral medial rectus resections
- Unilateral combined operation: lateral rectus muscle recession and medial rectus muscle resection

Symmetrical surgery is usually preferred over a monocular recession/resection procedure because bilateral surgery produces a comitant result. A large recession/resection procedure on the other hand can cause lateral incomitance, inducing an esotropia and diplopia on gaze to the side of the recession/resection. The incomitance usually dissipates over time, but adults may complain of diplopia in side-gaze for several months.

Intermittent exotropia can be classified into three types based on the difference between the distance and near deviation:

- *Basic:* The distance and near deviations are similar, within 10 PD. The target angle is the distance deviation.
- Divergence excess: Approximately 60% of intermittent exotropia patients have a divergence pattern, with the distance being at least 10 PD larger that the near deviation. If a divergence pattern is identified, then the "patch test" is needed to determine the target angle. Surgery is based on the average of the distance and near deviation after the "patch test".
- Convergence insufficiency: This occurs when the near deviation is larger than the distance deviation, and there is deficient convergence. The treatment are convergence exercises such as pencil push-ups (20 repetitions, 3 times a day), then bilateral rectus recessions with the target angle between the distance and near deviation. Postoperative convergence exercises are recommended.

Postoperative Management

The immediate postoperative goal is to achieve a small consecutive esodeviation approximately 8 to 10 PD. This initial consecutive esotropia usually causes diplopia. Preoperatively, it is important to inform patients that transient diplopia frequently occurs after surgery.

Sensory Exotropia

Sensory exotropia results when poor vision of one eye causes the eye to drift exotropic. Treat by performing monocular surgery on the poor vision eye: lateral rectus recession or medial rectus resection.

Congenital Exotropia

A congenital exotropia is very rare. The onset is usually present at birth. Very often it is associated with craniofacial anomalies, albinism, or other systemic syndromes. There can be found a large and constant angle > 40PD with a poor fusion potential.

The treatment is a surgery after 6 months of age, preferable bilateral lateral rectus recessions. After surgery don't forget a correct amblyopia treatment.

MAXIMAL DOSAGE OF THE RECTUS EYE MUSCLES IN STRABOLOGICAL SURGERY

During the planning of strabological surgery it is important that the upper and lower dosage limitation has to be kept in mind.

An over correction leads to unwanted and for the patient detrimental effects as long-term over correction, angle incomitance, mobility limitations, enophthalmus or a decrease of palpebral fissure.

For prevent this undesirable effects following maximal dosage have to be kept:

	Recession (mm)	*Resection (mm)*
• Superior rectus muscle	> 5-8	> 5-10
• Medial rectus muscle	> 5-8	> 5-10
• Inferior rectus muscle	> 5-8	> 6-8
• Lateral rectus muscle	> 5-10	> 6-10

REFERENCES

1. de Decker W. Fadenoperation als Standardeingriff bei frühkindlichem Innenschielen. Z Prakt Augenheilkd 1984; 5: 275-80.
2. de Decker W. Möglichkeiten und Grenzen der Frühbehandlung des Innenschielens. Z Prakt Augenheilkd 1986; 7: 238-42.
3. de Decker W. Langzeitresultate früher Fadenoperationen bei frühkindlichem Innenschielen. Z Prakt Augenheilkd 1997; 18: 257-62.
4. Deller M. Why should surgery for early-onset strabismus be postponed? Br J Ophthalmol 1988; 72:110-5.
5. Esser J, Gieseler A, Waubke THN. Die Prognose der funktionellen Heilung des frühkindlichen Schielsyndroms. Klin Monatsbl Augenkeilkd 1981; 179: 85-9.
6. Kaufmann H. Results of Cüppers Fadenoperation (Posterior fixation suture). van Balen ATM, Houtman WA, (Eds). Docum Ophthalmol Proc Series. The Hague 1982;32:143.
7. Kaufmann H, Krzizok T, Scharwey K. Ergebnisse sogenannter Frühoperationen beim frühkindlichen Innenschielen. Z Prakt Augenheilkd 1997; 18: 250-6.
8. Klainguti G, Chamero J, Deller M. Résultats angulaires à court et moyen terme de la myopexie rétroéquatoriale de Cüppers, avec et sans adjonction d'une technique d'affaiblissment conventionnelle. Klin Monatsbl Augenheilkd 1991;198:382-5.
9. Klainguti G, Strickler J, Presset C. Traitement chirurgical de l'excès de convergence accommodative. Etude de 50 cas opérés. Klin Monatsbl Augenheilkd 1998;212:291-3.

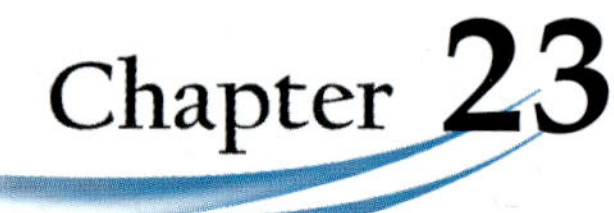

Möbius Syndrome (Sequence): Strabismus Surgery

LO Ventura, SB Travassos, HC Almeida (Brazil), MT Miller (USA), PA Jorge, BV Ventura (Brazil)

INTRODUCTION

In 1880, von Graefe and Saemisch described the "congenital facial diplegia" syndrome.[1] Subsequently, Harlan and Chisolm published cases of congenital paralysis of the abducens and facial nerves.[2,3] However, it was the German neurologist Paul Möbius who reported the association between congenital facial diplegia and bilateral abducens palsy in 1888.[4]

Since then, this entity has been known as Möbius syndrome; it is a rare condition, having an estimated prevalence of 0.0002-0.002% of births. Both sexes are affected equally.[5,6]

ETIOPATHOGENESIS

The most accepted etiopathogenic mechanism for the Möbius syndrome was proposed by Bouwes-Bavinck and Weaver.[7] They suggested that a disruption of the blood flow on a specific portion of the subclavian, basilar, vertebral and internal thoracic arteries early during morphogenesis causes ischemic alterations in the brainstem, especially around the sixth and seventh cranial nerve nuclei. The result is a wide range of mesenchymal and ectodermally-derived defects, depending on the specific location of the vascular insufficiency, the developmental stage in which the insufficiency occurred and its intensity and duration. This explains the different phenotypic expressions of the Möbius syndrome.[8]

The term "syndrome" implies a combination of developmental defects sharing a common etiology, while "sequence" refers to multiple causes resulting in an initial insult at some time in the morphogenesis determining subsequent events. Therefore, the term "Möbius sequence" better describes this condition.[9]

The Möbius sequence has a multifactorial etiology. It is usually sporadic, although some cases of familial occurrence have been described: autosomal dominant, autosomal recessive and X-linked recessive inheritance, and karyotypic changes.[10-12]

Several environmental agents have been associated with Möbius sequence when used in the first trimester of pregnancy, such as thalidomide,[13] benzodiazepine,[14] cocaine,[15] alcohol[16] and misoprostol.[17-20] Other cases have been described associating this syndrome with infections, hyperthermia, vasculites and abdominal trauma.[16,21]

CLINICAL FEATURES

The main findings of the Möbius sequence are congenital uni-or bilateral palsy of the abducens and facial cranial nerves (peripheral palsy), the latter being a peripheral palsy and resulting in the mask-like facies. The sixth and seventh cranial nerves have important ophthalmologic implications.[22,23] The most frequent eye signs are convergent strabismus and lagophthalmus.[24] The most common eye deviation in these patients is large angle esodeviation, but there are cases of orthotropia or exodeviation either isolated, or associated with vertical strabismus (Figs 1 and 2).

Frequently these cases show apparent gaze paresis with marked abduction deficit (6th nerve involvement), causing head turn, which results in cross fixation. In addition, there might be a smaller limitation of adduction.[22,24] Patients show limited conjugated horizontal eye movement, while the conjugated vertical movement is usually normal and there is some degree of ocular convergence.[25] Aberrant tearing is also a common finding in these patients, with dry eye in some cases specially when there is association with abnormal eye closure of palpebral fissure[26] (Figs 3 A and B).

Involvement of other cranial nerves may occur, such as trigeminal, glossopharyngeal and hypoglossal nerves. Associated craniofacial and limb malformations are also frequent. Mental retardation and autism have been reported.[9,10,20,27,28] (Fig. 4).

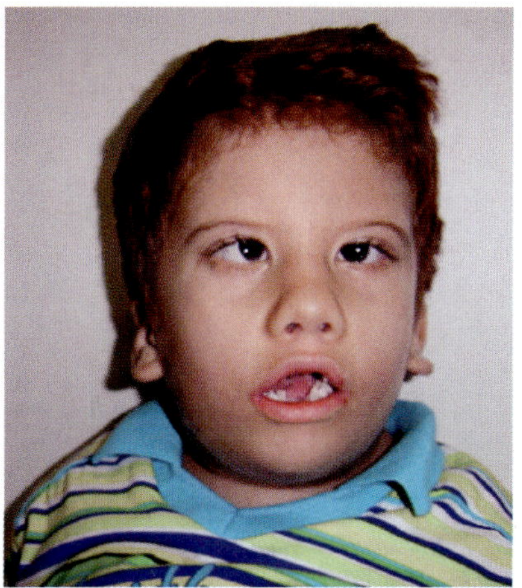

Fig. 1: Combined vertical and horizontal strabismus in a patient with Möbius sequence

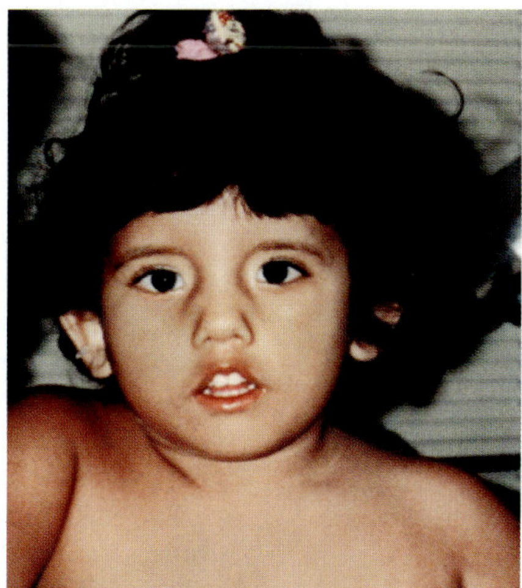

Fig. 2: Möbius patient with orthotropia

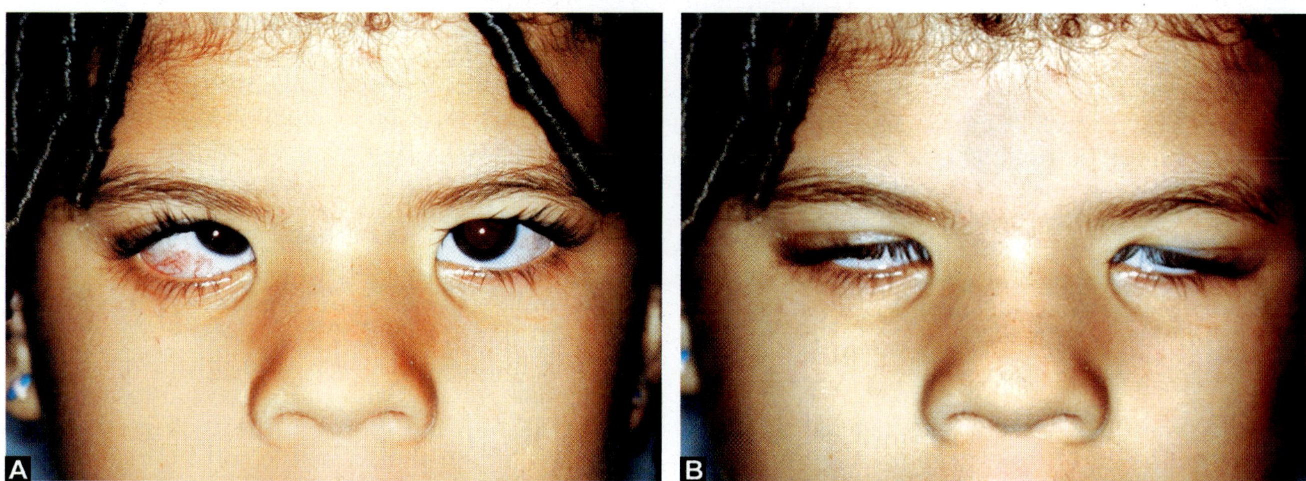

Figs 3A and B: (A) Dry eye in right eye. (B) Bilateral lagophthalmus

Table 1: Long-term surgical results in Möbius sequence.n = 10

Cases	**Strabismus in primary position**			**Deviation Pattern**		
ES	*Pre- operatory*	*90th day*	*2nd year*	*Pre-operatory*	*90 day*	*2nd year*
1	ET 35 PD HTD/E 10 PD	ET 4 PD	ORTHO	V	-	-
2	ET 50 PD HTD/E 10 PD	ET 10 PD	XT 6 PD	V	-	-
3	ET 50 PD HT E/D 10 PD	XT 8 PD	XT 35 PD HT D/E 4 PD	V	-	V
4	ET 50 PD HT E/D 10 PD	ET 10 PD	XT 10 PD	-	-	-
5	ET 85 PD HT D/E 16 PD	ET 26 P	ET 40 PD	-	-	-
6	ET 30 PD HT D/E 4 PD	ORTHO	ORTHO	A	-	-
7	ET 50 PD	HT E/D 4 PD	XT 6 PD HT E/D 2 PD	-	-	V
8	ET 50 PD HTE/D 4 PD	ET 16 PD	ET 10 PD	-	-	-
9	ET 50 PD	ORTHO	ET 5 PD	-	-	V
10	ET 15 PD HT E/D 10 PD	ET 16 PD	ET 10 PD	V	V	-

* PD = Prismatic Diopter.

TREATMENT

The appropriate treatment for patients with Möbius sequence depends on their major births defects and dysfunctions. It requires a multidisciplinary team, including pediatricians, ophthalmologists, plastic surgeons, orthopedists, neurologists, psychiatrists, psychologists, dentists, speech and language therapists and physiotherapeutic specialists.[10,20,29,30] Möbius sequence is initially evaluated and treated by the pediatric ophthalmologist and strabismus specialist during the early years of life.[31] The ophthalmologic approach of these patients consists on early detection and treatment of the corneal exposure, refractive errors, amblyopia and strabismus.[32] It is crucial to treat suppression and strabismic amblyopia.[31]

In cases with severely compromised seventh cranial nerve, with exposed cornea, especially in sleep, the eyes must be lubricated. Refractive errors and a lack of corneal clarity may exacerbate strabismic amblyopia. Besides lagophthalmos and entropion, corneal surface diseases may be aggravated by cornea anesthesia secondary to dysfunction of the fifth cranial nerve.

STRABISMUS MANAGEMENT

The management of strabismus in patients with Möbius sequence is difficult. No single approach is successful in all patients. A good surgical result aligns the eyes in primary position, but full ocular rotations cannot be restored.[29]

In these patients a fibrous tissue band has been observed and its histological exam revealed the paucity or absence of muscle tissue.[33] This paucity or absence of muscle tissue leads to restriction of the eye and makes the surgery approach a challenge. It is important to perform a forced passive duction test on each eye, trying to identify tight medial recti (MR)[31,33] (Figs 5A and B).

Experience has shown that standard MR recession alone is rarely effective in this condition because of the lack of abduction ability and by the frequently observed secondary MR muscle contraction.[34] However, Ventura et al 2007[35] have shown that this procedure corrects the esotropia satisfactorily and, sometimes, even hypercorrect it. In Table 1, it is reported ten cases of Möbius sequence operated on for the esotropia with medial recti recession and in cases with A or V pattern the MR was dislocated either inferiorly (V pattern) or superiorly (A pattern).

In two year-follow-up, 8/10 cases showed adequate results with residual deviation smaller than 10 Prismatic Diopter (PD) (Figs 6A and B; 7A and B; 8A and B; 9A and B).

Möbius patients should always be operated by recession of medial recti (Figs 10 to 13).

Since the abducens nerves are already dead in intra-uterine life, the medial recti may be contracted, tight at birth (Figs 14A and B). It has already been known that surgery in a contractured muscle, corrects more deviation than in a normal muscle. Therefore, the weakening of medial recti must be smaller than in a case of traumatic abducens palsy. Extra care must be taken in case of Möbius

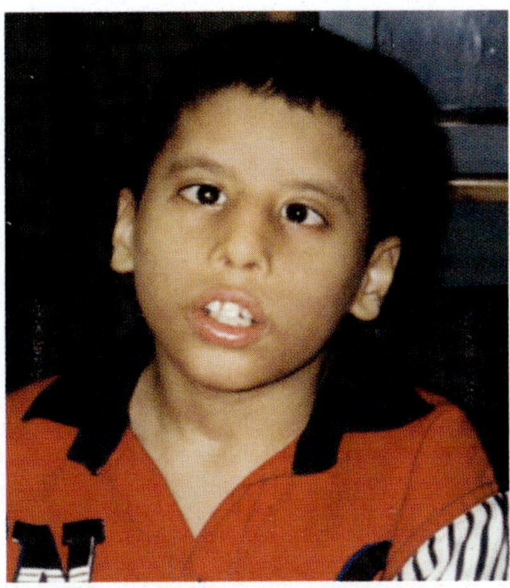

Fig. 4: Patient with Möbius sequence associated with autism disorder

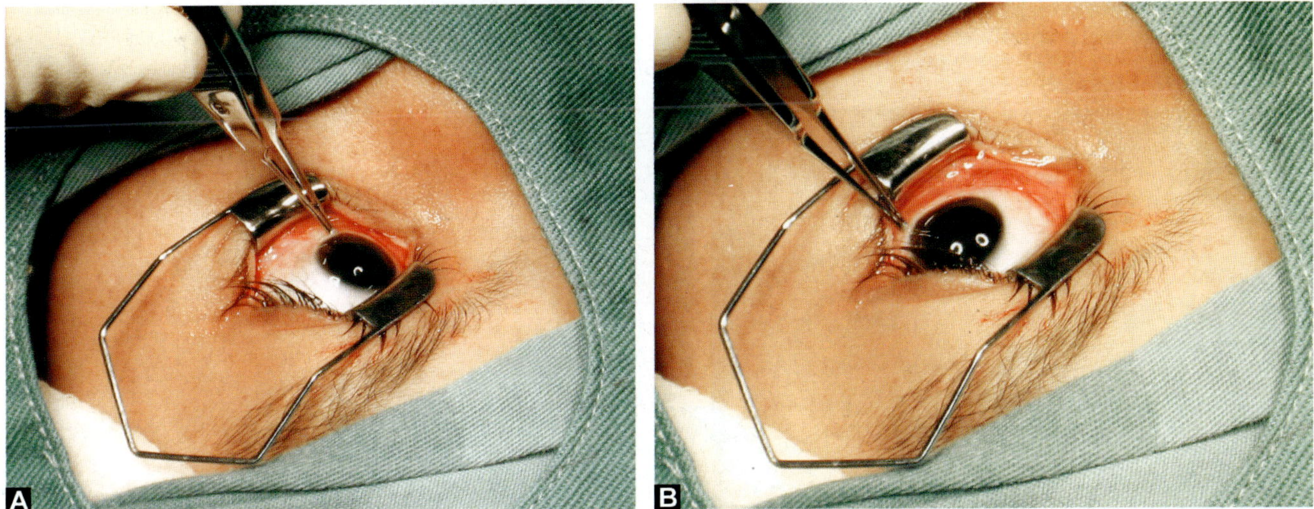

Figs 5A and B: Forced passive duction test positive A, with marked ocular limitation of adduction and B, mild limitation of abduction

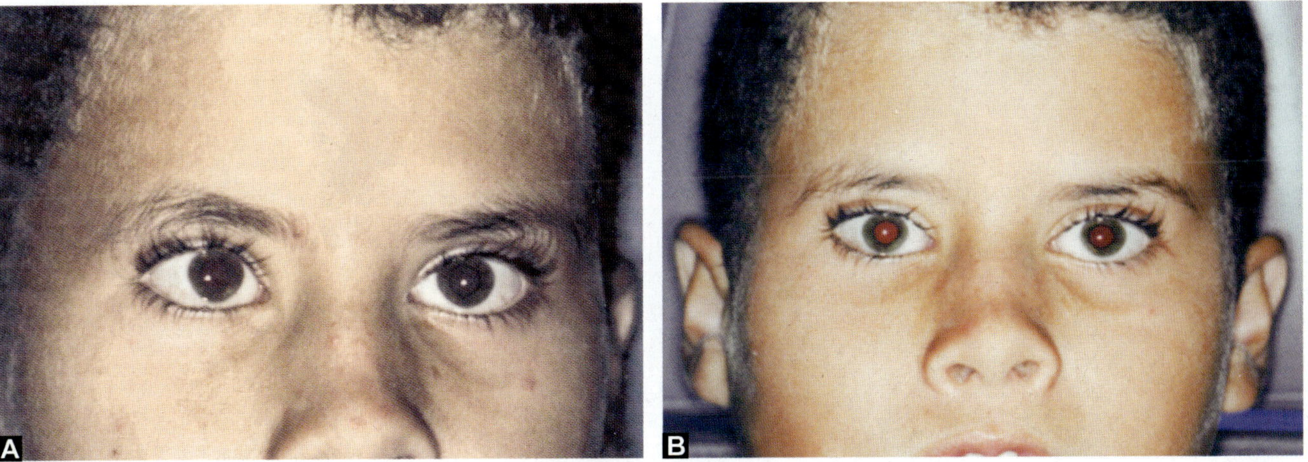

Figs 6A and B: Pre-and post-operatory findings of strabismus surgery for esotropia in Möbius sequence patient. (A) Pre-op ET 50 PD HT D/E 10 PD; (B) Post-op XT 6 PD

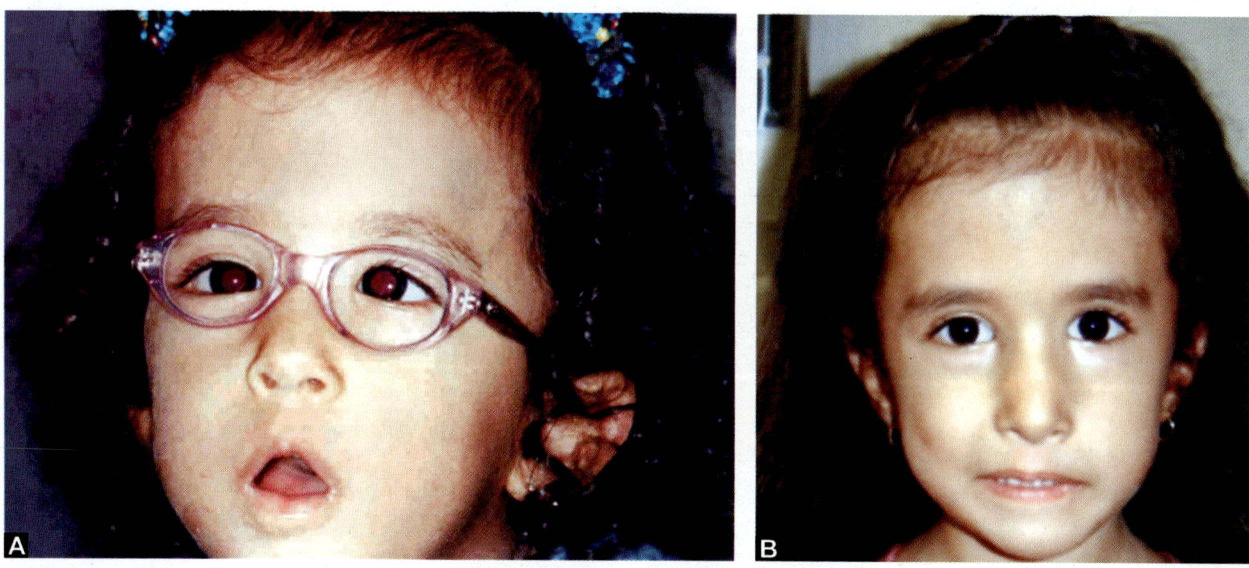

Figs 7A and B: Pre- and post-operatory findings of strabismus surgery for esotropia associated with left hypertropia in Möbius sequence patient. (A) Pre-op ET 50 PD HT E/D 4 PD. (B) Post-op ET 10 PD

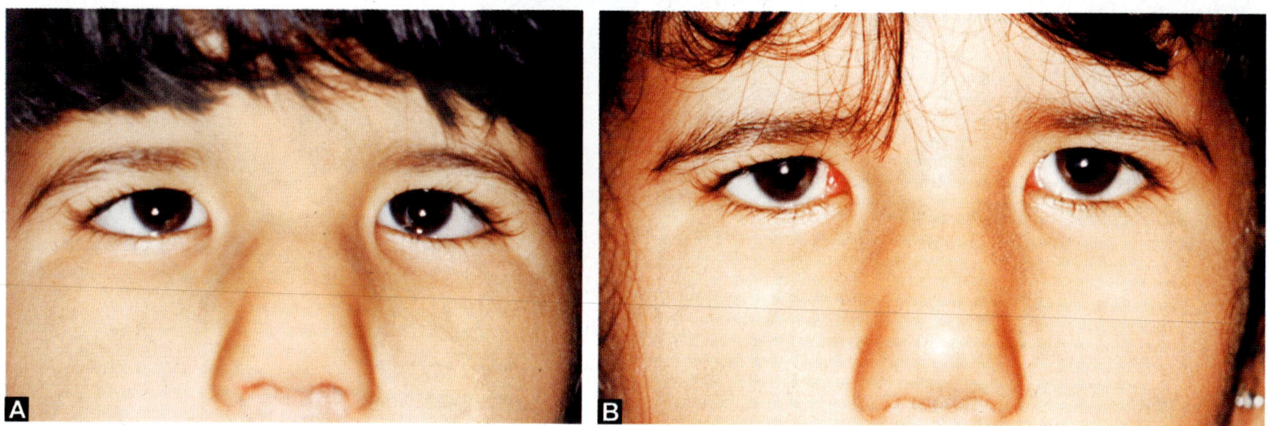

Figs 8A and B: Pre- and post-operatory findings of strabismus surgery for esotropia associated with right hypertropia in Möbius sequence patient. (A) Pre-op ET 50 PD (B) Post-op ET 5 PD

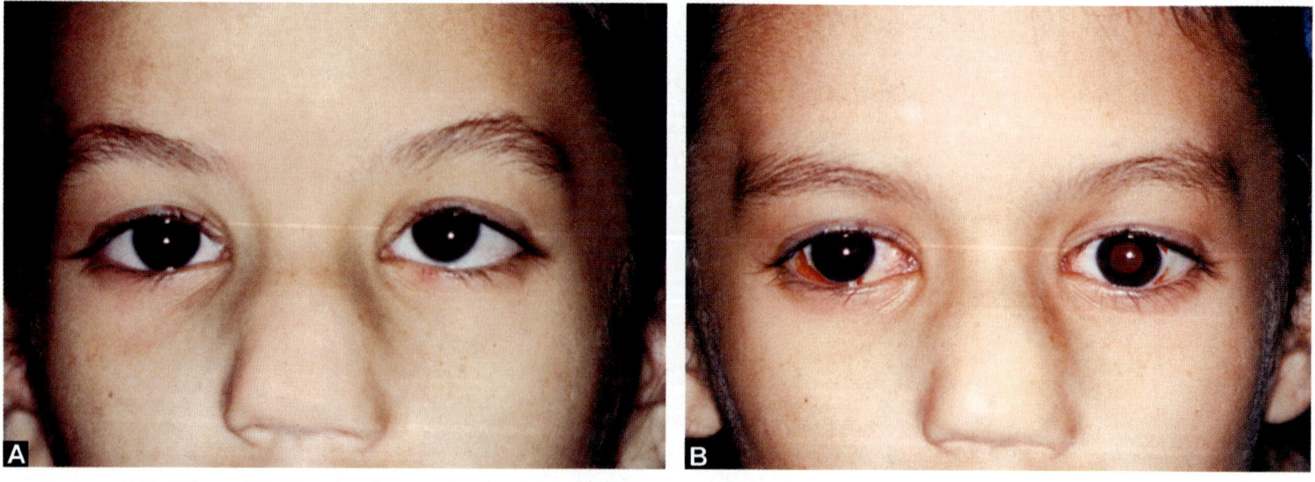

Figs 9A and B: Consecutive exotropia secondary to esotropia surgery, associated with hypotropia of left eye

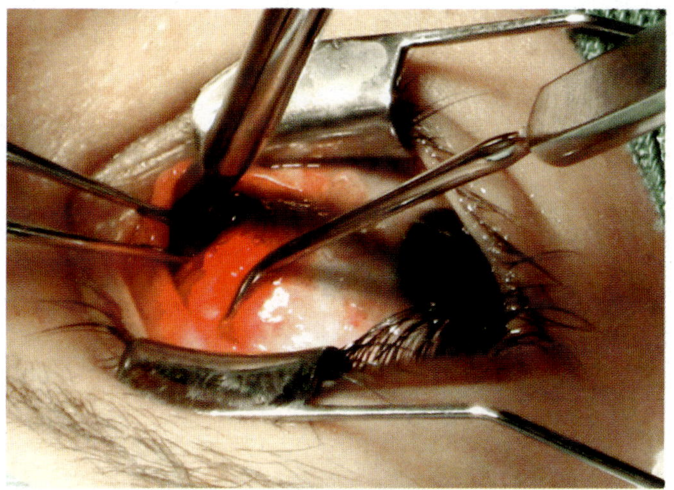
Fig. 10: Muscle isolation and hook exposition

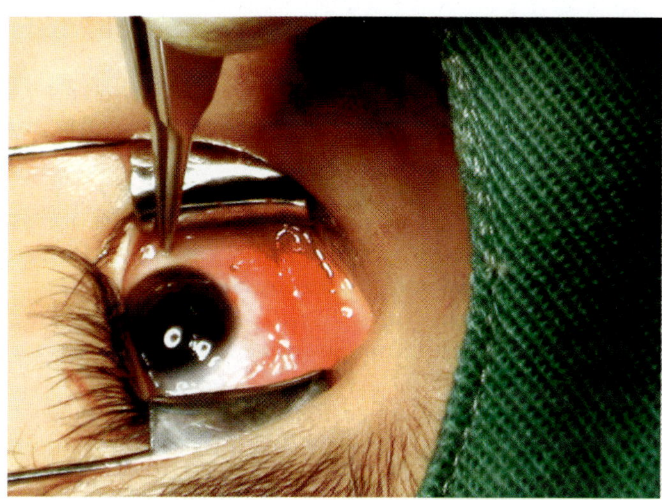
Fig. 13: Conjunctival suture with Vycril 7-0

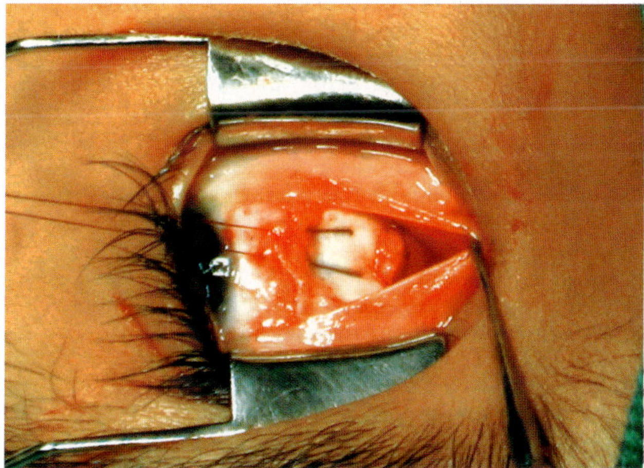
Fig. 11: Muscle suture, scleral insertion and anchor security suture on incision

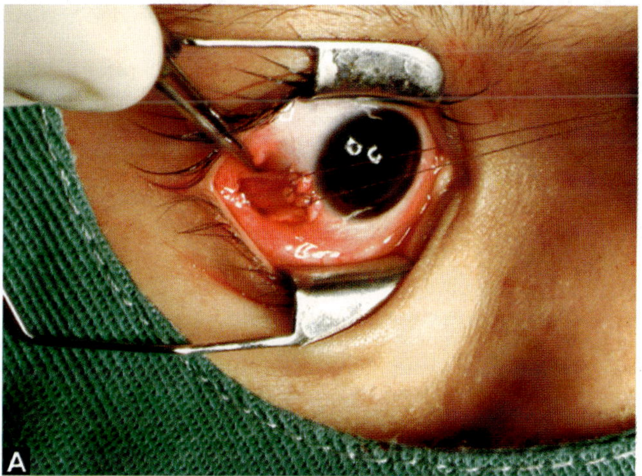

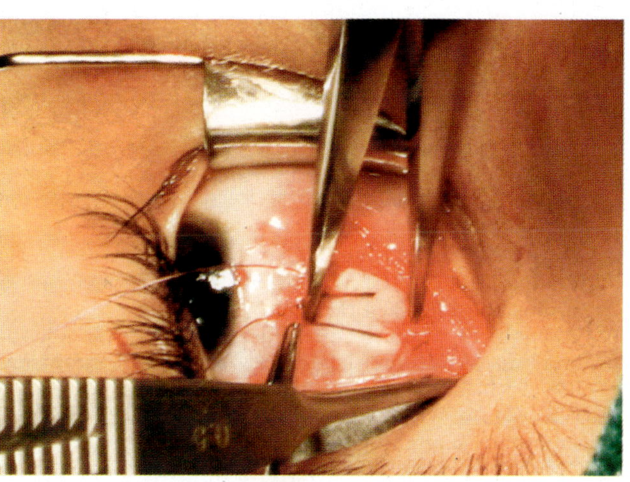
Fig. 12: Medial rectus recession measuring

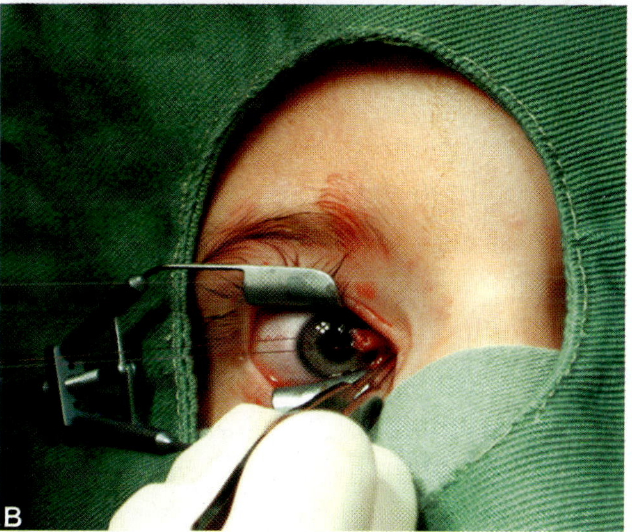
Figs 14 A and B: Lateral and medial rectus contracture. Queré test

patients with small angle esotropia, which might disappear spontaneously and gradually.[9,32]

It is not expected to gain abduction with medial rectus recession, but the goal is to correct the deviation in primary position. If any abduction occurs, it implies that the lateral recti were not dead muscles.

Some authors advocate vertical recti muscles transposition to the lateral recti (LR) insertions, followed by graded MR weakening (either by recessing the muscles or injecting botulinum toxin for any remaining esodeviation). This technique enhances the abduction of the eye in some cases.[31]

In these patients, when there is one dominant eye, occlusion of this eye should be performed until 10 years of age.

REFERENCES

1. Von Graefe A, Seamisch T. In: Handbuch der gesamtem Augenheikunde, Leipig: 1880;v.6.
2. Harlan GC. Congenital paralysis of both abducens and both facial nerves. Trans Am Ophthalmol Soc. 1880;3:216-8.
3. Chisolm JJ. Congenital paralysis of the sixth and the seventh pairs of cranial nerves in an adult. Arch Ophthalmol. 1881;11:323-5.
4. Möbius PJ. Üeber angeborene doppelseitige Abducens-Facialis-Lähmung. Munch Med Wochenschr. 1888;35(6):91-108.
5. Verzijl HT, van der Zwaag B, Cruysberg JR, Padberg GW. Möbius syndrome redefined: A syndrome of rhombencephalic maldevelopment. Neurology. 2003;61(3):327-33.
6. Briegel W. Neuropsychiatric findings of Möbius sequence: A review. Clin Genet. 2006;70(2):91-7.
7. Bavinck JN, Weaver DD. Subclavian artery supply disruption sequence: Hypothesis of a vascular etiology for Poland, Klippel-Feil, and Möbius anomalies. Am J Med Genet. 1986;23(4):903-18.
8. D'Cruz OF, Swisher CN, Jaradeh S, Tang T, Konkol RJ. Möbius syndrome: Evidence for a vascular etiology. J Child Neurol. 1993;8(3):260-5.
9. Miller MT, Strömland K. The Möbius sequence: a relook. J AAPOS. 1999;3(4):199-208.
10. Strömland K, Sjögreen L, Miller M, Gillberg C, Wentz E, Johansson M, et al. Mobius sequence: a Swedish multidiscipline study. Eur J Paediatr Neurol 2002;6(1):35-45.
11. McKusick VA. Mendelian inheritance in man. Catalog of autosomal dominant, autosomal recessive and X-linked disorders. 8. ed. Baltimore: Johns Hopkins University Press; 1988.
12. Baraitser M. Genetics of Möbius syndrome. J Med Genet. 1977;14(6):415-7.
13. Strömland K, Miller MT. Thalidomide embryopathy: Revisited 27 years later. Acta Ophthalmol (Copenh). 1993;71(2):238-45.
14. Courtens W, Vamos E, Hainaut M, Vergauwen P. Moebius syndrome in an infant exposed in utero to benzodiazepines. J Pediatr. 1992;121(5 Pt 1):833-4.
15. Kankirawatana P, Tennison MB, D'Cruz O, Greenwood RS. Möbius syndrome in infant exposed to cocaine in utero. Pediatr Neurol 1993;9(1):71-2.
16. Lipson AH, Webster WS, Brown-Woodman PD, Osborn RA. Moebius syndrome: animal model-human correlations and evidence for a brainstem vascular etiology. Teratology. 1989;40(4):339-50.
17. Pastuszak AL, Schüler L, Speck-Martins CE, Coelho KE, Cordello SM, Vargas F, et al. Use of misoprostol during pregnancy and Möbius' syndrome in infants. N Engl J Med 1998;338(26):1881-5.
18. Gonzalez CH, Marques-Dias MJ, Kim CA, Sugayama SM, Da Paz JA, Huson SM, et al. Congenital abnormalities in Brazilian children associated with misoprostol misuse in first trimester of pregnancy. Lancet 1998;351(9116):1624-7.
19. Boudoux DD, Matos AG, Gonçalves ED, Rocha M, Ventura LO, Hinrichesen SL. Síndrome de Moebius relacionada à ameaça de abortamento. Rev Bras Oftalmol 2000;59(3):173-7.
20. Ventura LO. Seqüência de Möbius: estudo comparativo das anomalias e distúrbios funcionais em crianças com ou sem uso de misoprostol durante e gestação [Tese]. Belo Horizonte: Universidade Federal de Minas Gerais; 2001.
21. Amaya LG, Walker J, Taylor D. Mobius syndrome: A study and report of 18 cases. Binoc Vis Quarterly 1995;5:119-32.
22. Santos LP, Ventura LO, Almeida HC, Miller M, Colier AC. Achados oftalmológicos em 28 crianças portadoras da seqüência de Mõebius. Arq Bras Oftalmol. 2004;67(4):591-5.
23. Henderson JL. The congenital facial diplegia syndrome: Clinical features, pathology and aetiology. A review of sixty-one cases. Brain 1939;62:381-403.
24. Souza-Dias CR, Goldchmit M. Further considerations about the ophthalmic features of the Möbius sequence, with data of 28 cases. Arq Bras Oftalmol. 2007;70(3):451-7.
25. Kumar, D. Möbius syndrome. J. Med. Genet Feb. 1990;27(2): 122-6.
26. Miller MT, Strömland K, Ventura L. Congenital Aberrant Tearing: A Re-Look. Trans Am Ophthalmol Soc. 2008;106: 100-06.
27. Bandim JM, Ventura LO, Miller MT, Almeida HC, Costa AE. Autism and Möbius sequence: An exploratory study of children in northeastern Brazil. Arq Neuropsiquiatr. 2003;61(2A):181-5.
28. Johansson M, Wentz E, Fernell E, Strömland K, Miller MT, Gillberg C. Autistic spectrum disorders in Möbius sequence: A comprehensive study of 25 individuals. Dev Med Child Neurol. 2001;43(5):338-45.
29. Simon JW, Buckley EG, Drack AV, Hutchinson AK, Plager DA, Raab EL, et al (Editors): In: American Academy of Ophthalmology. Pediatric ophthalmology and strabismus. Basic and clinical science course 2005-2006. San Francisco: American Academy of Ophthalmology 2005;6:137-49.
30. Almeida HC, Ventura LMVO, Miller MT, Rego PRPS, Travassos SB. Seqüência de Möbius. Projeto Diretrizes Centro Brasileiro de Estrabismo 2007. [CD-ROM]. Centro Brasileiro de Estrabismo. Gestão 2005-2007.
31. Laby DM. Möbius syndrome. In: Rosenbaum AL. Santiago AP. Clinical strabismus management: principles and surgical techiques. Philadelphia: W. B. Saunders Company; 1999. p.358-62.
32. Miller MT, Ray V, Owens P, Chen F. Möbius and Möbius-like syndromes (TTV-OFM, OMLH). J Pediatr Ophthalmol Strabismus 1989;26(4):176-88.
33. Traboulsi EI, Maumenee IH. Extraocular muscle aplasia in Moebius syndrome. J Pediatr Ophthalmol Strabismus. 1986;23(3):120-2.
34. Waterhouse WJ, Enzenauer RW, Martyak AP. Successful strabismus surgery in a child with Moebius syndrome. Ann Ophthalmol 1993;25(8):292-4.
35. Ventura LO, Cruz CB, Almeida HC, Millar M, Lira AFC, Antunes DL. Seqüência de Möbius: resultados a longo prazo, da correção cirúrgica do estrabismo. Arq Bras Oftalmol 2007;70(2):195-9.

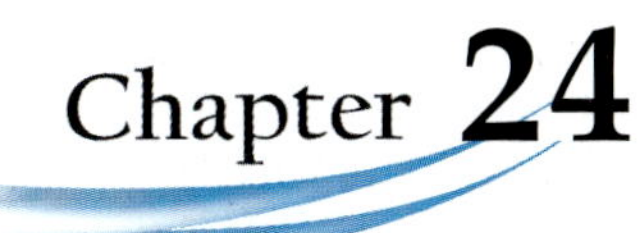

New Methods for the Analysis of Ocular Motility: 3D Video Oculography

Carlos Laria, Jorge L Alio (Spain)

For many centuries the study of ocular movements has been analyzed using different techniques and mathematical formulas, many of which are based on clinical analyses or theoretical studies. Currently a new system known as 3D video-oculography has been made available to analyze ocular motility. However, in order to understand the basis and possibilities of this equipment, we must first study the anatomophysiological bases of ocular motility.

ANATOMOPHYSIOLOGICAL BASES

Extraocular Muscles

There are six muscles responsible for ocular movement.[1-3] medial rectus, lateral rectus, superior rectus, inferior rectus, superior oblique and inferior oblique.

The four rectus muscles and the superior oblique originate at the vertex of the orbit, whereas the inferior oblique starts at the inferomedial part of the orbit. The four rectus muscles originate at a common tendon, the annulus of Zinn (Johann Gottfried Zinn, German anatomist, 1727-1759), which is inserted in the orbital vertex bones. From its insertion into the vertex of the orbit, all four rectus muscles move forward until they reach the ocular globe, defining a space known as the muscular cone, inside of which there are the optic nerve, ophthalmic artery, vessels and oculomotor nerves, oculomotor and sympathetic nerves, cilliary ganglion and all those covered in the orbital fat.

- The *medial rectus muscle* (Fig. 1) is 39 mm in length and extends over the medial wall of the orbit, being vertically inserted into the horizontal meridian of the eye, approximately 4.5 mm from the sclerocorneal limbus, establishing what is known as a contact arch with the sclera between 6 to 7 mm. It is innervated by the III cranial pair. Its contraction produces an inward rotation (adduction) horizontally.
- The *lateral rectus muscle* (Fig. 1) is 41 mm in length and extends in parallel to the lateral wall of the orbit being inserted at approximately 6 mm from the limbus, establishing a contact arch between 7 to 8 mm. Its innervation is by the VI pair and its contraction produces the outwards rotation (abduction) of the eye horizontally.
- The *superior rectus muscle* (Fig. 1) is 41 mm in length. It extends from the vertex forwards, laterally and slightly upwards, following the orbital axis and when the gaze is directed forwards, it forms an axis of approximately 23° with the eye. It is diagonally inserted by a tendon so that its middle part is inserted at approximately 7 mm and its lateral part at 9 mm from the sclerocorneal limbus. It runs below the elevator of the upper eyelid, being inserted above the superior oblique muscle. Innervated by the III pair, its contraction produces several combinations of vertical, horizontal and rotatory movements depending on the angle of the gaze. Since the muscle advances at an angle of 23° with respect to the internal wall of the orbit and is inserted in front of the center of the eye rotation, the movement produced by its contraction would be pure elevation if the eyes were in a horizontal abduction position of 23°. If in adduction the eye is at a position of 67°, its only movement when contracting will be that corresponding to incycloduction of the globe. With the eye in primary position of looking straight ahead, the contraction of the muscle produces elevation and incycloduction combined with slight adduction.
- The *inferior rectus muscle* (Fig. 1) is 40 mm in length, extending forward, downwards and laterally, forming an axis of 23° with the anteroposterior axis. It is diagonally inserted into the sclera so that its medial extreme is 6.3 mm from the limbus and its lateral extreme is 8.4 mm, establishing a contact arch with the ocular globe of 7 mm. It advances along the orbital floor being

separated by the orbital fat, the inferior oblique muscle (which crosses it transversally) and the Lockwood ligament. Its innervation is by the III pair and its contraction equally produces several combinations depending on the horizontal position of the eye. With the eye in a position of 23° of abduction, the only movement is depression. If the eye is in adduction at a position of 67°, the only movement is excycloduction, since the muscle is inserted in front of the point of rotation of the globe. When the eye is in primary position, the contraction of the inferior rectus produces depression and excycloduction with minimum adduction.

- The *superior oblique muscle* (Fig. 1) is the longest muscle, made up of two portions, one direct and one reflex. The direct portion goes from the vertex of the orbit to the superomedial angle of the orbit (trochlea), over the medial rectus. On leaving the trochlea, the reflex portion begins, changing direction and then the tendon is extended laterally backwards and downwards, forming a 54° angle with the direct portion thereby reaching the middle edge of the superior rectus and opening out as a fan. It is inserted underneath this one into the posterosuperolateral part of the eye, with a large variability in its insertion.[4,5] The innervation of this muscle is carried out by the IV pair. The contraction produces various combinations of vertical, horizontal and rotatory movements. With an initial abduction position of 39°, the only movement is incycloduction. With an initial adduction position of 51°, the only movement is infraduction. With the eye in primary position looking straight ahead, the movement combines a downwards rotation and incycloduction with minimal abduction. This last movement is due to the insertion of the muscle behind the center of ocular rotation when the eye is in primary position.
- The *inferior oblique muscle* (Fig. 1) is the only muscle which is inserted outside the annulus of Zinn, in the inferomedial angle of the anterior part of the orbit. It is 38 mm in length and it extends laterally, behind and above, between the inferior rectus and the floor of the orbit. After crossing the inferior rectus perpendicularly, it forms an extensive arch of contact until reaching the inferior edge of the lateral rectus. The inferior oblique muscle forms an angle of 75° with the axis of the orbit and of 50° with the anteroposterior axis of the eye. It is innervated by the III cranial pair and its contraction produces an equal combination of movements according to its position. Therefore, starting from a position of 39° of abduction, the only movement is excycloduction. From a starting position of 51° of adduction, the only movement is elevation. The contraction of the muscle with the eye in primary position produces excycloduction and elevation with minimal abduction, as a consequence of the insertion being behind the center of rotation when the eye is in primary position.

The Spiral of Tillaux

The spiral of Tillaux (Fig. 2) is an imaginary line that connects the insertions of the four tendons of the rectus muscles to the corneal limbus. As we have already been explaining on analysing the insertion of each muscle, as from the medial rectus and in a clockwise direction, the insertions move further away from the limbus.[6]

Ocular Movements

The movements of the ocular globe are carried out according to the so-called three axes of Fick, which cross over at a point known as the center of rotation of the ocular globe. These axes are:

- *Vertical axis (z) – Crosses the equator of the ocular globe (from top to bottom)*, and originates the horizontal movements.
- *Anteroposterior axis (y)* – Passes through the center of the pupil (from the front to the back) and originates the torsional movements.
- *Transversal axis (x)* – Passes at the height of the equator and originates the movements of elevation and descent.

The combination of this ocular dynamics over the different axes confirms the different positions of the gaze that we can resume as:

- *Primary position:* Looking forward with the head straight.
- *Secondary positions:* Looking up, down, to the right and to the left.
- *Cardinal positions:* There are six: (A) up and right; (B) sideways to the right; (C) down and to the right; (D) up and to the left; (E) sideways and to the left, and (F) down and to the left. In each of these positions the action of the muscle and of its contralateral synergist is assessed.

Individual Action of the Ocular Musculature

In the clinical practice the cardinal positions to study the action of the different muscles must be distinguished; as with the physiological actions of such muscles which are variable according to the position of the globe, as mentioned earlier, but we believe it necessary to clarify such muscular actions in a unified way.[7]

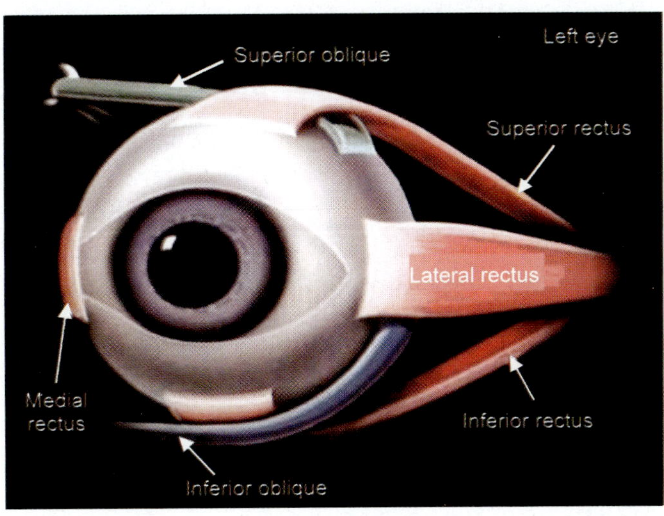

Fig. 1: Left eye

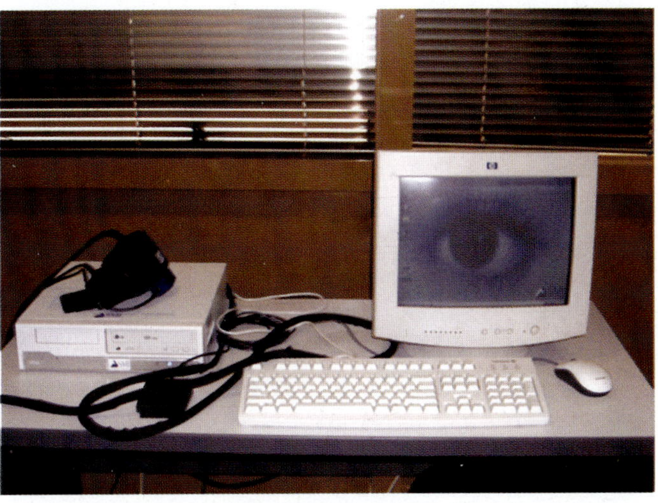

Fig. 4: VOG system

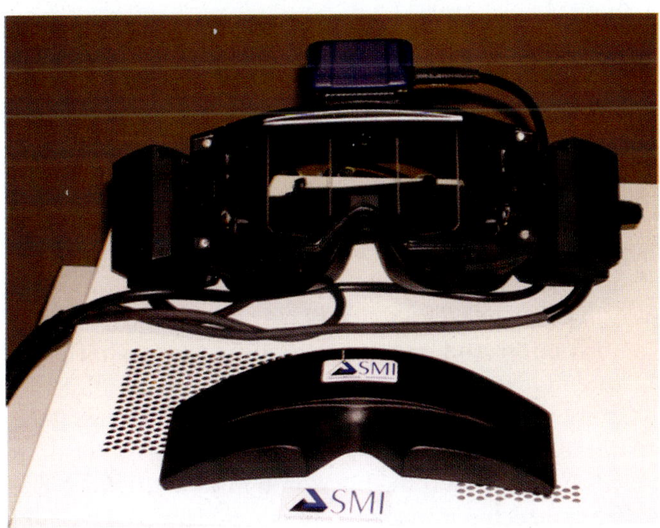

Fig. 5: VOG system

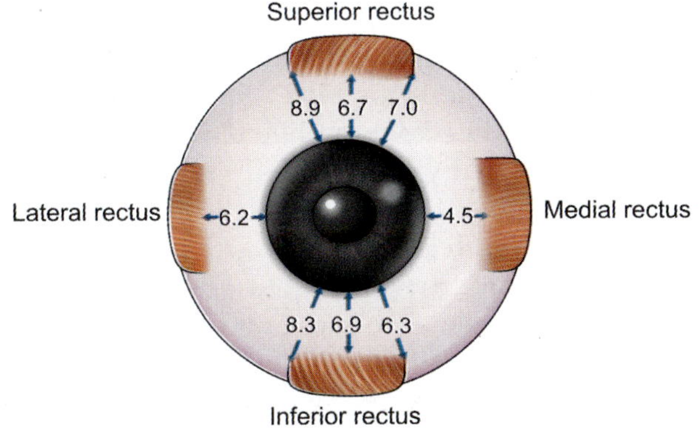

Fig. 2: Spiral of Tillaux

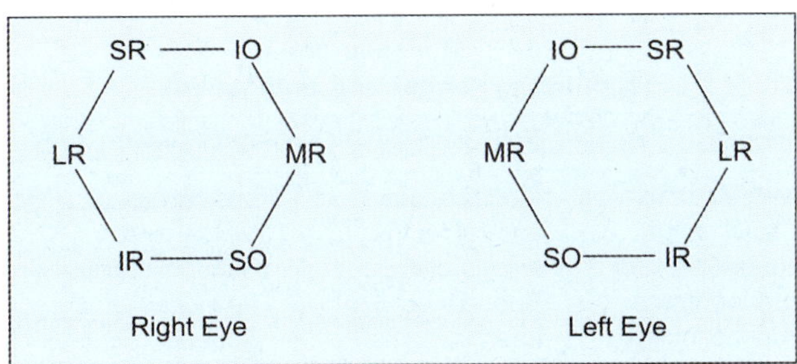

Fig. 3: Diagram of Pascal: Diagnostic positions of the gaze in both eyes

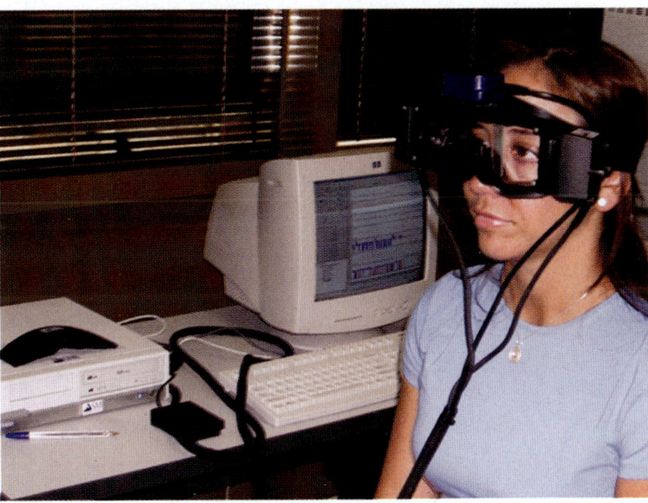

Fig. 6: VOG system

Therefore, in the primary position, the actions of the different muscles are shown in Table 1.

Table 1: Actions of the muscles in the primary position

Muscle	*Primary action*	*Secondary action*	*Third action*
Lateral rectus	Abduction		
Medial rectus	Adduction		
Superior rectus	Elevation	Intorsion	Adduction
Inferior rectus	Depression	Extorsion	Adduction
Superior oblique	Intorsion	Depression	Abduction
Inferior oblique	Extorsion	Elevation	Abduction

However, if we vary the position of the gaze, the action of the different muscles also varies, in this way:

- *Superior rectus:* In a 23 ° abduction, the action is pure elevation, whilst in adduction the elevating force diminishes and it reaches its maximum in intorsion and adduction.
- *Inferior rectus:* The same as with the superior rectus, its vertical action (depressive) reaches its maximum in abduction, while the extorsion and adduction actions are greater in adduction.
- *Superior oblique:* The muscle is purely depressive in adduction, whilst this action is minimal in abduction and intorsion and abduction are maximal.
- *Inferior oblique:* The action of elevation is maximum in adduction and minimal in abduction, where the extorsion action is greater.

In short, according to the diagram of Pascal[8] (Fig. 3) the vertical rectus are evaluated in abduction; the Superior in supra-abduction and the Inferior in infra-abduction. The horizontal rectus muscles are evaluated in a horizontal gaze; the medial in adduction and the Lateral in abduction. The oblique muscles are evaluated in adduction; the Superior in infra-adduction and the Inferior in supra-adduction.

The diagnostic position in the vertical action muscles (vertical and oblique rectus), does not coincide with the muscle action (for example, the oblique ones are abductors, but they are studied in adduction).

Homolateral Synergists and Antagonists

A primary motor muscle exists in each movement, fundamentally controlling such an action together with the so-called homo-lateral synergists which collaborate in these movements with secondary and tertiary actions. The homo-lateral antagonists are opposed to such action.[7] (Table 2).

Table 2: Muscular actions

Agonist	*Action*	*Synergists*	*Antagonists*
Lateral rectus	Abductor	Oblique	Medial rectus Vertical rectus
Medial rectus	Adductor	Vertical rectus	Lateral rectus Oblique
Superior rectus	Elevator	Inferior oblique	Inferior rectus Superior oblique
Inferior rectus	Depressor	Superior oblique	Superior rectus Inferior oblique
Superior oblique	Depressor	Inferior rectus	Inferior oblique Superior rectus
Inferior oblique	Elevator	Superior rectus	Superior oblique Inferior oblique

Classification of Ocular Movements

Ocular movements can be divided into monocular movements and binocular movements:[7,9]

- *Ductions:* Ductions refer to the movements of each eye separately without taking into account what is happening in the other eye. They are monocular movements on three axes: abduction, adduction, intorsion and extorsion.
- *Versions:* These are movements of both eyes while maintaining them in parallel. They are conjugated movements of the eyes in the different positions of gaze. The muscles that take part in a version are called: Agonists (primary agent muscle of movement), Antagonists (muscle of contrary action in the same or opposite eye), and Synergists (muscles that collaborate in the same movement). The contralateral synergist is also known as the yolk muscle. A primary motor muscle exists in each movement, fundamentally in charge of such an action and the so-called homo-lateral synergists that collaborate in such a movement with secondary and tertiary actions contrary to such an action are the homo-lateral antagonists. This can be seen in Table 3.

Table 3: Muscular actions (agonist, synergist and antagonist)

Agonist	*Synergist (yolk)*	*Antagonist*
Lateral rectus	Medial rectus	Lateral rectus
Medial rectus	Lateral rectus	Medial rectus
Superior rectus	Inferior oblique	Superior oblique
Inferior rectus	Superior oblique	Inferior oblique
Superior oblique	Inferior rectus	Superior rectus
Inferior oblique	Superior rectus	Inferior rectus

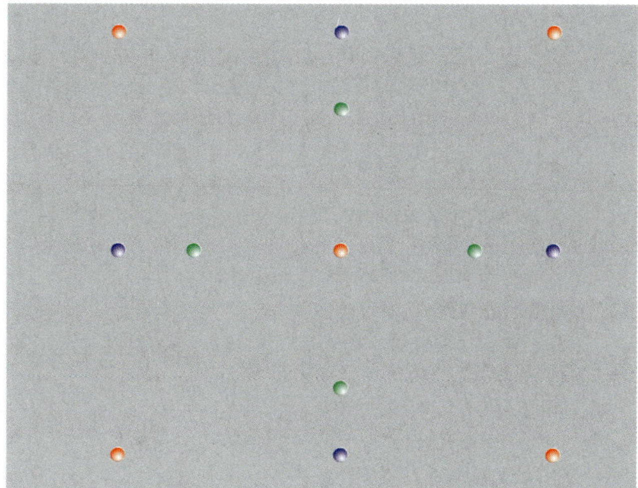

Fig. 7: Target point for calibration

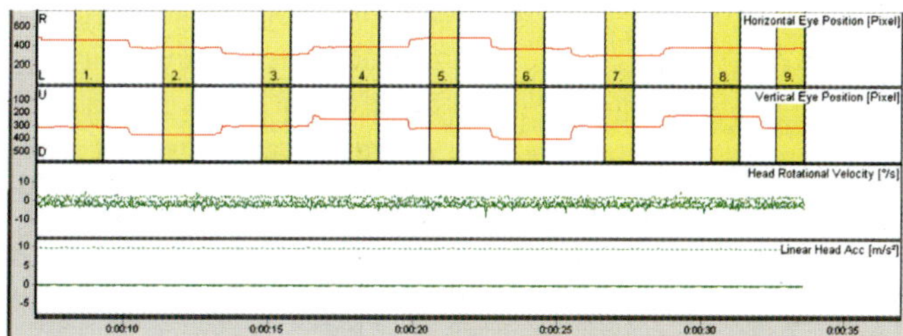

Fig. 8: Standard pattern which will be used as a reference for the ocular deviations

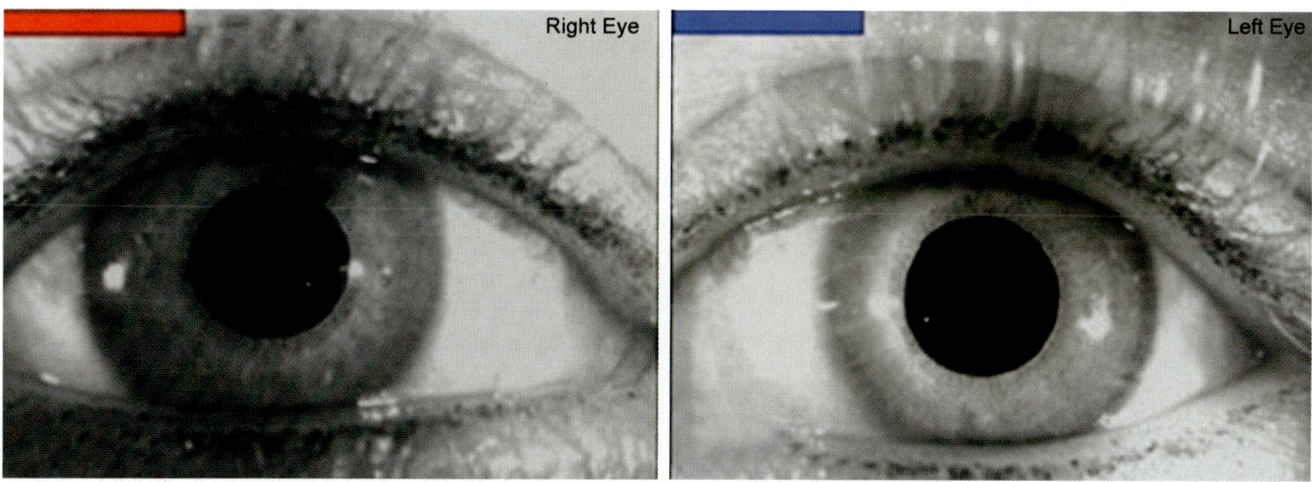

Fig. 9: Reference pattern of the iris of each eye

- *Vergences:* These are a disjunctive binocular movement, that is to say in the same direction but the opposite way around, on the vertical axes. They are slow movements. Their aim is to allow sensory fusion: making the relative position of the eyes suitable in order to allow images of objects situated at different distances from the individual to be captured in the corresponding areas of the retina (for example the two maculae). They are:
  - Convergence: Nasal deviation (adduction) of both eyes. Obeys 5 stimulations: 1. accommodation, 2. fusion, 3. innervational tone, 4. near reflection and 5. Willingness. It is related to near vision fixation and downward gaze.
  - Divergence: Eyes are deviated to temporal direction (abduction). This takes place in distance vision fixation. It is synergic with distance gaze and its elevation.

Ocular Motility Laws

The action and therefore the dynamics of ocular muscle contraction are guided by two laws:[1,7]

1. *Sherrington's law (Charles Scott Sherrington, English physiologist, 1857-1952) or the reciprocal innervation*[10] - When one eye moves in a certain direction, the agonists contract while the antagonists relax in the same proportion. When a muscle receives a contraction impulse, its homo-lateral antagonist receives an impulse of equal intensity, but in reverse (relaxation). If this did not occur, instead of a rotation, there would be a retraction as occurs in the retraction of Duane's syndrome.
2. *Hering's law (Heinrich Ewald Hering, German physiologist, (1866-1948) or law of motor correspondence or of innervation equality.* The nervous influxes sent by the oculomotor centers to the ocular muscles in order to carry out movement in a certain direction are symmetrical for both eyes. The motor central impulses are distributed equally between the yolk muscles of both eyes, their intensity being determined by the fixing eye; therefore the secondary deviation (fixation with the pathetic eye) is always greater than the primary deviation (fixation with the healthy eye).

EXPLORATORY TECHNIQUES: 3D VIDEO-OCULOGRAPHY (VOG-3D) SENSOMOTORIC INSTRUMENT®

Over the years different techniques have been developed searching for the register of ocular movements[11] in the horizontal and vertical axes, such as Electro-oculography and other photo-electric techniques, but which have been limited in their accuracy (around 2° in EOG and 0.25° in photo-electric techniques) and sometimes by the axes of measurement. The development of the photographic image as a technique for registering ocular movement has signified an important scientific advance.

The beginning of registering systems using small high resolution cameras for registering ocular motility began with horizontal and vertical movements (2D),[12] with an accuracy of between 0.1 and 0.5°.

But the most important development in the last years has been of techniques that allow the register of ocular movements not only in horizontal and vertical displacements but that also take into account torsional movements,[13-17] that is to say, a 3D register. Initially, these techniques were semi-invasive carried out through systems of rings linked to contact lens, of which the cost and managing complexity made them practically inaccessible and limited their use.[18-22] Thus, the idea arose of using non-invasive video-oculography techniques that allowed a 3D register of ocular movement,[12,23-42] and therefore between 1989 and 1991 in the University of Berlin, prototypes were designed that later on in 1991 led to the Foundation of Sensomotoric Instrument, a company with the object of developing these techniques and achieving the design of a system called 3D-VOG (Figs 4 and 5) and which has continued with different versions up to the latest 5th version, on which we will base our analysis and which allows the following aspects to be registered:

- Non-invasive binocular online tracking of horizontal, vertical and torsional eye movements.
- 6D Head Motion Sensor for measurement of 3D rotational head velocity (°/s) and 3D linear acceleration (ms^2).
- Automatic nystagmus detection.
- Much improved torsional eye tracking algorithm featuring
  - Multiple iris segment tracking.
  - Automatic iris segment selection.
  - Automatic pupil threshold setting.
  - Automatic geometric distortion compensation.
  - Automatic video parameter settings.
- Comfortable to wear VOG mask offering.
  - Very high contrast eye images
  - Invisible IR Illumination (950 nm)
  - Stroboscope IR-illumination eliminating motion blur.
  - Magnetically attached cover allowing quick change between recordings under free-field-of-view and light-occluding conditions
  - Bite bar.

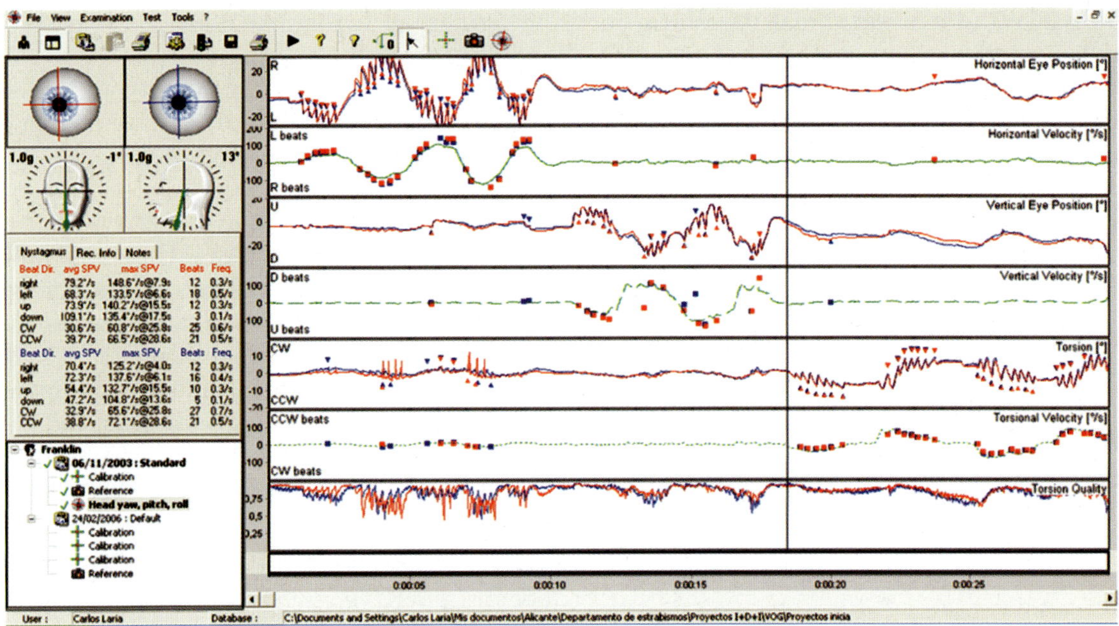

Fig. 10: Register of movements and nystagmus

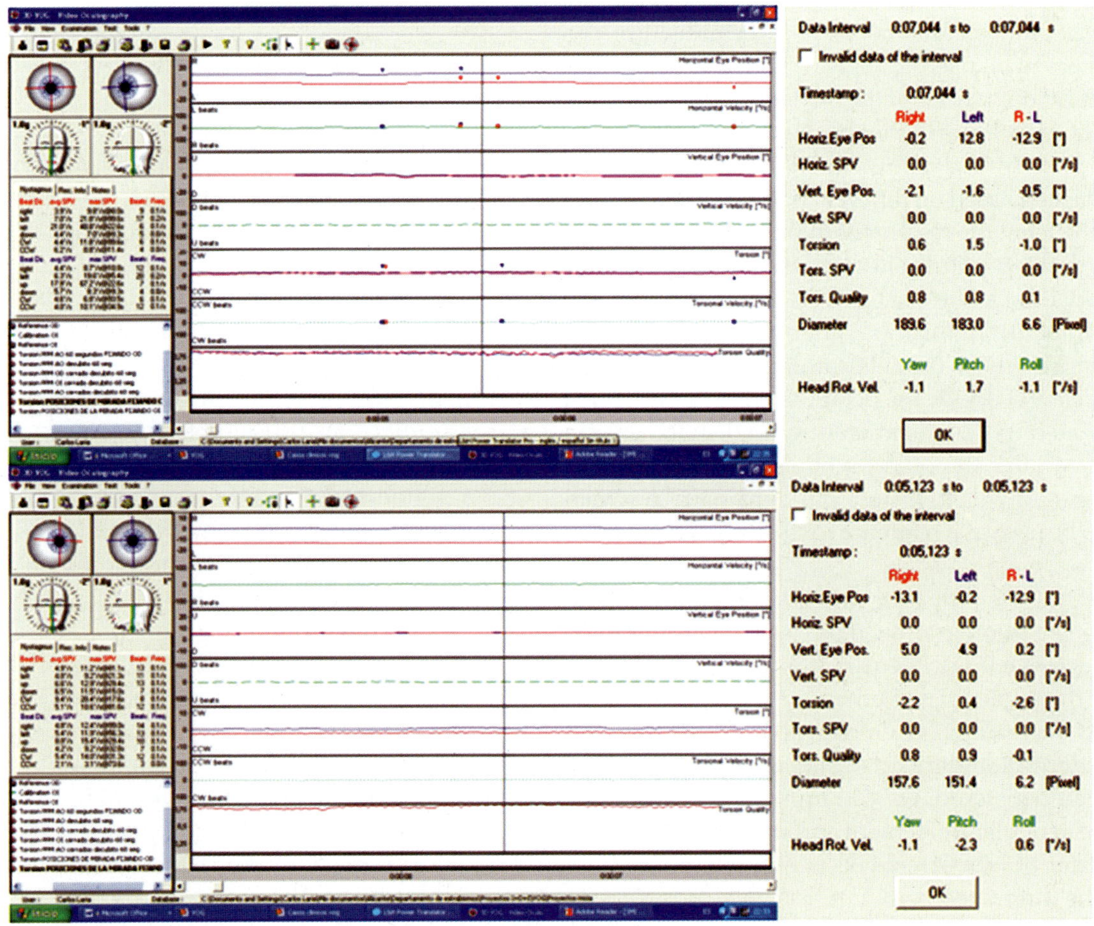

Fig. 11: Alternating esotropia

- Easy to use Windows graphical user-inter-face including.
  - Eye movement data presentation in head centered Listing or eye centred, Fick coordinate system.
  - Animated replay of eye and head movement data.
  - Examination template designer.
  - Subject database.
- Analog (8) and digital (8) auxiliary input channels (optional)

The registering technique of VOG-3D basically consists of the following steps:

- *Position of the 3D-VOG mask:* Attach the mask in front of the patient's eyes by using the rubber bands so as to allow a firm enough hold that will prevent the mask from slipping out of place with different movements or due to the law of gravity, since any slight movement of the mask could contradict the results of the registers (Fig. 6).
- *Centring of the figures:* The figures of both eyes are centered horizontally and vertically as well as the focusing of the iris monocularly.
- *System calibration:* This consists in establishing the parameters to be used to register both the horizontal and vertical deviations of the ocular movements. This system of register can either be done automatically by using a projector that allows the ocular movements to be established based on different patterns of images, or manually using the register of the eye positions joined to co-ordinated points situated at a certain distance (corresponding to the distance between the patient and the equipment). In this case, after having established the distance where the measurements will be taken and which will decide the position of the target points on the wall (Fig. 7), the patient should then look at the points one after the other, while such deviations in both eyes allow us to form a standard pattern which will later be used as a reference for the ocular deviations (Fig. 8).
- *Establishing the reference pattern:* This consists in registering a photographic figure of the pattern of the iris of each eye (Fig. 9), based on which we can later analyze the torsional movements.
- *Torsional studies (Fig. 10):* Once the parameters that can be considered standard according to ocular deviation have been registered, we can immediately carry out any type of ocular movement and dynamically obtain the register of movements occurring in both eyes, in any of the three axes.

A number of fundamental aspects must be considered while carrying out these tests:

- The mask must fit perfectly in order to avoid displacements and incorrect measurements.
- Avoid moving the head while carrying out the different tests.
- Do not take off the mask while carrying out the different tests nor re-adjust it without new calibrations.
- Remember that deviations are registered based on previous calibrations so that any factor that modifies the calibration will be erroneous.
- Carry out registers of calibration and of monocular form reference when dealing with strabismus.
- Keep the equipment clean as well as the prisms that are used to focus the Figure in the cameras.

TECHNICAL CHARACTERISTICS OF 3D-VOG

The technical characteristics of the equipment are as follows:

Measures and Resolution

- Temporal resolution: 50 Hz (PAL systems)/60 Hz (NTSC systems)
- Eye movement measurement
  - Measurement method: Optical, non-invasive using infrared video cameras (PAL/CCIR or NTSC/EIA)
  - Acquisition parameters: Horizontal (h), vertical (v), and torsional (t) eye rotation
  - Number of channels: Two (binocular)
  - Spatial resolution (h/v/t) 0.05° / 0.05° / 0.10°
  - Measurement range (h/v/t) ±25° / ±20° / ±18°
  - Measurement area for torsional ±20° Around the primary gaze position eye movement measurement
  - Torsion analysis method: Cross-correlation of iris segments
  - Iris segment selection: Automatic
  - Geometric compensation: Automatic
  - Calibration
    - Active 9 point
    - Fixation recognition: Automatic or manual
  - Torsion eye position coordinates: Fick or Listing
- Pupil measurements
  - Pupil detection method: Dark pupil
  - Pupil diameter determination: Automatic
- Head motion sensor (optional)
  - Number of dimensions: 6 (3 rotational + 3 translational)

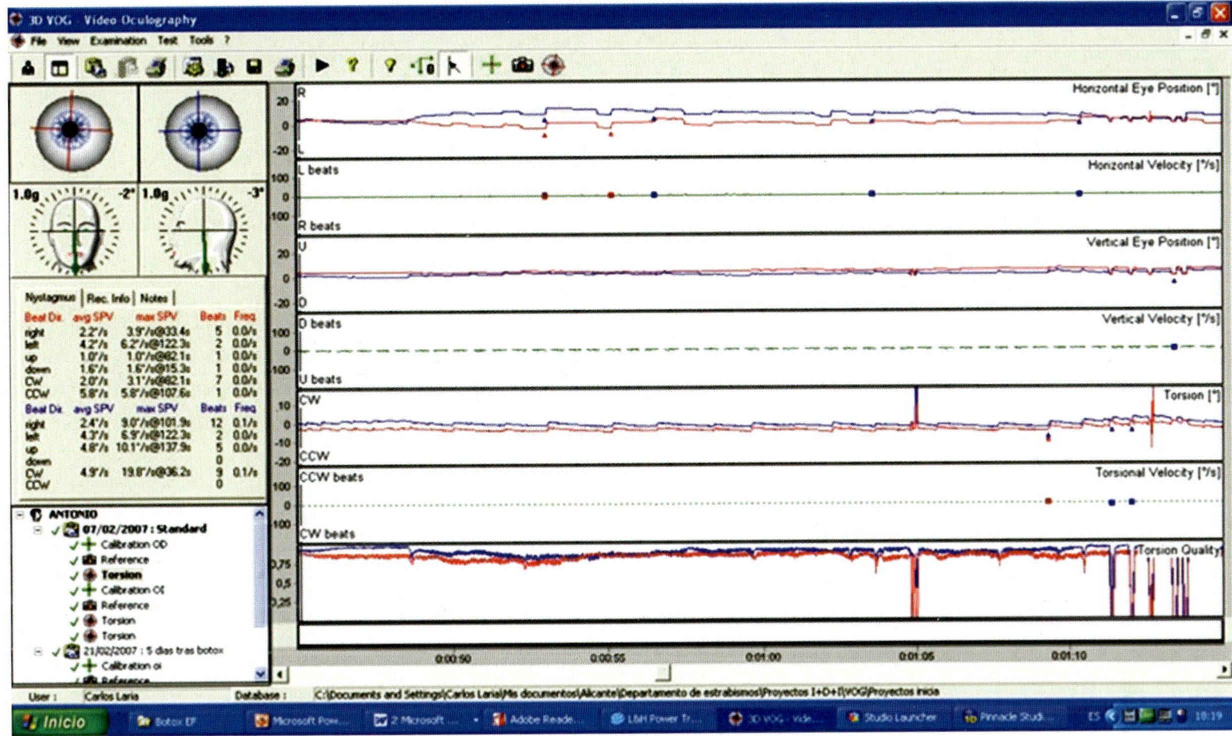

Fig. 12: Analysis of a phoria

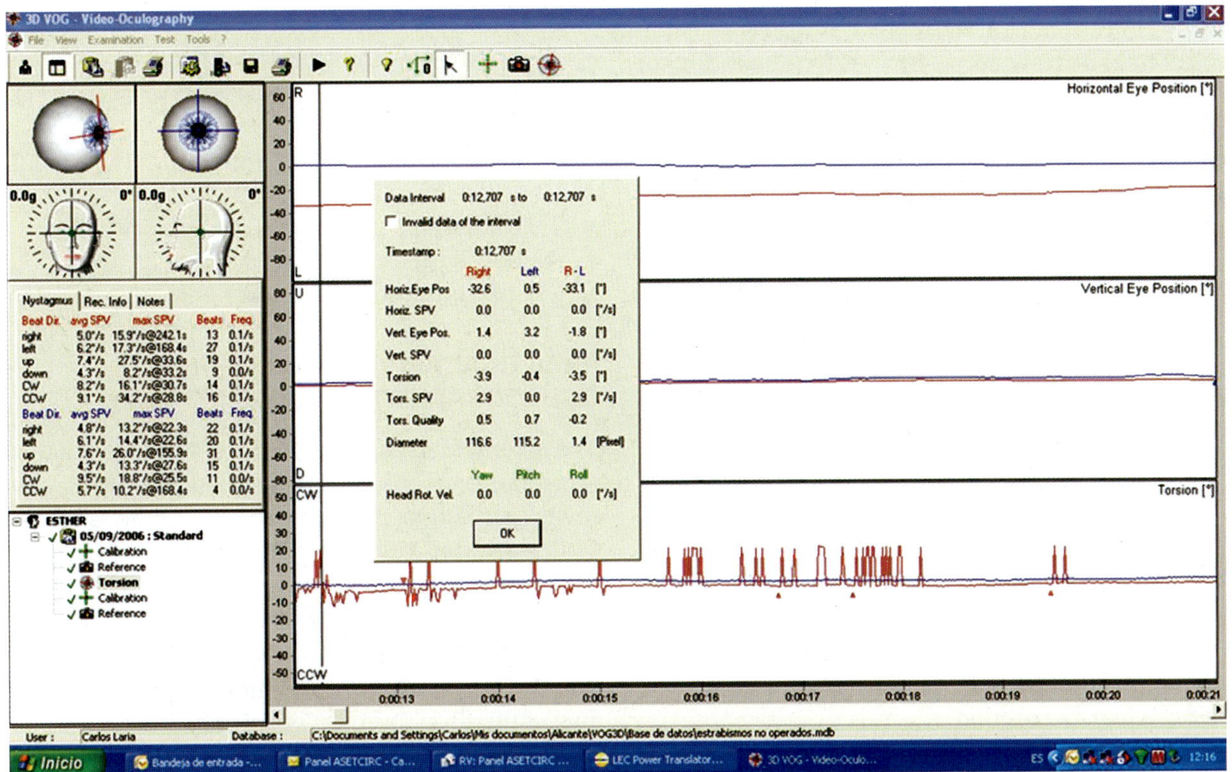

Fig. 13: Esotropia fixing the left eye

  - Measurements
    - Rotation Speed [°/s]
    - Translation Linear acceleration [m/s^2]
- Spatial resolution
    - Rotation app. 1 °/s
    - Translation app. 0.05 m/s^2
  - Measurement range
    - Rotation ± 900 °/s
    - Translation ± 20 m/s^2
  - Sensor position: Centred on top of VOG goggles
  - Weight app. 40 g
- Analog input channels (optional)
  - Number of channels 8
  - Resolution 12 bit
  - Voltage range ± 10 V
- Digital input channels (optional)
  - Number of channels 8
  - Signal type TTL

VOG Goggles

- Construction: Combination goggles for measurement in free-field of-view and light occluding conditions
- Cameras 2 (binocular)IR-CCD cameras PAL/CCIR or NTSC/EIA
- Wavelength of IR illumination 950 nm
- IR radiation strength at the eye < 1.35 mW
- Subject field of view app. ±40° / ±25° (depending on subject)
- Weight app. 400 g (+40 g when optional head motion sensor is added)
- Supply voltage 12 V
- Options:
  - Lens holder
  - Half covers for monocular coverage of subject's field of view.

Visual Stimulus (Visual LabTM)

- Stimulus generation Digital
- Resolution 640 x 480 pixels
- Projection Video projection on white wall
- Typical projection angle (h/v) app. ±25°/±20° gaze angle (depending on choice of projector and projection options)
  - Stimulus types Saccades/Calibration, smooth pursuit, optokinetic
  - Saccades/Calibration
    - Projection pattern Single point (customizable color and size) or bitmap (smiley face)
    - Adjustable parameters Positions, projection times, and projection breaks
  - Smooth pursuit
    - Projection pattern Single point (customizable color and size) or bitmap (smiley face)
    - Adjustable parameters Orientation (horizontal, vertical, diagonal), speed, linear/sinusoidal movement and amplitude
  - Optokinetic
    - Projection pattern Stripe pattern with customizable color and width, as well as bitmap
    - Adjustable parameters Orientation (horizontal, vertical), direction, and speed

Analysis

- Nystagmus analysis
  - Automatic detection and marking in the output data file (online)
  - Automatic calculation of slow phase velocity (online)
    Separate nystagmus pattern data display for horizontal, vertical, and torsional eye movements
- Squint angle between left and right eye channel

VOG Workstation

- Operating system: Windows 2000
- CPU Intel Pentium 4, 2.4 GHz (1)
- Memory 256 MB (1)
- Screen resolution 1024 x 768 pixels, 24 bit color (1)
- Interfaces 2 x COM, 1 x LPT, 1 x USB (1)
- Hard disk space 40 GB (1) and CD RW
- Network Ethernet 10/100 MBit/s
  (1) minimum configuration

PRACTICAL APPLICATION OF VIDEO-OCULOGRAPHY TO OCULAR MOTILITY

The use of video-oculography in analysing ocular motility is fundamental, given that the cycloducting analysis often reveals situations that are very difficult to analyse. Many studies exist revealing the advantages of video-oculography in different aspects of ocular motility. This demonstrates that such systems are clearly highly efficient and as an example of this, we can show a series of registers obtained from different patients with varying degrees of strabismus that could be analysed perfectly thanks to video-oculography, cases of diplopia, a stiff neck, dissociated strabismus, muscular paralysis, essential esotropia, etc.

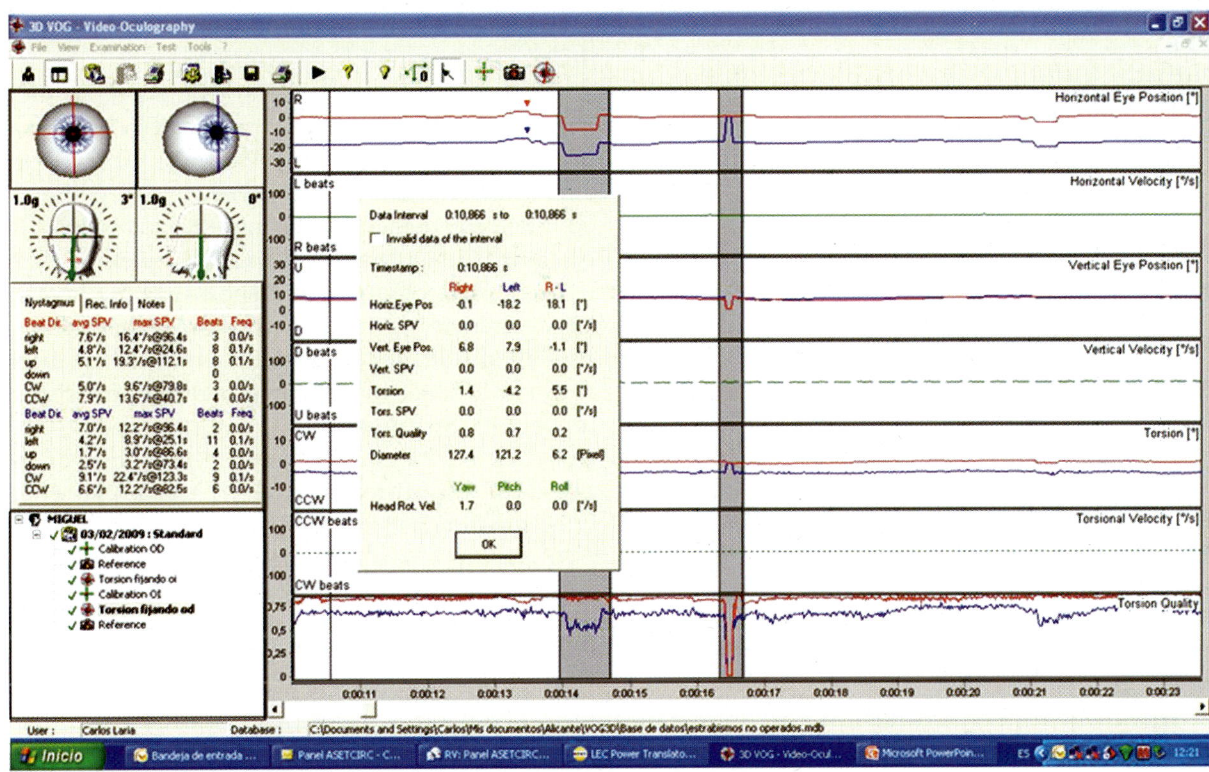

Fig. 14: Exotropia fixing right eye

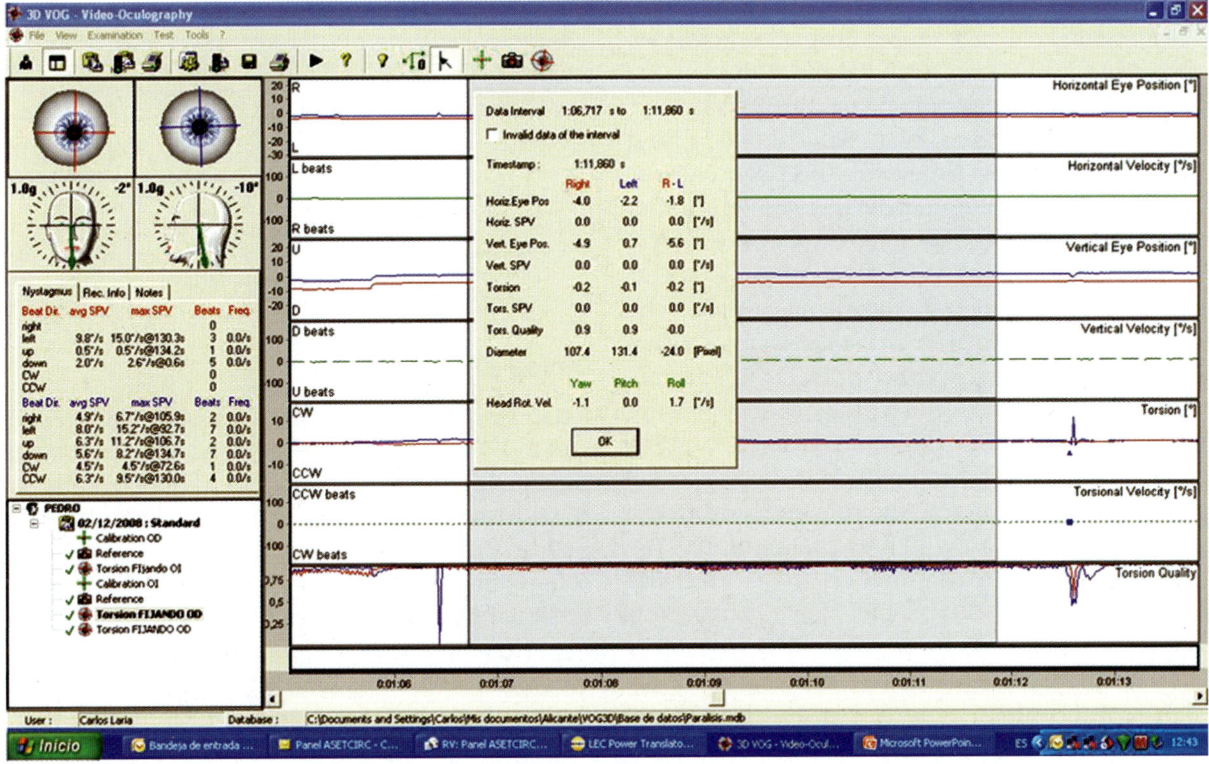

Fig. 15: Left hypertropia

Analysis of Different Types of Strabismus

- Alternating esotropia: The case is presented of an esotropia with an equal degree of deviation fixing the right eye (12.9°) compared to the left eye (12.9°), showing no evidence of secondary deviation and therefore showing no presence of muscular paralysis, but of an essential esotropia (Fig. 11).
- Dynamic analysis of a phoria (Fig. 12):
  We can see the typical dynamic movement of a phoria of the left eye with a deviation between 13° and 0° in primary position.
- Esotropia: Here we present the case of an esotropia of (33.1°) fixing the left eye without significant vertical deviation (Fig. 13).
- Exotropia. The next patient has an exotropia of 18,1° fixing the right eye, without vertical deviation in primary position (Fig. 14).
- Hypertropia. In this case we can observe a left hypertropia of 5.6° after cataract surgery with retrobulbar anesthesia (Fig. 15).

Analysis of Dissociated Strabismus; Dissociated Vertical Divergence (DVD)

- Asymetrical DVD
  Patient with asymmetrical DVD (Figs 16 and 17): The case is presented of congenital esotropia, associated to asymmetrical DVD, with 16° in RE and 4° in LE.
- Analysis of Bielschowsky Phenomenon in DVD.
  Even though Schweigger (1894)[43] Stevens (1895)[44] and Duane (1896) were the first to describe this phenomenon, Bielschowsky[45,46] made the first detailed description of this particular form of behavior of the oculomotor system and he called it Dissociated Vertical Divergence (DVD). Nevertheless, it was studied by numerous authors who gave it different denominations,[47] such as, alternating hyperphoria, alternating hypertropia,[45,48,-50] double hypertropia, occlusion hypertropia[50,51] alternating sursumduction,[52-55] hyperdeviation dissociated,[56] etc.

Among its clinical characteristics, it is distinguished by its permanent association to the congenital esotropia and latent nystagmus (LN) with a frequency of 92% (by authors), conforming in conjunction the Congenital Esotropia Syndrome.[57-63]

Inspite of being rare, it can be associated with other types of strabismus, such as sensorial strabismus.[64-67] Its main sign is intermitent hypertropia, but horizontal deviation (DHD) and/or torsional (DTD) could also be present. These deviations are called strabismus with a dissociated complex.[68]

Its principal characteristic is its slow elevation movement, of 2 to 40 degrees per second (%/sec). The DVDs movements do not follow Hering´s Law, because on alternating the cover, both eyes elevate while they are occluded and descend when they are uncovered. The DVD is bilateral, usually asymmetric and the magnitude of the hypertropia is variable. It also shows incommitance among lateroversions, normally a bit more in abduction, when combined with superior oblique muscle hyperfunction; and in adduction when combined with inferior oblique muscle hyperfunction.[68] It could be associated with torticolis in 35% of cases[69] where the tilting of the head over the shoulder of the fixating eye (which is intorsionating) is more frequent.

In Table 4, we can see the vertical and torsional components at the moment of occluding left eye with VOG.

In Table 5, we can see the variation of the evolution of DVD in a summarized way when the filters are put in front of the right eye (VOG). In graph 1 we can see the torsional changes of both eyes.[70]

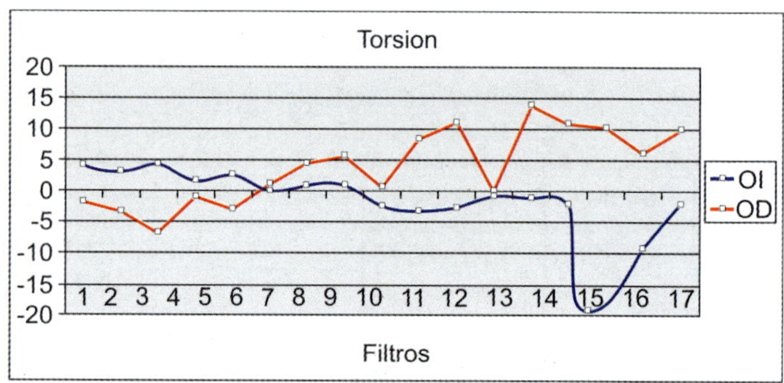

Graph 1: Torsional changes of both eyes

Diplopia Analysis

Patient with vertical diplopia in levo/dextroversion (Figs 18A to 19B). As we can see, evidence of hypertrophy of the right eye (RE) in dextroversion and hypertrophy of the left eye (LE) in levoversion, which did not show in the primary position and together with the difficulty of patient collaboration due to old age and to the evaluation of the torsional components and of cross-fixation, allowed the hyperfunction of both superior oblique muscles, which is very difficult to analyze by other means that would allow the vertical and torsional alterations that justify the diplopia to be registered.

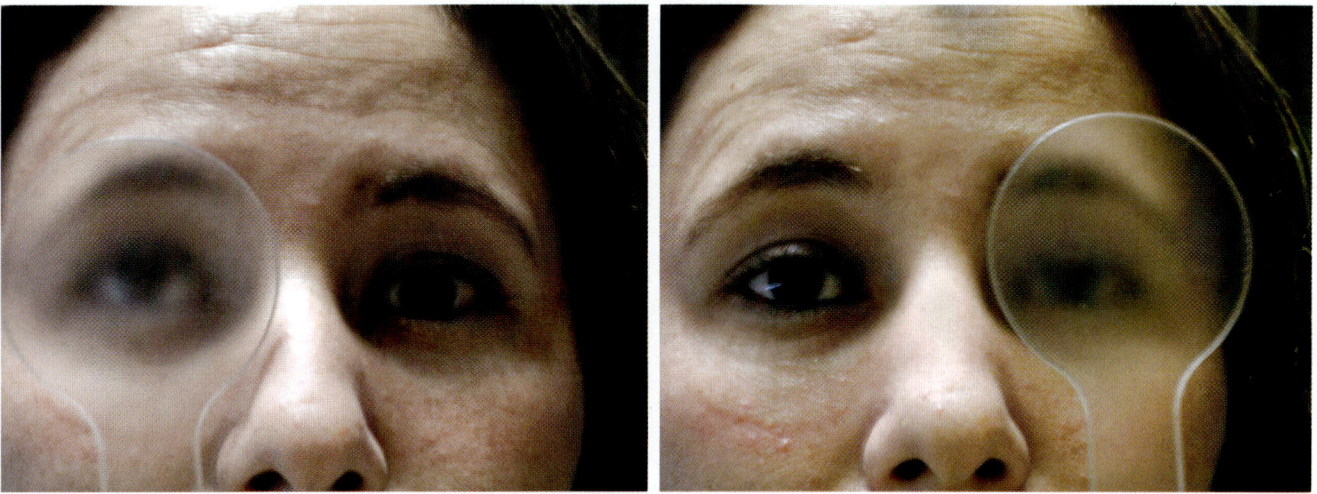

Fig. 16: Asymmetrical DVD

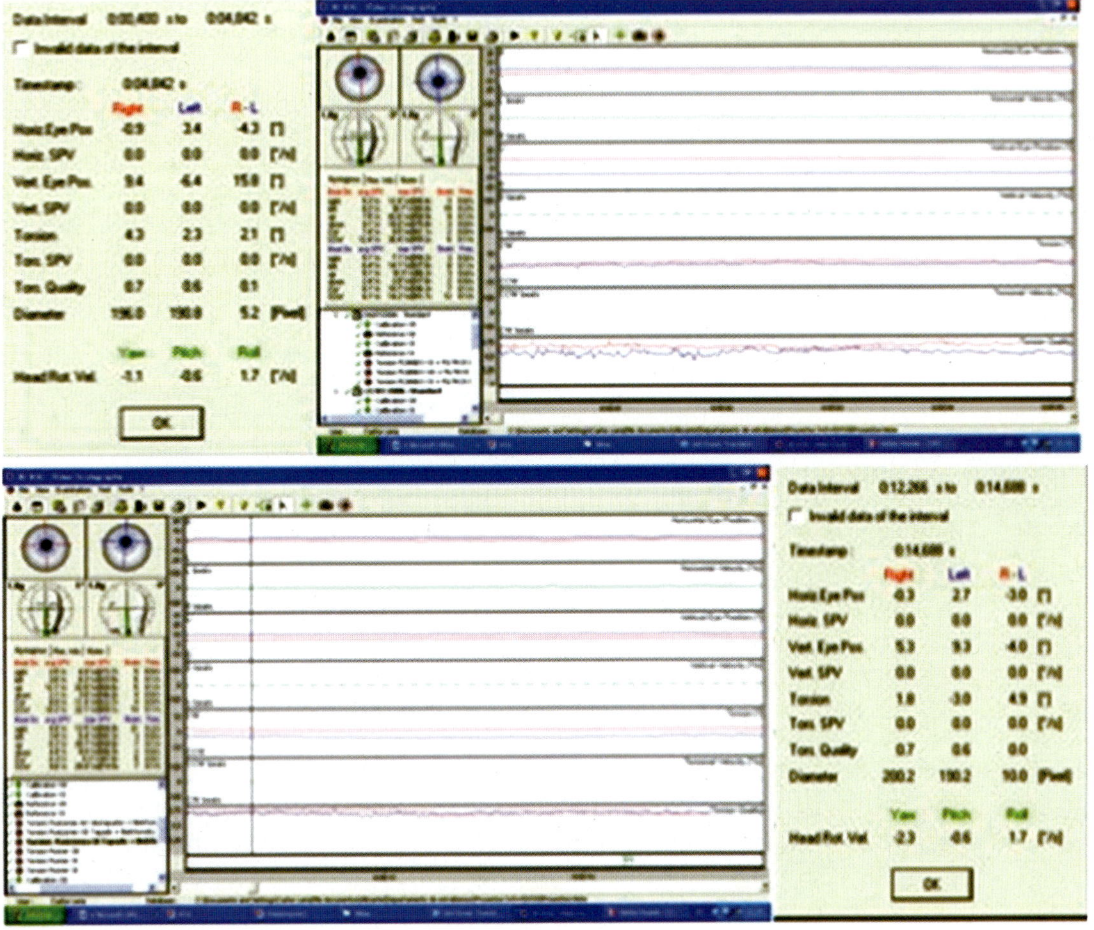

Fig. 17: Asymmetrical DVD

Table 4: Vertical and torsional components occluding left eye in DVD

LE OCCLUDED	*Right*	*Left*	*Right-Left*
Vertical eye position Torsional eye position	Hypotropia – 0.3º Inciclotorsion – 0.6º	Hypertropia +7.4º Exciclotorsion – 1.4º	DVD –7.7º –0.8º
FILTER # 1 R.E. / LE OCCLUDED			
Vertical eye position Torsional eye position	Hypertropia +0.4º Inciclotorsion –1.7º	Hypertropia +6.7º Exciclotorsion -4.3º	DVD –6.3º +2.6º
FILTER # 2 R.E. / LE OCCLUDED			
Vertical eye position Torsional eye position	Hypertropia +1º Inciclotorsion –1.4º	Hypertropia +7.2º Exciclotorsion –3.2º	DVD -7.2º +1.8
FILTER # 3 R.E. / LE OCCLUDED			
Vertical eye position Torsional eye position	Hypertropia +2.6º Inciclotorsion –6.8º	Hypertropia +6.7º Exciclotorsion –4.4º	DVD –4.2º –2.4º
FILTER # 4. R.E. / LE OCCLUDED			
Vertical eye position Torsional eye position	Hypertropia +2.1º Inciclotorsion –0.9º	Hypertropia +7.5º Exciclotorsion –1.7º	DVD –5.5º +0.8º
FILTER # 5 R.E. / LE OCCLUDED			
Vertical eye position Torsional eye position	Hypertropia +2.4º Inciclotorsion –2.9º	Hypertropia +8.5º Exciclotorsion –2.7	DVD –6.1 –0.1º
FILTER # 6 R.E. / LE OCCLUDED			
Vertical eye position Torsional eye position	Hypertropia +3.8º Exciclotorsion +1.3º	Hypertropia +9.3º Exciclotorsion –0.1º	DVD -5.5º +1.4º
FILTER # 7 R.E. / LE OCCLUDED			
Vertical eye position Torsional eye position	Hypertropia +5.2º Exciclotorsion +4.5º	Hypertropia +8.6º Exciclotorsion –1.1º	DVD –3.4º +5.6º
FILTER # 8 R.E. / LE OCCLUDED			
Vertical eye position Torsional eye position	Hypertropia +8º Exciclotorsion +5.8º	Hypertropia + 9º Exciclotorsion –1.3º	DVD –1,1º +7.1º
FILTER # 9 R.E. / LE OCCLUDED			
Vertical eye position Torsional eye position	Hypertropia +2.6º Exciclotorsion +0.8º	Hypertropia + 8.4 Inciclotorsion +2.4º	DVD –5.7º –1.6º
FILTER # 10 R.E. / LE OCCLUDED			
Vertical eye position Torsional eye position	Hypertropia +7.5 Exciclotorsion +8.6º	Hypertropia +9.6º Inciclotorsion +3.1º	DVD –2.1º +5.5º
FILTER # 11 R.E. / LE OCCLUDED			
Vertical eye position Torsional eye position	Hypertropia + 8.2º Exciclotorsion +11.2º	Hypertropia +9.5º Inciclotorsion +2.5º	DVD –1.3º +8.8º
FILTER # 12 R.E. / LE OCCLUDED			
Vertical eye position Torsional eye position	Hypertropia +8.3º Exciclotorsion +0.1º	Hypertropia +9.5º Inciclotorsion +0.8º	DVD –1.2º –0.7º

Contd.

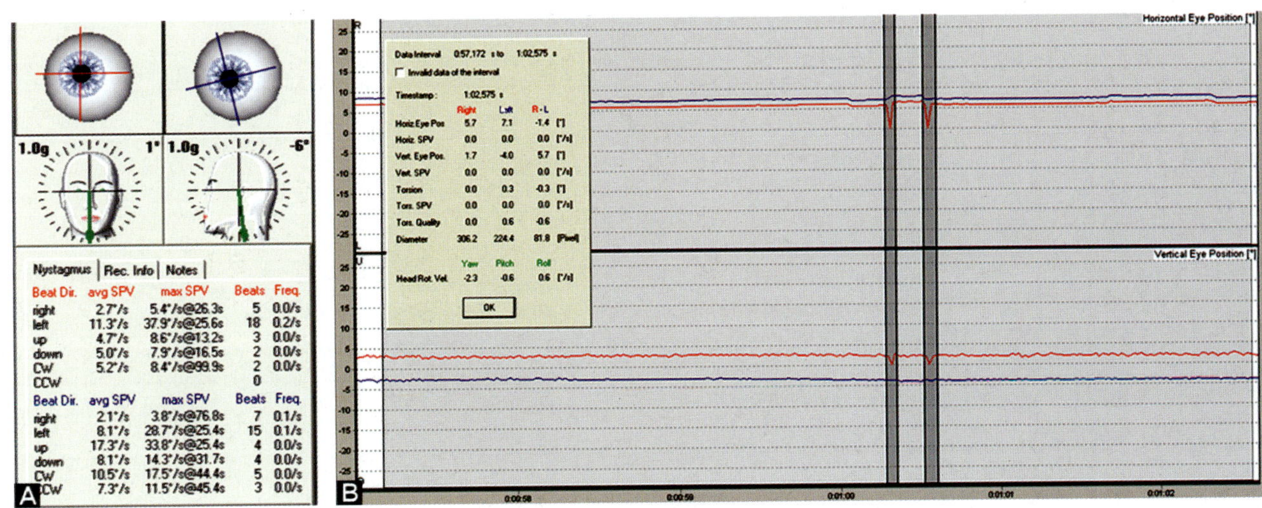

Figs 18A and B

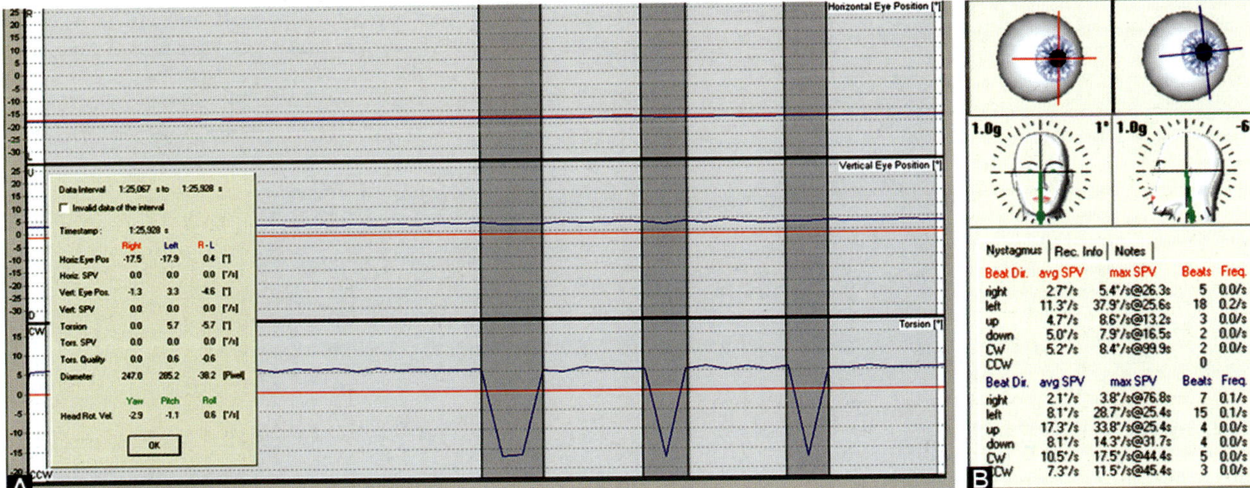

Figs 19A and B

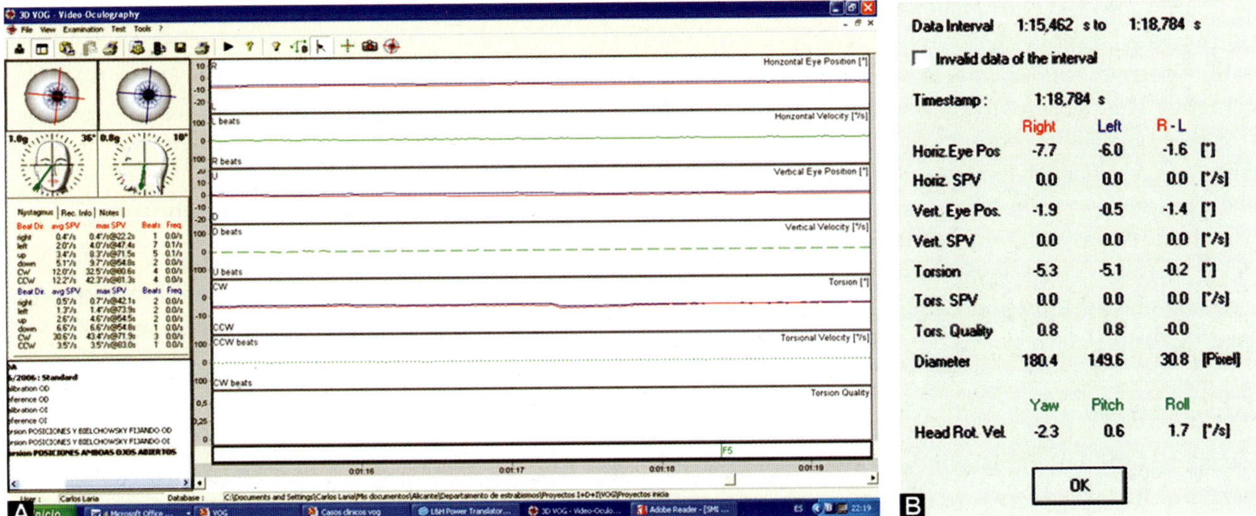

Figs 20A and B

Contd.

LE OCCLUDED	*Right*	*Left*	*Right-Left*
FILTER # 13 R.E. / LE OCCLUDED			
Vertical eye position Torsional eye position	Hypertropia +9.3 Exciclotorsion +14.0°	Hypertropia +11.8° Inciclotorsion +1.1	DVD –2.5° +12.9°
FILTER # 14 R.E. / LE OCCLUDED			
Vertical eye position Torsional eye position	Hypertropia +9.4° Exciclotorsion +11.1°	Hypertropia +10.1° Inciclotorsion +2.1°	DVD –0.7° +9.0°
FILTER # 15 R.E. / LE OCCLUDED			
Vertical eye position Torsional eye position	Hypotropia –3.7° Exciclotorsion +10.3°	Hypotropia –6.7° Inciclotorsion +18.3°	DVD +3.0° –8.0°
FILTER # 16 R.E. / LE OCCLUDED			
Vertical eye position Torsional eye position	Hypotropia –6.2° Exciclotorsion +6.3°	Hypotropia –7.1° Inciclotorsion +9.2°	DVD +0.9° –2.9°
FILTER # 17 R.E. / LE OCCLUDED			
Vertical eye position Torsional eye position	Hypertropia +9.7° Exciclotorsion +10.1	Hypertropia +8.6° Inciclotorsion +2.0°	DVD +1.1 +8.1

Table 5: Variation of the evolution of DVD

	LE occluded		# 1	# 2	# 3	# 4	# 5	# 6	# 7	# 8
DVD	–7.7°		–6.3°	–7.2°	–4.2°	–5.5°	–6.1°	–5.5°	–3.4°	–1.1°
	# 9	# 10	# 11	# 12	# 13	# 14	# 15	# 16	# 17	
DVD	–5.7°	–2.1°	–1.3°	–1.2°	–2.5°	–0.7°	+3.0°	+0.9°	+1.1°	

Analysis of Muscular Paralysis

IV Nerve Paralysis; Analysis of Stiff Neck

Patient with paralysis in the Superior oblique of the left eye (Fig. 20A and B). The 3D-VOG allows us not only to register the ocular movements in the three axes, but at the same time permits such an analysis together with the head movements. This is useful to analyze the stiff neck as is the Test of Bielschowsky in this case, where as seen in this patient with a stiff neck over the right shoulder, a lesser vertical component can be seen compared to when carried out on the left shoulder due to the conduct of the left superior rectus to compensate the excyclotorsion of the eye, whose elevating action cannot be balanced by the depressive action of the paralytic superior oblique.

VI Nerve Paralysis

A case is presented of paresis of the VI nerve of the RE in primary deviation, being shown that as the endotropia in levoversion (Figs 21A and B) is significantly less (8°) than that shown in dextroversion (58.4°) (Figs 22A and B), where the action of the lateral rectus innervated by the right VI nerve is needed.

III Nerve Paralysis

The next case presents the VOG study of paresis of the III nerve of the RE (Fig. 23) in dextroversion, levoversion and primary position.

Analysis of Duane´s Retraction Syndrome

The next patient has a Duane´s retraction syndrome in the left eye with esotropia in primary position (Fig. 24). There is a limitation in abduction of left eye (Fig. 25).

5. NYSTAGMOGRAPHY

The word nystagmus comes from the Greek nystagmos (νιδταγμοξ) and refers to the slow forward movements carried out by a person who falls asleep whilst sitting down.[71] They are defined by Kestembaum[72] as

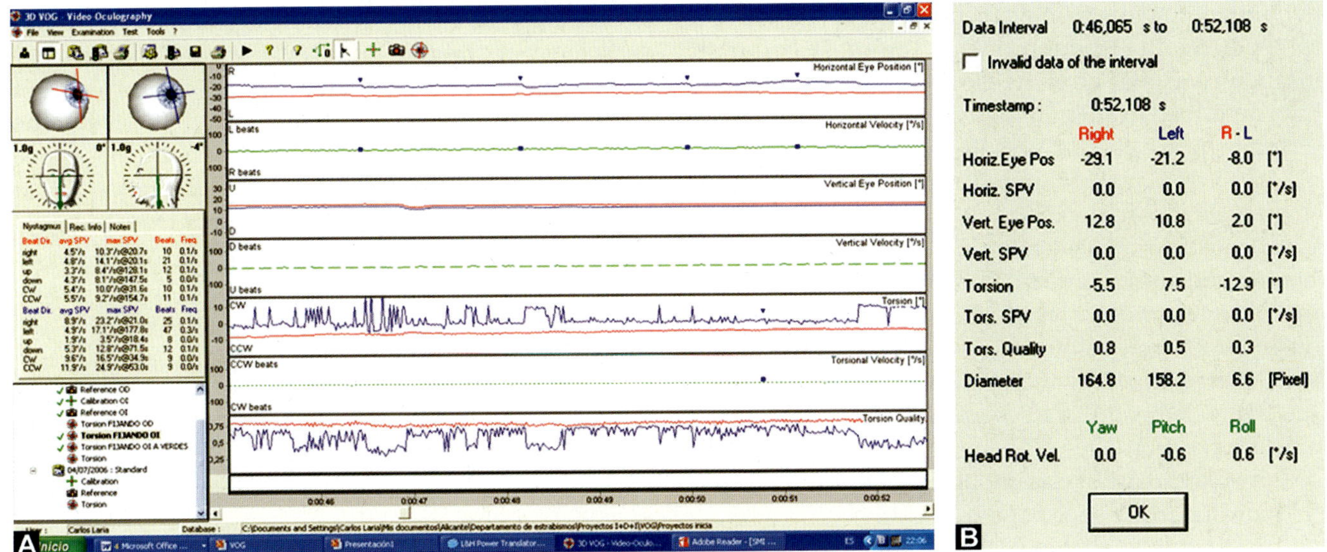

Figs 21A and B

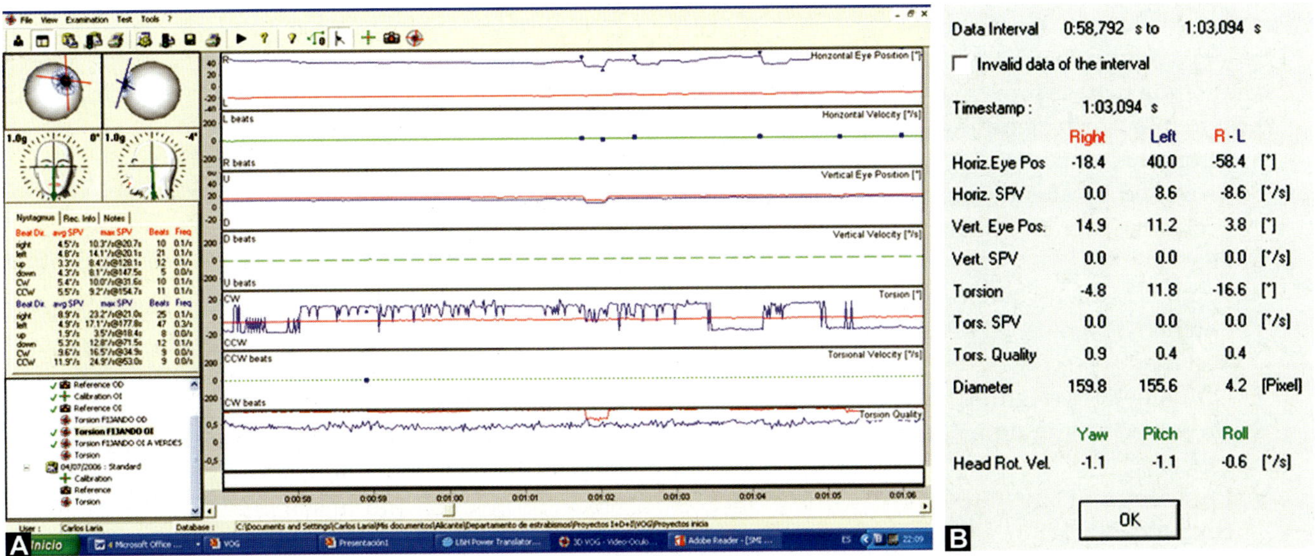

Figs 22A and B

"involuntary to-and-fro movements of the eyes, rhythmic and repetitive", although one of the most complete definitions was that given by Goddé-Jolly y Larmande[73] which described nystagmus as a "tremor associated with the ocular bulbs, characterized by rhythmic succession, more or less regular of conjugated movements, alternatively changing direction, pendular or dysphasic movements, spontaneous or provoked, normal or pathological, usually synchronized and congruent, unconscious, nearly always unintentional and which do not disturb the normal movement of the eyes. This is a disorder of the ocular statics, characterized by the stimulation or the alteration of one of the elements of the cybernetic system that controls the ocular position".

Many ways exist of classifying nystagmus;[71]

- According to the speed of the phases:
  - Nystagmus "shaking", "spring like" o "saccadic": It has a slow phase and a quick phase, of different speeds.
  - Pendular nystagmus: Equal rate in both phases.
  - Mixture of both with pendular nystagmus in one position and shaking in the rest.
- According to the form of occurrence:
  - Spontaneous nystagmus: Appears without specific stimulation to have provoked it. Pathological. The most frequent are cognitive that can be:
    - Idiopathic or motor.
    - Provoked by alterations resulting from visual problems (cognitive cataracts, retinitis, aniridia, etc.).
  - Nystagmus as a consequence of specific conditions:
    - Latent nystagmus: occurs only when one eye is occluded.
    - Optokinetic nystagmus.
    - Provoked vestibule nystagmus: Thermic or rotatory.
    - Pathological nystagmus of the lateral conjugated gaze.
    - Voluntary nystagmus.
- According to its frequency: By the number of oscillations per unit of time. If we use the second, the unit is the Hertz (one oscillation/second). It is more adequate to use the minute in order to avoid small oscillations of temporal frequency. Normally it is situated between 100 and 300 oscillations/minute.
- According to the direction: it can be horizontal, vertical, rotatory or retractory or a combination of these.

In order to detect them sometimes a simple observation is sufficient but different techniques are available, such as:

1. Electro-physiological methods; Electro-oculography (EOG)—This allows us to register the frequency, amplitude and the relative speed of both phases of the nystagmus, but its most important limitation is that it does not allow the register of rotatory movements.
2. Optical methods—This allows the register of not only the horizontal and vertical movements, but also the rotatory. Included in this method is video-oculography.[26,74,75]

The 3-DVOG system allows us the register as nystagmogram, discriminating the following components for each eye independently and in the different positions of the gaze[11] (Fig. 26).

- Direction of the beats.
- Average speed of the slow phase.
- Maximum speed of the slow phase and the moment when it occurs.
- Number of beats.
- Frequency of the beats.

In this way, we can establish fundamental aspects at the time of deciding upon a surgical intervention, as are:

- Discriminate the predominance of the horizontal, vertical or torsional components.
- Existence of blocking positions that make us take up compensatory stiff necks and which are essential in surgery
- Congruency of a stiff neck according to the fixating eye.

Following surgery, it is equally fundamental to analyze:

- Diminution of the stiff neck in primary position.
- Alteration of the frequency and/or speed of the nystagmus according to the type of intervention.
- Nystagmus in dextroversion. A case of nystagmus with blocking position (no nystagmus) in levoversion is presented (Fig. 27) and primary position (Fig. 28) and nystagmus in dextroversion (Fig. 29).

The study of nystagmus is a problem that up to now we have not been able to offer a definite solution, perhaps because we are not able to fully understand the complications of its mechanisms, but with the help of video-oculography as the one mentioned here we can begin to study its analysis in depth and perhaps we are at the beginning of a new era both in the analysis of nystagmus as in strabismus in general.

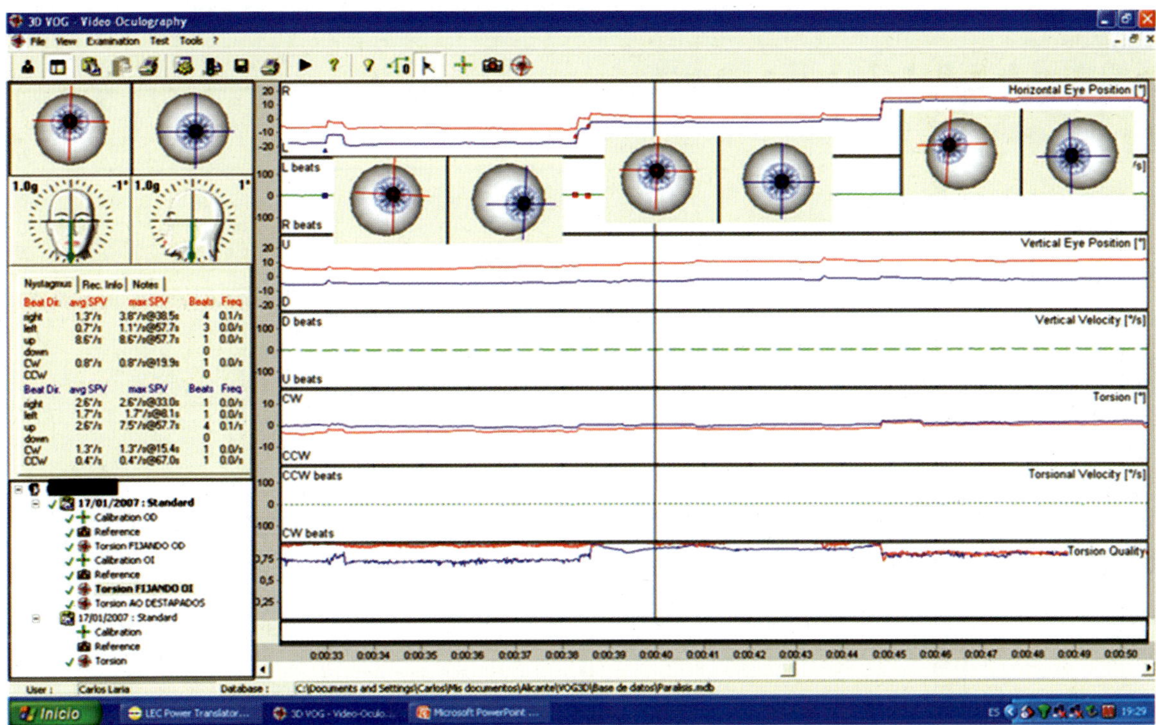

Fig. 23: III nerve paralysis of the right eye

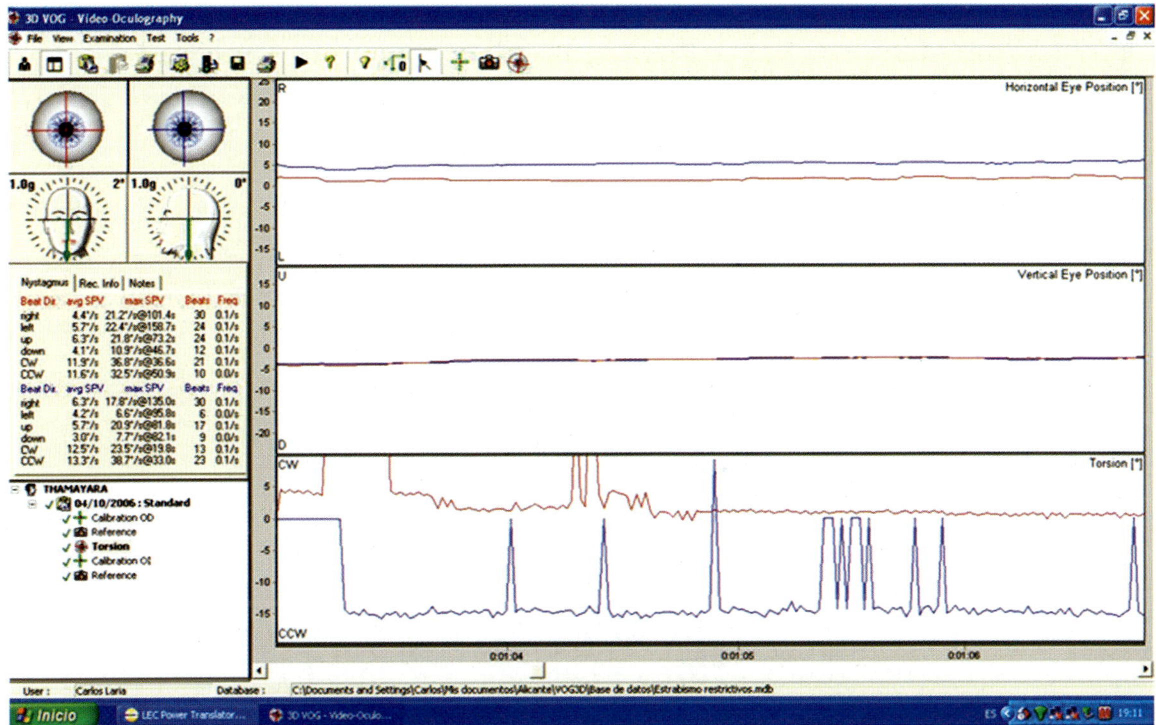

Fig. 24: VOG of Duane´s syndrome of left eye. Primary position

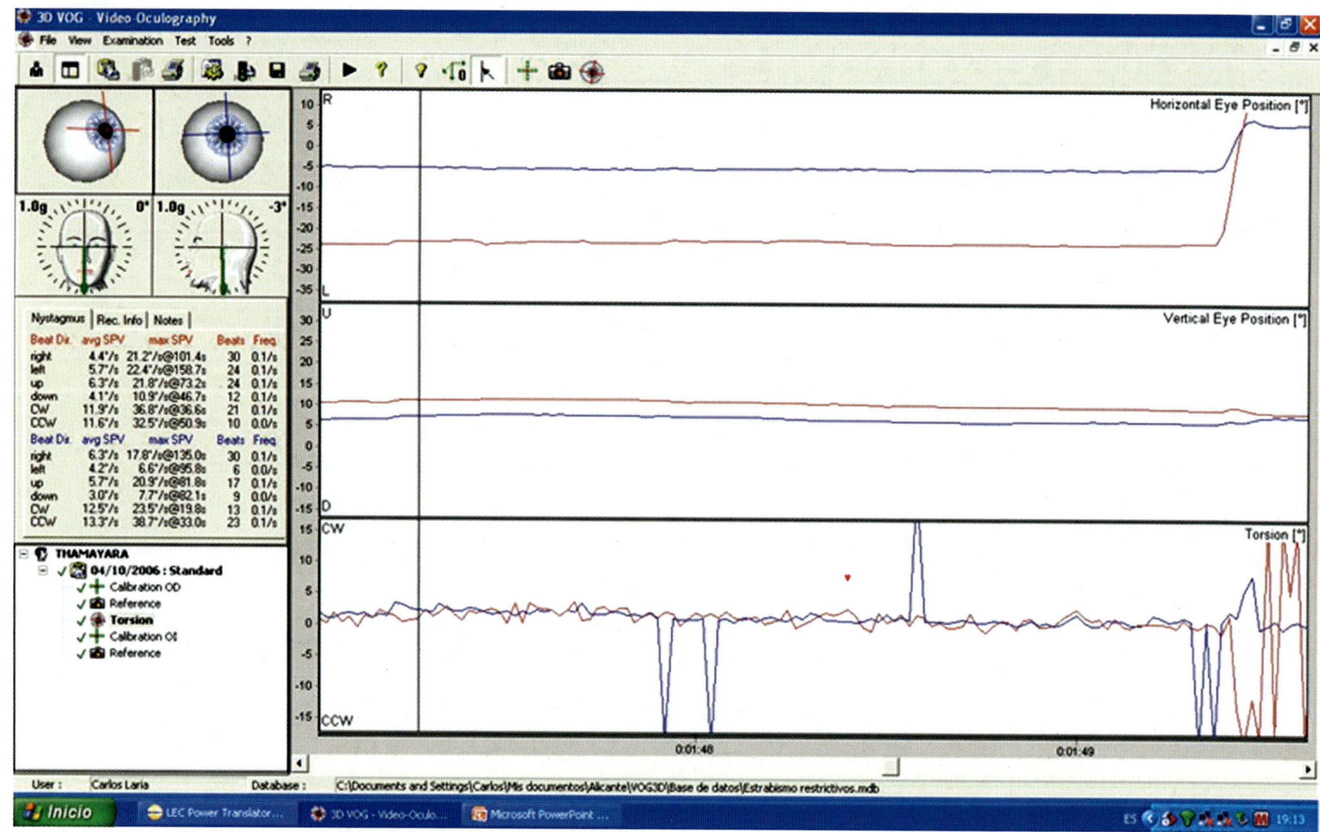

Fig. 25: VOG of Duane´s syndrome in left eye. Levoversion with limitation of abduction in left eye

Nystagmus | Rec. Info | Notes

Beat Dir.	avg SPV	max SPV	Beats	Freq.
right	57.7°/s	124.6°/s@32.3s	69	0.3/s
left	59.2°/s	108.6°/s@75.4s	55	0.3/s
up	5.9°/s	10.6°/s@47.2s	9	0.0/s
down	7.8°/s	16.0°/s@142.4s	10	0.0/s
CW	8.7°/s	13.4°/s@125.3s	8	0.0/s
CCW	18.6°/s	42.5°/s@60.6s	4	0.0/s
Beat Dir.	**avg SPV**	**max SPV**	**Beats**	**Freq.**
right	55.6°/s	102.6°/s@32.3s	74	0.3/s
left	51.2°/s	89.3°/s@160.8s	102	0.5/s
up	8.4°/s	15.0°/s@32.1s	19	0.1/s
down	7.0°/s	9.7°/s@33.5s	7	0.0/s
CW	19.4°/s	34.8°/s@25.3s	28	0.1/s
CCW	18.2°/s	38.4°/s@149.0s	9	0.0/s

Fig. 26: Analysis of nystagmus

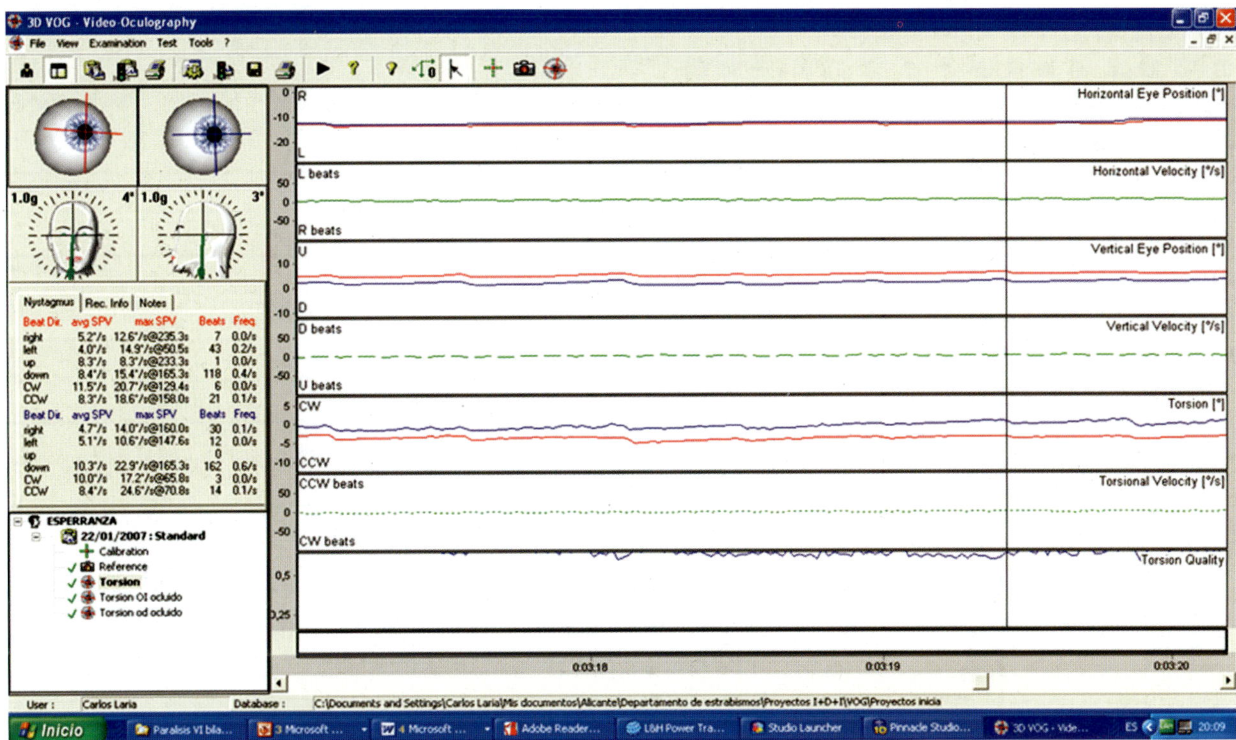

Fig. 27: VOG in levoversion, without nystagmus

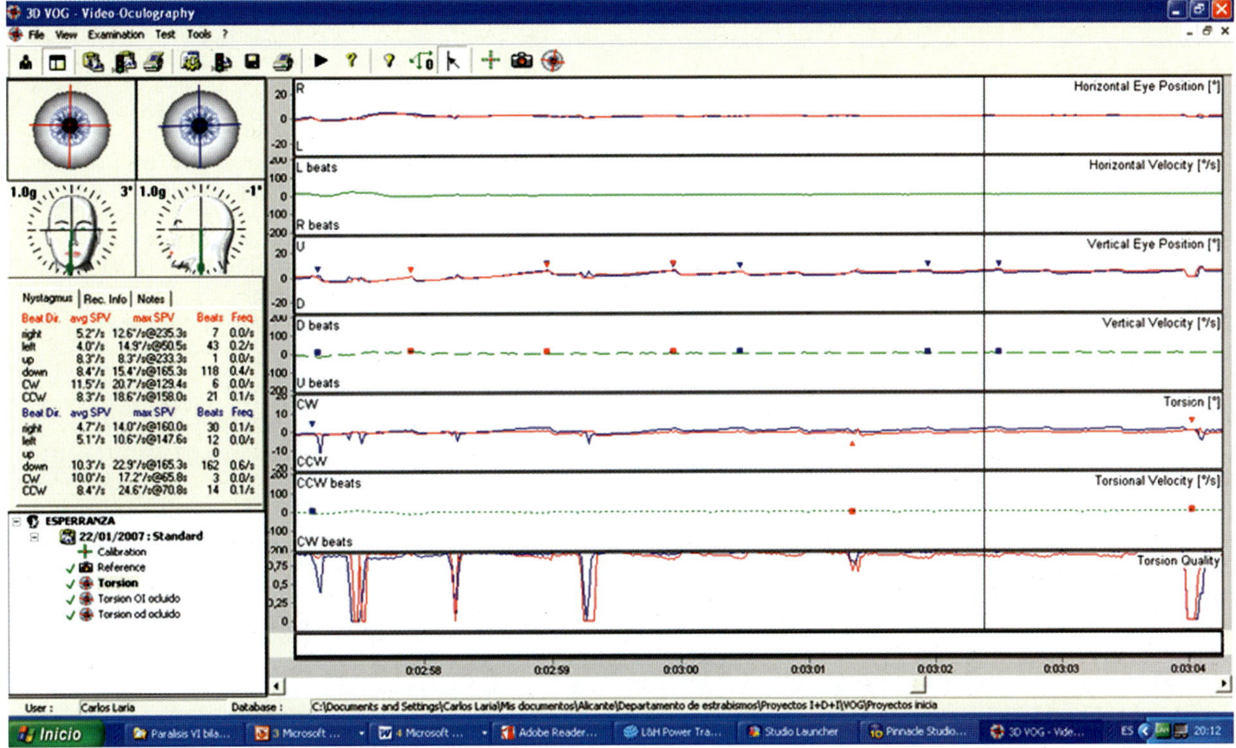

Fig. 28: VOG in primary position, without any beats of nystagmus

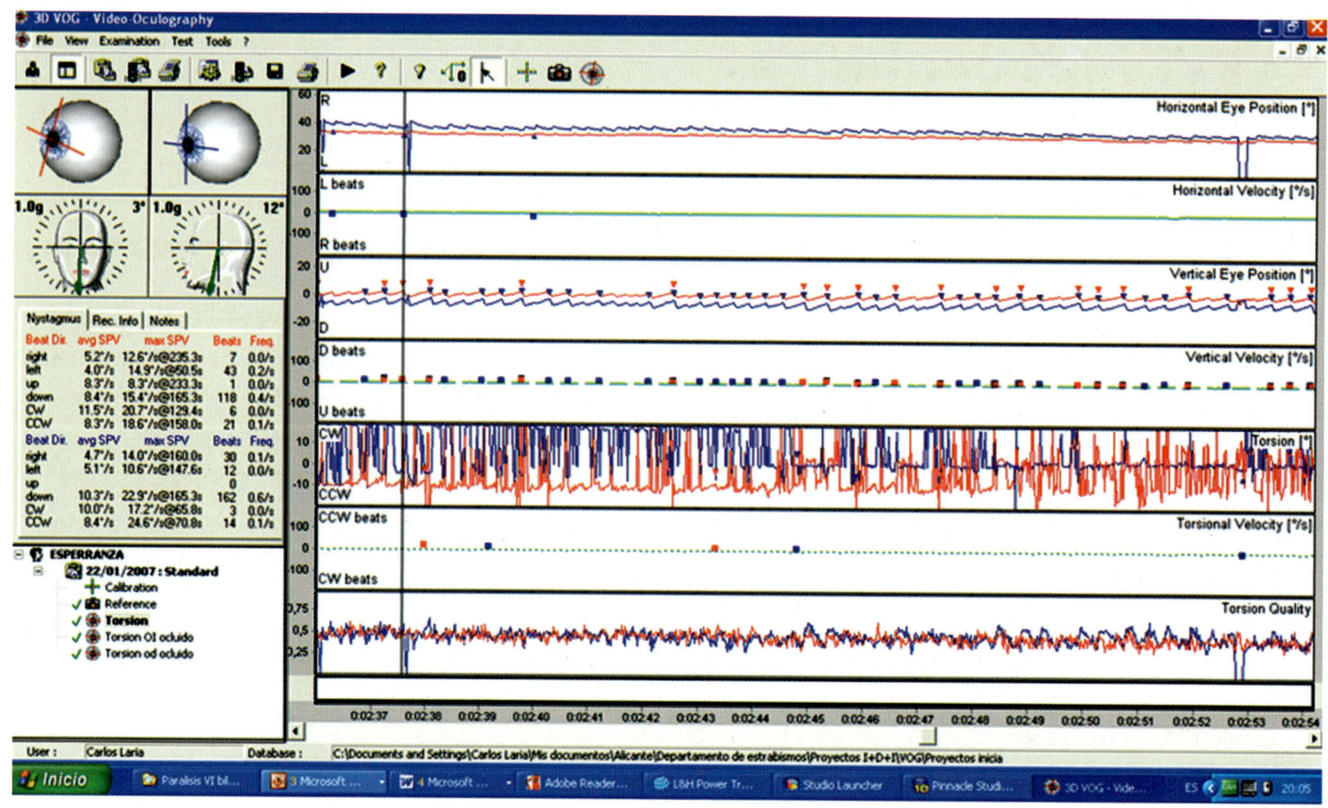

Fig. 29: VOG in dextroversion, with beats of nystagmus (triangles blues and reds)

REFERENCES

1. Prieto-Díaz J, Sousa-Diaz C. Motilidad ocular. En: Estrabismo. (Ed): Científicas Argentinas. Buenos Aires 2005;1-90.
2. Pavan Langstom D. Músculos extraoculares, estrabismo y nistagmo: En: Manual de Diagnóstico y terapéutica oculares. Ed. Científicas y Técnicas S.A. Barcelona 1993;349-86.
3. Saraux H, et al. Anatomía e Histología del ojo. Ed. Masson. Barcelona 1985;367.
4. Fink W. Surgery of the bolique muscles of the eye. St Louis: CV Mosby 1951.
5. Sousa-Dias C, Prieto-Diaz J, Uesugui C. Topographic aspects of the insertions of the extraocular muscles. J. Pediatr Ophthalmol Strabismus 1986;23:183.
6. Anatomías de los músculos extraoculares. En: Curso Semiología de las desviaciones oculares. [Campus virtual] Hospital Italiano de Buenos Aires. Argentina. 2006.
7. Ferrer J. Estrabismos y ambliopía. Práctica razonada. Doyma ed. Barcelona 1991;243.
8. Funciones de los músculos extraoculares. En: Curso Semiología de las desviaciones oculares. [Campus virtual] Hospital Italiano de Buenos Aires. Argentina 2006.
9. Ducciones, Versiones, Cover Test En: Curso Semiología de las desviaciones oculares. [Campus virtual] Hospital Italiano de Buenos Aires. Argentina 2006.
10. Sherrington CD. Observations on the sensual role of the proprioceptive nerve suplí of the extrinsic eye muscles. Brain 1918;41:332.
11. 3D VOG Video-Oculography® Versión 5. System Manual SensoMotoric Instruments. Alemania. 2004;202 pags.3D VOG
12. Fioravanti F, Bruno P, Inchingolo P, hart RT, Power H. Bidimensional eye position measurement using video-oculographic systems: close form solution and error analysis. In: Brebbia CA (Ed): Simulations in Biomedicine. Computational Mechanics Publications, Southampton 1994.
13. Peterka RJ, Merfeld DM. Calibration techniques for video-oculography. J Vest Res 1996;6:S75.
14. Ott D, Gehle F, Eckmiller R. Video-oculographic measurement of 3-dimensional eye rotations. J Neurosci Meth 1990;35: 229-34.
15. Scherer H, Teiwes W, Clarke AH. Measurig three dimensions of eye movement in dynamic situations by means of videooculography. Acta Otolaryngol 1991;111:182-7.
16. Sung K, Anderson DJ. Analysis of two video eye tracking algorithms. In: AnonymousProceedings of the Annual International Conference of the IEEE Engineering in Medicine and Biology Society 1991;1949-50.
17. Van der Glas M, Bosman J, de Jong I, Bovendeerd PHM, van Campen, DH, Kingma H. Real time data processing with the video eyetracker. 1999:99. (Conference Proceeding: Castelvecchio, I)
18. Teiwes DM, Merfeld LR. Young, and AH. Clarke. Comparsion of scleral search coil and video-oculography techniques for three-dimensional eye movement measurement. In: Three-dimensional kinematics of eye, head and limb movements, edited by M. Fetter, T. Haslwanter, H. Misslisch, and D. Tweed, Harwood Academic Publishers, 1997;429-44.

19. Murphy PJ, Duncan AL, Glennie AJ, Knox PC. The effect of scleral search coil lens wear on the eye. Br J Ophthalmol 2001 Mar;85(3):332-5.
20. van der Geest JN, Frens MA. Recording eye movements with video-oculography and scleral search coils: A direct comparison of two methods. J Neurosci Methods 2002 Mar 15;114(2):185-95.
21. Imai T, Sekine K, Hattori K, Takeda N, Koizuka I, Nakamae K, Miura K, Fujioka H, Kubo T.Comparing the accuracy of video-oculography and the scleral search coil system in human eye movement analysis. Auris Nasus Larynx. 2005 Mar;32(1):3-9.
22. Houben MM, Goumans J, van der Steen J. Recording three-dimensional eye movements: scleral search coils versus video oculography. Invest Ophthalmol Vis Sci 2006 Jan;47(1):179-87.
23. Clarke AH, et al. Registering eye movements using digital Figure processing. Biomed Tech (Berl). 1989;34 Suppl:22-3. German.
24. Clarke AH, Lennerstrand G, Figure processing techniques for the measurement of eye movement. In: Ygge J (Ed): Eye movements in reading. Pergamon 1994;21-38.
25. Clarke AH, Teiwes W, Scherer H, Zambarbieri D. Videooculography–an alternative method for measurement of three-dimensional eye movements. In: Schmid R (Ed): Oculomotor Control and Cognitive Processes. Elsevier, Amsterdam 1991;431-43.
26. Clarke AH, Waldmann K, Scherer H. Three-dimensional aspects of caloric nystagmus in humans. II. Caloric-induced torsional deviation. Acta Otolaryngol 1993a;113: 693-8.
27. Curthoys IS, Moore ST, Haslwanter T, Black RA, Smith ST, Lennerstrand G. Video procedures for the measurement and display of the three dimensions of eye movements. In: Ygge J (Ed): Eye movement in reading (Proceedings of the Wenner Gren Center International Symposium). Pergamon Press, Oxford 1994;39-49.
28. Curthoys IS, Moore ST, McCoy SG, Halmagyi GM, Markham CH, Diamond SG, Wade SW, Smith ST. VTM - A new method of measuring ocular torsion using Figure processing techniques. Annals New York Academy of Sciences 1992;826-8.
29. DiScenna AO, Das V, Zivotofsky AZ, Seidman SH, and Leigh RJ. Evaluation of a video tracking device for measurement of horizontal and vertical eye rotations during locomotion. J Neurosci Meth 1995;58:89-94.
30. Fioravanti F, Bruno P, Inchingolo P, Brebbia CA, Cislkowski RD, Power H. Spatial resolution enhancement and Figure restoration for high speed video-oculographic systems. In: Held KD (Ed): Computational Medicine. Computation Mechanics Publications, Southampton 1990b;301-08.
31. Fioravanti F, Bruno P, Inchingolo P, Rabischong P. Video oculography: High resolution motion estimation for fast eye movements. An algorithm for real time reconstruction of high resolution binary Figures In: Pedotti A (ed) 3rd European Conference on Engineering and Medicine — A bridge between Engineering and Medicine 1990a;394.
32. Groen E, Bos JE, Nacken PF, and de GB. Determination of ocular torsion by means of automatic pattern recognition. IEEE Trans Biomed Eng 1996;43:471-9.
33. P Guillemant, E Ulmer, G Freyss, "3D eye movement measurements on four Comex's divers using video CCD cameras, during high pressure diving", Acta Otolaryngol, (Stockh), 1995, suppl 520, pp 288-292, Scandinavian University Press.
34. Haslwanter T, Moore ST. A Theoretical Analysis of Three-Dimensional Eye Position Measurement Using Polar Cross-Correlation. IEEE Trans Biomed Eng 1995;42:1053-61.
35. Hatamian M, Anderson DJ. Design considerations for a real-time ocular counterroll instrument. IEEE Trans Biomed Eng 1983;30:278-88.
36. Imai T, Takeda N, Morita M, Koizuka I, Kubo T, Miura K, Nakamae K, Fujioka H. Rotation vector analysis of eye movement in three dimensions with an infrared CCD camera. Acta Oto-Laryngologica 1999;119(1):24-8.
37. Jampel RS, Shi DX. Retinal micromovements, the visual line, and Donders' law. Am.J Ophthalmol 2000;129(2):224-34.
38. Kingma H, Gullikers H, de J, I, Jongen R, Dolmans M, Stegeman P. Real time binocular detection of horizontal vertical and torsional eye movements by an infra red video-eye tracker. Acta Otolaryngol Suppl (Stockh) 1995;520 Pt 1: 9-15.
39. Moore ST, Curthoys IS, and McCoy SG. VTM—An figure-processing system for measuring ocular torsion. Computer Methods and Programs in Biomedicine 1991;35: 219-30.
40. Moore ST, Haslwanter T, Curthoys IS, Smith ST. Measurement of three dimensional eye position using figure processing: A geometric approach. In: Anonymous Proceedings of the IEEE - International Conference on figure Processing 1994;pp 436-40.
41. Moore ST, Haslwanter T, Curthoys IS, Smith ST. A geometric basis for measurement of three-dimentsional eye position using figure processing. Vision Res 1996;36: 445-59.
42. Nishihira O, Matsunaga K, Tokumitsu S, Ikeda K, T Uemura . TV eye tracker using first and fourth purkinje Figures 1991. (Conference Proceeding: 6th ECEM).
43. Schweigger C. Die Erfolge der Schieloperation. Arch Augenheilkd 1895;30:165.
44. Stevens GT. Du strabisme vertical alternant et des deviations symetriques moins pronounce que le strabisme. Ann Oculist 1895;113:225-385.
45. Bielschowsky A. Disturbances of the vertical motor muscles of the eyes. Arch Ophthalmol 1938;20:175.
46. Bielschowsky A. Die einseitigen und gegensinnigen ("dissoziierten") Vertikalbewegungen der Augen. Graefes Arch Clin Exp Ophthalmol 1931; 125: 493.
47. Von Noorden GK, Campos EM. Cyclovertical Deviation. In Mosby (editor). Binocular Vision and Ocular Motility. St Louis. 2002;378-84.
48. Anderson JR. Latent nystagmus and alternating hyperphoria. Br J Ophthalmol 1954;38:217-31.
49. Crone R. Alternating hyperphoria. Br J Ophthalmol 1954; 38: 591.
50. Houtman WA, Roze JH, De Vries B, Letsch MC. Alternating hyperphoria. Dissociated vertical deviation (DVD) occlusion hyperphoria. Doc Ophthalmol 1991: 78:135-40.
51. Billet E, Ehrilich M. Occlusion hypertropia: A contralateral fixation phenomenom. J Pediatr Ophthalmol Strabismus 1966;3:39.
52. Lancaster WB. Factors underestimated, features overemphasized, and comments on classification. In Allen JE, (editor): Strabismus Ophthalmic Symposium, II. Sgt Louis, Mosby-Year Book 1958;430.
53. Varn MM, Saunders RA, Wilson ME. Combined bilateral superior rectus muscle recession and inferior oblique muscle weaking for dissociated vertical deviation. J Am Assoc Pediatr Ophthalmol Strabismus 1996; 1:134.

54. Helveston EM. A exotropia, alternating sursumduction and superior oblique overaction. Am J Ophthalmol 1969;67:377.
55. Jones BA. Alternating sursumduction. Am Orthoptic J 1965; 15:117.
56. Sargent RA. Surgical correction of dissociated hyperdeviations. Am Orthoptic J 1976;26:89.
57. Nelly D, Helveston E, Thuente D, Plager D. Relationship of dissociated vertical deviation and the timing of initial surgery for congenital esotropia. Ophthalmology 2001;108:487-90.
58. Keiner GB. New viexpoints on the origin of the squint. The Hague: Nijhoff, 1951.
59. Lang J. [Letter] To the editor. J AAPOS 2000; 4: 254.
60. Mesker RP. De optische Localisatie onder envolved van optische en Houndingsfactoren [tesis]. Ámsterdam, 1953.
61. Rüssmann W, Albrecht J. Aufmerksamkeitsverlagerung und dissoziiertes Höhenschielen. Klin Mbl Augenheilk 1986;188: 245-7.
62. Schweigger C. Die Erfolge der Schieloperation. Arch Augenheilkd 1985;30:165.
63. Tychsen L. Pediatric motility disorders of neuro-ophthalmic significance. Neuro-Ophthalmol 1991; 4:615.
64. Kutluk S, Avilla CW, Noorden GK von. The prevalence of dissociated vertical deviation in patients with sensory heterotropia. Am J Ophthalmol 1995;119:744.
65. Metz HS, Norris H. Cyclotorsional diplopia following retinal detachment surgery. J Pediatr Ophthalmol Strabismus 1987; 24:287.
66. Sidikaro Y, Noorden GK von. Observations in sensory heterotropia. J Pediatr Ophthalmol Strabismus 1982; 19: 12.
67. Wilson ME, Saunders RA, Berland JE. Dissociated Vertical deviation and accommodative esotropia: Treatment options when an eso- or exodeviations co-exists. J Pediatr Ophthalmol Strabismus 1995;32:228.
68. Wilson ME, McClatchey SK. Dissociated Vertical deviation. J Pediatr Ophthalmol Strabismus 1991;28: 90.
69. Prieto-Diaz J, Sousa-Dias C. Divergencia vertical disociada. En: Estrabismo. Ediciones científicas argentinas 5th ed. Buenos Aires. 2005;219-42.
70. Laria C, Gamio S, Prieto-Díaz J, Alió JL, Miranda M. Análisis del fenómeno de Bielschowsky en la divergencia vertical disociada mediante Videooculografía".Acta Estrabológica. Vol. XXXVII, Septiembre-Diciembre 2008;3:117-124.
71. Prieto-Díaz J, Sousa-Diaz C. Nistagmo. En: Estrabismo. Ed. Científicas Argentinas. Buenos Aires 2005;495-510.
72. Kestenbaum A. Une nouvelle operation du nystagmus. Bull Soc Ophthalmol Fr 1953;6:599.
73. Goddé-Jolly D, Larmande A. Les nistagmus. Paris: Masson, 1973;705.
74. Clarke AH, Teiwes W, Oelhaffen P, Scherer H. Three-dimensional aspects of caloric nystagmus in humans: I. The influence of increased gravitoinertial force. Acta Otolaryngol 1993b;113: 687-92.
75. Enright JT. Estimating peak velocity of rapid eye movements from video recordings. Behavior Res Meth and Instr 1998;30: 349-53.

Chapter 25

Sutureless Closure in Strabismus Surgery

CS Dhull, Sumit Sachdeva (India)

Strabismus surgery traditionally involves weakening and strengthening of muscles by recession and resection respectively. The incision is usually placed at the limbus, thus a creating large wound which ultimately requires the closure of conjunctival wound with the help of 6-0 or 8-0 vicryl suture.

The main disadvantage of sutures is that they cause extreme foreign body sensation, inflammation, watering and discomfort because of the exposed suture knots. These symptoms are more pronounced in young children because of their thicker conjunctiva and Tenon's capsule Besides all this, suturing itself is a time consuming process.

To overcome this many surgeons have started performing strabismus surgery through a different cul-de-sac incision which requires no sutures to close the conjunctival wound. The wound if small can be left as such and if slightly large, can be closed with the help of commercially available fibrin glue.

PROCEDURE

Although slightly difficult to master, the conjunctival cul - de-sac incision allows the surgery to be performed through a smaller incision than the conventional limbal incision and the wound to be closed without sutures.

1. Although called cul-de-sac or fornix incision, it is a misnomer as the incision is placed in between the limbus and fornix. Normally either 4'o clock or 10'o clock site is chosen for the incision about 5 mm away from the limbus, midway between fornix and limbus. (Fig. 1).
2. The Tenon's capsule and the conjunctiva are incised with the help of Westcott's scissors and after separating intermuscular membrane, the muscle is hooked with the help of muscle hook (Figs 2A and B)
3. The conjunctiva and Tenon's is then moved so that muscle is brought out through the opening.
4. The muscle is then resected (Fig. 3) or recessed as in traditional strabismus surgery, using 6-0 vicryl sutures.
5. Finally after completion of surgery, the conjunctiva and Tenon's capsule are pulled back upon the muscle and the conjunctiva can now be left as such tucked in the fronix (Fig. 4) or may be sealed with the help of fibrin glue.

Fibrin glue is a blood-derived product that is absorbable, relatively easy to use, and can be kept at room temperature or in a refrigerator. It is a biological tissue adhesive which imitates the final stages of the coagulation cascade when a solution of human fibrinogen is activated by thrombin (the two components of fibrin glue). Fibrin glue includes a fibrinogen component and a thrombin component, both prepared by processing plasma.

The procedure of fibrin glue application is as follows:

The fibrinogen is taken in a 1cc disposable syringe, while thrombin and calcium are taken in another 1cc syringe in 1:1 ratio. The area to be glued is dried with a swab stick or cellulose sponge. One drop of each component was applied simultaneously on bare sclera, just below the free margin of conjunctiva. The conjunctival edge is then pressed gently over the glue for about 1 minute for firm adhesion.

The advantages of glue include, lesser wound closure time, reduced inflammation and reduced chances of infection. Further no special technique of application is required. There have been no reported cases of any complications or side effects due to the use of this glue.

Although many surgeons are trying to use various adhesives to anchor the muscle to sclera without the need of sutures, in animal models, but little success has been met as the glue with appropriate tensile strength is yet to be developed. But till such a discovery is made, sutureless closure in strabismus surgery is being increasingly followed by various surgeons, to not only reduce the surgical time, but also to make the patient comfortable and speed up recovery in the postoperative period.

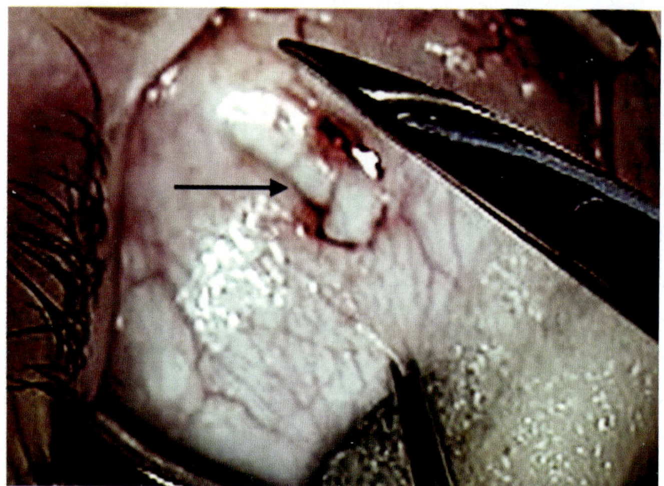

Fig. 1: Conjunctival cul-de-sac incision (arrow)

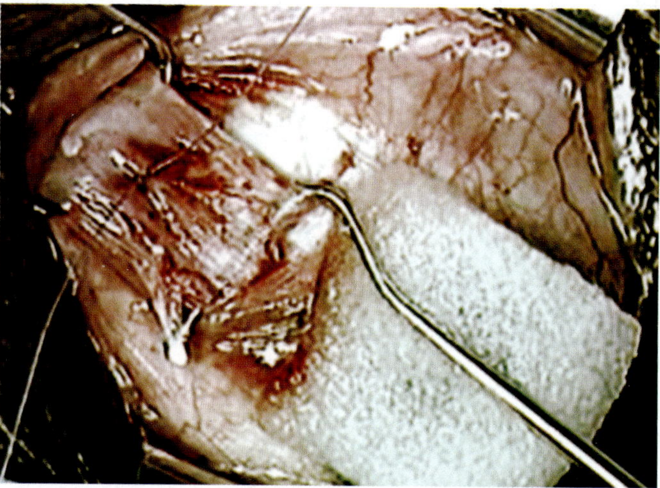

Fig. 3: Muscle being resected

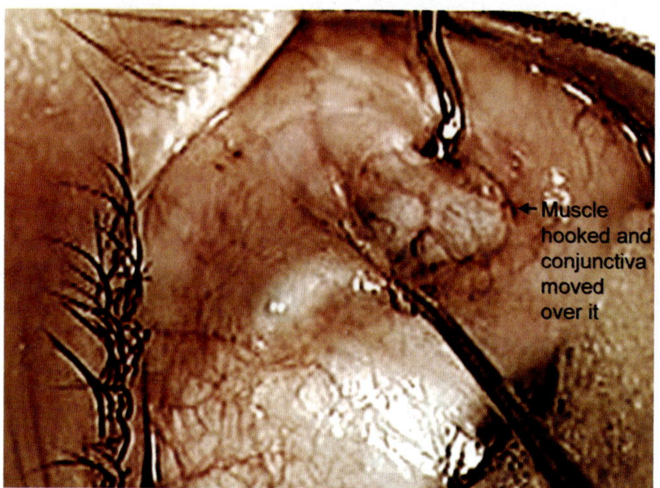

Fig. 2A: Hooking the muscle

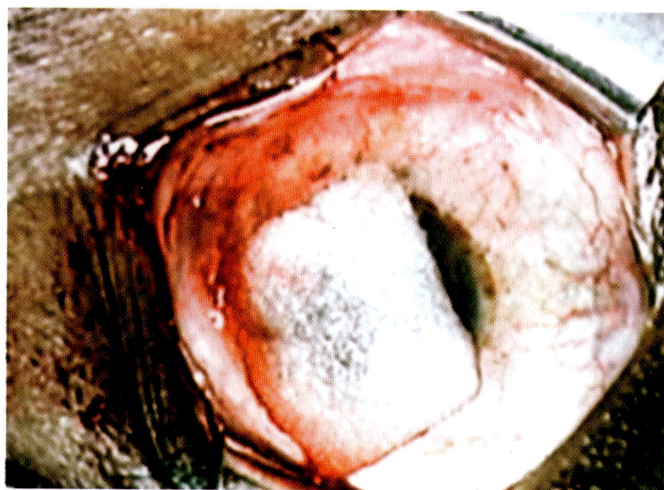

Fig. 4: Conjunctiva tucked in fornix

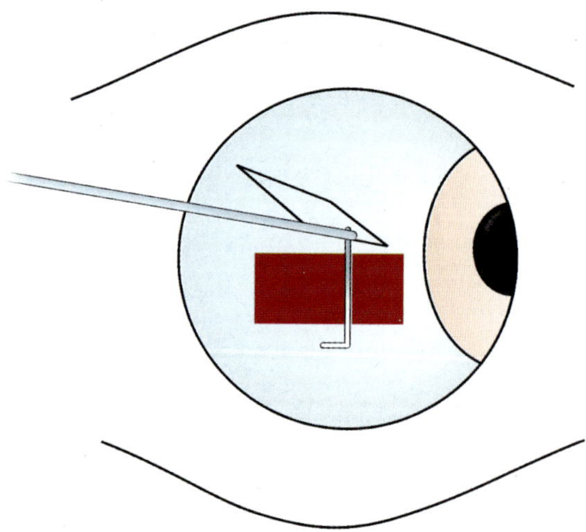

Fig. 2B: Schematic representation of how muscle is hooked from conjunctival opening

FURTHER READING

1. Anita Panda, Sandeep Kumar, Abhiyan Kumar, Raseena Bansal, Shibal Bhartiya. Fibrin glue in ophthalmology : Indian J Ophthalmol 2009;57:371-9.
2. Biedner B, Rosenthal G. Conjunctival closure in strabismus surgery:Vicryl versus fibrin glue. Ophthalmic Surg Lasers 1996;27:967.
3. Chabbat J, Tellier M, Porte P, Steinbuch M. Properties of a new fibrin glue stable in liquid state. Thromb Res 1994;15:525-33.
4. Ibrahim Erbagci, Necdet Bekir. Sutureless closure of the conjunctiva with a commercial fibrin sealant in extraocular muscle surgery for strabismus. Strabismus 2007;15:89-94.
5. Spierer A, Barequet I, Rosner M, Solomon AS, Matinowitz U. Reattachment of extra-ocular muscles using fibrin glue in a rabbit model.Invest Ophthalmol Vis Sci. 1997;38:543-6.
6. Subhash Dadeya, MS Kamlesh. Strabismus surgery: Fibrin glue versus vicryl for conjunctival closure: Acta Ophthalmol Scand. 2001:79:515-7.

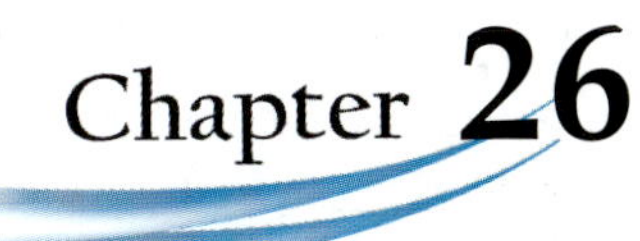

Chapter 26

Accommodative Esotropia—An Update

Arturo Pèrez-Arteaga (Mexico)

DEFINITION AND INITIAL CONSIDERATIONS

The term Esotropia refers to a type of Strabismus characterized by an inward deviation of one eye relative to the other eye. There are different kinds of Esotropia all depending upon the cause. When referring to Accommodative Esotropia (AE) we are talking about an esodeviation due to normal accommodation reflex in an uncorrected refractive error, that most of times, corresponds to hyperopia. The patient with a refractive defect (uncorrected hyperopia) must accommodate to clear a blurred retinal image. This process of accommodation will stimulate convergence and strain fusional divergence, because of a strong stimulus from the oculomotor nerve. This pathology is also known as Refractive Accommodative Esotropia (RAS). At the end the amount of convergence is generated by a given amount of accommodation; it is named by some authors the "focusing effort". One of the main issues of this pathology is the increase possibility of the development of amblyopia that means the reduced visual acuity of one eye due to an abnormal visual experience early in life (it is also known like "lazy eye". With some luck the patient is able to alternate, and so decrease the risk of developing amblyopia; unfortunately the most frequent cases do not correspond to alternate strabismus. The main physiopathologic presentation is the vision of a single blurred image or a double image in which one image is clear and one image is blurred, and subsequently the blurred image is suppressed and amblyopia develops.

EPIDEMIOLOGY

Because the "world" of a small child is almost at near, fixation efforts begin early in life. When a refractive defect is present this effort is manifest as convergence; so this condition usually presents by the age of 2 years. There is no gender or racial predilection to accommodative esotropia. Frequently a history of strabismus or hyperopia in the closest family is found. It may be the most common cause of strabismus during childhood.

SIGNS AND SYMPTOMS

The main symptom that causes consultation in this disease is that the patient's parents may notice an inward or upward deviation of one eye relative to the other eye. The age of onset of strabismus might vary, but almost the frequency is between 2 and 3 years of age. As was mentioned before, during the taking of medical records, a family history of strabismus or related diseases is common. In some particular cases, the physician can ask direct questions regarding the vision of the patient; they may see either a single blurred image or a double image in which one image is clear and one image is blurred; nevertheless sometimes this kind of description is difficult to address.

The main physical finding in AE is hyperopia. This should be determined by examinations and the method may vary according the age of the patient.

1. The measure of visual acuity is very important for the determination of a refractive error and also because of the possibility of amblyopia. For patients younger than 1 year, visual acuity is measured by objective means. For patients between 1 and 3 years of age the objective methods are also useful but the subjective methods, such as Allen cards, can be used in addition to address information. For patients between 3 and 5 years of age the letter or Figures chart can be very useful. For patients older than 5 years of age, the Snellen alphabet chart can be used in almost all cases.
2. Subjective refractive test can be performed once the adequate method to measure the visual acuity has been established in each particular patient. Test lenses can be used and the subjective refraction can be performed; as older the patient, more cooperation is expected in the subjective refractory tests. Frequently one eye

possesses more hyperopia in comparison with the another; frequently the deviated eye corresponds to one of higher refractive defect.

3. Once the subjective tests have been performed as much as possible in each particular patient, cycloplegic refraction should be performed on all children by using autorefractor, retinoscope and loose lenses. Cycloplegia can be achieved with Mydriacyl 1% if the patient is younger than 1 year and with Cyclogyl 1% if the patient is 1 year or older. Some physicians like to perform cycloplegia until the complete eye examination has been finished.
4. Frequently stereoacuity is altered. It might be measured using polarized glasses and Titmus test or Randot stereogram.
5. The angle of deviation should be estimated. It can be measured by centration of the corneal light reflex in each eye, while the patient fixes on objects at distance or near and if possible, the alternate cover test can be performed.
6. The complete eye exam should be finalized (extraocular movements, the anterior segment to assess the cornea, anterior chamber, and lens funduscopic examination).

At the Figures 1 and 2 of this chapter we can see Ricardo, a 9-year-old patient of our clinic, who has the diagnosis of AE since he was 2 years of age. In the Figure 1 we can see him actually without glasses, and we are able to observe the esotropia of the left eye. In the second picture we can see him again with test glasses, and we are able to see the correction of the esotropia when testing in a subjective mode, the total cycloplegic refraction. Notice that the angle of deviation decreases when using the test refraction.

DIFFERENTIAL DIAGNOSIS

It must be done with some other causes of strabismus, like Duane syndrome, infantile esotropia, pseudoesotropia, abducens nerve palsy, congenital fibrosis syndrome, and development of neurological disorders.

TREATMENT

Glasses prescription for the refractive error is the treatment of choice for Accommodative Esotropia. Mainly the refractive error is hyperopia, or can be combined with some degree of astigmatism. Also frequently, one eye is more hyperopic than the fellow one; the eye with higher refractive error is the one who is in risk to develop amblyopia. Sometimes it is not possible to start the first refractive correction with the total amount of the refractive error; so in some patients a partial correction for a limited period of time is the correct route to start. Prescription of the full amount of hyperopic correction provides adequate treatment for this disease in 75% of cases. At the Figure 3 of this chapter we can see again to Ricardo, our patient, with his full corrective glasses and we are able to notice the complete correction of the esotropia with their use; compare the degree of deviation with Figure 1, when he is not using correction.

Patching therapy (penalization of the eye with less refractive error) can be done with the objective to avoid or decrease amblyopia. This kind of treatment is adequate at less age of the patient, it means before the critical period of eye function development (4 to 6 years of age); once amblyopia has been established penalization therapy is not useful. This is the importance of avoid the delay onset of treatment; Early treatment of amblyopia may result in improved vision, leading to a better prognosis for binocular vision development and a more stable alignment in cases when surgery is required.

Surgery may be required if the esodeviation becomes refractory to optical treatment. Surgery often is needed when treatment is delayed, but unfortunately it is not able to correct the visual defect –it means that the patient still needs the use of refractive correction and also it does not improve amblyopia when it has been well established. Surgery is performed for the no accommodative component only; it means the residual deviation that can persist after an adequate long-term use of glasses. Surgery is often limited to only the amblyopic eye by performing a recession of the medial rectus and a resection or strengthening of the lateral rectus.

PROGNOSIS AND FOLLOW-UP

The main fact of this disease is that permanent vision loss can occur if strabismus and amblyopia are not treated before patients are 4 to 6 years of age. After this critical age any effort to improve the visual acuity in the amblyopic eye is not useful. So, the physician must emphasize to parents of young patients that regular follow-up care is necessary to avoid, evaluate and treat amblyopia. In cases when amblyopia is being treated (during the critical period) frequent visits are needed (from 1 to each 3 months), while stable patients can be seen by the doctor twice a year.

If glasses are worn faithfully and fusional patterns are established, many patients with refractive esotropia can maintain straight eyes without wearing glasses by the time they are teenagers. So, the early treatment of amblyopia, is the key factor in this disease, and can result in improved

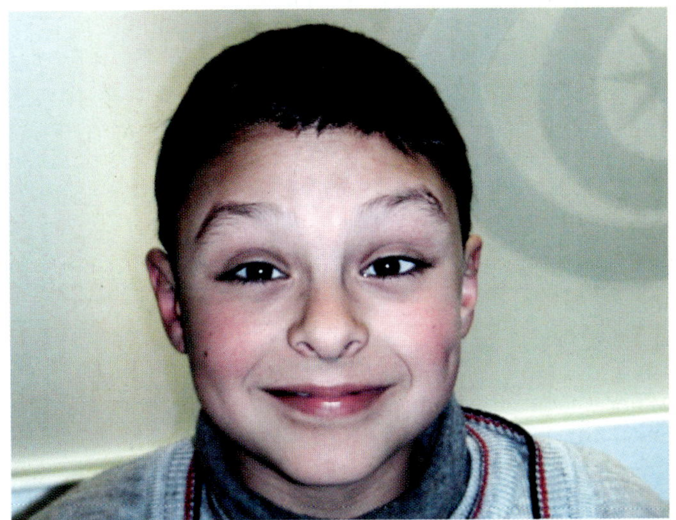

Fig. 1: Ricardo without glasses. Notice the Esotropia LE

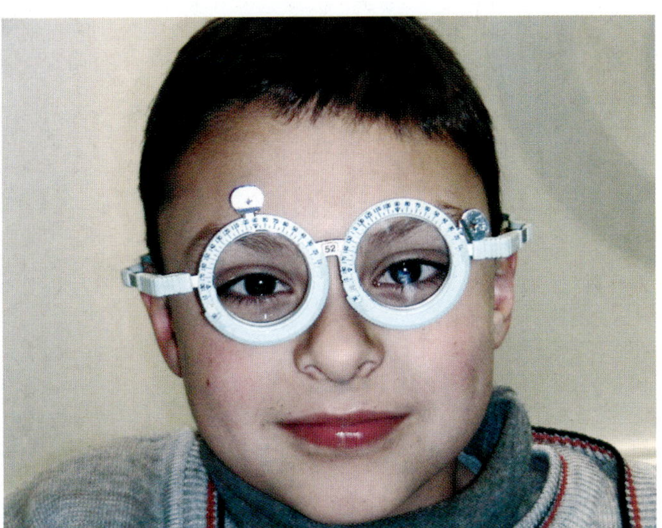

Fig. 2: Ricardo with test glasses. Notice the correction

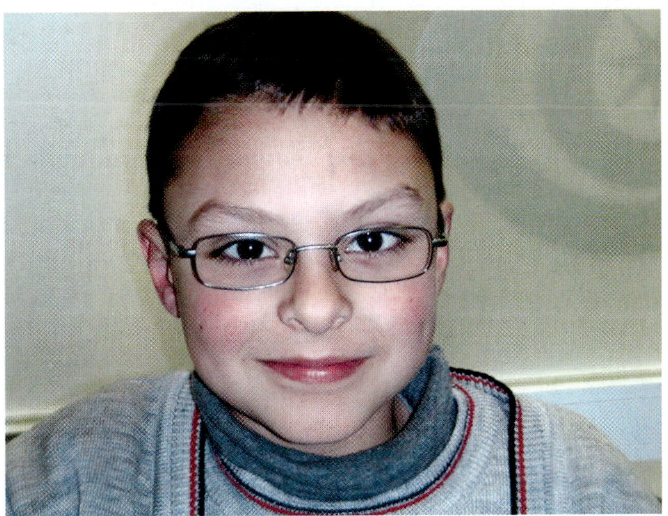

Fig. 3: Ricardo with definitive glasses. Notice the correction

vision, leading to a better prognosis for binocular vision development and a more stable alignment if surgical treatment is decided.

FURTHER READING

1. A Data-Driven Approach to the Management of Accommodative Esotropia, 25 May 2009. Ashvini K. Reddy, Cary H. Freeman, Evelyn A. Paysse, David K. Coats. American Journal of Ophthalmology 2009;148(3):466-70.
2. AE Kertesz, J Kertesz. Wide-field fusional stimulation in strabismus. Am J Optom Physiol Opt 1986;63(3):217-22.
3. Ashok Garg, Jerome Bovet, Bojan Pajic, et al. Surgical and medical management of Pediatric ophthalmology. Jaypee Brothers Medical Publishers. New Delhi, India, 2007.
4. Berson FG. Basic Ophthalmology for Medical Students and Primary Care Residents 1993.
5. Catalano RA, Nelson LB. Pediatric Ophthalmology: A Text Atlas 1994.
6. F Koc, H Ozal, H Yasar, E Firat. Resolution in partially accommodative esotropia during occlusion treatment for amblyopia. Eye 2006:20(3):325-8.
7. Helveston EM, Ellis FD. Pediatric Ophthalmology Practice 1980.
8. PV Berard, A Tassy, JC Deransart-Ferrero, N Mouillac-Gambarelli. Value of pursuit motor electro-oculography in the investigation of esotropia from strabismic amblyopia (author's transl)] . J Fr Ophtalmol 1980;3(12):719-30.
9. Surgical complications in accommodative esotropia. A Putteman Bull Soc Belge Ophthalmol. 1994;253:119-25.
10. The value of press-on prisms in the management of partially accommodative esotropia and surgically overcorrected esotropia. I Jacobucci. Am Orthopt J. January 1977;27:91-5.
11. Wright KW, et al. Pediatric Ophthalmology and Strabismus 1995.

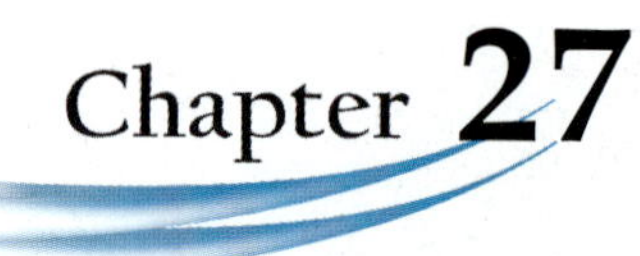

Functional Brain Imaging of Suppression

Marcel PM Ten Tusscher (Belgium)

ABSTRACT

When the two eyes are exposed to dissimilar images, these images either lead to binocular rivalry in which two percepts alternate in dominance or they appear simultaneously. In both conditions, for every point in the visual field, one of two monocular stimuli is finally suppressed. By way of functional magnetic resonance imaging rivalry and simultaneous perception were compared with each other and with reference images that were almost similar between the eyes in order to test which neural structures correlate with binocular differences. It showed that it is not alternation but dissimilarity between the images that correlates with increased activation in the lateral extrastriate, superior parietal and frontal areas. Perceptual suppression is most likely realized in the lateral extrastriate cortex while frontal and parietal areas modulate this process.

Keywords: Binocular vision, binocular rivalry, visual cortex, suppression, functional MRI.

INTRODUCTION

In normal binocular vision images presented to both eyes are integrated into a single interpretation of the visual world: the binocular percept. Hubel and Wiesel provided physiological evidence of convergence of inputs from the two eyes onto the same cortical cells.[8] Each of these binocular cells has two receptive fields, one in each eye. The two receptive fields have similar characteristics which allows the visual system to match the images in the two eyes.[7,8]

If the images in the two eyes do not match either binocular rivalry may occur or a stable binocular mosaic in which both images are superimposed in one composition (simultaneous perception) is perceived. During binocular rivalry the image perceived most often alternates between each monocular view. Single-cell recordings showed that this competition not only occurs in the primary visual cortex (V1) but also after V1.[11,12] A large number of neurones in the early visual areas remain active during the perceptual suppression of the stimulus. Therefore, most likely it is not the images presented on the retina of both eyes, but neural representations of stimuli that compete during rivalry.[11,12] A functional magnetic resonance imaging (fMRI) study in humans, focussing on transitions during rivalry, showed an increase in activation in frontal and parietal areas during transitions while there was no increase during a passive replay of the same scenes. This experiment suggests that during rivalry higher cortical areas regulate the alternation of binocular percepts .[13]

In the present study, functional magnetic resonance imaging was used to investigate, more generally, which cortical areas are involved when images projected on the two retinae do not match both during binocular rivalry, in which interocular competition gives rise to perceptual transitions and during simultaneous perception, in which interocular competition leads to a stable mosaic without transitions. Both conditions were individually matched to reference viewing conditions that were more similar between eyes.

MATERIALS AND METHODS

Subjects and Images FMRI scans were performed in seven individuals (four males and three females) in four viewing conditions: simultaneous perception and binocular rivalry both contrasted with appropriate reference conditions. Experiments were undertaken with the understanding and written consent of each subject according the tenets of the declaration of Helsinki. Prior to imaging, individuals were tested as to their ability to notice simultaneous perception and rivalry with slides comparable to the ones used during the experiments. Participants wore non-metallic red-green glasses. A mirror placed in front of the eyes brought to view a screen onto which every 15 seconds a new slide was projected. A uniform background and surrounding were presented in all slides during both test and reference conditions. The center was made up of green and red elements in the active viewing conditions, while the same

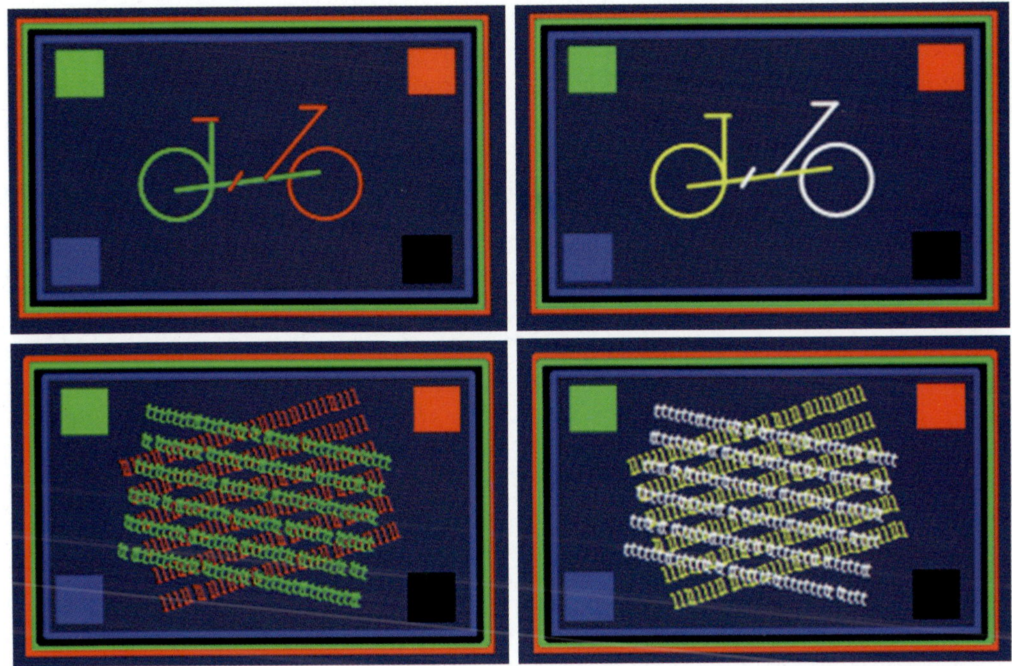

Fig. 1: Examples of images presented during fMRI scanning. Viewing through red and green filter glasses created dichoptic conditions. The images on the left show examples of test conditions during simultaneous perception (top) and binocular rivalry (down). On the right are examples of reference conditions for simultaneous perception (top), binocular rivalry (down)

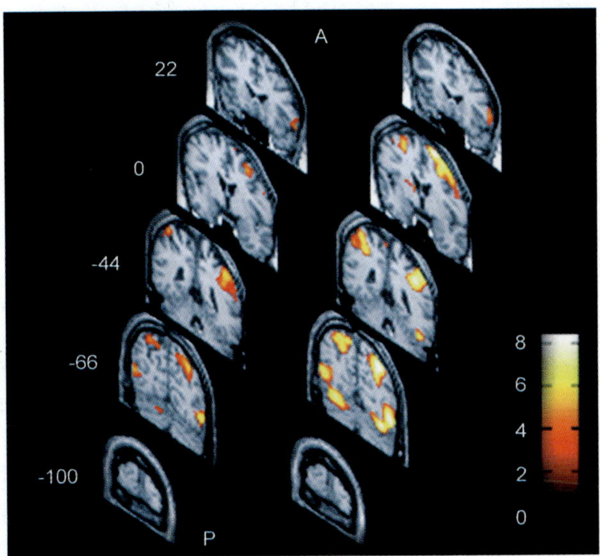

Fig. 2: Cortical areas engaged in simultaneous perception (left) and binocular rivalry (right). The colored areas represent activation foci with significant Z-values (P<0.05, corrected for multiple comparisons) from seven subjects superimposed on the normalised MR image of one subject. The co-ordinates of the coronal slices are given in mm with respect to the Talairach co-ordinate system. L: left; R: right; A: anterior; P: posterior. During both simultaneous perception and rivalry the lateral extrastriate area and frontoparietal areas showed increased activation. Note that there is a higher activation rise during rivalry as compared to simultaneous perception and only during rivalry the fusiform area shows more activation

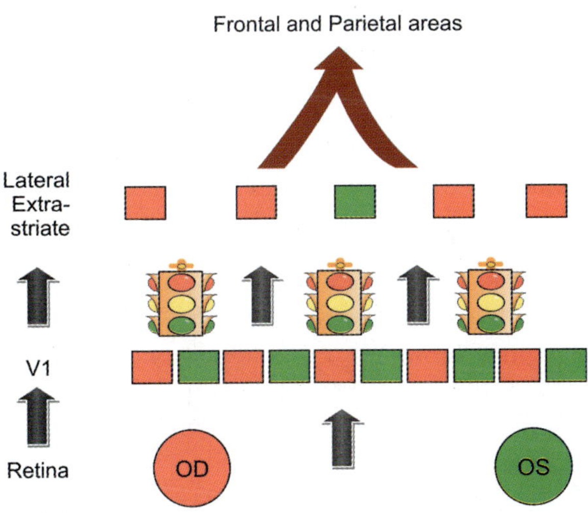

Fig. 3: Binocular melting. The diagram suggests how images projected on the retina of both eyes, that do not match appear in the striate columns. By way of timing a temporal solution is found up till the lateral extrastriate area where a choice between monocular inputs is made. Frontal and parietal cortical areas modulate the melting process. OD: right eye; OS: left eye.

elements were used in yellow and white during reference viewing. One example of all four conditions are given in Figure 1. While viewing these red-green dichoptically presented stimuli the uniform surrounding upholds peripheral fusion. So, simultaneous perception will not give rise to rivalry due to loss of fusion. As a consequence also reference conditions contain binocular differences. Nevertheless, although differences between test and reference conditions were very subtle highly significant results could be obtained. During simultaneous perception and its reference the images used were line drawings of objects and faces. In binocular rivalry gratings, red perpendicular to green, or white to yellow, were presented.

MRI Protocol

Images were acquired on a 1.5 Tesla Philips ACS-NT scanner (Philips, Medical systems, Best, The Netherlands), which was equipped with the standard receiver head coil. Head fixation was accomplished by two foam cushions and by a tape across the subject's forehead. On the basis of T1-weighted survey scans in three orthogonal directions, an approximately 12 cm thick stack of slices was defined, encompassing transversal slices that covered the entire cerebrum and as much as possible of the cerebellum. The functional scan session consisted of a single shot multiple slice T2 sensitive echo planar imaging (EPI) sequence, with parameters TR 5600 ms, TE 40 ms, flip angle 90°, matrix dimension 64 × 64, 32 continuous slices and an isotropic voxel size of 3.5 mm. This functional pulse sequence is sensitive to the blood oxygen level .[9,15] Before the acquisition of functional images started, two dummy full brain scans were acquired to run the system into a stable stationary mode. For anatomical reference, a 3D T1-weighted fast-field echo scan succeeded the functional scans with parameters TR 11 ms, TE 3.5 ms, flip angle 90 °, matrix dimensions 256 × 256, typically 150 continuous slices and an isotropic voxel size of 1 mm.

Data Analysis

The imaging data were analyzed using the Statistical Parametric Mapping (SPM 96; Wellcome Department of Cognitive Neurology, London, UK) software package implemented in MATLAB (Mathworks, Inc., Sherborn, MA) and run on a Ultra SPARC workstation (Sun Microsystems, Mountain View, CA). The scans were corrected for small motion artefacts by 3D rigid-body realignment to the first volume scan of the time-series. Subsequently, the images were normalized[1] by transformation into standard space, using the EPI template image of the MNI (Montreal Neurological Institute) as a reference to the stereotaxic atlas of Talairach and Tournoux.[19] To enhance the spatial signal to noise ratio and to facilitate intersubject averaging normalized images were smoothed with a Gaussian filter with a full-width at half maximum of 8 mm. For each subject as well as for the whole group, all dichoptic conditions and control conditions were specified in the appropriate design matrices.[2] Fluctuations of global activity were corrected by proportional scaling to a mean value. In the SPM design signal deflections due to activation from the baseline level were modelled by a boxcar function, of which the amplitude was statistically assessed by calculating Z-values. Temporal smoothing and a low-pass filter were applied to enhance the part of the hemodynamic response correlating to the stimulus time course.[3]

RESULTS

Table 1 summarizes the significance and localization of cortical activation in different viewing conditions. Cortical activation during conditions is visualized in Figure 2.

Table 1: Significant Z-scores and Talairach co-ordinates of cortical areas engaged in different viewing conditions are given. Only the most significant peaks (P<0.001) within areas of increased activation are reported. sup: superior; mid: middle; inf: inferior

	Z-score	*x,y,z (mm)*			*Cortical area*
Simultaneous perception					
	7.3	32	-66	52	right sup. Parietal
	5.4	-42	-44	60	left sup. Parietal
	5.6	-42	56	-4	left mid. Frontal
	4.8	-38	22	-2	left inf. Frontal
	5.4	32	0	54	right sup. Frontal
	5.1	60	22	-2	right inf. Frontal
	7.2	50	-72	0	right mid. Occipital
	5.6	-50	-72	2	left mid. Occipital
Binocular rivalry					
	8.3	36	-64	52	right sup. Parietal
	7.7	-34	-54	56	left sup. Parietal
	8.0	60	-4	60	right sup. Frontal
	7.2	-26	-4	52	left sup. Frontal
	7.7	61	10	28	right mid, inf. Frontal
	5.9	-52	8	30	left mid, inf Frontal
	8.0	50	-66	-4	right mid. Occipital
	7.9	-48	-70	-2	left mid. Occipital
	7.9	35	-70	-18	right fusiform
	7.5	-34	-64	-20	left fusiform
Rivalry>Simultaneous					
	6.5	32	-76	-16	right fusiform
	6.3	20	0	66	right sup. Frontal
	6.2	-42	-78	14	left mid. Occipital
	5.5	-12	-66	60	left sup. Parietal

Simultaneous perception. Areas that were more activated during superimposition were the middle occipital gyrus (lateral extrastriate area; Brodmann area 19), superior parietal (Brodmann area 7) and frontal areas. These areas showed activation in all individuals tested except for the frontal areas which showed increased activation only in five of them. The largest rise in activation was found in the right superior parietal lobe. Overall activation during this condition was less than during rivalry.

Binocular rivalry. In addition to the areas activated during simultaneous perception the fusiform gyrus (Brodmann area 19) showed increased activation during rivalry. The results were comparable throughout all subjects.

Rivalry compared with simultaneous perception. In order to compare conditions active rivalry –reference rivalry> active simultaneous perception- reference simultaneous perception was studied. The fusiform area, the lateral extrastriate and frontoparietal areas again showed more activation. A significant difference between rivalry and simultaneous perception did not appear in the striate cortex.

DISCUSSION

During presentation of images that do not match between the eyes, both in stable simultaneous perception and binocular rivalry, the middle occipital gyrus (lateral extrastriate area), the superior parietal lobe and frontal areas show highly significant increased activation in the present experiment (Fig. 2, Table 1). This means that superimposition of two dissimilar images correlates with the same cortical areas engaged during alternation from one image to another in rivalry. Lumer et al[13] showed that transitions compared to passively changing scenes correlate with an activation increase in frontoparietal areas. This experiment suggested that alternation itself is regulated by frontoparietal areas. The present study shows that also by probing the rivalry-state, without explicitly selecting transition events, results were virtually the same for the locations and strength of activities as in the experiment by Lumer et al.[13] These same areas, however, were presently found activated during the whole process of rivalry and also during stable simultaneous perception. During simultaneous perception there are no transitions. Both during binocular rivalry and simultaneous perception conflicting stimuli are presented to binocular neurones in V1. Suppression was found to occur as early as in the lateral geniculate body.[6] Lumer et al, however, did not compare transitions during rivalry with episodes between transitions but with a replay. During the replay there were no binocular dissimilarities. Somewhere a choice is made between the input of both eyes. Since there is no direct correlation between what we perceive and the image presented in V1 the choice between inputs must be made after V1.[11,12] Results of human event-related brain potentials to transitions from rivalrous to non-rivalrous stimulation suggested that rivalry is resolved at the latest in extrastriate areas.[9] At the level of V1 the final choice is likely postponed by way of timing of action potentials.[14] The present study corroborates these suggestions since conflicting stimuli both during rivalry and simultaneous perception reveal the same activation in V1. If a choice between stimuli would be made in V1 no activation was found in the present experiment after V1. The visual area that showed increased activation during both simultaneous perception and binocular rivalry is the lateral extrastriate area. The activation increase found in the lateral extrastriate area evoked during rivalry was higher than during simultaneous perception (Z=6.17). So, the site in the occipital lobe where alternating retinal monocular inputs change into a percept must be the lateral extrastriate area. Earlier visual areas did neither show differences in activation between rivalry and simultaneous perception nor differences between active and reference conditions. Apparently stimuli that do not match have the same hemodynamic consequences in these earlier visual areas. It was suggested that integration and rivalry are solved by co-ordination of actionpotential timing in V1.[14] We therefore, assume that non-matching stimuli alternate with one another from the binocular neurones in V1 till the lateral extrastriate area. The superfluous stimulus is suppressed (or the perceptual stimulus gets the attention) in the lateral extrastriate area. Most likely, this process is modulated by frontal and parietal neurones.

Besides similarities in cortical activation for simultaneous perception and binocular rivalry, we found two striking differences. First, in all subjects only during rivalry there was activation in the fusiform gyrus. This corroborates the experiment by Lumer et al[13] in which the fusiform gyrus appeared to show increased activation during rivalry. However, this activation was found also during passive replay when visual scenes change all the time. So, the fusiform gyrus reacts to, but not initiates, changes of scenes. The exclusive activation during rivalry in the present experiment agrees with the fact that transitions did not occur during simultaneous perception. The second difference obtained was the much higher activation in all areas involved during rivalry than during simultaneous perception. Obviously, generating alternations during rivalry puts higher demands on the hemodynamic response than stable perception does.

Why do frontal and parietal areas correlate with binocular rivalry and more generally with non-matching stimuli? In the present study the superior parietal cortex appeared to be the area with the highest activation both during rivalry and simultaneous perception. It has been suggested that the frontoparietal areas play a central role in conscious perception and are specifically related to perceptual transition.[13] We demonstrate with simultaneous perception that these areas are also engaged when there are no transitions. It was found recently that units in the posterior parietal cortex contribute to attending to and remembering shape features.[16] Neurophysiological experiments in monkeys revealed that neurones in this area may play a role in redirecting visual attention.[18] By using event related potentials (ERP) in humans it was shown that visual-spatial attention modulates neural activity in the lateral extrastriate cortex but does not affect the initial evoked response in striate cortex.[4] So, possibly in the lateral extrastriate cortex (middle occipital gyrus) parts of both images are selected by way of directed attention. This also is in accordance with an ERP and fMRI study[15] that revealed attention-related increases in blood flow in the posterior fusiform and middle occipital gyri in the hemisphere contralateral to attended visual stimuli. A possible function during binocular blending for frontal cortical areas is even more speculative. A change in the selection of a fragment from one eye's image to the other is complicated by differences in the subjective visual directions of both eyes. However, areas in the frontal cortex of the macaque monkey turned out to contain neurones with visual receptive fields that remain in the same location, even when the monkey is not fixating or is moving the eyes.[5]

In conclusion, increased activation of the lateral extrastriate, parietal and frontal cortical areas during both stable simultaneous perception and binocular rivalry is explained by a sequence of processing in which both monocular images that do not match remain available after the primary visual cortex. The choice between monocular inputs is most probably made in the lateral extrastriate areas while frontal and parietal areas modulate this choice (Fig. 3).

REFERENCES

1. Friston KJ, Ashburner J, Frith CD, Poline JB, Heather JD, Frackowiak RSJ. Spatial Registration and Normalization of Images, Hum Brain Mapping 1995;2:165-89.
2. Friston KJ, Holmes AP, Worsley KJ, Poline J-B, Frith CD, Frackowiak RSJ, Statistical Parametric Maps in Functional Imaging, Hum Brain Mapping 1995;2:189-210.
3. Friston KJ, Jezzard P, Turner R. Analysis of Functional MRI Time-Series, Hum Brain Mapping 1994;1:153-71.
4. Gomez-Gonzalez CM, Clark VP, Fan S, Luck SJ, Hillyard SA. Sources of attention sensitive event-related potentials. Brain Topogr 1994; 7: 41-51.
5. Graziano MS, Gross CG. Visual responses with and without fixation: neurons in premotor cortex encode spatial locations independently of eye position, Exp Brain Res 1998;118: 373-80.
6. Haynes JD, Deichmann R, Rees G. Eye-specific effects of binocular rivalry in the human lateral geniculate nucleus, Nature 2005;438:496-9.
7. Hammond P, Fothergill LK. Interocular comparison of length summation and end-inhibition in striate cortical neurones of the anaesthetized cat, Proc. Physiol. Soc. 1991; 446:232-8.
8. Hubel DH, Wiesel TN, Receptive fields of single neurones in the cat's visual cortex, J. Physiol 1959;148:574-91.
9. Kaernbach C, Schroger E, Jacobsen T, Roeber U. Effects of consciousness on human brain waves following binocular rivalry, NeuroReport 1999;10:713-6.
10. Kwong KK, Belliveau JW, Chesler DA, et al. Dynamic magnetic resonance imaging of human brain activity during primary sensory stimulation, Proc Natl Acad Sci 1992;89:5675-79.
11. Leopold DA, Logothetis NK. Activity changes in early visual cortex reflect monkeys' percepts during binocular rivalry, Nature 1996;379:549-53.
12. Logothetis NK, Leopold DA, Sheinberg DL. What is rivalling during binocular rivalry?, Nature 1996; 380:621-4.
13. Lumer ED, Friston KJ, Rees G. Neural correlates of perceptual rivalry in the human brain, Science 1998;280:1930-34.
14. Lumer ED, A neural model of binocular integration and rivalry based on the coordination of actionpotential timing in primary visual cortex, Cereb. Cortex 1998;8:553-61.
15. Mangun GR, Buonocore MH, Girelli M, Jha AP. ERP and fMRI measures of visual spatial selective attention, Hum. Brain. Mapping 1998;6:383-9.
16. Ogawa S, Tank DW, Menon R, et al. Intrinsic signal changes accompanying sensory stimulation: Functional brain mapping with magnetic resonance imaging, Proc Natl Acad Sci USA 1992;89:5951-5.
17. Sereno AB, Maunsell JH. Shape selectivity in primate lateral intraparietal cortex. Nature 1998;395:500-03.
18. Steinmetz MA, Constantinidis C. Neurophysiological evidence for a role of posterior parietal cortex in redirecting visual attention. Cereb Cortex 1995;5:448-56.
19. Talairach J, Tournoux P (Eds). Co-planar stereotaxic atlas of the human brain. Stuttgart: Georg Thieme Verlag 1998.

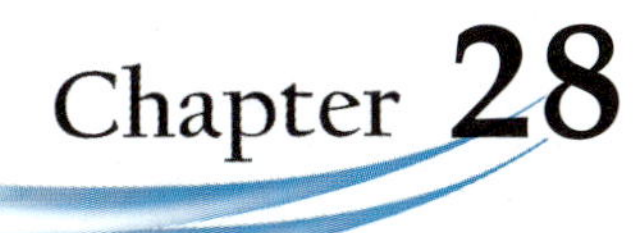

Managing Amblyopia with Corneal Wavefront-guided Lasik in Children

Keiki R Mehta, Cyres K Mehta (India)

Amblyopia is the most common cause of visual impairment in childhood. The condition affects approximately 2 to 3 out of every 100 children.

Unless it is successfully treated in early childhood, amblyopia usually persists into adulthood, and is the most common cause of monocular (one eye) visual impairment among children and young and middle-aged adults.

The American Academy of Ophthalmology, in its preferred pattern, gives the prevalence estimates range from 1 to 5 percent depending on the population studied and the definition used.[3-6,8-11] It states that 2 percent is generally accepted to be a conservative estimate based on surveys of school children and selected adult populations (military recruits) in the United States and abroad.[3-6] Over half of the amblyopic children in one study had visual acuity of 20/80 or worse in the amblyopic eye.[11]

The visual pathways continue to develop from birth to approximately age 10, with the most rapid progression occurring in infancy. Based on cases of amblyopia detected in infancy but treated suboptimally, it appears that the potential for the development of amblyopia persists to approximately age 10, at which time plasticity of the visual pathways ceases. The visual impairment from amblyopia will become permanent and will result in lifelong visual loss if it is untreated or insufficiently treated in early childhood.

Pattern deprivation, or severe blurring due to media opacities, through the first 3 postnatal months produces profound and permanent reductions in spatial (e.g. grating or optotype) acuity, typically to the level of legal blindness in the affected eye(s). Similar deprivation after 3 months of age but before 30 months can lead to less profound visual acuity reduction but still in the range of 20/200 or less.[20-23]

Deprivation commencing between the ages of 30 months and 8 years differs only in that vision is reduced at a slower rate and is more likely to respond to subsequent therapy.[20]

The progression of amblyopia in early childhood is inversely proportional to the child's age: the younger the child, the faster the progression. Amblyopia is a risk factor for the development of strabismus and reduction of binocularity, and strabismus is a risk factor for the development of amblyopia. In young children, treatment improves the visual deficit and can foster the redevelopment of binocular vision more rapidly and completely.

CAUSES OF AMBLYOPIA

Animal and human research conducted over the last several decades has shown that amblyopia is associated with maldevelopment of the visual pathways in the brain.[27-32]

The three primary causes of amblyopia, all associated with abnormal visual input, are pattern deprivation, strabismus, and optical defocus.

Pattern deprivation is the most amblyogenic. Pattern deprivation patients at greatest risk for visual acuity reduction are infants who experience early pattern deprivation, and the effect on visual development is compounded when only one eye is affected. Pattern deprivation is the result of media opacities such as a dense cataract, uncorrected aphakia, large uncorrected refractive errors, or a dense corneal opacity. The visual acuity outcome may be excellent in some young children who have binocular or monocular cataract surgery that is followed by rapid optical correction and properly administered occlusion of the nonamblyopic eye.[38, 39]

Patients with high degrees of axial ametropia in one eye often have relatively resistant amblyopia.

Strabismus

Strabismus (ocular misalignment) deprives the visual cortex of the synchronous stimulus of corresponding images from the two foveas.

Optical Defocus

Optical defocus generally causes milder amblyopia that is relatively amenable to therapy. It is the result of a refractive error that selectively removes fine details (high spatial frequencies) from the retinal image with a relative preservation of low frequencies. Optical defocus can be uni- or bilateral and can be related to astigmatism and/or differences in the spherical refractive error between the eyes.

The prevalence and severity of amblyopia also increases with increasing amounts of anisometropia.[50-54] Amblyopia generally occurs in the more hyperopic eye, except in cases of high axial myopia where the highly myopic eye is at greater risk. Studies of anisometropic patients indicate an amblyopia prevalence of 100 percent in hyperopes with 4.0 diopters (D) of anisometropia and in myopes with 6.0 D of anisometropia, and 50 percent for hyperopes with 2.5 D of anisometropia and myopes with 4.0 D of anisometropia.[50,51]

Rationale for Treatment

The value of normal visual function and the effectiveness of treatment justify the difficulty and inconvenience of managing amblyopia in children. Successful treatment of amblyopia improves visual acuity and binocularity, and binocular vision makes work-related activities, activities of daily life, and recreational activities easier to perform.

Normal vision in each eye and binocular vision may have a beneficial effect or be required for a variety of visually demanding career fields.[61]

The difficulties of treatment must be weighed against the potential lifetime benefit of successful treatment.

How is amblyopia treated in children?

Treating amblyopia involves making the child use the eye with the reduced vision (weaker eye). Currently, there are two ways used to do this:

Atropine

Instilled in the stronger eye once a day to temporarily blur the vision so that the child will prefer to use the eye with amblyopia. Treatment with atropine also stimulates vision in the weaker eye and helps the part of the brain that manages vision develop more completely.

Patching

An opaque, adhesive patch is worn over the stronger eye for weeks to months. This therapy forces the child to use the eye with amblyopia. Patching stimulates vision in the weaker eye and helps the part of the brain that manages vision develop more completely.

Previously, eye care professionals often thought that treating amblyopia in older children would be of little benefit. However, surprising results from a nationwide clinical trial ATS 3 : NEI Study shows that many children age seven through 17 with amblyopia may benefit from treatments that are more commonly used on younger children. This study shows that age alone should not be used as a factor to decide whether or not to treat a child for amblyopia

For patients 7 to <13 years old, prescribing 2 to 6 hours per day of patching with near activities and atropine can improve visual acuity even if the amblyopia has been previously treated.

For patients 13 to <18 years old, prescribing patching 2 to 6 hours per day with near activities may improve visual acuity when amblyopia has not been previously treated but appears to be of little benefit if amblyopia was previously treated with patching.

Amblyopia treatment study: A randomized trial to evaluate 2 hours of daily patching for amblyopia in children 3 to < 7 years old with moderate to severe amblyopia

Results

1. Refractive correction alone improves visual acuity in many cases and results in resolution of amblyopia in *at least one third* of 3 to <7-year-old children with untreated anisometropic amblyopia.
2. Following a period of treatment with spectacles, two hours of daily patching combined with one hour of near visual activities modestly improves moderate to severe amblyopia in children 3 to 7 years old still further.

- No of children 16
- Ages 2 year to 11 years
- Sex ratio 11 females/ 5 males

• Power	No
• -5.00 to 7.75	5
• -8.00 to -11.00	6
• +3.00 to +4.75	3
• +5.00 to +7.00	2

Fig. 1: Demographics

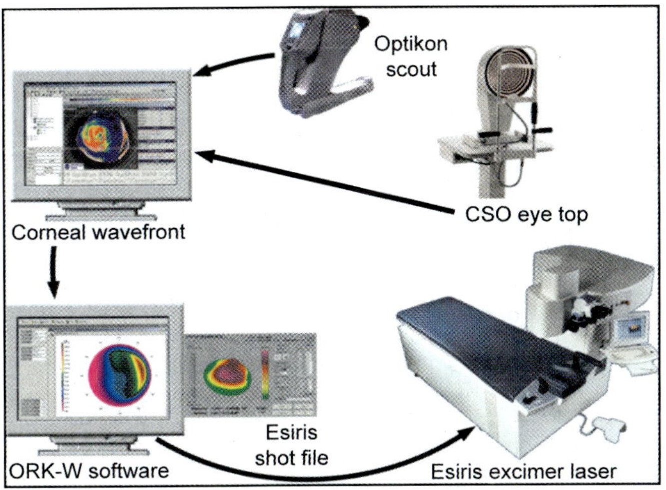

Fig. 2: The Schwind platform

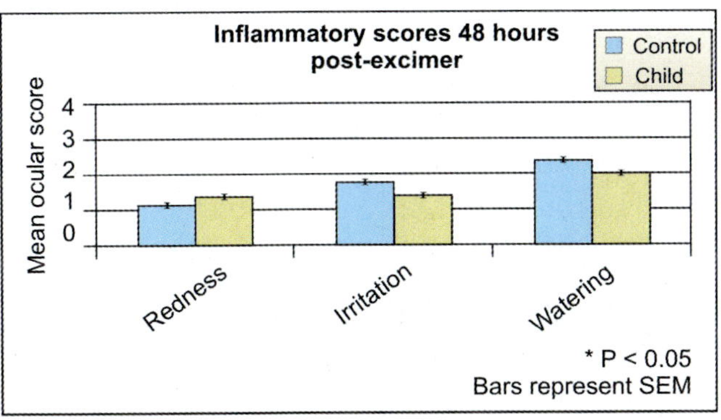

Fig. 3: Eye settling down under therapeutic contact lens

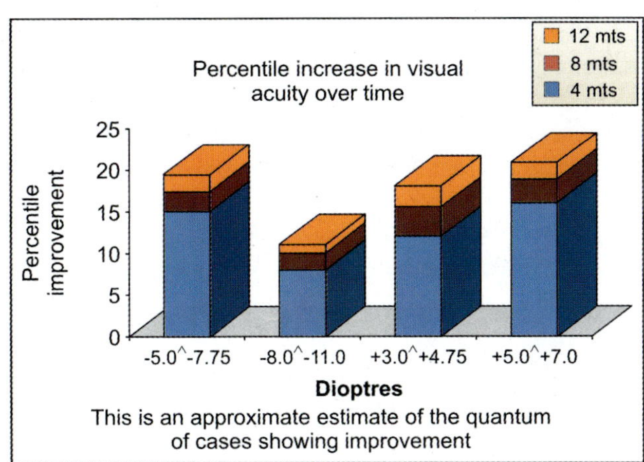

Fig. 4: Estimated visual acuity following excimer

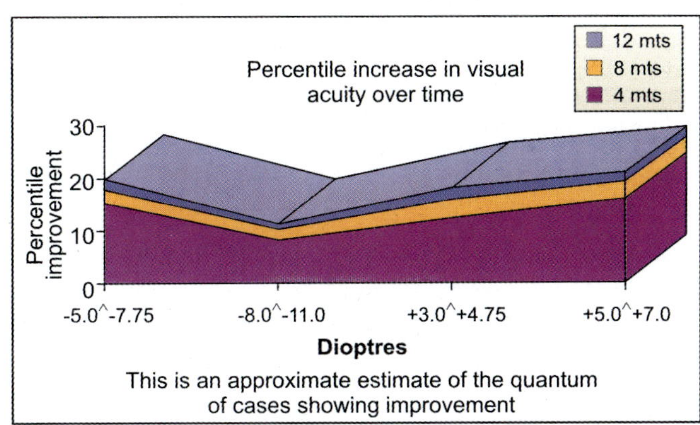

Fig. 5: Estimated visual acuity following excimer

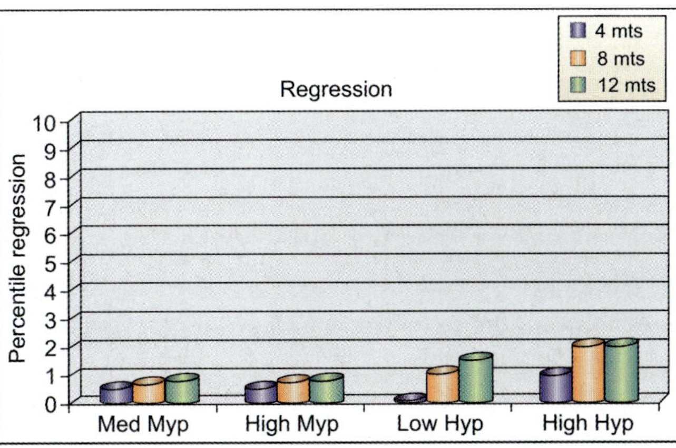

Fig. 6: Regression following Lasik

In the Amblyopia Treatment Study, 215 children were randomly assigned to receive patching, and 204 were assigned to receive atropine eyedrops. *Researchers found that 79 percent of those receiving the eye patch were treated successfully, and that 74 percent of those receiving the atropine were treated successfully.* This difference is clinically insignificant. Although researchers found that vision in the amblyopic eye improved faster in the patching group, the *difference in the two groups at six months* was small and not significant.

This study shows that *one drop a day of atropine* works as well as patching the eye for some children with amblyopia. Since both patching and atropine work equally well, the choice of treatment can be made by the eye care professional in consultation with the parent."

Problems for excimer laser refractive surgery with children:

- Children need GA for refractive surgery
- Lack of fixation can interfere with pupil centration
- Difficult in managing post excimer care
- Children are inveterate eye rubbers.
- Difficulty in keeping safety glasses.

Standard treatment for anisometropia amblyopia

- Spectacles
- Contact lenses

With occlusion or penalization (atropine) of the sound eye

Children non-compliant because:

Intolerant to spectacles if the anisometropia is severe because of resultant aniseikonia and diplopia caused by the refractive correction.

Customary tolerance limit is 5 to 6 percent aniseikonia (2-3D anisometropia) after which image disparity is intolerable.

Children non-compliant because:

- Child has one good eye and perceives no benefit from glasses or contact lenses and rejects them
- Contact lens insertion and removal is traumatic for child and parents.

Our criteria for Lasik in children

- Anisomyopia of at least 5 D or anisohyperopia of at least 3 D
- Poor compliance with spectacles or contact lenses and occlusion therapy.
- Total disinclination of parents despite counseling
- Amblyopia of the eye with the better vision at least 3 Snellen lines better than the BCVA of the amblyopic eye.

Refractive goals in the child

- Emmetropia or reduction of anisometropia to less than 3 D up to a max of 9 D myopia or 6 D hyperopia.
- All Lasik patients to have a 1 hour post Lasik occlusion *on moving image format* for 6 months.

Follow-up schedule

- Every alternate week for 2 months
- Every 2 months for 6 months
- Every 4 months subsequently

Examination schedule

- Corneal haze
- Topography
- Visual acuity
- Sterioacuity
- Change in ocular alignment

Caution with our study

- Small sample size
- Short follow-up
- Inability to pick and choose children from alter cohort
- Selection bias is a weakness in all studies

Examination protocol

- VA charts as applicable
- UCVA/BCVA
- Cycloplegic refraction
- Sterioacuity testing
- Ocular motility
- Airpuff IOP
- Biomicroscopy
- Funduscopy.
- Scout Keratometry
- Non-contact pachymetry

CONCLUSION

- Up to 16 month follow-up demonstrated improvement in UCVA and BCVA and steriopsis in children.
- Refractive errors seem to be stable after 9 months.
- Only moderate improvements in VA, probably because amblyopia may be long-standing, deeply ingrained and severe.
- At the last follow-up visit 86 percent of our cases were within 1.00 diopter (SE) of the target.

- Up to 16 month follow-up demonstrated improvement in UCVA and BCVA and stereopsis in children.
- Refractive errors seem to be stable after 9 months ?
- Only moderate improvements in VA, probably because amblyopia may be long standing , deeply ingrained and severe

Fig. 7: Conclusion

- At the last follow-up visit 86% of our cases were within 1.00 diopter (SE) of the target .
- Stereoacuity improved in 8 of 11 children where it could be elicited
- High myopic children had a poorer initial and final visual acuity as compared to the other groups and occlusion did not significantly help this subgroup.

Fig. 8: Conclusions

Let me describe two cases from our one of our "outstanding series" group.

Fig. 9

- These two cases occurred in the last 14 months when we , having our new Schwind Esiris Laser with the Corneal topographer and aberrometer were better able to analyze the cases.
- The first case straight from 6/36 to 6/9 part in 3 days falt..

Fig. 10

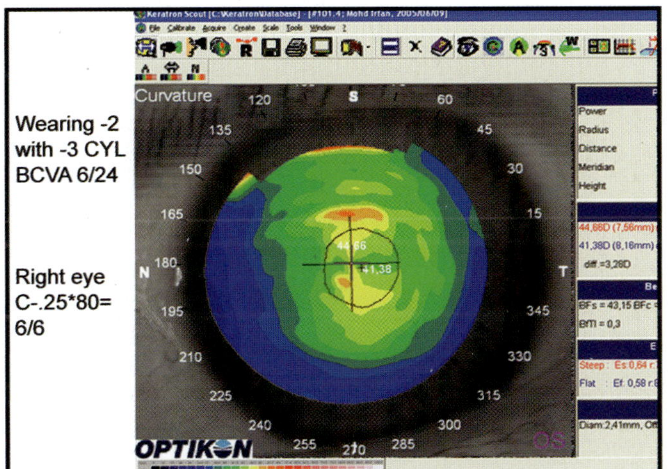

Fig. 11: Anisometropic amblyopia—27/M

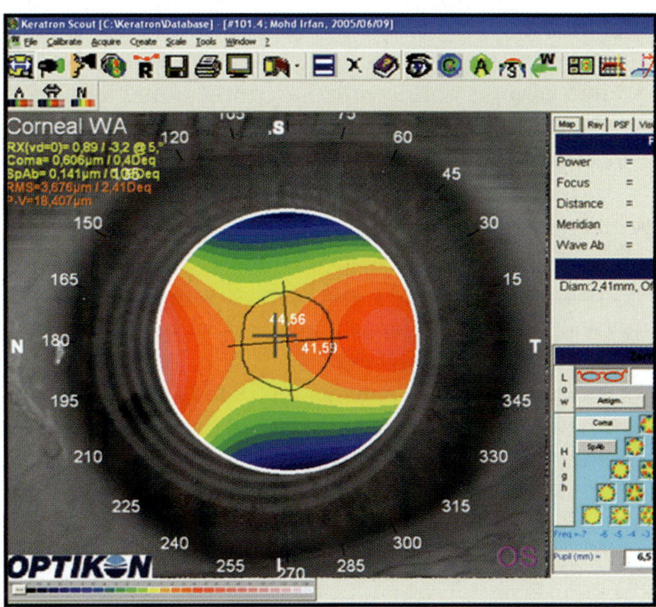

Fig. 12: Corneal wavefront

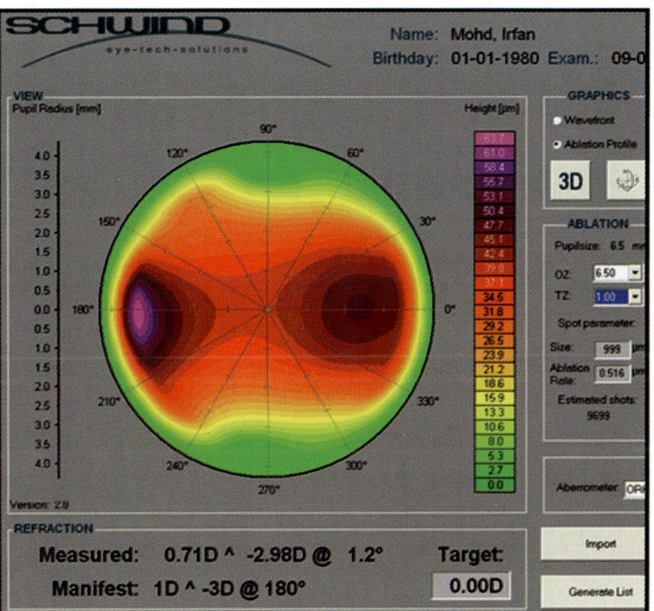

Fig. 13: Shotfile—ablation pattern

- Sterioacuity improved in 8 of 11 children where it could be elicited
- High myopic children had a poorer initial and final visual acuity as compared to the other groups and occlusion did not significantly help this subgroup.

And how does our data compare with international results published.

Nucci P; Drack AV refractive surgery for unilateral high myopia in children J *AAPOS. 2001; 5(6):348-51.* University of Milan, Department of Ophthalmology, San Paolo Hospital, Milan, Italy.

Fourteen eyes of 14 patients aged 9 to 14 years received refractive surgery. The vision of 5 of 14 patients improved 1 or 2 lines after refractive surgery. Two patients who had 20/80 vision preoperatively improved to 20/60. No patients lost any lines of vision. All 4 patients demonstrated stereopsis preoperatively, and all retained postoperatively.

O'Keefe M; Nolan. L LASIK surgery in children. Br J Ophthalmol. 2004; 88(1):19-21: Mater Private Hospital and Children's University Hospital, Temple Street, Dublin 1,

Six children with high myopia ranging from -5.00DS to -16DS were treated. Five children had improved refraction and visual acuity post-LASIK. Stereopsis improved in 4.

Baylor College of Medicine, Texas Children's Hospital, Houston, Texas 77030, USA.

Eleven children, 2 to 11 years old, with anisometropic amblyopia who were noncompliant with conventional therapy with glasses or contact lenses and occlusion therapy were treated with PRK. Five (71 %) of the 7 children had uncorrected VA improvement of at least 2 lines, and 4 (57 %) of 7 had best spectacle-corrected VA improvement of at least 2 lines, with 1 improving 7 lines. Five (55 %) of 9 children had improvement of their stereoacuity at last follow-up.

Phillips CB; Prager TC; McClellan G; Mintz-Hittner HA. Laser in situ keratomileusis for treated anisometropic amblyopia in awake, autofixating pediatric and adolescent patients. J Cataract Refract Surg 2004; 30(12):2522-8.

Department of Ophthalmology and Visual Science, University of Texas-Houston Medical School, Houston, Texas, USA.

Seventeen patients were treated in the amblyopic eye only to correct anisometropia, followed for a mean of 18.0 months. Anisometropia decreased uniformly to less than 2.00 D in all patients (mean 1.52 D). The percentage of patients with stereoacuity increased from 63.0 percent preoperatively to 84.0 percent postoperatively.

Conclusion: The value of normal visual function and the effectiveness of treatment justify the difficulty and inconvenience of managing amblyopia in children. Successful treatment of amblyopia improves visual acuity and binocularity, and binocular vision makes work-related activities, activities of daily life, and recreational activities easier to perform. Normal vision in each eye and binocular vision may have a beneficial effect or be required for a variety of visually demanding career fields.[61]

Obviously we need to rethink the entire concept. There would seem to be a hope now for amblyopes which earlier were simply left unattended. One of us (CKM) has named this concept as "Corblyopia" which we now feel is a viable subset of Amblyopia. We now do feel that every patient should undergo a corneal wavefront analysis as a routine examination. Considering that we have now done Corneal wavefront Lasik on children as small as 8 and that too with good results, we do feel that a cut off age now no longer applies.[63] The difficulties of treatment must be weighed against the potential lifetime benefit of successful treatment.

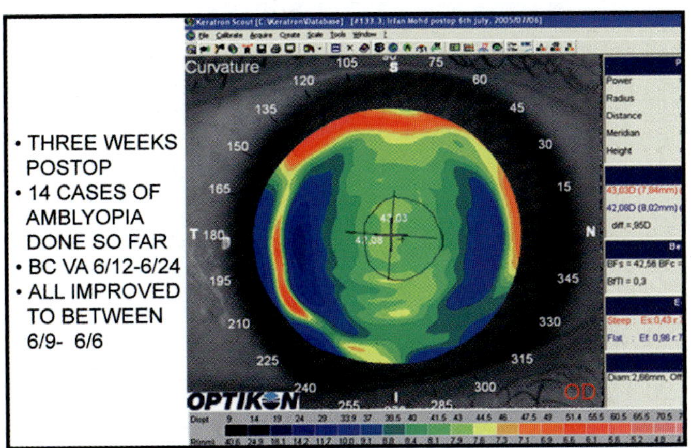

Fig. 14: Postoperative topography and wavefront—UCVA 6/6

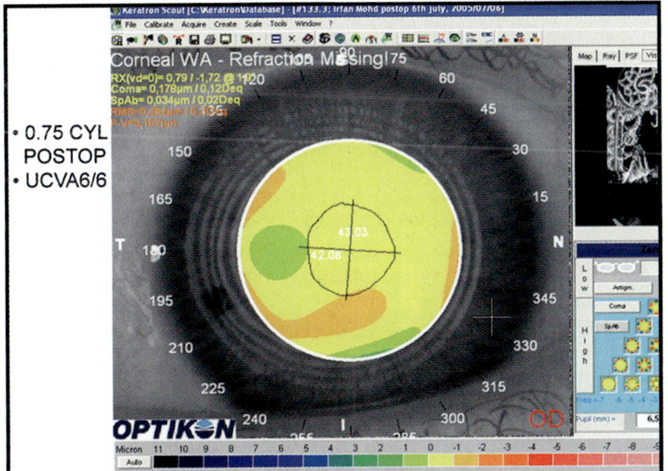

Fig. 15: Postoperative wavefront, minimal aberrations 3 wks postoperative

An yet another. We felt he was a simple amblyopia. Told the father he "may" improve by one or two lines and that to after 6-8 months of penalization. We were surprised to see the improvement to almost 6/9 Snellen.

Fig. 16

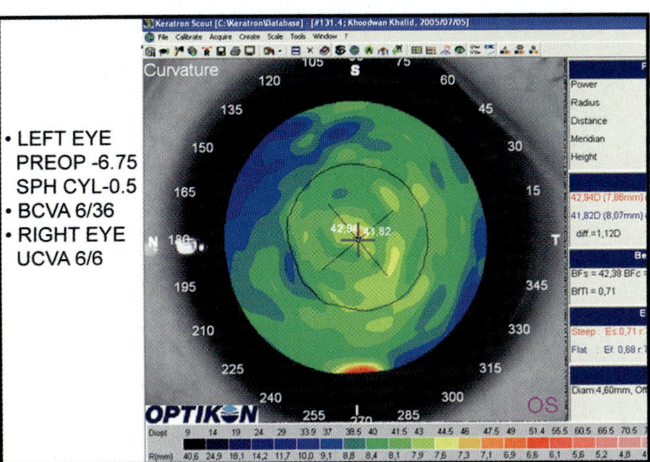

Fig. 17: 11-year-old boy,anisometropic amblyopia

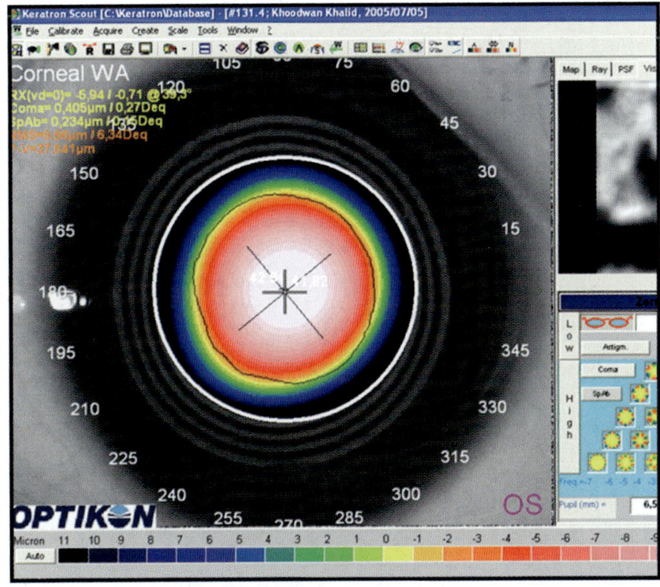

Fig. 18: Corneal wavefront

REFERENCES

1. Sachsenweger R. Problems of organic lesions in functional amblyopia. In: Arruga A (Ed): International Strabismus Symposium. Basel and New York: S. Karger, 1968;63.
2. Evens L, Kuypers C. Incidence of functional amblyopia in Belgium. Bull Soc Belge Ophthalmol 1967;147:445-9.
3. National Society to Prevent Blindness. Vision problems in the U.S. Data analysis. Definitions, data sources, detailed data tables, analysis, interpretation. Publication. New York: National Society to Prevent Blindness, 1980;10
4. Simons K, Reinecke RD. Amblyopia screening and stereopsis. In: Helveston EM (Ed): Symposium on Strabismus: Transactions of the New Orleans Academy of Ophthalmology. St. Louis: CV Mosby Co., 1978;15-50.
5. Oliver M, Nawratzki I. Screening of pre-school children for ocular anomalies. II. Amblyopia. Prevalence and therapeutic results at different ages. Br J Ophthalmol 1971;55:467-71.
6. Sorsby A, Sheridan M, Leary G. Vision, visual acuity, and ocular refraction of young men. Br Med J 1960:1394-8.
7. Hillis A, Flynn JT, Hawkins BS. The evolving concept of amblyopia: A challenge to epidemiologists. Am J Epidemiol 1983;118:192-205.
8. Flom MC, Neumaier RW. Prevalence of amblyopia. Public Health Rep 1966;81:329-41.
9. Williams C, Harrad RA, Harvey I, Sparrow JM. Screening for amblyopia in preschool children: Results of a population-based, randomised controlled trial. ALSPAC Study Team. Avon Longitudinal Study of Pregnancy and Childhood. Ophthalmic Epidemiol 2001;8:279-95.
10. Leibowitz HM, Krueger DE, Maunder LR, et al. The Framingham Eye Study monograph: An ophthalmological and epidemiological study of cataract, glaucoma, diabetic retinopathy, macular degeneration, and visual acuity in a general population of 2631 adults, 1973-1975. Surv Ophthalmol 1980;24:335-610.
11. Frandsen AD. Occurrence of Squint: A Clinical Statistical Study on the Prevalence of Squint and Associated Signs in Different Groups and Ages of the Danish Population. Copenhagen: HK Kristensen, 1960;64.
12. National Advisory Eye Council. Vision Research: A National Plan. Report of the Strabismus, Amblyopia, and Visual Processing Panel, vol 2, part 5. Bethesda: US DHHS, NIH Publ No. 83-2475., 2001.
13. Castren J. The significance of prematurity on the eye. With reference to retrolental fibroplasia. Acta Ophthalmol Suppl 1995;44:19-31.
14. Fledelius H. Prematurity and the eye. Ophthalmic 10-year follow-up of children of low and normal birth weight. Acta Ophthalmol Suppl 1976;128:3-245.
15. Kushner B. Strabismus and amblyopia associated with regressed retinopathy of prematurity. Arch Ophthalmol 1982;100:256-61.
16. Pigassou-Albouy R, Fleming A. Amblyopia and strabismus in patients with cerebral palsy. Ann Ophthalmol 1975;7:382-4, 6-7.
17. Abrahamsson M, Magnusson G, Sjostrand J. Inheritance of strabismus and the gain of using heredity to determine populations at risk of developing strabismus. Acta Ophthalmol Scand 1999;77:653-7.
18. Pike MG, Holmstrom G, de Vries LS, et al. Patterns of visual impairment associated with lesions of the preterm infant brain. Dev Med Child Neurol 1994;36:849-62.
19. van Hof-Van Duin J, Evenhuis-van Leunen A, Mohn G, et al. Effects of very low birth weight (VLBW) on visual development during the first year after term. Early Hum Dev 1989;20:255-66.
20. Vaegan, Taylor D. Critical period for deprivation amblyopia in children. Trans Ophthalmol Soc U K 1979;99:432-9.
21. Kitchen WH, Richards A, Ryan MM, et al. A longitudinal study of very low-birthweight infants. II: Results of controlled trial of intensive care and incidence of handicaps. Dev Med Child Neurol 1979;21:582-9.
22. Hoyt CS. The long-term visual effects of short-term binocular occlusion of at-risk neonates. Arch Ophthalmol 1980;98:1967-70.
23. Mohindra I, Jacobson SG, Thomas J, Held R. Development of amblyopia in infants. Trans Ophthalmol Soc U K 1979;99:344-6.
24. Awaya S, Miyake S. Form vision deprivation amblyopia: further observations. Graefes Arch Clin Exp Ophthalmol 1988;226:132-6.
25. Tychsen L. Binocular Vision. In: W Hart (Ed): Adler's Physiology of the Eye. St. Louis: Mosby, 1992; chap. 24.
26. Rentschler I, Hilz R, Brettel H. Spatial tuning properties in human amblyopia cannot explain the loss of optotype acuity. Behav Brain Res 1980;1:433-43.
27. Hubel DH, Wiesel TN. Binocular interaction in striate cortex of kittens reared with artificial squint. J Neurophysiol 1965;28:1041-59.
28. Hubel DH, Wiesel TN. Receptive fields and functional architecture of monkey striate cortex. J Physiol 1968;195:215-43.
29. Tigges M, Boothe RG, Tigges J, Wilson JR. Competition between an aphakic and an occluded eye for territory in striate cortex of developing rhesus monkeys: cytochrome oxidase histochemistry in layer 4C. J Comp Neurol 1992;316:173-86.
30. von Noorden GK. Amblyopia: A multidisciplinary approach. Proctor lecture. Invest Ophthalmol Vis Sci 1985;26:1704-16.
31. von Noorden GK, Crawford ML. The lateral geniculate nucleus in human strabismic amblyopia. Invest Ophthalmol Vis Sci 1992;33:2729-32.
32. Horton JC, Stryker MP. Amblyopia induced by anisometropia without shrinkage of ocular dominance columns in human striate cortex. Proc Natl Acad Sci U S A 1993;90:5494-8.
33. Movshon JA, Van Sluyters RC. Visual neural development. Annu Rev Psychol 1981;32:477-522.
34. Wiesel TN. Postnatal development of the visual cortex and the influence of environment. Nature 1982;299:583-91.
35. Boothe RG, Dobson V, Teller DY. Postnatal development of vision in human and nonhuman primates. Annu Rev Neurosci 1985;8:495-545.
36. Hess RF, Pointer JS. Differences in the neural basis of human amblyopia: The distribution of the anomaly across the visual field. Vision Res 1985;25:1577-94.
37. Yu M, Brown B, Edwards MH. Investigation of multifocal visual evoked potential in anisometropic and esotropic amblyopes. Invest Ophthalmol Vis Sci 1998;39:2033-40.
38. Gelbart SS, Hoyt CS, Jastrebski G, Marg E. Long-term visual results in bilateral congenital cataracts. Am J Ophthalmol 1982;93:615-21.

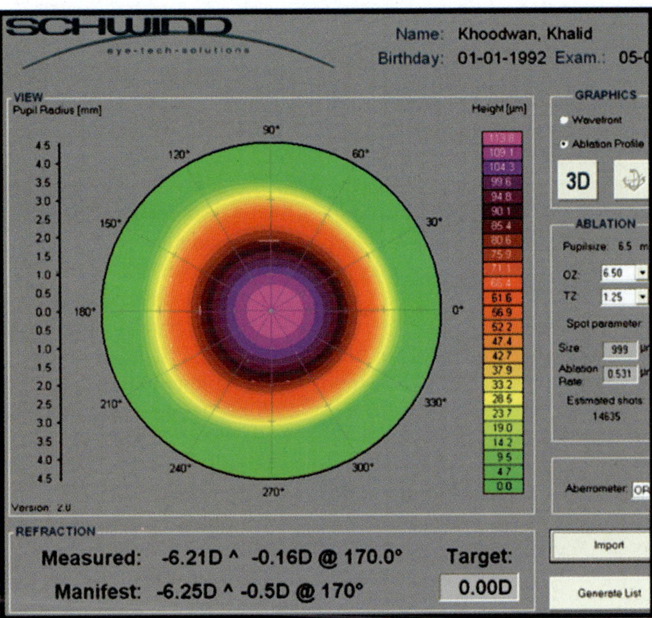

Fig. 19: Shotfile

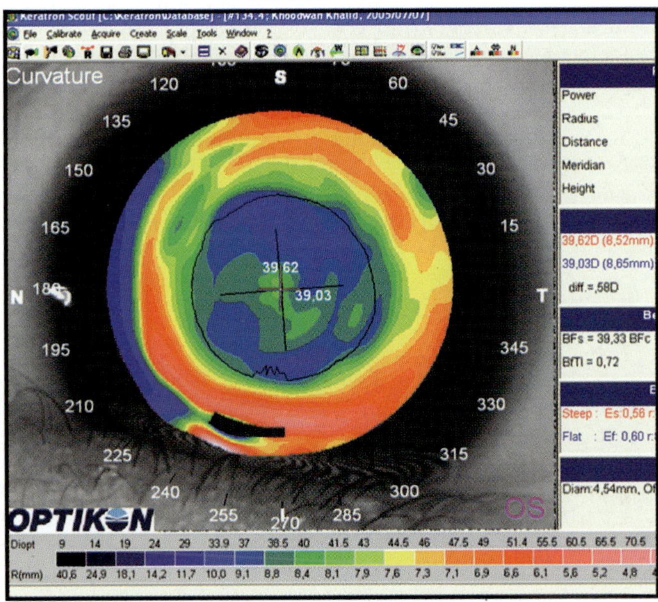

Fig. 20: One day postoperative topography—6/9p UCVA

39. Beller R, Hoyt CS, Marg E, Odom JV. Good visual function after neonatal surgery for congenital monocular cataracts. Am J Ophthalmol 1981;91:559-65.
40. Kushner BJ. Functional amblyopia associated with organic ocular disease. Am J Ophthalmol 1981;91:39-45.
41. Summers G, Phelps DL, Tung B, Palmer EA. Ocular cosmesis in retinopathy of prematurity. The cryotherapy for retinopathy of prematurity cooperative group. Arch Ophthalmol 1992;110:1092-7.
42. Von Noorden GK, Dowling JE. Experimental amblyopia in monkeys. II. Behavioral studies in strabismic amblyopia. Arch Ophthalmol 1970;84:215-20.
43. Baker FH, Grigg P, von Noorden GK. Effects of visual deprivation and strabismus on the response of neurons in the visual cortex of the monkey, including studies on the striate and prestriate cortex in the normal animal. Brain Res 1974;66:185-208.
44. Ikeda H. Is amblyopia a peripheral defect? Trans Ophthalmol Soc U K 1979;99:347-52.
45. Birch EE, Stager DR. Monocular acuity and stereopsis in infantile esotropia. Invest Ophthalmol Vis Sci 1985;26:1624-30.
46. Dickey CF, Metz HS, Stewart SA, Scott WE. The diagnosis of amblyopia in cross-fixation. J Pediatr Ophthalmol Strabismus 1991;28:171-5.
47. Day SH, Orel-Bixler DA, Norcia AM. Abnormal acuity development in infantile esotropia. Invest Ophthalmol Vis Sci 1988;29:327-9.
48. Mitchell DE, Freeman RD, Millodot M, Haegerstrom G. Meridional amblyopia:Evidence for modification of the human visual system by early visual experience. Vision Res 1973;13:535-58.
49. Gwiazda J, Scheiman M, Held R. Anisotropic resolution in children's vision. Vision Res 1984;24:527-31.
50. Tanlamai T, Goss DA. Prevalence of monocular amblyopia among anisometropes. Am J Optom Physiol Opt 1979;56:704-15.
51. Kivlin JD, Flynn JT. Therapy of anisometropic amblyopia. J Pediatr Ophthalmol Strabismus 1981;18:47-56.
52. Townshend AM, Holmes JM, Evans LS. Depth of anisometropic amblyopia and difference in refraction. Am J Ophthalmol 1993;116:431-6.
53. Fielder AR, Moseley MJ. Anisometropia and amblyopia—chicken or egg? Br J Ophthalmol 1996;80:857-8.
54. Abrahamsson M, Sjostrand J. Natural history of infantile anisometropia. Br J Ophthalmol 1996;80:860-3.
55. The natural ocular outcome of premature birth and retinopathy. Status at 1 year. Cryotherapy for Retinopathy of Prematurity Cooperative Group. Arch Ophthalmol 1994;112:903-12.
56. Maumenee IH, Alston A, Mets MB, et al. Inheritance of congenital esotropia. Trans Am Ophthalmol Soc 1986;84:85-93.
57. Chew E, Remaley NA, Tamboli A, et al. Risk factors for esotropia and exotropia. Arch Ophthalmol 1994;112:1349-55.
58. Rantakallio P, Krause U, Krause K. The use of the ophthalmological services during the preschool age, ocular findings and family background. J Pediatr Ophthalmol Strabismus 1978;15:253-8.
59. Miller M, Israel J, Cuttone J. Fetal alcohol syndrome. J Pediatr Ophthalmol Strabismus 1981;18:6-15.
60. Hakim RB, Tielsch JM. Maternal cigarette smoking during pregnancy. A risk factor for childhood strabismus. Arch Ophthalmol 1992;110:1459-62.
61. Laby DM, Rosenbaum AL, Kirschen DG, et al. The visual function of professional baseball players. Am J Ophthalmol 1996;122:476-85.
62. Tommila V, Tarkkanen A. Incidence of loss of vision in the healthy eye in amblyopia. Br J Ophthalmol 1981;65:575-7.
63. Yang LL, Lambert SR. Reappraisal of occlusion therapy for severe structural abnormalities of the optic disc and macula. J Pediatr Ophthalmol Strabismus 1995;32:37-41. American Academy of Ophthalmology, Preferred Practice Pattern Amblyopia 2005.

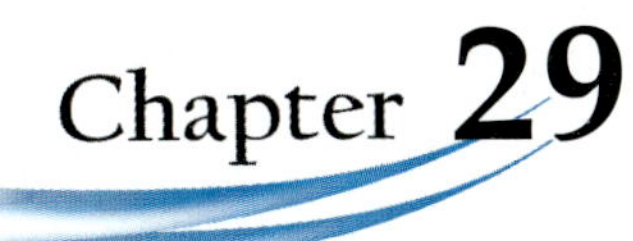

Strategies for Amblyopia: Rehabilitation Orthoptics and Refractive Surgery

Roberto Pinelli, Fabrizio Gabas, Ilaria Sireno (Italy)

The term "amblyopia" literally means "dullness of vision" and derives from the Greek *amblyos* meaning "dull". The synonym "lazy eye" is commonly used; often the eye does not have anatomical problems and its structural maturation is comparable to that of the other eye. However, the difference lies in the maturation of the visual structures of the cortex with which it is connected.

Modern medicine has made great strides and achieved much in this field. Nonetheless we firmly believe that the definitive chapter on ambylopia has yet to be written. We therefore ask the reader to read this in a pioneering spirit, critically, and with an open mind.

Amblyopia strikes approximately 5% of children and often it is not clinically diagnosed until school age, as they do not have any visual comparisons enabling them to alert anyone to their difficulties. At the Istituto Laser Microchirurgia Oculare in Brescia (Italy), we always recommend that children of a minimum of three years of age be brought for an eye test, since timely diagnosis and treatment are fundamental for a successful restoration of sight (Fig. 1).

HOW DOES AMBLYOPIA ARISE?

When we receive a visual message, the occipital cortex of the brain analyses the information contained within it, giving us a visual sensation; it is this which may be considered the means enabling sight, as the eyes themselves do not see.

At birth, visual acuity is reduced; both the anatomical structure (retina) and above all the nervous structure (lateral geniculate body cells and occipital cortex cells) have yet to mature.

It is only as a result of the continuous stimulus of the visual apparatus that these processes are initiated, continuing up to the first six months of life. It is also the case that the cerebral processes continue to be refined for several years, until they are complete. This period is commonly referred to as the "period of plasticity".

If during this initial, highly delicate, period an eye does not permit the passage of the visual message or if this image is not amenable to analyses by the brain because it is "distorted", a defence mechanism comes into play whereby the message is not read or is only partially analyzed by the brain. The cells of the lateral geniculate body connected to the amblyopic eye atrophy, as do the cells responsible for the analysis of binocular stimuli. The result is a more or less marked visual deficit in the amblyopic eye which can become permanent if not treated quickly, whereas the degree of sensory deficit will depend on the period of stimulation insufficiency.

CLASSIFICATION OF AMBLYOPIAS

There are several classifications of amblyopia in existence and every ophthalmologist will have, over the years, probably developed their own personal classification. We do not believe in employing unduly complex classification schemes, but prefer one which is simpler, clearer and easy to use.

ETIOLOGICAL CLASSIFICATION

- *Sensory deprivation amblyopia:* this is caused by reduced sensory stimulation of the retina with a consequent reduction of neurocerebral afference. This may be due to:
  1. the presence of a visual defect which has not been adequately rectified (anisometropia) with the result that the image is blurred.
  2. the absence of visual stimulation at the retinal level caused by an "obstacle" such as congenital cataract, ptosis etc (Fig. 2).

3. stimulation which varies in quantity and quality such as for example in nystagmus
4. incorrect stimulation caused by the incorrect use of glasses, eye patches etc.

It must be remembered that deprivation amblyopia may be accompanied by manifestations of strabismus, which are the consequence, and not the principal cause, of the clinical picture.

- *strabismus amblyopia:* when one of the eyes is deviated it is no longer possible for the fusion mechanism to occur; this may result in diplopia, which, however, does not become manifest, since the brain, involuntarily, tends to eliminate the afferent impulses from the non-fixing eye in order to avoid confusion in analyzing the visual message. It affects the majority of strabismics and strikes the deviated eye. Depending on the level of deviation we may determine different levels of amblyopia: in microstrabismus, suppression occurs with a small central scotoma, in medium-level strabismus, anomalous retinal correspondence occurs with stimulation of the non-macular cells thereby leading to the creation of a pseudofovea, leading to a wide degree of suppression in high-level deviation.
- *Mixed or combined amblyopia:* all those cases in which it can be ascertained that several factors contribute simultaneously to visual deprivation (anisometropia and strabismus, ptosis and strabismus, etc.)

It is always recommended to assess whether children with visual defects above 2.50 D of myopia or hypermetropia and above 1.50D of astigmatism have a similar degree of visual acuity in both eyes.

In this case the phenomenon of crowding in this type of amblyopia should be noted: the visual acuity of a child calculated by presenting different symbols simultaneously (optotype line) will be lower with respect to the calculated visual acuity when a single symbol is shown.

In amblyopia the brain cannot discriminate between different symbols if they are positioned close together. The clinical visual acuity will obviously remain that which was obtained by presenting one line of the optotype, but the visual acuity determined by means of a single symbol can give us some idea of the hidden potential of the amblyopic eye and of the possibility of recovery after appropriate treatment (Figs 3A and B).

PROGNOSIS OF AMBLYOPIA

It is never an easy matter to offer a prognosis of visual recovery in the amblyopic eye, since it is dependent upon many factors such as the child's capacity for adaptation, the cooperation of the parents, the possibility of eliminating visual impediments, etc (Fig. 4).

The rule always holds true that the sooner treatment commences (and the younger the child), the greater is the probability of a good degree of recovery.

Until the age of six years it is reasonable to believe that the cerebral system responsible for sight is able to restore its lost functionality. Over the age of six the possibility for a total recovery becomes less and often a partial recovery occurs of the visual acuity in the amblyopic eye. It also depends on the fact that the amblyopigenic factors have remained unaltered for a long time. Nevertheless, it is worth making every attempt at recovery. Finally amblyopia is considered unlikely to be reversible if it is still persisting at the end of the period of plasticity. At the end of this period the visual cerebral structures are considered to have matured.

Our advice is, however, to leave nothing untried. Adult patients with a high visual deficit and amblyopia in one eye have, after refractive surgery, shown a greater improvement in visual acuity, with improved correction which is not fully explicable by the resolution of lens aberrometries.

DIAGNOSIS

As stated earlier, many cases of amblyopia are discovered when the child is of school age, since sight difficulties do not manifest themselves inasmuch as one eye sees well and compensates for the other. Parents should be advised to take the child for an eye check-up as soon as possible.

At pre-school age, eyesight problems are often associated with particular ways of behaving, such as difficulties in grasping objects or a surly or even uncooperative or defensive attitude towards peers. All these situations could suggest the presence of amblyopia.

The examination of the child should be undertaken as soon as such events appear: note how the child relates to the environment, head position (exclude the abnormal head position) and their degree of interest in specific stimuli.

EXAMINATION OF THE CHILD

During the examination it is important to reduce the interference of external factors that could distract the attention of the observer, especially if the patient is very young. Many colleagues in such cases even advise against the parents being present. In our view, the parents should play an active role in the examination, and be suitably

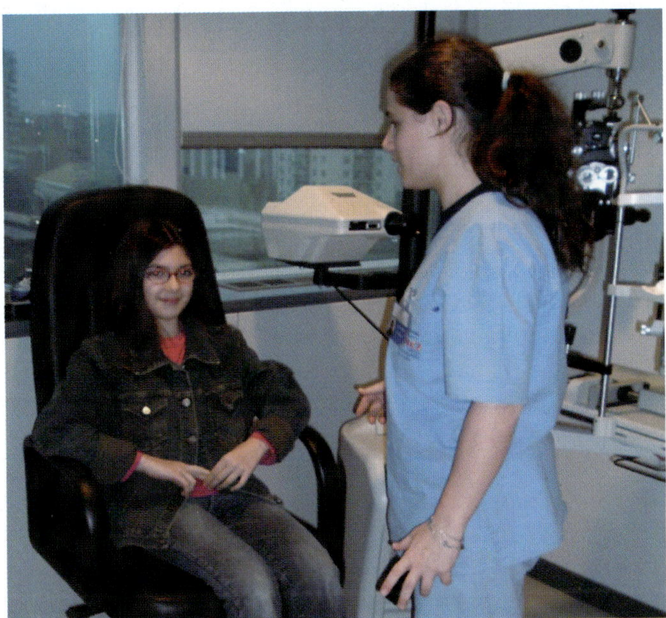

Fig. 1: Time and early diagnosis are factors of primary importance for a successful restoration of sight

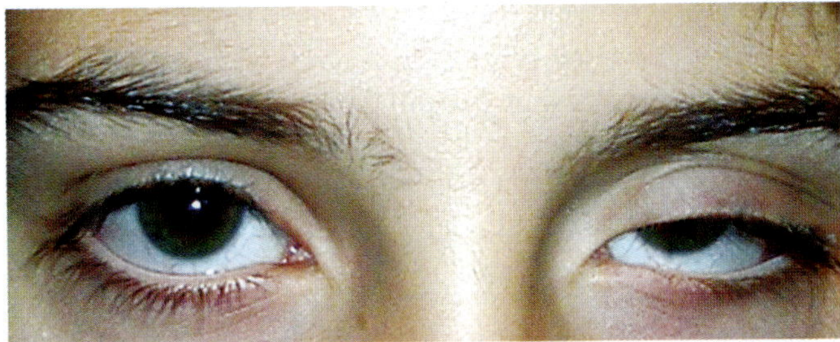

Fig. 2: Ptosis can be a cause for a reduced sensory stimulation

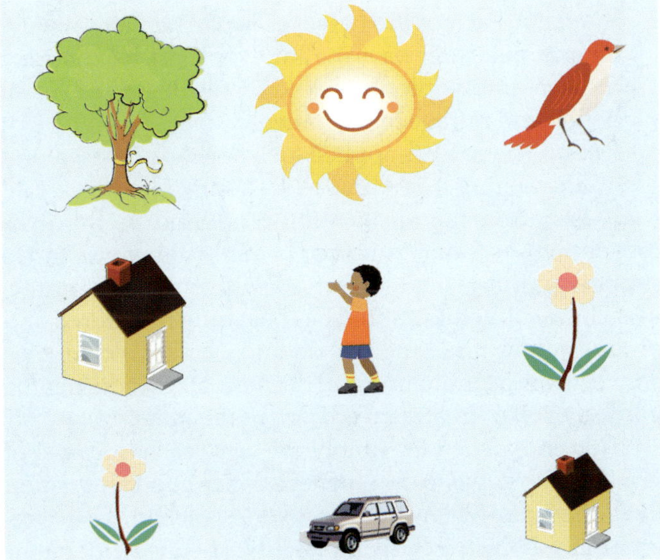

Fig. 3A

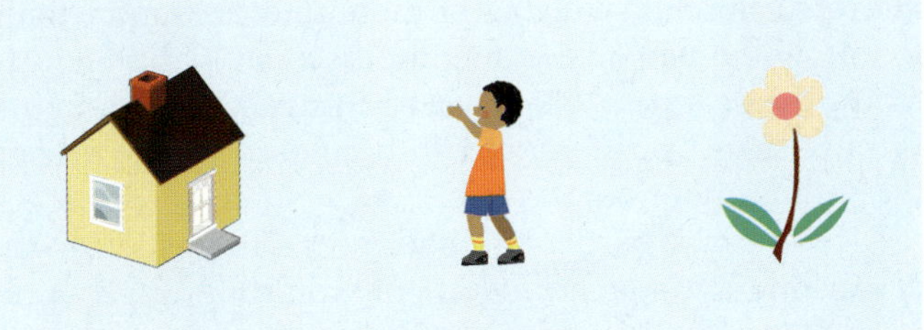

Fig. 3B

Figs 3A and B: The potential of the amblyopic eye can be discovered by means of when they are close together

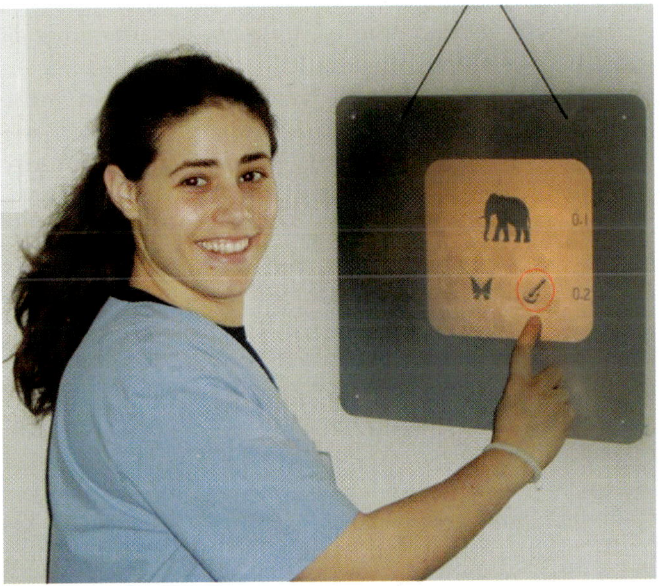

Fig. 3C

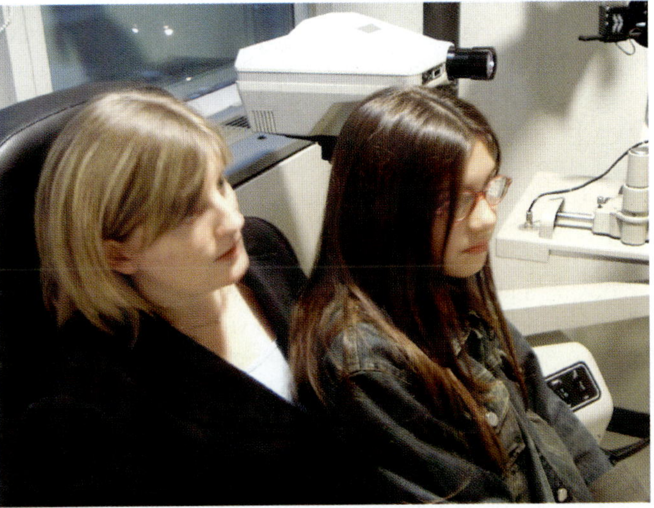

Fig. 4: Parents' cooperation is an important factor for the visual recovery of the amblyopic eye

informed; the child will then be more amenable and willing to follow the person conducting the examination and to follow the treatment which will be entrusted to the parents. We advise using different brightly colored objects to keep the child's attention.

There are no particular differences with respect to the eye examination an adult patient would undergo, apart from the need to consider time factors in order not to tire the child. The first examination is extremely important and the impression the child forms of you will have a bearing on all subsequent examinations and treatment itself. Having ascertained the poor visual acuity in one or both eyes, search for possible causes:

from the examination of the globe and its adnexa, evaluate the dioptric media transparency (Fig. 5). As mentioned previously, opacity or even a ptosis in the pupillary field may provoke amblyopia. We advise using the direct ophthalmoscope taking advantage of any cyclopegia in order to evaluate the possible visual defect. (Fig. 6A). Another important examination during the visit to assess amblyopia is the skiascopy, we usually perform it at the Istituto Laser Microchirurgia Oculare together with direct and indirect ophthalmoscopy (Fig. 6B). To assess the normality of the afferent routes make maximum use of the stimulation of the retina with a light (not in cycloplegia) which produces a direct pupillary constriction (direct light reflex) and a consensual pupillary constriction (indirect light reflex). If you stimulate an eye in which the afferent routes are damaged, you will receive no response.

The orthoptic assessment remains an essential aspect of the child's eye examination: the ocular motility examination, alternate cover test, cover-uncover test, papillary reflex assessment (asymmetric in the presence of strabismus) can shed much light on any visual deficit that has been determined. Pay particular attention to the possibility of small or very small angle strabismus, which can be difficult to diagnose, but highly amblyopigenic (Figs 7A to E).

If you do not detect any anomalies, examine the fundus with the indirect ophthalmoscope to assess the state of health of the retina.

If during the examination you ask the child to look at an object held in your hand, while you use the other hand to cover one eye, the child will have no problem if you have covered the amblyopic eye. However if you cover the non-amblyopic eye the child will become agitated and try to break free from your hand. (Figs 8A and 8B). In order to ascertain that the child is not suppressing, employ the test for single binocular vision, polarised tests (e.g. the Titmus test) or random points (e.g. the Lang test and TNO test) (Fig. 9)

HOW TO TREAT AMBLYOPIA

The most commonly used method to treat amblyopia is undoubtedly the orthoptic method. Its aim is to improve the visual acuity of the amblyopic eye so that it becomes closer, if not equal, to that of the visual deficit-free eye. Treatment varies in accordance with the age of the child, onset, the type of amblyopia, whether there are any refractive errors, and the possibility of eliminating amblyogenic factors such as ptosis or congenital cataract. For successful treatment outcome it is useful to speak with, and fully explain to the parents what the aims are and what methods will be used, since it is they who will have the task of following the child most of the time.

First of all any visual defects must be eliminated unless they are of benefit to the treatment: for example, we would not correct the defect in a child with slight hypermetropia and exophoria which manifests as tropia since we could exploit the child's natural accommodation and stimulation of convergence.

In cases of elevated anisometropia, prescribe glasses which are not difficult to wear by the child, otherwise one runs the risk of an amblyopigenic factor. In addition to correcting the visual defect one must also consider the possibility of occlusion therapy.

Occlusion is applied by means of an eye patch over the fixing eye with the better visual acuity in order to rehabilitate the amblyopic eye.

1. *Total:* When the fixing eye is closed all day during waking hours. This is recommended in serious amblyopia, but not with patients under one year of age for whom occlusion should not exceed half the waking hours.
2. *Alternate*: Each of the two eyes is patched alternately, for example, three days the amblyopic eye and one day the non-amblyopic etc., based on the degree of visual deficit and the age of the patient.
3. *Partial:* The patch is applied for a portion of the waking hours ranging from three to six hours (Fig. 10).

Alternating the application is a good method for preventing secondary amblyopia in the fixing eye and is strongly recommended in children under six years of age. In each case the child should be constantly monitored and no more than three months should be allowed to pass between one examination and the next, at least during the initial period of treatment efficacy assessment.

This ends when the amblyopic eye reaches a level of visual acuity equal to the other eye with a good alternating fixation. Even when the objective is reached, however, occlusion should not be completely suspended, but rather the number of hours should be gradually diminished.

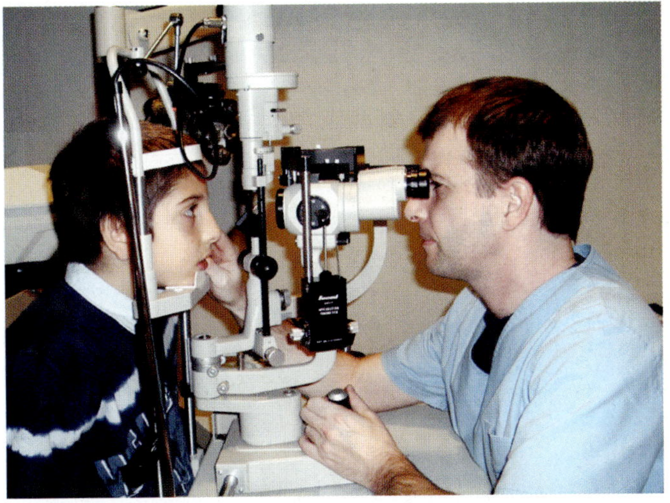

Fig. 5: The slit lamp examination represents an important moment during the visit

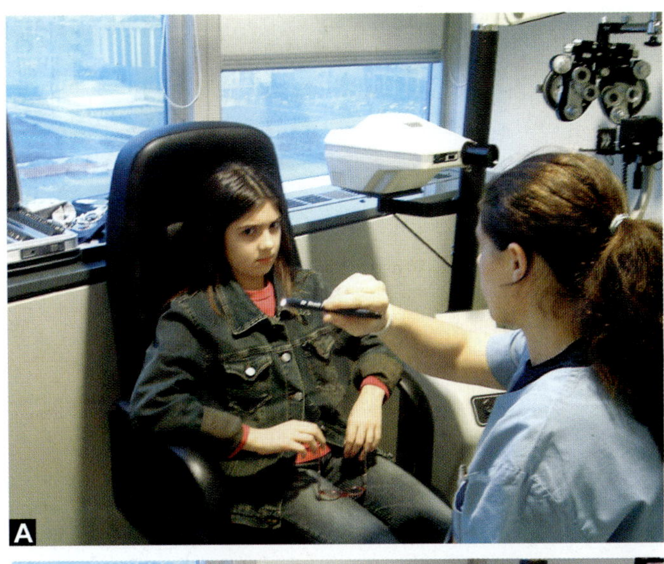

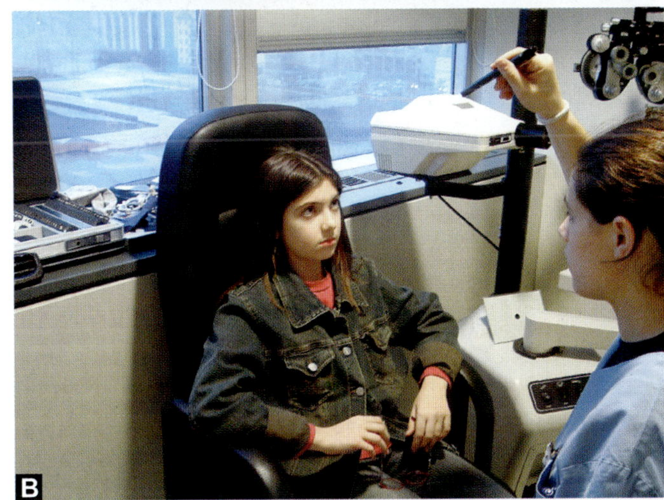

Figs 7A and B: ocular motility examination

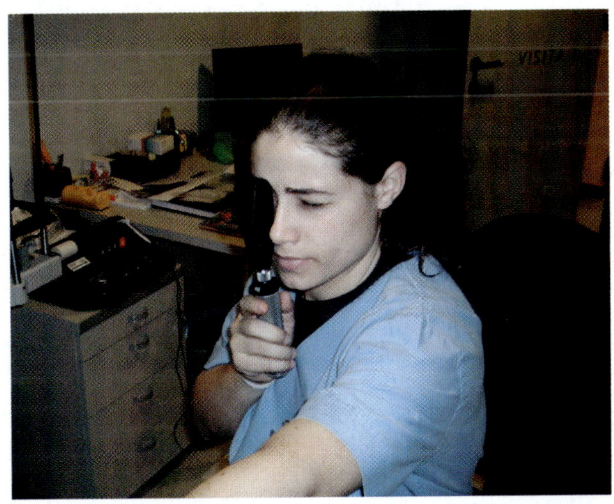

Fig. 6A: Skiascopy

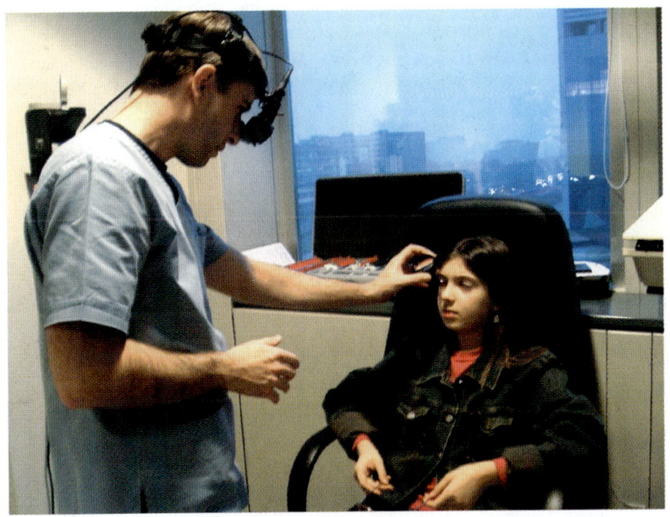

Fig. 6B: Indirect ophthalmoscopy

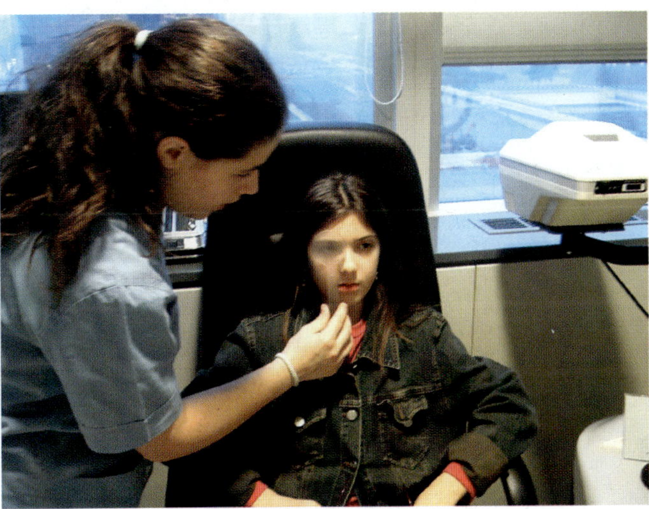

Fig. 7C

Some describe the use of a red filter in front of the amblyopic eye, to provide greater stimulus of the macular cones, in combination with occluding the other eye.

Another method is penalization: This consists in defocusing the image in the non-amblyopic eye to compel the child to use the other eye. This is usually conducted by prescribing high-power negative or positive lenses and the instillation of cycloplegic eye drops in the non-amblyopic eye.

1. *Total penalization*: The non-amblyopic eye can see neither far nor near distance.
2. *Far penalization*: The amblyopic eye is corrected for optimal vision whilst the non-amblyopic eye is myopised.
3. Near penalization: The amblyopic eye may only be used for near diatance by means of a suitable prescription, while the other eye is put under cycloplegia.

TREATMENT FROM A SURGICAL VIEWPOINT

Surgery can represent a staunch ally in the treatment of amblyopia. It is undoubtedly necessary when certain amblyopigenic factors are to be eliminated such as cataract or ptosis. In addition, strabismus surgery is beneficial in that it leads to a good recovery of visual acuity and so is employed subsequent to amblyopia treatment. Refractive surgery on the other hand can be of great benefit in those amblyopias in which the principal cause is a refractive error. We normally treat adult patients with already-diagnosed amblyopia, who have visual defects and in some cases even nystagmus.

They are treated by the LASIK technique and the treatment with the excimer laser is carefully adjusted to the specific characteristics of each individual. All patients have shown an increase in visual acuity in the amblyopic eye which cannot be accounted for by the sole resolution of the visual defect or of lens aberrations. All have superseded the limits of visual acuity with the corrective lens to such an extent that we are inclined to speak of refractive subamblyopia. The treatment in children therefore could represent a quick and safe method to obtain excellent results and therefore qualitatively and quantitatively improve sight in patients who by reason of their age are not treated any more.

The manufacturing of pediatric microkeratomes or the evolution of the femtosecond laser technology could improve the quality of life of amblyopic children, allowing them to gain access to refractive surgery. Only few literature exists on this topic, but it theoretically represents an exciting option. The anesthesia in children must be taken into consideration and discussed, in particular considering that keratomileusis is nowadays performed simply with topic anesthesia.

BIBLIOGRAPHY

1. Agarwal A, Agarwal A, Agarwal T, Azim Siraj A, Narang P, Narang S. Results of pediatric laser in situ keratomileusis, Journal of Cataract and Refractive Surger 2000;26(5):684-9.
2. Rutstein RP, Corliss DA. Long-term changes in visual acuity and refractive error in amblyopes. Optom Vis Sci 2004; 81(7):510-5.
3. Cotter SA, Edwards AR, Wallace DK, Beck RW, Arnold RW, etc. Treatment of anisometropic amblyopia in children with refractive correction, Ophthalmology 2006;113(6);895-903.
4. Gusek-Schneider GC, Martus P. Stimulus deprivation ambliopya in human congenital ptosis: A study of 100 patients, Strabismus 2000;8(4);261-70.
5. Menon V, Chaudhuri Z, Saxena R, Gill K, Sachdeva MM. Factors influencing visual rehabilitation after occlusion therapy in unilateral ambliopya in children, Indian J Med Res 2005;122,(6);497-505.
ambliopya prevalence and severity of ambliopya, J AAPOS 2000;4(4)194-9.
7. Wu C, Hunter DG, Ambliopya diagnostic and therapeutic options, Am J Ophthalmol 2006;141(1)175-84.

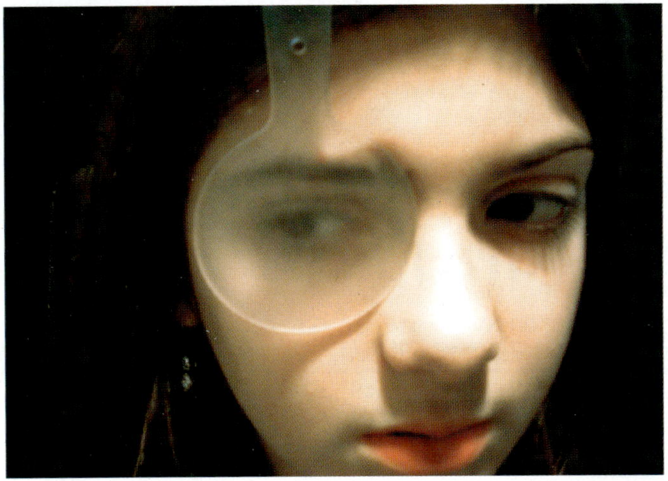

Fig. 7D

Figs 7C and 7D: Cover test

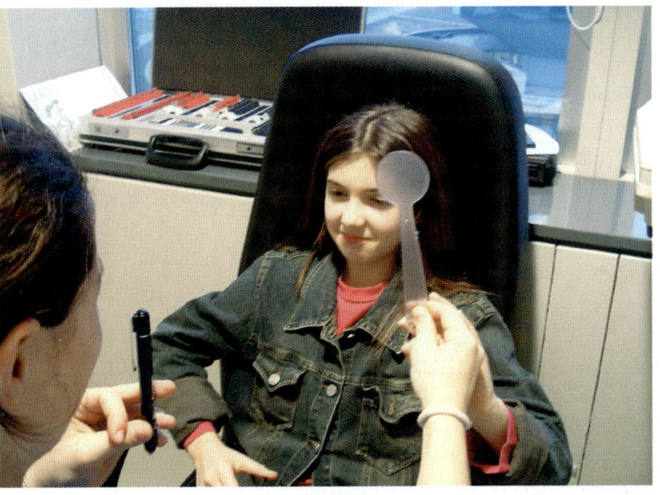

Fig. 8B

Figs 8A and B: The child reacts in different ways if the amblyopic eye is covered during the examination

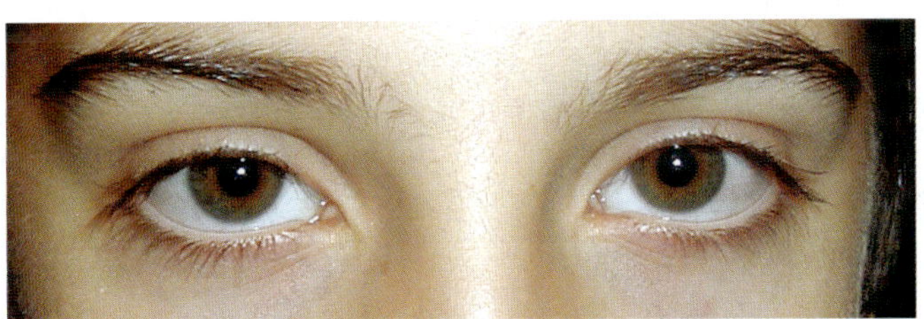

Fig. 7E: Papillary reflex assessment

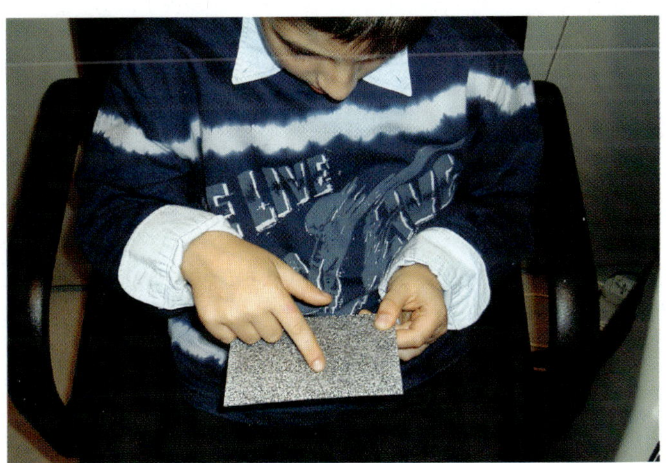

Fig. 9: Lang test

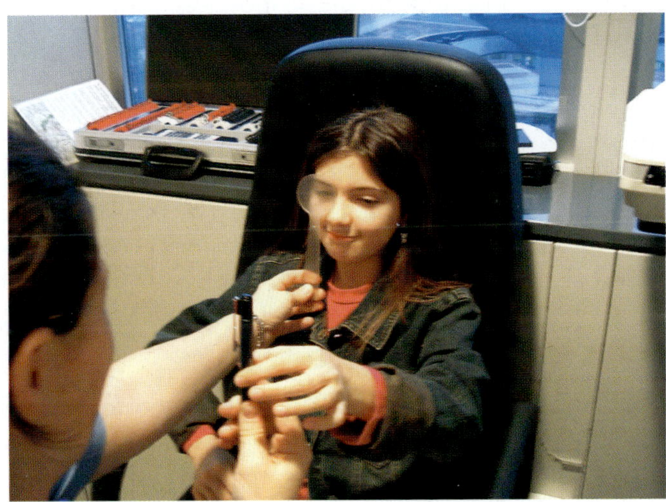

Fig. 8A

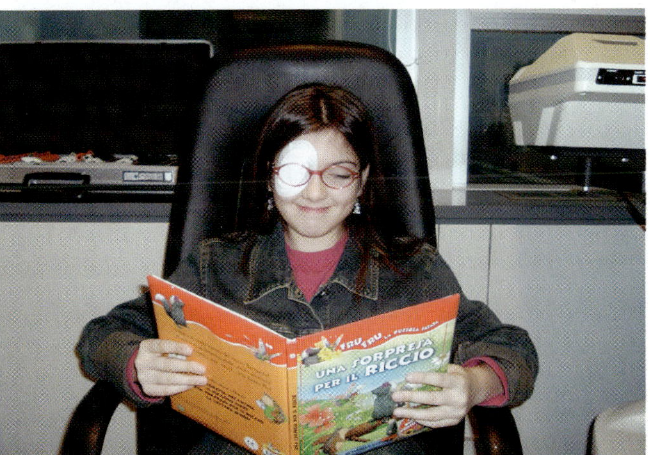

Fig. 10: Occlusion for the rehabilitation of the amblyopic eye

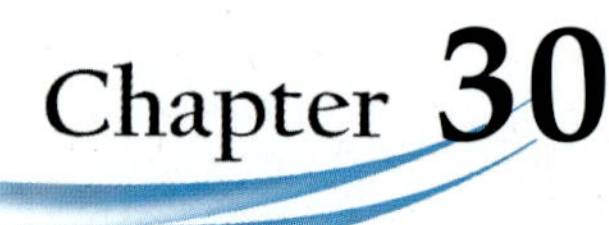

Double Elevator Palsy (Monocular Elevation Deficit): An Update

Sneha Kataria (USA), Sunil Moreker, Mayur Moreker, Rashmi Shukla, Sheetal Kharatmal (India)

INTRODUCTION

Double elevator palsy presents a unique situation to a squint specialist due to the presence of ptosis in some of the patients and the unpredictability of outcomes. Double elevator palsy is a monocular elevation deficit in abduction and adduction due to reduced function of the superior rectus (SR) and inferior oblique muscles.[1] The Figures 1 to 4 show the straight gaze, upgaze and the elevation deficit of the left eye in left and right gazes. The forced duction test shows restriction.

Moreker Kataria Classification of Monocular elevation deficit (Modified Ziffer Rosembaum[2] classification of Double elevator palsy)

A. Monocular elevator deficit with pseudoblepharoptosis
   a. **Congenital**: These were in the past further subclassified into:
      i. primary inferior rectus restriction –with normal upward saccadic speeds
      ii. primary superior rectus paresis –with reduced upward saccadic speed
      iii. congenital supranuclear elevator deficiency

   These can further be classified further as
   1. with forced duction positive
   2. with forced duction negative

   b. **Acquired:** seen with pineacytoma[3]

B. Monocular elevator deficit with true blepharoptosis

Investigations

i. ENG: Saccadic velocity assessments
ii. MRI: A volume scanning technique has been used by some authors where the MRI showed decreased volume of the superior rectus muscle on the affected side. This probably meant that there was congenital hypoplasia or paresis of the involved superior rectus muscle. MRI may be a useful in assessing various types [4]

Treatment

A. Inferior rectus recession is usually the surgery of choice in cases with positive forced duction.[5] Most patients recover satisfactorily by this procedure alone.
B. Knapp's procedure:[6] Full tendon width vertical transposition of the horizontal recti is an established treatment for double elevator palsy. The Knapp procedure had an increasing effect over time.
C. Combination of Both:[7] Transposition surgery has excellent results according to the authors but the surgical effect of transposition surgery may be enhanced by inferior rectus recession.
D. Vertical rectus recession and superior oblique tenectomy.
E. Moreker Kataria procedure—combination of inferior rectus recession with partial knapp's with frontalis sling.

The Figures 5 to 8 show isolation of the lateral and medial recti and splitting of the muscles midway in the muscle and transposing the split half parts of both muscles by suturing them to the superior rectus. Then the inferior rectus is recessed. Extreme care is taken to operate the eye under the microscope and isolate the vessels supplying the muscles and preserving them so as to prevent anterior segment ischemia. The ptosis corrected by frontalis sling. This can be done by either autologous fascia or by non-absorbable suture material.

POSTOPERATIVE RESULTS

The Figures 9 to 11 show the immediate postoperative results of the transposition suture and inferior rectus with ptosis being corrected by sling surgery and the result at the end of one week with orthophoria in straight gaze, equal lid position and complete eye closure.

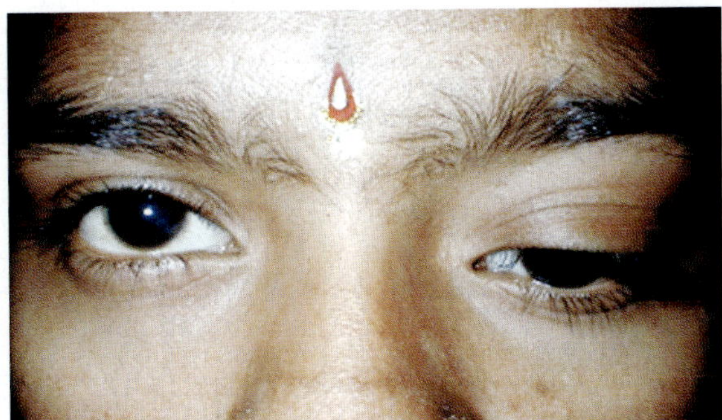

Fig. 1: Straight gaze

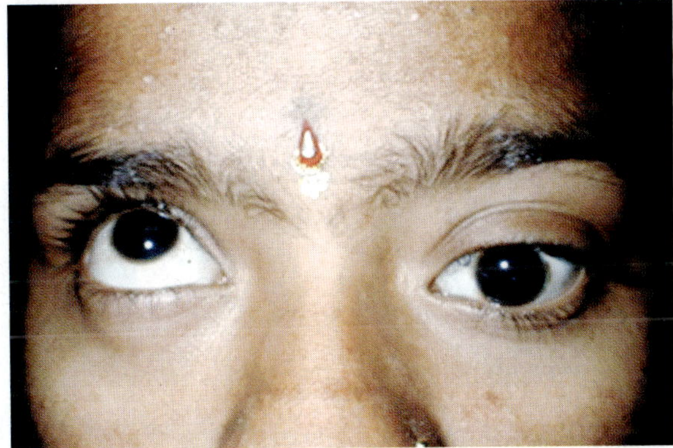

Fig. 2: Upgaze

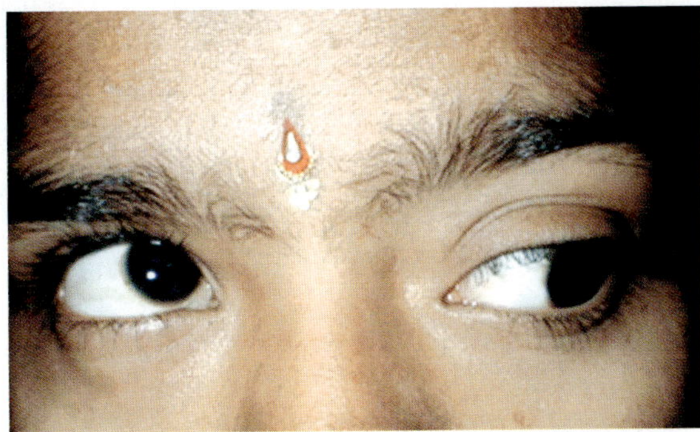

Fig. 3: Elevation when looking left

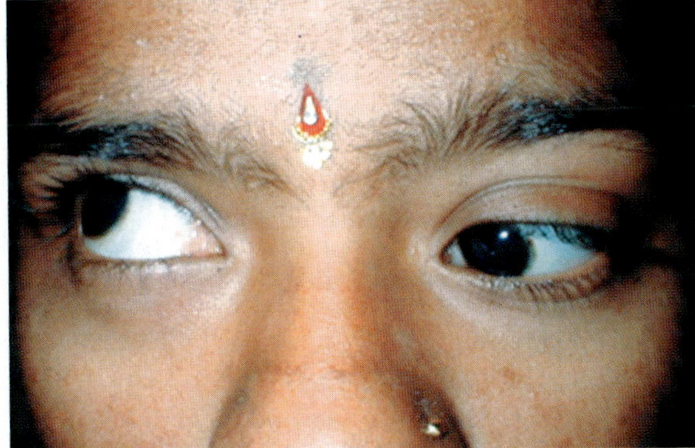

Fig. 4: Elevation when looking right

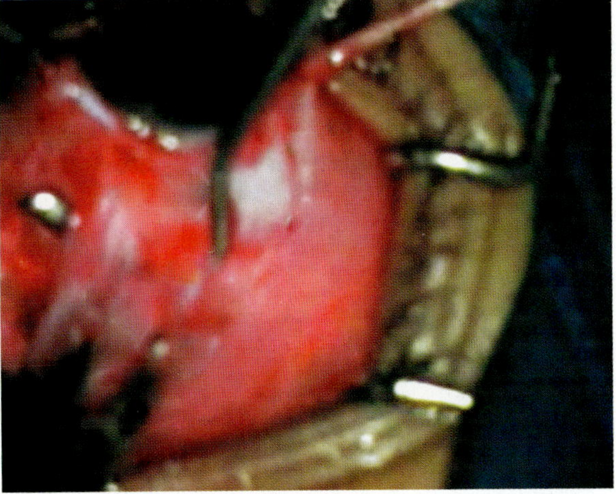

Fig. 5: Hooking and splitting lateral rectus

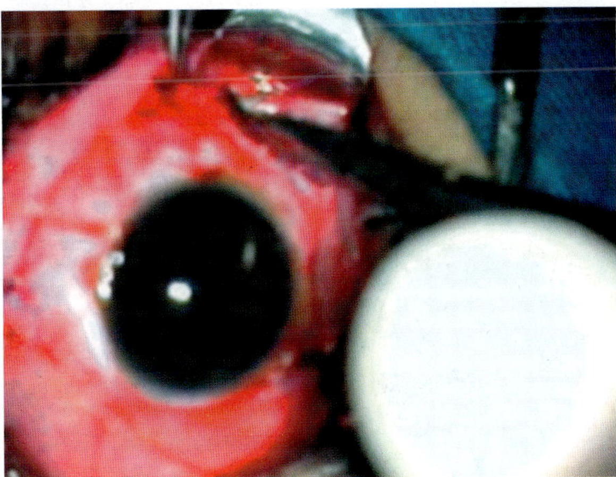

Fig. 6: Suture through medial rectus split part

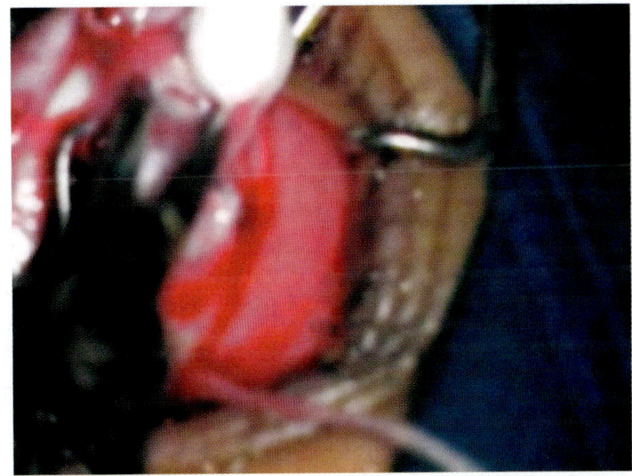

Fig. 7: Non-traumatic splitting of medial rectus along the length

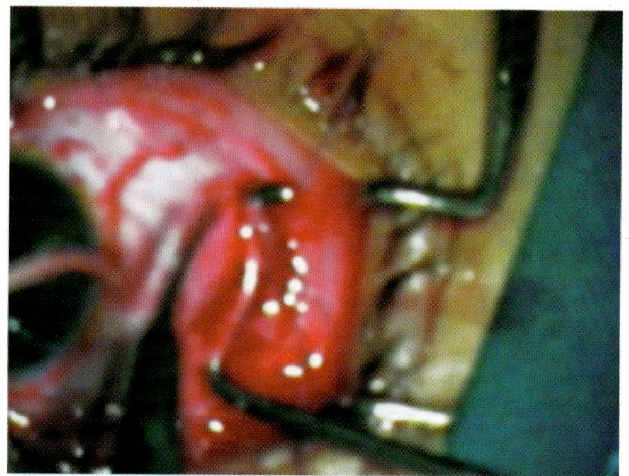

Fig. 8: Suturing the split parts to superior rectus

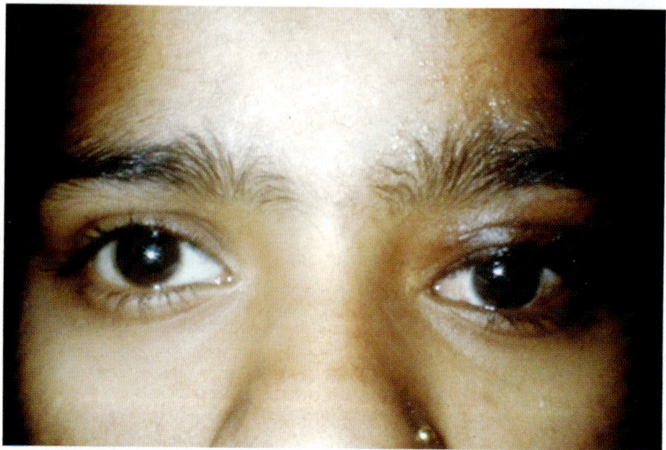

Fig. 10: Week later figure

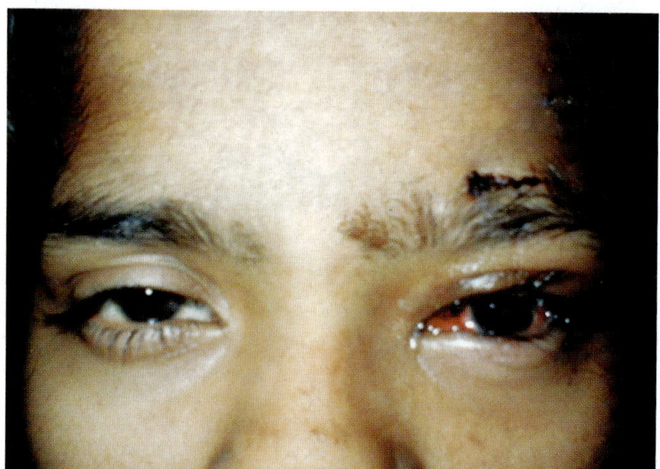

Fig. 9: Immediate postoperative figure

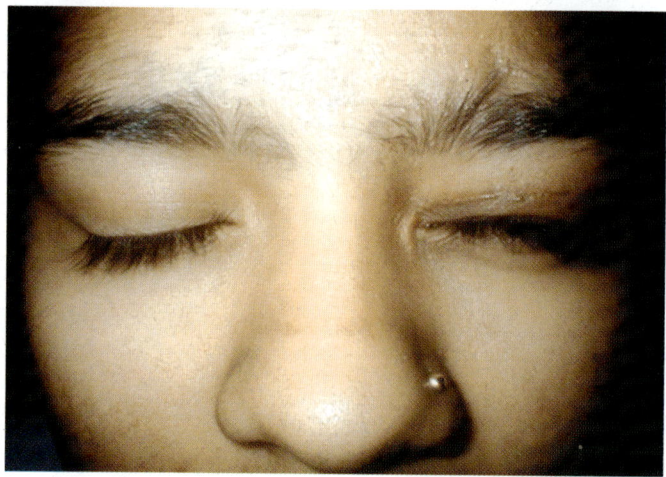

Fig. 11: Complete lid closure

Most reports suggest that there may be a relapse in the late postoperative period but in one of the authors experience there have not been relapses when a combination of modified Knapp's procedure and inferior rectus recession has been used.[8]

REFERENCES

1. Xiao MY, Shou JY, Li YP. Clinical features and surgical treatment of congenital ocular muscle palsy characterized with double elevator dysfunction. Zhonghua Yan Ke Za Zhi 2004;40(10):652-4.
2. Ziffer AJ, Rosenbaum AL, Demer JL, Yee RD. Congenital double elevator palsy: Vertical saccadic velocity utilizing the scleral search coil technique. J Pediatr Ophthalmol Strabismus 1992;29(3):142-9.
3. Muñoz M, Page LK. Acquired double elevator palsy in a child with a pineocytoma. Am J Ophthalmol 1994;15;118(6):810-1.
4. Cadera W, Bloom JN, Karlik S, Viirre E. A magnetic resonance imaging study of double elevator palsy. Can J Ophthalmol 1997;32(4):250-3.
5. Barsoum-Homsy M. Congenital double elevator palsy. J Pediatr Ophthalmol Strabismus. 1983;20(5):185-91.
6. Burke JP, Ruben JB, Scott WE: Vertical transposition of the horizontal recti (Knapp procedure) for the treatment of double elevator palsy: Effectiveness and long-term stability. Br J Ophthalmol 1992;76(12):734-7.
7. Kocak-Altintas AG, Kocakkkk-Midillioglu I, Dabil H, Duman S. Selective management of double elevator palsy by either inferior rectus recession and/or knapp type transposition surgery. Binocul Vis Strabismus Q. 2000;15(1):39-46.
8. Sunil Moreker. Surgical Audit of Double elevator palsy. Proceedings of the Joint Congress.The xth meeting of the international strabismological Association and the First meeting of the Latinamerican Council of Strabismus. Brazil.Feb 2006(Edited by Jan-Tjeerd de Faber and Carlos Souza-Dias,Mauro Goldchmit.

Index

T

U

V

W

X

Y

Z